How To Be a Nurse Assistant

Creating Awareness and Understanding of Those in Your Care

JEANNE A. BOSCHERT, RN

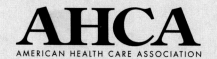

AMERICAN HEALTH CARE ASSOCIATION

Project Managers: Jon-Patrick Ewing and Danielle Levitan
Developmental Editor: Tom Lochhaas
Design: Westbound Publications, Inc.
Cover Design: A. Tomlinson/Sims Advertising, Inc.

ISBN 978-0-9765147-3-2

Printed in the United States of America by H. G. Roebuck & Son, Inc.

American Health Care Association
1201 L St. NW
Washington DC 20005-4015
www.ahca.org

Dedication

I would like to dedicate this book to all the caregivers who make it their mission to provide the best quality care possible. Their commitment and dedication cannot be honored enough. Although the tasks they perform may seem thankless at times, they are rewarded and sustained by the smiles on the faces of their residents and by the tender touch of those who say, "You have made my day better by being here for me." To these caretakers, I say: Be proud of what you do because you truly make a difference to every life you care for.

I want to acknowledge my family at Signature Healthcare for once again graciously allowing me the flexibility to write this sixth edition. There is no way that I could ever give all the credit that is due to each of you. I especially want to thank our CEO, mentor, and leader, Joe Steier. Joe, you inspire me with your vision and passionate commitment to the revolution of health care. You motivate me to grow as a person, both personally and professionally. Your dedication is contagious.

I also want to thank my own family members for their continued support and understanding. To my husband Bill and my children Jarrad, Justin, Blakely, and Ashton: Thank you for sharing me with my work. It means so much to me that you understand and appreciate what is in my heart and how important it is to me to make a difference.

To my twin grandchildren, Hadley and Harrison: Thank you for letting me type with you on my lap. Your innocence and zeal for life inspire me.

From the CNA to the CEO, you have taught me so much. For each lesson I have learned, I am humbled and grateful. All of you have helped to write my life story.

Jeanne Boschert

About the Author

Jeanne A. Boschert has been a registered nurse since 1986 and has held a variety of leadership roles within health care. Since 1999, Jeanne has written and developed programs and training materials for a variety of health care providers, including a 40-hour case management training program, a feeding assistant program, and a competency-based curriculum for both nurse assis- 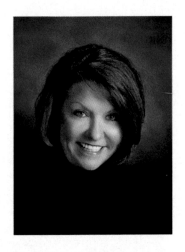 tants and licensed staff in long term care. These materials focus on providing quality of care to the whole person while continuing to enhance the individual's quality of life.

As the Director of Clinical Education for Signature Healthcare in Louisville, Kentucky from 2009 until 2013, Jeanne was responsible for the development of clinical education and professional development programs for facilities throughout seven states. She managed the CEU certification program and worked closely with the educa-tion department on content development and training for all clinical staff within the organization.

Currently, she serves as the Director of Operations for the Homecare Division of Signature Healthcare. She is responsible for the daily operations for the state of Tennessee and for the implementation of private duty serv-ices into Signature HomeNow divisions in Florida.

In 2010, AHCA selected Jeanne as the author of the fifth edition of *How To Be a Nurse Assistant*. The opportunity allowed her to apply her knowledge of clinical education and her experience in health care within a complete pro-gram including the textbook, workbook, and instructor's manual. Jeanne is once again honored to partner with AHCA and excited to contribute to the sixth edition of *How To Be a Nurse Assistant*.

"Never get tired of doing little things for others. For sometimes, those little things occupy the biggest part of their hearts."

IDA AZHARI

Acknowledgments

How To Be a Nurse Assistant is the centerpiece of the educational resources published by the American Health Care Association (AHCA). The development of the 5th Edition has truly been a collaborative effort involving dedicated individuals and organizations that share our unwavering commitment and recognition of the preeminent role of nurse assistants in long term care.

Long term care professionals from across the country have dedicated their talent and energy to this significant undertaking. They include subject matter experts, nurse assistants, administrators, directors of nursing, residents, and member facilities.

AHCA is indebted to this legion of volunteers and to our members for their generous and selfless contributions. Their passion and dedication has allowed us to develop the finest nurse assistant training program in the country, a program that provides both the professional skills and knowledge as well as the critical competencies that ensure and sustain caregiving excellence.

AHCA STAFF CONTRIBUTORS

AHCA extends sincere appreciation to these staff for sharing their talents.

Jennifer Shimer, Chief Operating Officer & Senior VP, Member Relations
Dianne DeLa Mare, VP of Legal Affairs
Jon-Patrick Ewing, Senior Director of Marketing
Danielle Levitan, Director of Marketing

OTHER CONTRIBUTORS

Developmental Editor
Tom Lochhaas, Newburyport, Massachusetts

Design
Cynthia Merrifield, Merrifield Graphics & Publishing Service

Cover Design
A. Tomlinson/Sims Advertising, Inc.

CHAPTER CONTENT REVIEWERS

To ensure the quality and accuracy of the textbook content, each chapter underwent a thorough review by two or more independent subject matter experts. Our reviewers were selected for their specific expertise and reputations in their respective fields. Their highly responsive, thoughtful, and well-documented feedback was greatly appreciated. Responsibility for the final text is the authors'.

Reviewers for Chapters 31 and 32 of the 5th Edition:

Gail Clarkson, RN, Chief Executive Officer, Medilodge, Washington, Michigan

Linda Jennings, RN, NHA , Director of Clinical Services, Tennessee Health Care Association, Nashville, Tennessee

Jodi L. Vanderpool, NHA, MBA, Chief Operating Officer. Covenant Dove, LLC, Bartlett, Tennessee

Reviewers for the subacute sections of the 4th Edition:

Eileen T. Doll, RN, BS, NHA, Efficiency Driven Healthcare Consulting, Baltimore, Maryland
Laura Tubbs, RN, BSN, MS, Director of RCQS-Clinical, Evangelical Lutheran Good Samaritan Society, Sioux Falls, South Dakota

PHOTOS, DRAWINGS, AND VIDEO

Many AHCA member facilities opened their doors to allow us to conduct on-site photography and video filming. Their willingness to participate ensures that student training is grounded in portrayals based on actual long term care settings. We are especially grateful to the management staff of these facilities for the extra work that needed to be done to coordinate staff schedules and to ensure that our presence did not disrupt resident care. We also want to thank all the residents and staff who agreed to participate in the project.

for the 5th Edition:
Marilyn Feree, RN, photography coordinator
Scott McIntyre, photographer, Scott McIntyre
  Photography, Louisville, Kentucky
Donna Whistler, RN, photography coordinator

Four Courts of Cherokee Park, Louisville, Kentucky,
  Steve Robeson, Administrator
Redstone Village, Huntsville, Alabama, Zach Jacobsen,
  Executive Director
Signature HealthCARE of Memphis, Memphis,
  Tennessee, Betty "Corky" Rodman, Administrator
Signature HealthCARE of South Louisville, Louisville,
  Kentucky, Charlie Meyer, Administrator
Signature HealthCARE of St. Francis, Memphis,
  Tennessee, Renee Tudor, Administrator
Signature HealthCARE of St. Peter Villa, Memphis,
  Tennessee, Pam Jowers, Administrator

for the 4th Edition:
Adam Motyl-Szary, Mass Monopoly Media Productions,
  Worcester, Massachusetts
Baker Katz, Haverhill, Massachusetts,
  Barbara Galaza, PTA
Penacook Place, Haverhill, Massachusetts,
  Maureen F. Blake, Admissions Coordinator and
  Beth Torla, PTA
Elder Service Plan, Winthrop, Massachusetts,
  Ann Connaughton, Admissions Coordinator

Stock photos
www.photos.com
www.bigstockphotos.com
www.shutterstock.com
www.istockphotos.com

Drawings
Jack Pardue, Pardue Studio, Alexandria, Virginia

Video
Cal Covert, Silver Ridge Productions

Ellen T. Kurtzman, RN, MPH, technical advisor
Mount Vernon Nursing Center, Alexandria, Virginia,
  Ms. Betty G. Solomonson, Administrator

Note on English Style and Readability

STYLE

This book has been edited using a modified Associated Press (AP) Style and *Webster's New World College Dictionary*, Fourth Edition.

One of the most difficult problems is how to handle the "he/she" issue. Using the traditional "he/his/him" in a profession where both the residents and caretakers are predominantly women is not acceptable; nor is it in keeping with the trends of the last 40 years. Also unacceptable would be the equally exclusive "she/her." Using "he/she," "his/her," and "him/her" quickly becomes very awkward. Fowler, long an authority on English usage, calls the "he/she" usage an "abomination." We agree. That only leaves using "they," "their," and "them" to refer to either masculine or feminine singular. Some readers may interpret this as a "mistake." However, most authorities on English usage today not only permit it, but recommend it. The best and most educated speakers and writers in English have used it for centuries. All native speakers use it, but its popular acceptance as "correct" is much more widespread outside the United States.

AP style also uses a single apostrophe instead of apostrophe s ("Mrs. Jones' bed" rather than "Mrs. Jones's bed").

We have used numerals instead of words for numbers if they are used in some type of measurement ("5 cc of water" not "five cc of water," for example), or if it is part of a range ("after 5-10 minutes..."), but we have used words rather than numerals for time ("four hours later...") for the numbers 1-9 in other places. In particular, we tried to use numerals rather than words in boxes and tables.

AHCA does not hyphenate "long term care."

READABILITY

The readability of this book, as measured by the Flesch-Kincaid formula, is grade 8. The 32 chapters break down by grade level as follows:

grade 6	2 chapters
grade 7	12 chapters
grade 8	15 chapters
grade 9	3 chapters

We understand that a great many students do not speak English as a native language. We have tried to make this book as reader-friendly as possible by:

- providing a list of medical terms at the beginning of each chapter (these are repeated in footnotes as they occur and are gathered together in Appendix A, which can be used as a mini-dictionary).
- footnoting words that are used in a special sense in long term care ("Autonomy," for example is not a medical term, but it is a term used in a technical way in long term care, and it is a word that non-native speakers might not know).
- providing a list of words in the Instructor's Manual that non-native speakers might find difficult (similar to the footnoted non-medical terms, but easier).
- providing glossaries of medical terms and English-Spanish/Spanish-English words

Finally, we often faced the issue of either repeating an explanation given elsewhere or simply referring to it (for example, "See page 243"). Generally, we decided to repeat information rather than simply referencing it. Since this is a textbook for students, we felt that constantly turning back and forth would be distracting, and as the Romans said, "Repetition is the mother of education." Except they said it in Latin!

Introduction

Welcome and thank you for purchasing *How To Be a Nurse Assistant*. You have chosen a great text to help you learn everything that you will need to know to pass your state nursing competency exam and become a nurse assistant. The text focuses on how to provide quality care to the residents you will care for. What makes this book unique is that it goes well beyond the technical skills needed to do the job. You will learn what it really means to care for another human being.

The role of the nurse assistant begins with supporting residents in their activities of daily living (ADLs). The nurse assistant must be the voice for the residents when they cannot communicate, eyes and ears for other interdisciplinary team members when they are not with the residents, and arms and legs for the residents when they cannot move. The nurse assistant must be with residents when they need someone to hold their hands. How the nurse assistant does this is key to whether the residents and their families feel that they are receiving the quality of care needed to enhance their quality of life.

How is this accomplished?

First, the best way to show that you care is to BE AWARE. The text helps create a culture of caring by introducing the concept of being aware at all times. It is important to be aware of and anticipate the resident's needs and all safety issues in the surrounding environment. Awareness leads to a sense of mindfulness during caregiving activities. You can become mindful by being open to change and new ideas as you care for your resident. It is important for nurse assistants to be honest and observant and to maintain a positive attitude. You can express this through a smiling face, a soothing tone of voice, and a gentle touch. A nurse assistant who remains both mindful and aware will not let routine activities become automatic and robotic. By staying attentive to details, a nurse assistant with a keen sense of awareness provides the best quality care.

Second, this text will teach you the key themes of care. These themes should be incorporated in all the tasks you perform. Themes help nurse assistants find a balance between the art of care giving and the technical skills needed to do their job. This balance results in quality care that also improves or maintains each resident's quality of life.

A theme is something repeated over and over. It's like a song you cannot get out of your head; the words may change in different verses, but the melody, the musical theme, stays the same and keeps repeating. The tasks that nurse assistants perform every day are like the song. The specific words may change throughout the day or may vary for different residents with different preferences, but the themes of care always stay the same. In every interaction with every resident, these themes are part of the care nurse assistants give. Staying aware of these eight themes and weaving them throughout every task you perform is vital for providing the best possible care.

Be Aware of Autonomy — residents make decisions for themselves

Be Aware of Respect — residents are worthy of high regard

Be Aware of Communication — quality care depends on an exchange of words, active listening, and positive nonverbal communication with residents and other health care workers

Be Aware of Maximizing Capability — care helps residents use their own capabilities to their fullest

Be Aware of Observation — watching residents and paying attention to details is important for quality care

Be Aware of Infection Control — care is given in ways that prevent the transmission of infection

Be Aware of Safety — residents must be free from harm or risk and secure from threats or danger

Be Aware of Time Management — nurse assistants organize their activities and perform them efficiently

The third key component of *How To Be a Nurse Assistant* is the organization of the text. The six sections help students to gain knowledge in a systematic way. Each section provides a foundation for the next section, contributing to the total picture of quality care.

Section 1: Your New Job As a Nurse Assistant

describes where nurse assistants work in long term care and what things a nurse assistant can expect to do and experience while working in each environment. The roles of the nurse assistant and others in the interdisciplinary team are described. The philosophy of mindfulness is introduced. This section has two chapters:

Chapter 1 Where You Work
Chapter 2 Starting Your Job: What to Expect

Section 2: Maintaining the Resident's Quality of Life teaches nurse assistants how to help maintain or improve each resident's quality of life. Nurse assistants will learn how to get to know and create a positive relationship with each resident. This section has four chapters:

Section 3: You Are Responsible for Quality Care presents the foundation of what nurse assistants need to understand before they learn the specific tasks for supporting residents in their ADLs. This section has five chapters:

Section 4: How to Give Quality Care teaches skills needed to support residents in their activities of daily living. This section covers most of the skills on the state competency evaluations. This section has 11 chapters:

Section 5: Advance Your Skills introduces other long term care environments and the residents who live in them. This section describes different opportunities to care for different residents other than the frail elderly. This section helps students understand that different groups and individuals have different specific needs, while the information students learned in earlier chapters can still be applied to these new populations. This section has five chapters:

Section 6: How To Be Successful gives nurse assistants information to help them be both personally and professionally successful. Being successful personally is critical for providing quality care. There are five chapters in this section:

Health care is a constantly changing environment. With new research and techniques, practices and guidelines change. The 6th edition of *How To Be a Nurse Assistant* has been updated to reflect changes within the health care system since 2010. Changes have occurred in CDC infection control guidelines, HIPAA standards, new reporting requirements in the Elder Justice Act, and standard of care updates. This edition also emphasizes the need to Be Aware of and Understand the needs of residents. This is critical in every aspect of providing their care.

This 6th edition is published by the American Health Care Association (AHCA). AHCA is the largest trade association for long term care and is proud to provide the most comprehensive and up-to-date text available for nurse assistants in long term care. AHCA'S commitment to quality is demonstrated daily through its work on behalf of over a million residents who reside in the more than 12,000 long term care facilities that AHCA represents. With AHCA'S support this text was developed through an endeavor embracing the whole profession. A team of individuals collaborated and reviewed the text under the oversight of an advisory committee. AHCA works to ensure that all information needed for state certification is included within the process. Every effort has been made to incorporate the most up to date and comprehensive information from each state. In addition, the very latest information about regulations affecting residents and nurse assistants is included along with everything students need to know to be safe in their practice.

Thank you again for purchasing *How To Be a Nurse Assistant*. I hope that it meets your needs for this training and that you will continue to use it as a reference tool in the future. I hope that you enjoy your learning experience.

Respectfully,
Jeanne A. Boschert, RN

Features of This Book

The **Chapter Opening** explains why the information in the chapter is necessary for a nurse assistant. When necessary, the relationship of material in the chapter to the Nursing Home Act of 1987 and OSHA regulations is explained here.

Objectives—This list corresponds to "In This Chapter You Learned How To" at the end of each chapter. These objectives represent the key knowledge and skills students should learn as they read the chapter.

Medical Terms—In the first chapter in which a medical term is discussed in depth, it is defined in a list at the beginning of the chapter and then highlighted and defined again in a footnote when the word is used. This list makes it easy to review the key terms in a chapter.

Chapter 13

GATHERING INFORMATION

In Chapter 8 you learned about your important role in gathering information that may be used in the Resident Assessment Instrument (RAI). Remember that the RAI is a data collection tool with five parts, one of which is called the Minimum Data Set (MDS). You will hear nursing staff refer to the MDS as the tool for collecting information about residents. It is important to accurately report or record your observations about your resident's physical, social, psychological, and recreational or relaxation activities for the accuracy of the MDS. All facility staff collect information about the resident. Much of it comes from the physical examination, including the resident's vital signs, height, and weight. Data collection begins when the resident is admitted to the long term care facility. Data collection is a continuous process in which you will play a critical role (Fig 13-1).

In this chapter you will learn how to assist with a physical examination, how to take vital signs, and how to measure the resident's height and weight. These important skills help determine a resident's health status and help all members of the health care team to provide resident care.

OBJECTIVES

- Explain the purpose of an accurate history
- Describe what information the health care team obtains about a resident's past medical history
- Define two interviewing techniques the health care team uses during the physical examination
- Describe two methods used by the health care team for collecting history data
- Describe questions asked by the health care team during the review of body systems
- Explain your role in the physical examination
- Explain techniques used by the physician to examine the resident
- Demonstrate how to take an oral temperature
- Demonstrate how to take a rectal temperature
- Demonstrate how to take an axillary temperature
- Demonstrate how to take a radial pulse
- Demonstrate how to take an apical pulse
- Demonstrate how to take count respirations
- Demonstrate how to take a blood pressure
- Demonstrate how to measure height and weight

MEDICAL TERMS

- **Auscultation** – a technique of listening through a stethoscope to sounds produced by organs (such as heart, lungs, or bowels) to evaluate a body area
- **Axillary** – armpit
- **Blood pressure** – pressure of blood in the arteries
- **Glaucoma** – disease of eye that can cause gradual loss of vision
- **History** – A record of a person's medical background, including lifestyle and social information
- **Macular degeneration** – eye condition that causes loss of central vision
- **Oral** – by mouth
- **Palpation** – an examination technique of touching the resident's body on the surface and more deeply in an organized manner
- **Percussion** – tapping on a body area and listening to the sound produced, used to determine if tissue is air-filled, solid, or fluid-filled
- **Physical examination** – an organized approach to learn about a resident's health status and needs by looking, listening, feeling, and smelling.
- **Pulse** – measure of heart rate
- **Rectal** – by rectum
- **Temperature** – a degree of heat that naturally occurs in the body
- **Temporal scan** – measurement of temperature of the forehead
- **Tympanic temperature** – measurement of temperature of the eardrum
- **Vital signs** – necessary for life: temperature, pulse, respiration, and blood pressure

230

Quotation—Each chapter begins with a quotation from a resident. These help show the real-life value of key points in the chapter—how the nurse assistant can really make a difference in the resident's life.

Introduction—Each chapter begins with a short introduction that challenges students to think and feel like residents. What experiences have students had that are similar to a resident's? How would students feel if they were in a resident's place? This helps students learn to always think of the residents first.

Quotation—Each chapter begins with a quotation from a resident. These help show the real-life value of key points in the chapter—how the nurse assistant can really make a difference in the resident's

"You constantly amaze me. You are so efficient and care for each of us as though we were your only focus."

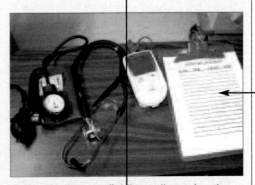

Fig. 13-1 – A blood pressure cuff, stethoscope, thermometer, and a resident's chart.

Photos and Illustrations—There are over 500 photos and 150 drawings in this book. These are designed to illustrate and help clarify key points in the chapter and give students a sense of what it is really like to be a nurse assistant.

life.

Highlighted Words are defined in footnotes on the same page. These include both key medical terms and other words that have a special meaning in the context of long term care.

Think about when you last had a physical exam. Maybe you were entering a new school or job, or you may have been ill. Now, think about how you felt during the exam. Was your privacy protected? Were you draped properly? Did the physician knock before entering the exam room? Was everything explained to you? Remember that your resident will have the exact same concerns when questioned by the physician about their medical history and during the physical exam.

PHYSICAL EXAMINATION AND HISTORY

To clearly understand a resident's total physical, psychological, and social needs, a physical examination must be performed. The examination is performed using an organized approach. As a nurse assistant your role is to assist the physician during the physical examination. Along with the physical examination, the resident's vital signs are taken, and height and weight are measured—these provide you with quick information about the person's health. Later in this chapter you will learn these skills.

A physical examination is always performed by a physician or designated health care provider when a resident is admitted to a facility. An examination is also done when a

Main Headings are in all caps and bold. These show the main topics in the chapter and are listed in the detailed Table of Contents.

Main Headings are in all caps and **bold**. These show the main topics in the chapter and are listed in the detailed Table of Contents.

Procedure List—Procedures that appear in a chapter are listed at the beginning. All the procedures in the book are listed at the end of the Table of Contents.

Medical History – A record of a person's medical background, including lifestyle and social information

Physical examination – an organized approach to learn about a resident's health status and needs by looking, listening, feeling, and smelling.

Footnotes give definitions of the highlighted words on the page.

A **Procedure** is a step-by-step description of how to perform a skill, usually how to give resident care. Procedures can be easily identified by their blue background screen. There are also several skills that are screened, but not numbered as procedures. This is because these activities do not have the same common preparation and completion steps—they are either emergency skills or skills that do not involve residents. Examples are handwashing; putting on and removing gloves, gown, and mask; and emergency skills such as CPR and the Heimlich manoeuver.

Items Needed—Supplies and equipment needed for a procedure are listed at the beginning of the procedure so you have them ready before starting.

Photos or Drawings illustrate the key steps of procedures. The illustration appears above the step pictured. Remember that the numbered steps are read down each column, not across.

Common Preparation Steps
A reminder to use the acronym BE AWARE appears at the start of each procedure and will help you remember all the necessary steps to begin each procedure. These steps should always be performed before the specific actions of the procedure, See more details in Table 12-1 on pp. 222.

PROCEDURE 13-6. TAKING A BLOOD PRESSURE

▶ **REMEMBER: BE AWARE**

Items Needed
* BP cuff of correct size
* sphygmomanometer
* stethoscope
* paper and pencil

Note: *To take a blood pressure you use a stethoscope, a blood pressure cuff, and a sphygmomanometer. You will learn the equipment used in your facility.*

1. Have the resident place their arm on the bed, bedside table, or arm of the chair, with their palm up and elbow at the same level as the heart. (If the arm is higher than the heart, the blood pressure can register too high. If the arm is lower than the heart, the blood pressure can register too low.)

2. Expose the resident's arm by rolling the sleeve up to the shoulder, taking care that the sleeve is not too tight on the arm, which might increase the blood pressure. Wrap the blood pressure cuff evenly around the upper arm 1 inch above the elbow. Make sure the arm is not lying on the tubing and the tub-

ing is not kinked. The tube that is attached to the bulb should be on the side closest to the resident's body. The tube to the sphygmomanometer gauge should be on the other side of the arm, away from the body. Be sure to use the correct size cuff for the resident. The wrong size cuff can give you an incorrect reading. The cuff should fit over the center of the resident's upper arm. It should not extend to the elbow or to under the resident's armpit.

3. Close the valve in the air pump by turning it clockwise. The valve is the little metal knob on the bulb.

4. Place the stethoscope earpieces in your ears.

5. Locate the pulsation in the brachial artery by placing your second and third fingers over the area. When you find the pulse, place the diaphragm of the stethoscope firmly over the area and hold it in place with your left hand. Use your right hand if you are left-handed.

6. With your right hand, pump air into the cuff by squeezing the bulb until the gauge measures 180-200.

Note: *If you hear the pulse immediately after stopping pumping, begin again and pump the cuff so the gauge reads higher than 200 mm Hg (Hg=symbol for mercury). One way to avoid pumping the cuff too high is to feel the pulse at the brachial artery and pump the cuff slowly until you no longer feel the pulse, making sure to remember where you last felt the pulse and to add 30 mm Hg when beginning to take the blood pressure.*

7. Slowly open the valve on the bulb and watch the cuff pressure decrease on the gauge.

8. Listen for the first thumping sound and note the pressure reading; remember this number. This is the systolic pressure.

9. Continue to listen for a distinct change in sound (muffled sounding) or the last sound and note the pressure reading. This is the diastolic pressure.

10. Record the results.

▶ **REMEMBER: UNDERSTAND**

Notes caution the student to beware of special situations or exceptions. These are found in the text as well as the procedures and are in blue letters.

Common Completion Steps that end each procedure are highlighted with the acronym UNDERSTAND. These steps are listed in detail and explained in Table 12-2 on p. 223.

Parenthetical expressions in procedures often explain the reason why an action in a step is needed.

Boxes and Tables present important information. Both have a yellow background screen.

Examples and Case Studies have a yellow background. They are used to illustrate concepts and show the consequences of a nurse assistant's actions.

In This Chapter You Learned– This list of key points corresponds to the objectives listed at the beginning of the chapter. These are the main points students should have learned.

BOX 28-1.
NURSE ASSISTANT
RESPONSIBILITIES

1. Recognize residents as individuals.
   • Learn their likes and dislikes.
   • Ask how they want things done. Get to know their routine.
   • Learn about their cultural background.
   • Find out if they have cultural preferences for their care.

2. Promote residents' autonomy and independence.
   • Know, respect, and support their rights.
   • Encourage and work with them to maintain their optimal level of functioning.
   • For personal care:
     – Be sure you give residents choices.
     – Let them participate in care decisions.
     – Maintain their privacy and dignity.

3. Provide mindful caregiving.
   • Balance the skill and the art of caregiving.
   • Observe residents closely.
   • Watch for any change in their attitudes, behaviors, or condition.
   • Let the residents determine their own routines.
   • Report any changes in their condition to the charge nurse immediately.

4. Be a good employee.
   • Be reliable.
   • Be accountable.
   • Be healthy.
   • Be considerate of others.
   • Be caring.
   • Cooperate with other team members.
   • Be efficient with your time and supplies.
   • Follow all personnel policies.
   • Dress appropriately: neat and clean.
   • Pay attention to personal hygiene.
   • Do not use drugs or drink alcohol.

Also think about Chapter 12, Themes of Care, where you learned the concept "It's not what you do, but how you do it." Think about the following:
• Who is the first person you see every day?
• Who is the last person you see before you go to sleep? Is it the same person?
• What kind of influence does this person have on your day, on how you sleep?
If you always saw the same person the first thing in the morning and the last thing at night, what would you want them to be like? Doesn't your day begin more pleasantly when someone says "Good morning!" and smiles at you (Fig. 28-3, next page)? Don't you find it easier to sleep if the last person you talk to treats you well? This is true also for residents. You influence the quality of their care like no other person in the facility because you are the one who spends the most time with them. You and other nurse assistants are the first person a resident sees each day, and the last. Read the following example and think about how that nurse assistant influences that resident's day.

It is 6 a.m. and most of the residents in the facility are just waking up. The night-shift nurse assistants are making their rounds, recording measurements on intake and output sheets and starting a.m. care for residents who want an early start. One of the nurse assistants, Mary, decides to weigh residents before the next shift arrives. She checks the weight chart and makes a list of residents to be weighed.
When Mary arrives at the first room on her list, she knocks on the door and introduces herself. As she walks in, she tells Mr. Sinclair she wants to weigh him. Without apologizing for waking him or even saying "Good morning," Mary again says that she wants to measure his weight. He hesitantly agrees and climbs out of bed onto the scale.

How would you feel if someone else awakened you this way? Would you think that the person who woke you this way cared about you? Is this a pleasant way to start the day?
Mary had good intentions: to help the day staff with some of their work, but she did not consider this resident's needs. Mary was not thinking of Mr. Sinclair as a person—but as a task to check off on a list. It cannot be overemphasized that residents should be treated with respect and dignity. Although Mary was trying to use her time wisely, she did not consider the resident's preferences or needs.

IN THIS CHAPTER YOU LEARNED:
• Your role in a resident's history and physical exam and why it is important
• Why a physical examination is important
• How and why it is important to measure and record vital signs
• How and why it is important to measure and record a resident's height and weight

SUMMARY
Gathering accurate information about a resident is one of the best ways to get to know them. It also allows the entire team to give the best possible care. As the person who spends the most time with the resident, you play a vital role in assuring that the resident receives necessary care and support. Taking and recording accurate information can make a big difference in the resident's life.

PULLING IT ALL TOGETHER
Just imagine what could happen if a resident is admitted to the facility and inaccurate information is recorded or valuable information is not documented. Most likely, the resident will not receive the proper care. In addition, reimbursement for services is based on information documented in the MDS, and part of this information comes from the history and physical examination.
Imagine that the resident or a family member gave you information and you forgot to document it or to tell other team members about it. This could result in the resident not receiving medication or an infection getting worse.
Accurate documentation and communication to other team members is critical for success when caring for residents.

The **Summary** brings together the main points of the chapter in paragraph form.

Pulling It All Together shows how students can use what they learned in the chapter in their careers as nurse assistants in long term care. Often a case study is used and a question asked to help students develop critical thinking abut an issue. It has a blue background screen.

Check What You've Learned–Each chapter concludes with a 10-question multiple choice review. Answers to the chapter review questions are in the Instructor's Manual. Students should think about why one answer is better than another. The Student Workbook and Instructor's Manual each have sample exams that cover the entire book.

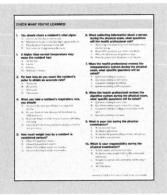

Table of Contents

Detailed Table of Contents

Procedures *

*In this book, a "procedure" is a multi-step activity that includes the "common preparation steps" and "common completion steps." There are many other multi-step activities (putting on gloves, mask, and gown, for example) that do *not* include the common preparation and completion steps, so we do not consider them procedures. Some other books do. There are other multi-step activities (making a bed, for example), where a simple change in one step (for example, turning down the top sheet or not) creates an entirely separate procedure in some books. We don't think you need an entirely new set of steps to turn down a sheet!

(See following page for activities without common preparation and completion steps.)

Multi-Step Activities Without Common Preparation and Completion Steps

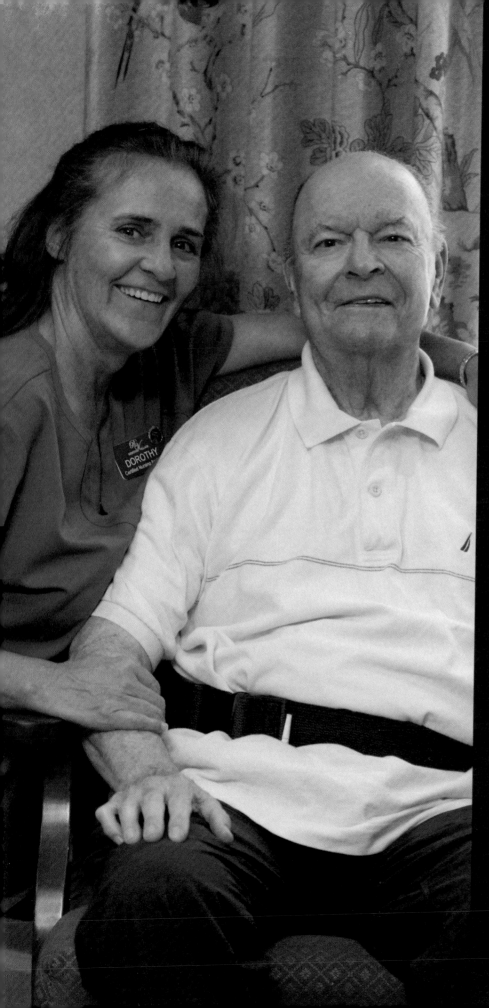

Your New Job As A Nurse Assistant

WHERE YOU WORK

Long term care providers serve the fastest growing age group: the elderly. As society changes, long term care is changing, too. Years ago, long term care facilities, called nursing homes, cared for only the elderly. Often care was given without a clear idea of this group's needs. Today, long term care includes a broad range of locations, services, and care. Long term care may include medical care, ongoing skilled nursing care, and care for the intellectually or developmentally disabled. Care and services are provided in many different settings in addition to facilities. Long term care includes adult day care, residential care, assisted living, and home-based care. Long term care is also given to very diverse people from children to elderly residents over 100.

Facilities providing these services are also changing to meet a variety of people's extended care needs. Long term care today is given in nursing facilities, subacute care centers, rehabilitation centers, and assisted living facilities. These changes happened for many reasons. More elderly people are alive than in the past, and many are living longer lives. More people also have chronic illnesses. Medical care has improved and is better able to meet their needs. Research continues to improve care.

This chapter introduces you to long term care facilities. The focus is mostly on the care of the elderly, the largest group that receives long term care. In later chapters you will learn also about other places you may work and other groups of people you may care for. You will learn why people enter long term care and what services they receive. You will learn about the members of the interdisciplinary care team, how care is typically paid for, and who oversees facilities.

OBJECTIVES
- Define what makes life worth living
- Describe a long term care facility
- List the four basic services provided in long term care
- Give two reasons why people are admitted to long term care
- List the types of care offered in long term care facilities
- Define the role of the members of the interdisciplinary health care team
- Explain how care is paid for
- Describe the agency that oversees long term care

MEDICAL TERMS
- **Biologicals** – medical products made from living organisms, such as vaccines or blood components
- **Chronic** – an ongoing illness or condition that does not have a cure, usually has a gradual onset, and lasts for a long time
- **Convalescent** – recovering health and strength gradually after sickness or weakness
- **Intellectually disabled** – a person with impaired mental skills, characterized both by a significant below average score on a test of mental ability or intelligence and by limitations in the ability to function in areas of daily life; sometimes called cognitive disability or mental retardation
- **Interdisciplinary team** – a group of caregivers from all departments in a facility
- **Intravenous** – entering through a vein
- **Occupational therapist** – works with fine motor skills to help residents to keep using their hands and arms for activities
- **Physical therapist** – works with residents to improve functional mobility so residents can maintain or increase their physical abilities, such as walking
- **Rehabilitative** – restoring to former health
- **Restorative** – designed to help one return to health and be as independent and functional as possible
- **Speech therapist** – works with residents who have difficulty with speech
- **Subacute care** – care provided to residents who do not need to be in the hospital but are not ready to be at home

"I feel better knowing that I have so many choices to meet my needs."

If you ask 10 people what makes life worth living, you will get 10 different answers. One may say, "Life is worth living when I'm with my family." Another might say traveling to new places makes it all worthwhile. Although living is defined simply as being alive, to each person it means something different to really be alive. How you think about what makes your own life worth living may be very different from how a resident of a long term care facility feels about life. You may share some ideas, but what is true for one person may not be true for another.

As a nurse assistant, you need to understand and respect how a resident feels about life. Things that a resident feels make life worth living do not change when they enter a long term care facility. Their own feelings are important to them. This is important for you to understand in order to give quality care. You must get to know residents and learn what life means to them. Never try to convince them of what you think is or is not important. If a resident cannot tell you their feelings, you must work with family members and others to learn how to make the best life for the resident.

WHAT IS LONG TERM CARE?

Long term care is a part of our health care system. It is care given over a long time on a daily or ongoing basis. The health care system includes many different types of facilities, such as hospitals, home health agencies, clinics, mental health centers, hospices, and alcohol and drug addiction facilities. Long term care facilities are an important part of this system because of the growing number of elderly people whose medical, social, and psychological needs need continuous support.

Gerontology is the study of older adults. This growing field has shown how important long term care is. Long term care facilities are also important because of growing health care costs. Because of costs, society is exploring different ways to provide long term care. Now, more nurse assistants than ever work in long term care jobs.

There are many names for long term care facilities.

There are nursing facilities, nursing homes, convalescent homes, assisted living centers, rehabilitation centers, and residential care facilities. The facility may be a separate building, a unit in a hospital, or a home that has been modified to provide long term care (Figs. 1-1 and 1-2). But all facilities provide services to people with special needs, such as nursing services that cannot or should not be given in the person's own home.

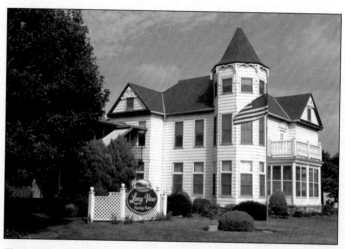

Fig. 1-1 – Long term care facilities include homes that have been converted into facilities.

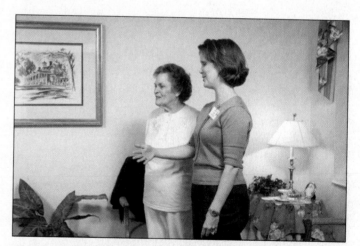

Fig. 1-2 – Facility staff make every effort to create a homelike environment for residents.

Convalescent – recovering health and strength gradually after sickness or weakness

The person usually needs the services for a long time. Some residents will need care the rest of their lives. Others may live in a long term care facility for a time, with their care focusing on their eventual return home. Four basic types of services are provided in long term care facilities. These are described in the next sections.

Medical Care

Residents in nursing facilities are under the care of a physician. In some states, the physician may have a physician assistant, nurse practitioner, or clinical nurse specialist give care. This is called delegating care. The physician and other members of the team are responsible for the resident's plan of care. When someone enters the facility as a resident, the physician writes orders for needed medications and helps develop their care plan. The care plan is a written guide used daily by the entire team. You can find the care plan in a separate notebook or the resident's individual **chart**. The care plan lists the resident's strengths, problems, and goals of care. It includes the actions the team takes to achieve these goals. The care plan can change over time. Care plan meetings are held regularly to update the resident's care plan. The plan may include **restorative** and **rehabilitative** procedures, special diets, and treatments. Every nursing facility also has a physician on staff or on call for emergencies.

Nursing and Rehabilitative Care

All nursing facilities use the professional skills of registered or licensed practical nurses. Nursing services include:
- assessment (collecting resident information to make a plan of care)
- coordination of care
- treatment
- medication administration

Residents may need rehabilitative services after a hospitalization for a stroke, heart attack, broken bone, or other condition. These services may include respiratory, physical, occupational, or speech therapy. Dental services are also available, along with dietary consultation and laboratory, X-ray, and pharmaceutical services.

Personal Care

Personal care is given to residents who need help with daily activities. These include bathing, dressing, transferring, toileting, and eating. These activities are referred to as the activities of daily living, or the ADLs. As a nurse assistant you will provide many of these services in your long term care facility.

Residential Care

Residential care services include supervising residents in a safe and secure environment. Many programs support the resident's quality of life and help meet their social and spiritual needs.

In most facilities, residents have various needs. Special units or wings may give special types of care. Other specialty facilities care for groups of residents, such as these:
- An **Alzheimer's disease** unit or facility cares primarily for residents with Alzheimer's disease or related disorders. These residents have problems with their memory. Because they may wander about, safety is a major concern. These facilities are structured for wandering, forgetful residents.
- A **pediatrics** unit or facility cares for children from birth to 22 years of age.
- A **traumatic head injury** unit or facility cares for people, often young adults, with traumatic head injuries. The focus is rehabilitation.
- A **rehabilitation** unit or facility has the primary goal of restoring residents to their **optimal** level of functioning. Residents are usually admitted directly from a hospital and remain for a specific time.
- A **subacute** unit or facility cares for residents needing high levels of nursing care. This may include **intravenous** therapy, respiratory or cardiac care, or treatment of wounds.
- An **HIV-AIDS** unit or facility cares for residents with the diseases that occur with HIV infection and AIDS.
- **Assisted living facilities** provide 24-hour supervision in a home-like setting. Support services are based on

---

Chart – a summary of the resident's medical records, routine care, treatments, drugs, etc.

Intravenous – entering through a vein

Optimal – most desirable or satisfactory, highest

Restorative – designed to help one return to health and be as independent and functional as possible

Rehabilitative – restoring to former health

Subacute care – care provided to residents who do not need to be in the hospital but are not ready to be at home

each resident's needs. Services may include help with eating, bathing, dressing, toileting, taking medicine, transportation, laundry, and housekeeping. Many assisted living facilities have dining rooms that are like restaurants. Social and recreational activities also are provided.

- **Continuing care retirement communities** have a full range of services. They provide care based on each resident's needs as they age. Care is usually given in three main categories: independent living, assisted living, and skilled nursing care.
- **Intermediate care facilities** for the intellectually disabled have a wide variety of services for mentally and developmentally disabled people. Care focuses on helping the person become as independent as possible. Staff work with the skills of each person and build success from that starting point. A whole range of health care services are also available.

WHY ARE PEOPLE ADMITTED TO LONG TERM CARE FACILITIES?

Each resident in a facility is a special person with a unique history. The only thing that residents have in common is that they live in the facility.

People enter long term care facilities for many different reasons. The facility or unit chosen depends on what support they need. For example, a person may decide to move to an assisted living facility because their house is too large, their children have moved away, and the stairs are too hard to climb. They choose an assisted living facility because they can live fairly independently. They receive the support of staff only when they need it.

Another person may have a health condition that requires medical and nursing support. It may affect their activities of daily living such as bathing, walking, and eating. In this case they may be admitted to a long term care facility.

The person's individual situation determines what type of facility and support they need. The goal is for the person to be in an environment that supports their quality of life. The benefits of living in a long term care facility include:

- help with activities of daily living: bathing, dressing, transferring, toileting, and eating
- security: knowing someone is just a call away if they fall, get sick, or just want to talk
- friendships: being around other people with similar interests, concerns, and problems (Fig. 1-3)
- independence: not having to depend on their family

Some people think that residents are "dumped" into

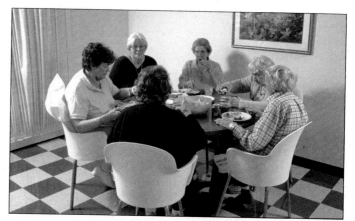

Fig. 1-3 – In long term care facilities residents can make new friendships with other residents who have similar interests.

facilities by families who no longer care for them. This is not true. Residents come to a long term care facility because it offers the kinds of care they need.

The reasons a resident lives in a long term care facility can change. For example, a resident may first come to a facility for nursing support for a cardiac (heart) condition. Later they may fall and break their hip, go to the hospital, and return to the long term care facility for rehabilitation services. But the goal of long term care is always the same: to maintain or restore each resident's level of optimal functioning. It helps all residents be the best they can be.

Residents in long term care receive one or more of these types of care:

- **Rehabilitation.** Residents who need rehabilitation often stay several weeks to several months. They usually have an illness or injury and need help to get back to their previous level of abilities before going home.
- **Skilled nursing care.** This is care for residents needing subacute care from both nursing and rehabilitation services. This care is provided by a team of many health professionals (Fig. 1-4, next page).
- **Continuous supportive care.** Most residents need ongoing help meeting basic needs such as eating, bathing, and movement. They also need basic health care. This involves the staff in giving them medications,

📖

Intellectually disabled – a person with impaired mental skills, characterized both by a significant below average score on a test of mental ability or intelligence and by limitations in the ability to function in areas of daily life; sometimes called cognitive disability or mental retardation

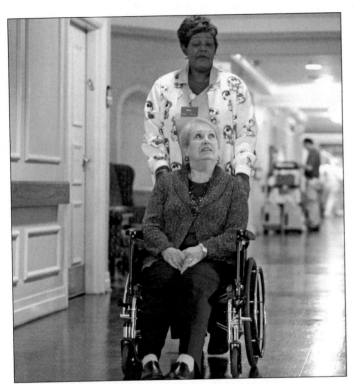

Fig. 1-4 – As a nurse assistant, you help ensure residents get the best care possible.

The Long Term Care Population

Long term care provides services to the fastest growing age group in our country. Residents over age 65 living in long term care will increase from 5.8% of the population in 1999 to an estimated 8.4% in 2050, when 20% of the population will be over 65. According to the U.S. Census Bureau, the number of residents in long term care facilities will rise to 2.9 million in 2020 and 6.6 million by 2050. Twelve million Americans now receive long term care services each year. Over 75% of nursing home residents are disabled to the extent that they cannot perform three or more ADLs. More than half are 85 years old or older.

WHO PROVIDES CARE IN A LONG TERM CARE FACILITY?

An interdisciplinary team cares for residents in long term care facilities. This means that staff from every department are involved in each resident's care.

All staff are members of the team. As in sports, the team players should respect each other and work together well. As a nurse assistant, you will be in contact with people from every service area. You will talk to them casually in the hallway and in team meetings. The team approach gives residents the highest quality care because information is shared, care is coordinated, and a care plan is based on each resident's needs. Following are the team members and their general responsibilities (Fig. 1-5, next page):

- **Resident.** The resident is always the most important person on the team. The resident is the primary customer purchasing the service. Every effort must be made to meet their individual needs and maintain their quality of life.
- **Resident's family.** A resident's family members and significant others support the resident in care decisions. They provide valuable information to staff. If a resident can no longer make decisions about care, the family usually has this role (Fig. 1-6, next page).

monitoring their vital signs, and counseling. This care may also include restorative care. The long term care facility is their home. You may become like family to them.
- **Respite care.** Individuals may come to a facility for temporary care when family members who normally provide care need a break or are away from home.
- **Hospice care.** Hospice care is special care given to individuals who are dying. Not all long term care facilities have a hospice. A hospice is usually a special unit that is very home-like. Visitors may come anytime, and meals can be prepared within the unit rather than the main kitchen. Every effort is made to ensure the resident's comfort. Hospice services may also be provided by an outside organization. In this case a team comes to the facility as needed.

Some residents are active and independent, while others need more help. Units, or special care areas, in the facility are often organized differently depending on how much care residents need. The level of care determines how a unit is staffed, including the number of nurses and nurse assistants. Residents are often very involved in their care and help staff develop their care plans.

📖

Interdisciplinary – involving two or more academic, scientific, or artistic disciplines

Respite – an interval of rest or relief (in this case, rest or relief for family who have been providing care)

Significant other – a person who is very close and important to another person, but who is not related by a traditional family relationship or marriage; usually refers to a sexual partner outside of marriage

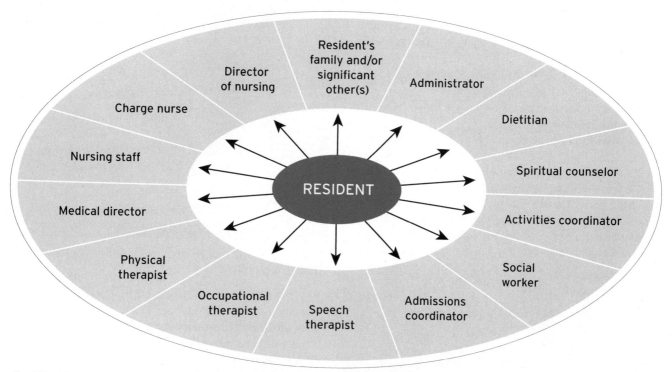

Fig. 1-5 — All members of the interdisciplinary team work to help the resident achieve optimal health. The resident is always the central focus.

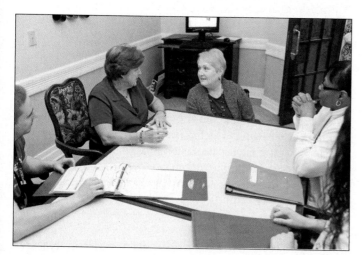

Fig. 1-6 — The resident's family participates in decisions about the resident's care.

- **Charge nurse.** The charge nurse reports directly to either the director or assistant director of nursing, depending on the facility. They have the day-to-day responsibility for supervising resident care. Charge nurses give the specific care assignments. They may also have some responsibility for staff education.
- **Nursing staff.** The nursing staff is the largest department. They help residents with the activities of daily living, medical treatments, medications, and health promotion. Staff include registered and licensed nurses and nurse assistants.
- **Medical director.** The staff physician treats residents' medical conditions and directs general medical care.
- **Physical therapist.** Physical therapists help residents maintain or improve their physical abilities, such as walking.

- **Director of nursing.** The director of nursing supervises the nursing staff and sets the philosophy and approach for caregiving.

Physical therapist – works with residents to improve functional mobility so residents can maintain or increase their physical abilities, such as walking

- **Occupational therapist.** Occupational therapists focus on fine motor skills. They engage residents in various activities to maintain or improve the use of their hands and arms.
- **Speech therapist.** Speech therapists work with residents who have difficulty speaking.
- **Admissions coordinator.** This person helps residents through the admission process.
- **Social worker.** Social workers counsel residents and their families. They might help residents apply for Medicaid. They might also arrange home care services for residents who are being discharged.
- **Activities coordinator.** The activities coordinator plans and directs activities that help improve quality of life. These may include shopping, going to plays or other outside events, games, and discussion groups (Fig 1-7).

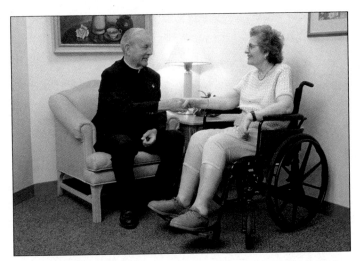

Fig. 1-8 – A resident's spiritual needs are still important when living in a long term care facility.

Other people too have important functions in different facility departments:
- **Building maintenance** maintains the physical structure, including the facility's grounds (area surrounding the buildings).
- **Housekeeping** keeps the inside of the facility clean.
- **Personnel** hires all staff.
- **Bookkeeping** manages accounting, payroll, and purchasing.
- **The laundry** cleans and maintains the linen and residents' clothing.

Each staff member in the facility has a special skill or knowledge. Each works with the team as a whole. Here's an example of how the team provides care for a specific resident. A person with a fractured hip is referred by their physician to the facility for rehabilitation services. The facility's social service department or admissions coordinator meets the family and resident. The social worker or

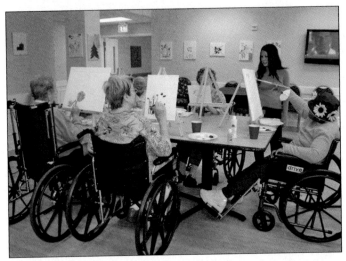

Fig. 1-7 – The activities coordinator plans all kinds of activities for the residents to enjoy.

- **Dietitian.** The dietitian or food supervisor plans and prepares meals, assesses a resident's likes and dislikes, and ensures good nutrition.
- **Spiritual counselor.** The spiritual counselor gives guidance, coordinates religious services, and counsels family members (Fig 1-8).
- **Administrator.** The administrator manages the facility and directs all staff. The administrator's goal is to make sure each resident's quality of life and care needs are met.

Admission – administrative procedure for entering a facility; opposite of discharge

Discharge – administrative procedure for leaving a facility; opposite of admission

Linen – bed linen: sheets, pillow cases, mattress covers

Occupational therapist – works with fine motor skills to help residents to keep using their hands and arms for activities

Speech therapist – works with residents who have difficulty with speech

admissions coordinator, physical therapist, and registered nurse review the referral. The resident, family, physician, and other team members together make a plan for rehabilitation and discharge. Rehabilitation services are ordered by the physician and recommended by the physical therapist. The rehabilitation and nursing departments provide services, and the social worker follows through on discharge.

All departments work together to help meet each resident's goals. Team members also help each other. For example, the housekeeping department helps you keep the resident's environment clean. You help the housekeeping department when you clean up a spill quickly so that no one will fall.

As a team member, you play a very important role. You spend more time with residents than anyone else. You will learn information about individual residents and develop relationships with them that no other team member may have. You can help each resident in long term care to feel that life is worth living.

HOW IS CARE PAID FOR?

Paying for long term care is often a challenge for residents and their families. The resident's payments may come from a variety of sources. These include state and federal aid, private insurance, and personal funds.

Medicare

Medicare, a federal health care insurance for the elderly, began in the 1960s. At that time, less was known about the special needs of the elderly, especially their **chronic** care needs. Today Medicare alone does not fully satisfy our society's needs, because people are living longer and longer.

Medicare covers limited long term care, but only after a three-day hospital stay. Medicare pays for a certain number of days in a facility. After that, the person must turn to Medicaid or their own resources to pay for care.

Medicaid

Medicaid is a state and federal program that pays the costs of a nursing home for people with limited income and assets. Eligibility varies by state. It was originally intended to meet the health care needs only of the poor. Today, Medicaid is a major part of the U.S. long term care system because so many people cannot pay in other ways. Many elderly middle-class residents rely on Medicaid to pay for

their long term care because they already have spent their life savings and assets paying for their care. Most use up their own financial assets during their first year in a facility.

Personal Resources

About half of all residents pay for long term care from their own savings. After their savings and other resources are spent, many people who stay in facilities a long time eventually become eligible for Medicaid.

Managed Care Plans

Managed care is a type of private insurance. A managed care plan pays for long term care if the facility has a contract with the plan. In such cases the managed care plan monitors caregiving to ensure it meets the resident's needs. These plans vary from state to state. Some plans also manage the resident's Medicare insurance and support the facility's staff in giving care.

Long Term Care Insurance

This is private insurance for which the resident or family has paid premiums. The benefits and costs of these plans vary widely. Long term care insurance is becoming more popular. Long term care insurance has some tax benefits.

WHO OVERSEES LONG TERM CARE?

The Centers for Medicare and Medicaid Services (CMS) provides health insurance for 74 million U.S. citizens through Medicare, Medicaid, and other programs. CMS oversees the surveying and certification of long term care facilities.

CMS requires that facilities follow government rules and regulations. Most facilities receive government Medicare and Medicaid funds. Facilities must follow CMS regulations to receive reimbursement.

These rules and regulations are the minimum requirements for a long term facility. They set service requirements for the facility and define staffing needs. They help residents know what to expect when they move into a facility. They state the rights of all persons living in long term care facilities. They outline how a facility determines

---

Chronic – an ongoing illness or condition that does not have a cure, usually has a gradual onset, and lasts for a long time

a resident's level of care and works with each new resident to develop a care plan.

Facilities must provide the services all residents need to maintain at least the level of ability they had when they were admitted. For example, if a person enters a facility walking with a cane, every effort must be made to help that person keep walking with a cane. Unless the person develops physical problems, they should not have to use a wheelchair or be confined to bed. Also, residents must be stimulated and motivated to stay active mentally. All staff must be aware of each resident's level of ability and work toward maintaining or improving that level.

Federal rules and regulations state that a long term care facility must have or provide the following:

- **Nursing services.** The facility must have enough staff to make sure the resident's assessment and care plan are effective. The resident must attain or maintain the highest practicable health. This includes their physical, mental, and psychosocial health. These services may include physical care (such as bathing), restorative care (such as providing range-of-motion exercises), and psychosocial care (such as support at the time of death). They should focus on all areas of health care, including health promotion, independence, and health maintenance.
- **Dietary services.** Each resident receives nourishing, well-balanced, good-tasting meals. Their meals must meet their daily nutritional and special dietary needs. The food choices available to each resident are based on their preferences, always considering taste.
- **Physician services.** Residents are admitted to a facility by a written order from a physician. While in the facility, the resident remains under their care. In some states the physician may delegate care to a nurse practitioner, physician assistant, or clinical nurse specialist.
- **Specialized rehabilitative services.** Special services include physical therapy, speech or language therapy, occupational therapy, and health rehabilitative services for mental illness and mental retardation. These services are available at the facility or at a nearby hospital or health center.
- **Dental services.** Facility staff must provide routine dental care.
- **Pharmacy services.** Facilities must follow safe procedures to accurately obtain, receive, dispense, and administer medications and biologicals to meet residents' needs.
- **Administration.** A facility must use its resources effectively and efficiently for each resident to attain or maintain their highest practicable physical, mental, and psychosocial well being. The administration must have the following:

    Licensure under state and local law
    Compliance with federal, state, and local laws and professional standards
    Compliance with other U.S. Department of Health and Human Services regulations
    Governing body
    Required training of nursing aides
    Proficiency of nurse aides
    Staff qualifications
    Use of outside resources
    Medical Director
    Level B requirement: Laboratory services
    Radiology and diagnostic services
    Clinical records
    Disaster and emergency preparedness
    Transfer agreement
    Quality assessment and assurance
    Disclosure of ownership
- **Social services.** This department coordinates admissions, discharges, and transfers of residents. It also gives financial guidance to residents and their families.
- **Infection control program.** The program is designed to provide a safe, sanitary, and comfortable environment. Infection control procedures must help prevent the development and transmission of disease and infection.
- **Healthy and safe physical environment.** The facility must be designed, constructed, equipped, and maintained to protect health and safety. This protection is for residents, staff, and the public.

Every facility is required to offer recreational therapy and planned activities. These encourage residents to stay involved and active in life. The state licensing body surveys all facilities every year to ensure that they comply with all rules and regulations.

Federal rules and regulations ensure that every resident receives the same high quality of care. This does not depend on how they pay for these services or whether they can request these services themselves.

📖

Biologicals – medical products made from living organisms, such as vaccines or blood components

Preferences – personal choices or favorites

Recreational therapy – working with residents to help them stay active

CMS requires nursing homes to be inspected at least once a year if they received Medicare or Medicaid payments. Surveys are conducted by teams of state surveyors at any time: day or night, weekdays or weekends. Surveyors do not give any advance warning of a survey. Appendix F explains the role of the nurse assistant in the survey process.

In addition to CMS, other organizations also oversee long term care facilities. The Joint Commission on Accreditation of Healthcare Organizations (JCAHO) evaluates and accredits health care organizations and programs in the United States. It is an independent, non-profit organization. Long term care facilities, including subacute care programs and rehabilitation centers, often seek JCAHO accreditation in order to receive managed care contracts. To earn and keep accreditation, an organization must have an on-site survey by a JCAHO survey team at least every three years.

In later chapters you will learn about other places where you may work as a nurse assistant. These include home care, assisted living facilities, hospitals, and community support homes.

IN THIS CHAPTER YOU LEARNED:
- What makes life worth living to each person
- What a long term care facility is
- The four basic services provided in long term care
- Reasons why people are admitted to long term care
- The types of care offered in long term care facilities
- The roles of the members of the interdisciplinary health care team
- How care is paid for
- Agencies that oversee long term care

SUMMARY
This chapter describes the changing focus of long term care to meet the needs of the growing numbers of elderly. You learned about different long term care settings, the services provided, the team that gives care, and the complexity of long term care financing. You also learned that long term care facilities must follow many rules and regulations. All this helps make sure all residents receive quality, individualized care.

PULLING IT ALL TOGETHER
Long term care has never been as exciting as it is today. Providers of long term care now understand better what care is needed for people who are aging. There are wonderful opportunities for nurse assistants. Because long term care involves such diverse activities and the role of nurse assistants keeps growing, you can happily make a lifetime commitment to your work. As a nurse assistant, you will support the fastest growing demographic group in the country, the elderly, as well as others with long term care needs. You will also be able to provide care in many different settings.

Accredit – to recognize or vouch for as conforming with a standard

CHECK WHAT YOU'VE LEARNED

1. **What is gerontology?**
   A. An interval of rest or relief.
   B. The study of older adults and aging.
   C. A type of speech therapy.
   D. The recovery of health and strength after illness or weakness.

2. **Which of these facilities is a long term care facility?**
   A. A dialysis center.
   B. A cancer treatment center.
   C. An assisted living facility.
   D. An outpatient surgery center.

3. **In the year 2050, what percentage of the U.S. population will be over 65?**
   A. 5%.
   B. 15%.
   C. 20%.
   D. 30%.

4. **What is a chronic illness?**
   A. An illness that has no treatment.
   B. An illness that causes a great deal of pain.
   C. An illness that usually lasts a long time.
   D. An illness that requires surgery.

5. **Who is the most important member of the resident care team?**
   A. The resident.
   B. The nurse assistant.
   C. The medical director.
   D. The director of nursing.

6. **Which interdisciplinary care team member counsels residents and their families about services such as Medicaid?**
   A. The bookkeeper.
   B. The administrator.
   C. The social worker.
   D. The director of nursing.

7. **Which of these is performed by nursing staff?**
   A. Prescribing medications.
   B. Giving medications.
   C. Planning menus for the whole facility.
   D. Repairing medical equipment.

8. **Which of these services is usually provided in a long term care facility?**
   A. Home health care.
   B. Radiation therapy.
   C. Rehabilitative care.
   D. Surgery.

9. **What is the role of the Centers for Medicare and Medicaid Services (CMS)?**
   A. To manage hospitals and surgical units across the U.S.
   B. To send monthly welfare checks to people who live in nursing facilities.
   C. To provide health insurance and oversee the surveying and certification of long term care facilities.
   D. To provide medications for residents with emergency needs.

10. **Which organization accredits long term care facilities?**
    A. HMO.
    B. AARP.
    C. CMS.
    D. JCAHO.

(Answers to "Check What You've Learned" are in the Instructor's Manual.)

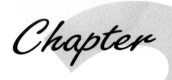

Chapter 2

STARTING YOUR JOB: WHAT TO EXPECT

There are more opportunities for nurse assistants in long term care today than ever before. That is because, according to the National Center for Chronic Disease Prevention and Health Promotion, people in the United States are living much longer than ever before. Between now and the year 2030, the number of older people in this country will double, to over 70 million. One out of every five people will be elderly. Long term care is a part of our health care system designed for people of any age, but it mostly serves the elderly.

Long term care meets both residents' medical needs and their need for help with the activities of daily living. This care is usually given over a long period of time. Long term care facilities have many staff, but most care is given by nurse assistants. Therefore, as a nurse assistant, you can have a great effect on the quality of care and the quality of life of residents in long term care facilities. Career opportunities in long term care are constantly growing. As you become involved today, you help shape the future of long term care.

This chapter introduces you to the role of nurse assistants in long term care. It has three main topics: caregiving, working with the interdisciplinary team, and job functions of the nurse assistant.

OBJECTIVES
- Explain what is meant by mindful caregiving
- List 10 questions to ask when learning about a resident's routine
- Define ethical decisions
- Describe the nursing team
- Explain the importance of developing a trusting relationship with the charge nurse and co-workers
- List four questions to ask when receiving an assignment
- Describe the four different approaches to care
- List at least three factors that influence care
- Describe four essential job functions common to nurse assistant job descriptions
- Describe two ways to take care of yourself

MEDICAL TERMS
- **Contracture** – deformity caused by a permanent shortening of a muscle or by scar tissue
- **Resuscitate** – to revive from apparent death

"I'm glad to be in a place where the people love what they do."

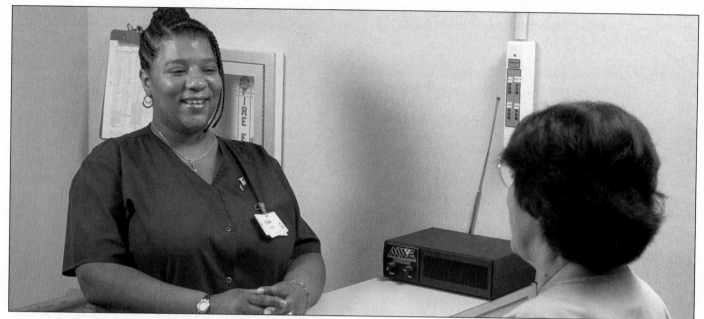

Fig 2-1 – Talking with the charge nurse will help you learn about other nursing roles.

Nurse assistants work in long term care for many reasons. Some of them plan to go on to become nurses someday, and working as a nurse assistant is great experience. Others like working with the elderly. Many have cared for family members in their homes and want to continue to care for others.

What are your reasons for wanting to be a nurse assistant? You should explore your own thoughts and feelings. Understanding why you want to be a nurse assistant will help you think about your role, seek guidance from other staff, plan your continuing education, and stay motivated.

For example, if you plan to become a registered nurse, you may pay special attention to the relationship between nurse assistants and the charge nurse. You may work on skills you can use both as a nurse assistant and later as an registered nurse (RN) (Fig. 2-1). If you are very interested in people, you can learn about residents' many experiences while giving them care. Learning about a resident's past helps you understand who they are now. You may want to become an expert in a type of care such as restorative nursing or wound care. You may want to be a senior nurse assistant who helps new staff in your facility. The key is to understand your own special reasons for working as a nurse assistant. This key will help unlock many opportunities for you.

PROVIDING CARE

What does it mean to provide care? Everyone has their own style of caregiving. As a nurse assistant, you will develop your personal caregiving style.

Nurse assistants help with about 80% of all residents' care. Other team members guide this care. For example, physicians write orders for treatments, and the charge nurse shows you how to give treatments and follow the plan of care. But you have more contact with residents than anyone else on the health care team. You have a very privileged role because you are in a position to give excellent care to residents.

If you or someone you love were ill, how would you want to be cared for? If you were with one person more than with anyone else, how would you want that person to behave or treat you? In long term care, residents rely mostly on nurse assistants. Think about how you would like to be treated yourself. Think about how you would want the most important person in your life to be treated. This is how you should care for residents, too. Your relationship with a resident can make a huge difference in how they view their quality of life and care.

Providing the Best Care Possible: Addressing Quality of Life and Care

You already know that a long term care facility is a place where people live and receive care. Your care should balance the science and skills of nursing, which are the tasks you must perform, and the art of caregiving, which is your personal caregiving style. These two are equally important and must work together. If either is missing, you cannot give quality care and meet the residents' needs for quality of life.

For example, a nurse assistant who focuses only on skills may be efficient, but also may seem cold and uncaring. A nurse assistant who focuses only on the art of caregiving may be caring and compassionate, but may be slow and inefficient. Both skill and art are important in themselves, but balancing them makes you the best caregiver. With both you care for residents in a thoughtful, efficient way—mindfully. Balancing the science and skills of nursing with the art of caring helps ensure that you meet residents' needs (Fig. 2-2).

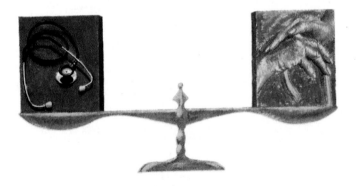

Fig. 2-2 – To give the best care possible you must balance the science of nursing with the art of caregiving.

Here are two examples of how you can achieve this balance:

While helping Mrs. Wallace prepare for breakfast, ask about her plans for the day. Ask how she's feeling, what she would like to wear today, and if she is expecting any visitors. By talking with her you show you care about Mrs. Wallace as much as you care about getting your job done.

Mr. Davis is sitting in his chair while you make his bed. You can say something like, "While I'm making the bed, will you tell me about your children who visited last night?" If Mr. Davis sees that you are really listening and truly interested, he will feel that you care about him (Fig. 2-3).

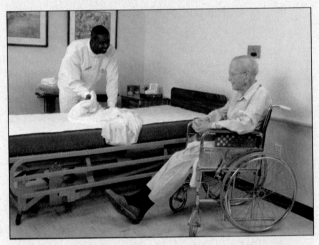

Fig. 2-3 – Talking with residents while you do various tasks shows you care about them, not just about getting the job done.

These examples show the key to successful caregiving. They show that you can "do your job" and at the same time create a caring atmosphere.

While you do your daily duties, remember to act mindfully and to balance the science and skills of nursing with the art of caregiving. This way you give the best care possible.

Mindful – continually being aware

Mindful Caregiving

What is mindful caregiving? It means paying attention to details, looking at situations openly, being observant, and being willing to change. When you care every day for the same residents, you may expect that everything about them will always be the same. Your actions might become automatic, and your caregiving may suffer. Consider this situation:

You have been caring for Mr. Jones for the last month. You know he likes to eat breakfast, then shave, and then bathe and dress. Every day seems the same. Today, you get his breakfast tray and prepare his shaving supplies. Later, you return to help him prepare for his shower and put away his shaving equipment. You help him take his shower and dress. Then suddenly you notice that he did not shave (Fig. 2-4).

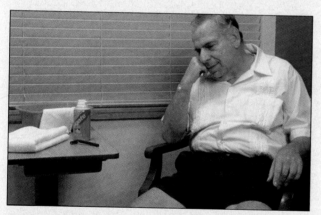

Fig. 2-4 – Paying attention to residents helps you identify changes in them.

Today Mr. Jones found out that his son is very ill and has been admitted to a hospital. He is so upset and worried that he did not eat or shave. You mindlessly assumed that today was the same as every other day. You didn't even notice at first that he hadn't eaten his breakfast or shaved and that he was quieter than usual. You are the person Mr. Jones spends the most time with. To Mr. Jones you are a friend, but today you were so busy, or so mindless, you didn't even notice him.

How would you feel if the person you spent most of your time with didn't notice something important to you? You might feel that person didn't care for you after all.

In a long term care facility you will care for several residents. Pay close attention to all your actions. Think about Mr. Jones again. One of your daily tasks is to help Mr. Jones shave. What should you have noticed that would show you something was wrong?

You had two chances to notice changes in Mr. Jones that should have alerted you that something was wrong. First, you should have seen the change in Mr. Jones' eating habits. You could have asked, "Mr. Jones, you didn't eat your breakfast today. Is there something wrong?" Second, you should have noticed that Mr. Jones, who shaves every day and cares about how he looks, didn't shave today. Paying attention to a resident's routine and noticing any changes help you to be a better caregiver. You can see signals that something is wrong. This is part of mindful caregiving.

You could also miss important signs and symptoms if you do not pay attention as you do your job. Mr. Jones might have skipped his breakfast and shaving because he felt ill rather than sad. What if you did not really look at him but just automatically removed his tray and shaving equipment? You would miss seeing that he is flushed and his skin feels hot. This information is very important, and you should report it right away. Mr. Jones could have a serious infection.

Whether he was sad or ill, either way you missed important signals from this resident. Mr. Jones needed you to listen to him, or to notice his condition and report it so that he could receive treatment.

Be mindful when you provide care. Never let **routine** care, such as eating, bathing, and dressing, become automatic or "routine." This helps you to be aware of problem situations like Mr. Jones'. Residents have a right to have their needs met. A nurse assistant who mindlessly does tasks for residents strips them of their independence and dignity and misses important clues and signals. Mindless caregiving leads to residents having a lower quality of care and a lower quality of life. But mindful caregiving leads to residents having a higher quality of care and a higher quality of life.

Routine – pattern of activities you set with each resident individually; something repeated on a schedule

Understanding Residents' Routines

New nurse assistants often wonder how they can know what a resident likes or dislikes. It is your responsibility to understand how residents and their families want to be cared for.

The best way to learn about residents is to ask questions (Fig. 2-5). Ask the resident, family, and other health care workers, especially the charge nurse. You can also review a resident's care plan and medical records to learn more about their preferences. Here are some questions you can ask residents:

- How do you like to start your day?
- Do you like to get up early and be ready for breakfast?
- How do you like to bathe?
- What do you need help with?
- What can I do to help make you more comfortable?
- What do you do in your spare time? Read? Watch television? Walk? Visit with friends?
- Describe the kind of day you like.
- Do you like to nap during the day?
- Does anything give you trouble when getting dressed?
- How much would you like me to help with your personal care?

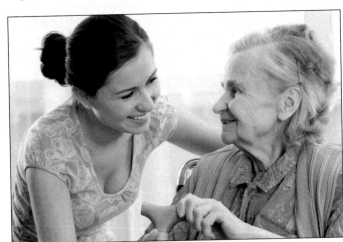

Fig. 2-5 – Taking the time to ask residents questions helps you learn about their likes and dislikes.

Think of other questions you would want someone to ask you if they were caring for you. You'll learn that all residents have preferences for their care. Every resident wants to be treated respectfully, but that may mean different things. For example, one resident feels that privacy is very important and thinks questions about their family are disrespectful. Another wants you to be interested in their family and to ask about them. Remember, no two people are the same. Everyone has different habits, preferences, and beliefs.

Asking questions is also important when you work together with residents to make a daily routine. This includes dressing, bathing, and grooming. Think about your own morning routine. Do you first drink coffee, or brush your teeth, or take a shower? You probably have a routine that you've followed for years. Think about times when your routine was disrupted. The coffee maker was broken, or you missed your bus, or one of your children was sick. At such times you miss the comfort of your personal routine.

The same is true for residents. They, too, like to do certain things at certain times and in certain ways. Remember that a change in routine can be very disruptive and upsetting to a resident. Routines involve residents' personalities. You might think it would be easier if you set the routine for residents, but that would take away their individuality and their choice.

Values and Culture

People's **values** guide how they choose to live their lives. Everyone's values are individual and very personal. Values are beliefs that come from a person's family, upbringing, religion, friends, education, and individual experience. Following are some examples of values:

- being healthy and active
- respecting persons with authority, such as parents, teachers, and police officers
- being able to take care of oneself
- making a lot of money
- practicing religious beliefs
- being useful
- having close friends

Try to understand the values of each resident you care for. Although this takes time, it's worth it. Residents' values help you understand what gives meaning to their lives and why they act as they do (Fig. 2-6, next page). For example, a resident who does not visit with other residents or take part in social events may value privacy more than friendship. You may feel the person is lonely because you would

---

Values – beliefs people have about what is important to them

be lonely if you spent so much time alone. But that is your own value, not this resident's. A resident may simply enjoy their solitude, or time alone.

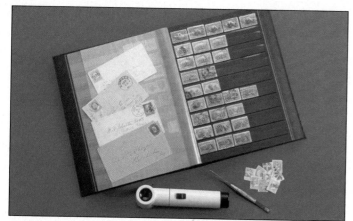

Fig. 2-6 – You need to learn about the resident's interests and how they like to spend their free time.

To learn a resident's values, ask questions like these:
- What is important to you?
- What did you do for a living?
- What was special about your job?
- Do you go to religious services?
- Is your family important to you?
- How do you like to spend your free time?

Sometimes a resident's values are very different from their friends' or family members', yours, and society's. But we cannot say that one person's values are right and another's are wrong. Values are not matters of right and wrong. It is very important to your job to accept the values of others, even if you do not agree with them.

Culture has a strong influence on values. Culture influences one's food preferences, personal care practices, clothing choices, and family relationships. For example, in some cultures, a "laying on of hands" is believed to cure illness. Some cultures expect women to dress in a certain way. Other cultures have special rituals for personal care practices like cutting hair or bathing.

Contracture – deformity caused by a permanent shortening of a muscle or ligaments, or by scar tissue
Culture – the customary beliefs, social forms, and traits of a racial, religious, or social group
Ethics – knowledge, awareness, or study of good and bad, right and wrong, and moral duty
Resuscitate – to revive from apparent death

Remember that your own values and culture might influence how you give care, just as residents' values and culture affect their preferences for care. You are not expected to know everything about every culture. But try to understand how the resident's culture influences their values. Ask the resident about any cultural preferences they have that might affect your caregiving. Some areas to consider are personal care, nutrition choices, pain management, spirituality, and end of life issues and concerns.

Ethics

There are no right or wrong values, although sometimes a decision must be made that favors one value over another. Decisions may also involve ethics. Ethical issues often arise in relation to values about the quality of life. People may value life differently, and make different ethical decisions based on those values. Table 2-1 presents examples of this.

TABLE 2-1 ETHICAL DECISIONS BASED ON INDIVIDUAL VALUES

VALUE	ETHICAL DECISION
Life is worth living only if there is some hope that you can take care of yourself.	• To choose not to be resuscitated if cardiac arrest happens, or if you are bedridden with severe contractures and a lot of pain • To choose not to have a feeding tube if you can no longer eat • To choose to remain in the facility if seriously ill, and not be moved to a hospital
Life is worth living no matter whether or not you can ever take care of yourself again.	• To choose to be resuscitated if cardiac arrest happens, regardless of your functional ability or amount of pain • To choose to have a feeding tube if you can no longer eat • To choose to go to the hospital for treatment of a life-threatening illness

Most decisions about care do not involve conflicting values. A resident and family usually make ethical decisions about care along with their physician without any conflict. However, if you ever feel someone is making a wrong decision on behalf of a resident, talk to the charge nurse.

Never argue with a resident or family member about their values or ethics. It is important for you to support residents and family members, especially in how they make decisions about important issues such as the end of life.

Developing Trust

It takes time to learn about residents. Some openly tell you about themselves and what they like and don't like. Others are slow to share this information with you. Try to develop a trusting, respectful relationship with all residents, even though with some of them this will take a little longer. Trust is the basis for any relationship: A relationship cannot grow without it. To develop a trusting relationship with your residents, follow these guidelines:

- Make sure residents feel safe. Support them when walking. Help them when they ask you. Answer their call lights.
- Listen to what residents want you to do and how they want things done (Fig. 2-7). Follow their exact instructions unless those instructions will endanger them, you, or others.
- Be clear with residents about what you can and cannot do for them. Be courteous at all times.
- Be honest and open with residents. If a resident calls you for help when you are on your way to help another resident, ask if they can wait 10 minutes until you finish helping the other resident. If the resident can wait, be sure to come back in 10 minutes as you promised. Be reliable.
- Be consistent. Help each resident with morning care and routines at the same time every day, based on their preferences. Remind residents who you are—give your name and say what you're going to do. Treat each resident respectfully.
- Dress professionally. This conveys your respect for residents. Residents will feel that if you do a good job taking care of yourself, you will also do a good job taking care of them.

Gaining a person's trust also involves keeping their confidence. When caring for and talking with a resident, you learn many personal things about them. An important part of being a caregiver is keeping this information confidential. Do not talk about a resident with other residents or with anyone not connected with a resident's care.

If you are uncomfortable or embarrassed about giving certain kinds of care (like helping with toileting), tell the charge nurse about your feelings. The resident may also feel uncomfortable, and discussing this might help the resident. If you are not open about your feelings, you may send mixed messages to a resident. For example, when a

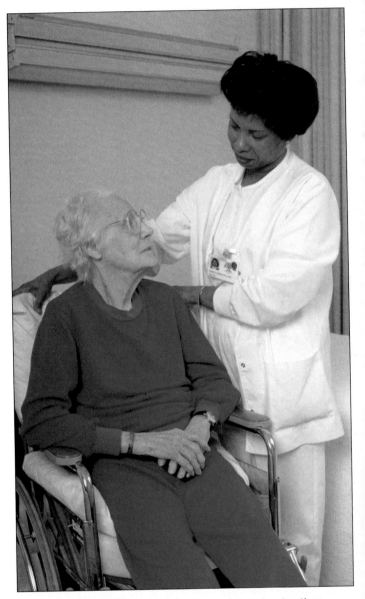

Fig. 2-7 – Listening to the resident helps you to create a trusting relationship.

resident asks for help with toileting, you may frown even though you try to answer positively, and the resident will see this. Work to overcome any negative feelings so that you do not react to a resident in ways that hurt your trusting relationship with them. You will learn more about nonverbal communication in Chapter 7, Communication.

THE INTERDISCIPLINARY TEAM

In Chapter 1 you learned that many different people provide services for residents in long term care. The largest department is the nursing department, led by the director of nursing. Nursing departments are typically organized as in Figure 2-8. All team members work together to provide the service. You will spend more time with nursing team members than anyone else on the interdisciplinary team.

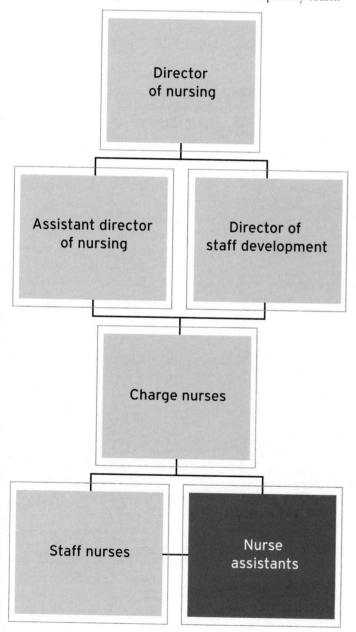

Fig. 2-8 – Typical organizational chart of nursing services.

- The **director of nursing** develops the philosophy (a belief about quality care) and approach for care. The nursing staff follows this approach. The director also determines staffing requirements.
- The **assistant director of nursing** helps the director of nursing put into action the philosophy and approach to care.
- The **director of staff development** usually reports directly to the director of nursing. This person oversees staff education in the philosophy and approach to nursing care.
- **Charge nurses** report directly to either the director or assistant director of nursing, depending on the facility. They have the day-to-day responsibility for supervising resident care. Charge nurses give the specific care assignments. They are a resource for problem solving and teaching, and they can help you with inservice education. (Fig. 2-9).

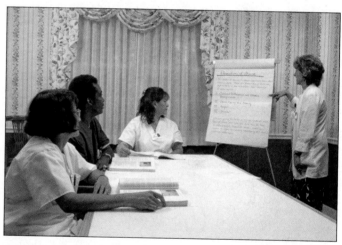

Fig. 2-9 – The charge nurse or the director of staff development may provide formal or informal inservice education.

- The number of **staff nurses** depends on the facility's staffing needs. Staff nurses are responsible for special treatments and medications. A staff nurse may act as a charge nurse on some shifts.
- **Nurse assistants** report directly to charge nurses or staff nurses. Nurse assistants give 80% of all resident care.

Shift – scheduled period of work for a group of people (day shift, evening shift, night shift)

Developing a Relationship With the Charge Nurse

Your relationship with the charge nurse will help you give quality care. You need to feel you are partners in order to reach the caregiving goals for all residents. The charge nurse can also help you understand how best to give care. They can help you with problem solving and inservice education. To develop a good relationship with the charge nurse, be reliable and trustworthy, and communicate openly.

Follow these guidelines to develop a good relationship with the charge nurse:
- Be on time for work every day (Fig. 2-10).

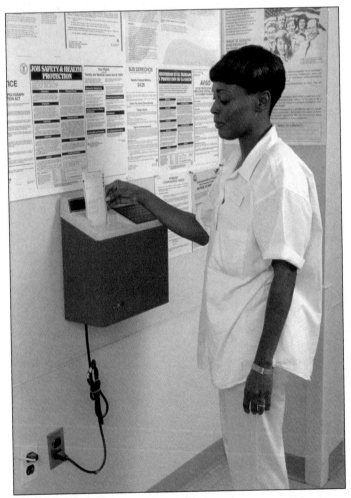

Fig. 2-10 – Being on time for work helps show you are a reliable team member.

- Be open-minded and flexible in accepting your assignment.
- Ask questions about things you do not understand.

Make sure you understand what the charge nurse expects of you.
- Be patient when you need the charge nurse's help. Remember, the charge nurse has many other responsibilities, too.
- Report any resident changes immediately to the charge nurse.
- Talk about any problems or concerns you may have.
- Be accountable and honest.

Developing Relationships With Co-workers

A positive relationship with your co-workers is also important. Every nurse assistant has their own assignment, but you should help each other and work together. For example, sometimes residents you are not assigned to will ask you for help with something. Residents expect their needs to be met when they ask. You must never say, "I can't do that. I'm not your nurse assistant." Instead, help the resident with their request and then report this to the nurse assistant assigned to them.

If the request is something you cannot do, simply tell the resident, "I cannot do that. Let me get the nurse assistant caring for you." You then can offer the assigned nurse assistant your help. Some tasks, such as moving a very weak resident, require help from another nurse assistant to prevent injury to you and the resident. You can do many nurse assistant skills on your own, but some others require help from your co-workers (Fig 2-11).

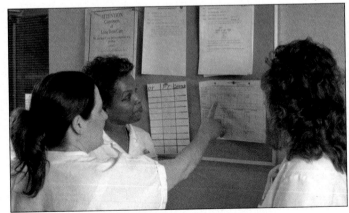

Fig. 2-11 – Before you begin your day, plan with the other nurse assistants when you can help each other.

Inservice – Educational programs taught to staff while on the job

Therefore, develop a good working relationship with your co-workers. Remember that working together with others on the caregiving team improves your ability to give residents good care. Here are some actions that help develop positive relationships:

- Offer to help to co-workers.
- Be supportive and available to help co-workers when needed, as long as it doesn't interfere with immediate care that you are giving to another resident.
- Go to lunch together (if staff scheduling allows).
- Share ideas about caregiving (but remember, respect the residents' rights to confidentiality).
- Call in sick only when you are ill.
- Attend inservice education classes together.
- Be honest and reliable.
- Be open to learn about and accept cultural differences.
- Respect others' opinions and beliefs.

Remember that although the charge nurse guides your activities, your co-workers are the ones who help you when needed. Try to get along with them. A supportive work environment is also a more pleasant one.

When everyone on the care team cooperates and works together, residents receive better care.

Daily Assignments

At the start of your shift every day, you will receive your assignment from the charge nurse. This assignment includes the residents you will care for that day. You might also meet with staff on the previous shift to hear their report about these residents, or you may get this information from the charge nurse. For example, you may learn that a resident who usually sleeps all night was awake and pacing the floor. You also learn about residents' treatments and medication status.

Carefully review your assignment and ask the charge nurse any questions. Always have all the information you need before you begin giving care. This includes the following:

- Do any residents have special needs today?
- Do I need help from the charge nurse at any time to give a resident a treatment?
- Does the charge nurse want any particular things done first?
- Do any residents have any special appointments today?

Review your assignment with the charge nurse (Fig. 2-12).

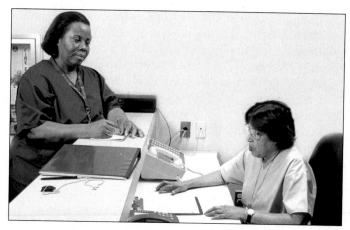

Fig. 2-12 – Be sure to ask any questions you may have when the charge nurse gives you your assignment.

This is a good time to talk about and ask questions about anything you feel uncomfortable doing. Always be honest with the charge nurse about this. Talking openly with the charge nurse about your assignment lets them know when you need help and when you can be independent. For example, a resident needs to go to the hospital for an x-ray, but you have never done this, and so you do not know about all the tasks that are involved in sending the resident. The charge nurse can teach you about the tasks you will be doing. Never try to do anything you have not learned to do. For example, if you do not talk with the charge nurse about how to send a resident for an x-ray, you might forget to send the resident's chart. Then the x-ray might not get taken and the resident will have to go back again later. You will find the charge nurse to be a great resource and educator.

APPROACHES TO CARE

Different approaches to nursing care are used in different facilities. The director of nursing usually determines the facility's approach based on a philosophy of caring, the residents' needs, available staff, and costs.

Team nursing is a common approach in long term care. The charge nurse is the team leader and makes assignments based on the needs for the shift. The team cares for a whole group of residents in a unit or a wing (sometimes called a neighborhood or a household). The charge nurse assigns team members to specific residents, but you work with other nurse assistants as a team to give care. For

Wing – separate section of a building attached to the central section example, nurse assistants may discuss how to feed a large number of residents. They may decide to change their own lunch breaks so everyone can help with feeding, regardless of who is assigned. They talk to the team leader about any problems or concerns they have about residents. With team nursing, a group of nursing team members is assigned to care for a group of residents, and together all the care is provided.

Another nursing approach is called functional nursing. With this approach, you have specific tasks rather than specific residents as the focus of care. For example, you might have the responsibility of helping with all the showers one day, while another nurse assistant makes all the beds. Sometimes this approach is used when there is a staffing shortage. If a nurse assistant calls in sick, the charge nurse may assign tasks to other nurse assistants so that all care activities are done on the shift.

A third nursing approach is called primary nursing. With this approach, a registered nurse or licensed practical nurse has the primary responsibility for residents' needs. You work with this nurse and care for the same residents each day. Together, you are responsible for residents' care 24 hours a day. On other shifts, other staff members carry out the plan of care that has been set by you, the nurse, and each resident. This approach is more common in hospitals and facilities where residents are assigned to nurse assistants for a long time.

You will learn which approach your facility uses when you start work. Regardless of which approach is used at your facility, always focus on giving quality care to residents. If you are unclear about which approach is being used, ask the charge nurse. Many factors influence caregiving. Be open to all approaches, and always keep residents' needs your primary concern.

FACTORS THAT INFLUENCE CARE

In addition to the facility's approach, these other factors influence care:

- **The resident's needs.** A resident's needs are always the primary focus of care. Always ask yourself, "Is this what this resident wants or needs?"
- **Philosophy of caring.** The director of nursing sets the direction for care activities. Different directors have different ideas about how to do things. You will learn your director of nursing's focus on care in the facility where you work.
- **New treatments and equipment.** Facilities are always looking for better ways to give care. Your facility may try new things, such as new products to treat skin breakdowns or new back-protection devices.

- **Federal and state regulations.** Federal and state regulations provide a framework for caregiving. These include the Code of Federal Regulations and the Occupational Safety and Health Administration (OSHA) standards. These rules and regulations influence how much care you give, how you give care, and how often. This helps ensure that residents receive quality care. For example, facilities are required to display the Residents' Bill of Rights. In many facilities, posters are displayed in bathrooms to remind staff to wash their hands.
- **Staffing.** The reliability of staff is a major influence on caregiving. If staff members often call in sick or resign, the team does not function as well and residents' care may suffer. The attitude of the nursing staff influences all the factors above.

These factors sometimes lead to changes in caregiving. You may not always know the reason for a change. But if you keep an open mind, ask questions, and keep residents' well being the highest priority, you will be more comfortable with changes.

JOB FUNCTIONS

As a nurse assistant, you are a member of the nursing team. You work closely with other nurse assistants, the charge nurse, and other members of the interdisciplinary team. Usually the facility gives you its written personnel policies as well as your job description, which includes this information:

- your department
- your title
- overview of your job
- list of your responsibilities
- description of your specific functions
- qualifications needed for your job

Carefully read your facility's job description for nurse assistants. Talk with the charge nurse about any questions or concerns you have. An example of a job description is shown here. Notice that it describes the qualifications needed for the job and outlines the job functions and requirements for being successful. Future chapters in this book will fully describe all the job functions listed here.

NURSE ASSISTANT JOB DESCRIPTION

Department: _____

Name: _____

Date of Hire: _____

GENERAL PURPOSE

To perform direct care duties under the supervision of nursing personnel and to assist in maintaining a positive physical, social, and psychological environment for the residents.

QUALIFICATIONS

- Pass the state competency evaluation.
- Be a state registered nurse assistant (certified or licensed) in good standing according to all applicable federal and state certification requirements, or be in training to become a state registered nurse assistant.
- Be at least 16 years of age.
- Be able to read, write, and follow oral and written directions, and have successfully completed elementary education.
- Speak and understand English.
- Have a positive attitude toward the elderly.

ESSENTIAL JOB FUNCTIONS

A. PERSONAL CARE FUNCTIONS
Duties:

Assist residents with: daily bath, dressing, grooming, dental care, and bowel and bladder functions; preparation for medical tests and exams; ear and eye care; and transferring into and out of beds, chairs, bathtubs, etc.

Physical and sensory requirements:

Walking; reaching; bending; lifting; grasping; fine hand coordination; pushing and pulling; and ability to distinguish smells, tastes, and temperatures.

B. NURSING CARE FUNCTIONS
Duties:

Provide nursing functions as directed by supervisor, including daily perineal care and catheter care; change dressings; turn residents in bed; give sponge baths; measure and record temperature, pulse, and respirations; weigh and measure residents; perform restorative and rehabilitative procedures; observe and report presence of skin breakdowns; review care plans daily; report changes in resident conditions to supervisor; record all necessary charting entries; and report all accidents and incidents.

Physical and sensory requirements:

Bending; lifting; grasping; fine hand coordination; ability to communicate with residents; ability to distinguish smells, tastes, and temperatures; and ability to hear and respond to resident requests.

C. FOOD SERVICE FUNCTIONS
Duties:

Prepare residents for meals and snacks; identify food arrangement, and assist in feeding residents as needed; record food and fluid intake; and perform after-meal resident care.

Physical and sensory requirements:

Lifting; grasping; fine hand coordination; ability to distinguish smells, tastes, and temperatures; and ability to write or otherwise record intake.

D. RESIDENTS' RIGHTS FUNCTIONS
Duties:

Maintain resident confidentiality; treat residents with kindness, dignity, and respect; know and comply with Residents' Bill of Rights; and promptly report all resident complaints, accidents, and incidents to supervisor.

Physical and sensory requirements:

Ability to communicate with residents and to remain calm under stress.

OTHER JOB FUNCTIONS

A. SUPPORT FUNCTIONS
Duties:

Assist as directed in proper admission, transfer, and discharge of residents; inventory residents' possessions and report food articles and medications found in residents' rooms; and report defective equipment to administration.

Physical and sensory requirements:

Ability to communicate with residents and to read and write in English.

B. SAFETY AND SANITATION FUNCTIONS
Duties:

Understand and use Centers for Disease Control and Prevention (CDC) Standard Precautions, OSHA's Occupational Exposure to Bloodborne Pathogens standard, and follow established infection control, hazardous communication, and other safety rules; ensure cleanliness of assigned residents' rooms; properly maintain and record residents' restraints; and promptly report all violations of safety and sanitation rules to supervisor.

Physical and sensory requirements:

Walking; bending; lifting; grasping; fine hand coordination; ability to read and write in English; and ability to distinguish smells.

C. STAFF DEVELOPMENT FUNCTIONS
Duties:

Attend and participate in orientation, training, educational activities, and staff meetings.

Physical and sensory requirements:

Ability to understand and apply training and inservice education.

D. ALL OTHER DUTIES AS ASSIGNED

Once you are on the job you will learn your specific job responsibilities. You will learn the facility's 24-hour routine and what happens during each shift. The day shift is usually 7 a.m. to 3:30 p.m., the evening shift 3 p.m. to 11:30 p.m., and night shift 11 p.m. to 7:30 a.m. These shifts ensure residents receive care 24 hours a day, seven days a week, including holidays, all year.

Your general responsibilities to residents and your employer include the following:

1. Recognize residents as individuals.
- Find out residents' likes and dislikes.
- Ask how they want things done. Get to know their routine.
- Learn about their culture (Fig. 2-13).
- Find out if they have cultural preferences regarding their care, and follow their preferences.

2. Promote residents' autonomy (self-determination).
- Understand residents' rights.
- Respect their rights when giving care.
- Encourage residents to maintain their highest level of functioning.
- Support their choices in personal care.
- Involve residents in all decisions about their care.
- Maintain their privacy.

3. Provide mindful caregiving.
- Balance the science and skills and the art of caregiving (Fig. 2-14).

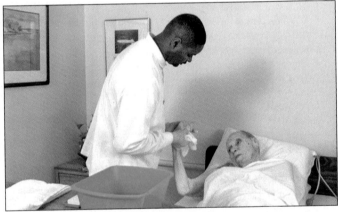

Fig. 2-14 – Take advantage of every opportunity to talk with your residents.

- Observe residents closely.
- Watch for any changes in their attitude or behavior.
- Report any changes to the charge nurse.

4. Be a good employee.
- Be reliable.
- Be healthy: Get enough sleep, eat a balanced diet, exercise.
- Be considerate of others.
- Cooperate with other team members.
- Be efficient with your time and supplies.
- Follow all personnel policies.
- Dress appropriately: neat and clean.
- Pay attention to personal hygiene.
- Do not use drugs or drink alcohol during work hours or before coming to work.

Box 2-1 lists tasks nurse assistants commonly perform.

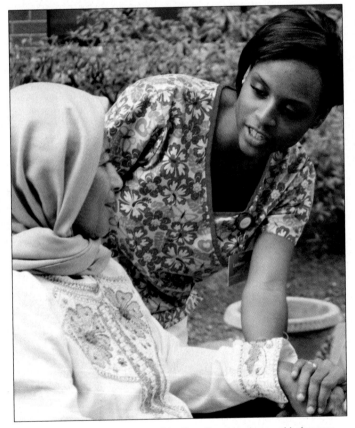

Fig. 2-13 – Learning about a resident's cultural background helps you understand their needs and give the best possible care.

BOX 2-1. COMMON TASKS OF NURSE ASSISTANTS

ASSISTING WITH PERSONAL CARE FOR RESIDENTS:
- bathing
- oral hygiene
- grooming (hair and nail care)
- dressing and undressing

ASSISTING RESIDENTS WITH MOBILITY (FIG. 2-15):
- walking
- positioning
- range-of-motion exercises

ASSISTING RESIDENTS WITH MEALS:
- transporting to dining room
- preparing the environment
- preparing residents
- feeding residents
- caring for residents after meals
- recording intake and output

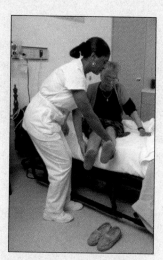

Fig. 2-15 – Helping residents stay mobile is an important nurse assistant task.

PROVIDING PHYSICAL COMFORT TO RESIDENTS:
- back rubs
- pillow fluffing
- hand-holding (if a resident desires)
- touching gently (if a resident desires)

PROVIDING EMOTIONAL SUPPORT FOR RESIDENTS:
- listening carefully
- working with family members
- holding a resident (if they desire)
- being with residents when they receive bad news
- sharing experiences

MAINTAINING EACH RESIDENT'S ENVIRONMENT:
- practicing infection control procedures
- cleaning residents' rooms
- making residents' beds
- preventing injuries

As you start your job, you will see that taking care of yourself is also important in order to be a successful employee. Chapter 30 discusses the skills and knowledge you need to be a successful employee.

TAKING CARE OF YOURSELF

Your role as a caregiver makes it important to learn to take care of yourself both physically and emotionally. Your work can be very demanding at times. You may feel you have too much to do or that residents ask for too much. You may feel stress.

Coping With Stress

If you are worried about things, not sleeping well, eating poorly or overeating, feeling moody, or drinking too much, these conditions could be signs that you are feeling stressed. Sometimes it is hard to cope with stress. Sometimes you do not even know what is causing your stress. Often people think that their job is causing stress when actually it is something else. To be able to deal with stress in your life, you must first figure out what is causing it. It might be:
- financial concerns
- your children
- a significant other, friend, or family member
- your job
- a combination of several factors

Thinking about these things will help you find the cause of your stress. If you conclude that your job is causing you stress, try these tips:
- Make a list of what you need to do. Start with the most important task, and cross off each task as you do it.
- Explain to a resident why you cannot spend more time with them. Say something like, "Mr. Jones, I want to hear what you are saying, but right now I have a lot to do. May I come back a little later? Let's set a time."
- Make time daily to do something relaxing for yourself, like reading, taking a walk, or spending time with a friend.
- Talk to a friend or spouse about your job and how you are helping others. It always feels good to talk about your work and things you experience, whether good or bad.
- If something besides your job is causing you stress, such as a death in your family or your marital problems, talk with your supervisor. In some cases you may need to take some time off to handle personal problems.

Here are some other things you can do to reduce the stress you feel:
- Spend time with a friend.
- Treat yourself to your favorite dessert.
- Exercise with a co-worker (Fig. 2-16).

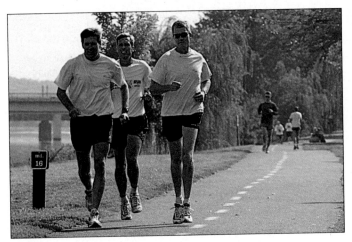

Fig. 2-16 – Exercise with friends can help you manage your stress.

- Do not abuse alcohol or other drugs.
- Eat a balanced diet.
- Get a good night's sleep.

Coping With Your Emotions

Some residents you care for may become like family. If they get sick, move away, or die, you may miss them and feel sad about losing them. To cope with your feelings of grief, you can:
- Talk about your feelings with co-workers or family members.
- Take time to think about why you miss that person and what they meant to you.
- Let yourself feel sad. This is a normal reaction when something bad happens to someone you care about.
- Sometimes when you're feeling sad or stressed, you need to get away from the situation for a while. You may need be alone to cry or scream.

In your job as a nurse assistant, you will not have to decide about resuscitating residents, starting tube feeding, or sending residents to the hospital. Even so, you will feel these things should be done or should not be done because of your own values. Sometimes you may be uncomfortable with a decision or feel it is wrong. To manage your feelings of discomfort, you can:

- Talk to your supervisor, who may give you information that helps you to better understand the decision (Fig. 2-17).

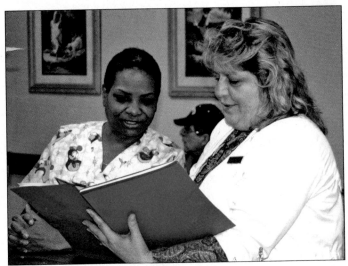

Fig. 2-17 – Talking with your supervisor will help you understand different decisions about residents.

- Talk to your minister, priest, rabbi, or religious leader about your feelings.
- Remember that although you need to talk about your feelings about a situation, all residents have a right to privacy. Once a decision has been made, do not try to talk a resident or their family member into changing their mind.

IN THIS CHAPTER YOU LEARNED:
- What mindful caregiving means
- Ten questions to ask when learning about a resident's routine
- How to make ethical decisions
- How the nursing team works together
- The importance of developing a trusting relationship with the charge nurse and co-workers
- Four questions to ask when receiving an assignment
- Different approaches to care used in facilities
- Factors that influence care
- Four essential job functions common to nurse assistant job descriptions
- Two ways to take care of yourself

SUMMARY
This chapter concerns your general role as a nurse assistant. It includes information you need to know to be successful in this role and important information about the philosophy you should adopt about mindful caregiving.

Creating positive relationships with your supervisor and other staff you work with is important as you grow as a nurse assistant. You will be learning a wide range of tasks to perform your job well.

PULLING IT ALL TOGETHER
Think about why you want to be a nurse assistant. This will help you be successful in your work. Being a nurse assistant is a career, not just a job. You should look forward to doing it because you can make a difference in residents' quality of life and care.

The keys to quality caregiving include adopting a philosophy of mindful caregiving; being open, observant, caring, and willing to change; and balancing the art of caregiving with the skills of nursing care.

In addition to creating your own style of caregiving, think about the skills you will be learning for your work, such as creating positive relationships and learning about your facility's organizational structure.

1. **What is "mindful caregiving"?**
   A. Wearing comfortable shoes and clothing to work.
   B. Storing soiled equipment and supplies in the clean supply room.
   C. Paying attention to details and being open, observant, and flexible.
   D. Sharing your opinions about a resident's care with their family members.

2. **What is an example of mindful caregiving?**
   A. Being on time for work.
   B. Encouraging residents to wear clothing you like.
   C. Observing changes in a resident's mood or routine.
   D. Requiring a resident to stick with the facility's schedule.

3. **Which of the following statements about values is true?**
   A. Some cultural groups have better values than others.
   B. Nurse assistants should teach their values to residents.
   C. Residents must accept that they cannot bring their own values along when they move into a long term care facility.
   D. It is important to respect the values of other people, even if we don't agree with those values.

4. **Which of these behaviors will help you develop a good relationship with the charge nurse?**
   A. Ask questions about things you do not understand.
   B. Always make it look like you know what you are doing.
   C. To show the charge nurse your eagerness, demand help for things immediately.
   D. Do not waste the charge nurse's time by reporting changes in residents.

5. **Which of the following is important for developing and maintaining a trusting relationship with a resident?**
   A. Hiding any mistakes you make from them.
   B. Making all important decisions for them.
   C. Providing care when they need it.
   D. Discussing the resident's business with other residents.

6. **How do you create a good relationship with a co-worker?**
   A. Call in sick if you think they would like some extra overtime work.
   B. Promise them you'll never tell the charge nurse if they accidentally hurt a resident.
   C. Tell them funny stories you learn about residents you care for.
   D. Offer them your help when needed.

7. **Mrs. Davies is a new resident with special needs you've never handled before. You should:**
   A. Simply do the best you can for her.
   B. Let Mrs. Davies take care of herself.
   C. Discuss your concerns with the charge nurse.
   D. Ask another nurse assistant to handle Mrs. Davies for you.

8. **What is "functional nursing"?**
   A. Nurse assistants are responsible for specific tasks, such as bathing or bedmaking, rather than for specific residents.
   B. Nurses and nurse assistants work in pairs to provide care each day.
   C. A group of nursing team members are assigned to care for a group of residents.
   D. Another term for primary nursing.

9. **What is a common task for a nurse assistant?**
   A. Taking residents out to the movies.
   B. Removing stitches from an incision.
   C. Helping a resident with personal care.
   D. Changing light bulbs in the dining room and hallways.

10. **Which strategy can help you deal with stress?**
    A. Call in sick for work as often as possible.
    B. Take time for yourself each day, to just relax.
    C. Exercise no more than an hour each month.
    D. To avoid feeling overwhelmed, never make a list of everything you need to do.

(Answers to "Check What You've Learned" are in the Instructor's Manual.)

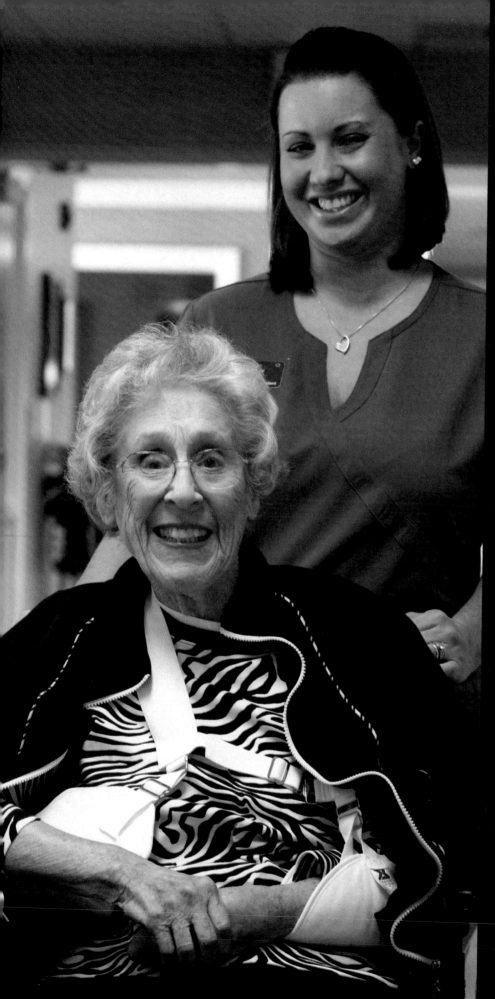

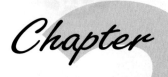

Chapter 3

UNDERSTANDING PEOPLE By the time you meet the residents you will care for, they will have lived many years. Some of their experiences over the years will have been positive, and others will have been negative, but they all add to who they are. Often, residents think moving into a long term care facility will be a negative experience. Even with negative experiences or feelings, however, residents still value their lives. You need to understand what residents have done, how they make decisions, how they deal with stress and conflict, and how they respond in their daily lives. This way you can better support the residents, help them meet their needs, and help them find meaning in their lives while living in a long term care facility.

This chapter is about understanding residents. This helps you meet their needs. It is about how residents develop into who they are, how you learn about them, and how people cope with changes in different stages of life.

OBJECTIVES
- Describe how you get to know a resident
- List Erikson's eight stages of psychosocial development
- Define Maslow's hierarchy of needs
- List ways to meet residents' needs
- Describe how residents' basic needs are similar to your own
- Describe how knowing a resident's history will help you understand them better

MEDICAL TERMS
- **Amputation** – cutting a limb (for example an arm or leg) from the body
- **Psychosocial** – involving psychological, emotional, and social aspects of mental health

"Know me for who I am and treat me like a special friend."

Think about what you consider important in your life. Maybe this includes being loved, looking your best, or choosing where you live and with whom you spend time. Think about important events that affected you. Think about things that have made you feel good, such as graduating from high school, having a child, or getting a job you really wanted—times when you were proud of what you had accomplished. Remember also times you were sad. Maybe someone you loved died, or you lost a job or had to move. Think about the impact of those experiences on you. Did they lead you to act in positive or negative ways? Did those actions cause problems? Does the experience still affect you in some way?

Now think about people with whom you work: residents, their families, and other staff. They have also had experiences that affected their lives. Maybe their experiences are similar to yours, or maybe different. Part of what makes an experience positive or negative for each of us has to do with how we deal with it and its outcome.

PSYCHOSOCIAL WELL-BEING

How do you help residents live their lives in your long term care facility? As you learned in Chapter 2, the best thing you can do for a resident is to get to know them. Understanding their **needs** and wants helps you give them the best care you can. Talking with them about their background, their personality, and their coping skills will help you to learn about them. These are all factors that can contribute to their **psychosocial** well-being.

For example, you may notice that a resident acts differently when one of their children visits than when another does. You may not know the history of that relationship, but you see the resident's reaction to the visit. Talk with the resident about this so you can offer support if needed. You may learn that one child met all the resident's expectations and the other did not. You may even encounter a situation in which either the resident or their child has been abusive to the other. Remember that it's important to remain neutral at all times when you communicate with residents and families about these relationships. Talk to the charge nurse about what you see, so that the entire team can plan for the resident's safety and psychosocial well-being.

Discovering the Resident

What do you have in common with residents?

All human beings have the same basic needs. Just becoming older does not mean that a person's needs change. Most people try to meet their needs the same way all of their lives. As you read the following descriptions of three different people, look for the same basic needs that all three have. Also notice the different ways they meet these needs.

Ellen is a 32-year-old divorced mother of three children who is now a nurse assistant in a long term care facility in her hometown. Although she comes from a large family, she has little daily contact with them. She receives little financial or emotional support from them. After her divorce two years ago, she needed welfare services and food stamps to give her children food, clothing, and housing. Then she took a nurse assistant course and got her current job. Her primary social outlet is her church.

Bruce is a 25-year-old disabled veteran who is partly paralyzed. He has been confined to a wheelchair since a car accident three years ago in the army. He was in a military hospital for 18 months for acute care and rehabilitation. He gets a military pension and lives in his own apartment, with a paid companion. His parents live in the same city and help out in emergencies, but he prefers to take care of himself. Before his accident he was active in sports, and he still has trouble accepting his limitations. He has joined a support group for people with spinal cord injuries. He is training to compete in wheelchair sports.

Maureen is a 67-year-old resident in a long term care facility in the city where her oldest daughter lives. She is diabetic and had a below-knee **amputation** of her right leg. She is in the early stages of Alzheimer's disease. She was admitted to the facility six months ago when her children realized her husband could no longer care for her. Her husband now lives with their oldest daughter. He visits every day for several hours. Maureen is often alert and fully oriented to her surroundings. She insists on doing everything she can for herself, and she wants her husband to help her with those things she cannot do for herself.

Amputation – cutting a limb (for example an arm or leg) from the body
Need – something necessary for a person
Psychosocial – involving psychological, emotional, and social aspects of mental health

What do you have in common with these three people? Do they remind you of anyone you know? Are their needs different from yours, your family's, or those of residents in your care? Everyone has the same basic human needs: to eat, to be safe, to be as independent as possible, and so on.

Can you identify the basic needs in each of these examples? Most people react to new situations in ways that have worked for them in the past. This is true also for residents in your facility. A resident who has always enjoyed new situations can cope with moving into the facility more easily than a resident who always hated change and lived in the same house for 50 years. Did you notice that each person in these examples wants to stay independent?

Our need for contact with other people also stays much the same throughout life. Being with others helps us meet our safety and social needs. However, being with others may also cause conflict and frustration. Some people try to avoid conflict by avoiding other people. You must respect the different ways people relate to other people. For example, you may get along well with someone who is outgoing and talkative, but how should you act with someone who is quiet and shy?

GAINING AN UNDERSTANDING OF RESIDENTS

How a resident acts in various situations is affected by a lifetime of experiences. Sometimes you will not understand a resident's reaction. You may think, "Where did that come from?" The key is to ask the resident questions to help you understand. If you are still troubled or concerned, then talk to the charge nurse.

There are many **theories** about how we grow and develop into who we are. This is part of our psychosocial development. Our psychosocial self involves our personality, how we react to things and interact with others, and how we develop relationships. Our social development also affects how we behave. The same is true for residents.

The following sections outline two theories about how we develop and meet our needs. The psychologist Abraham Maslow believed that people's needs fit into a **hierarchy**. Another psychologist, Erik Erikson, studied how our psychosocial development occurs in different age stages. Can you think of things that may have affected your own psychosocial development? We each have a lifetime of positive and negative experiences. They all contribute to who we are and how we think today. Indeed, many factors influence our growth.

Erikson's Eight Stages of Psychosocial Development

Erik Erikson's theory helps us understand how people develop and meet their needs. He believed that development occurs in stages, with critical milestones to achieve at each stage throughout our lives. This theory supports the idea that childhood problems can be healed in adulthood.

Table 3-1 outlines Erikson's eight stages of psychosocial development. Each stage involves a potential success or type of conflict. In each stage a person must accomplish something to meet their needs. The table also describes how you can support a resident at each stage.

Most of the residents you will care for are adults, but remember that previous stages of their lives still influence their behavior. You need to understand the stages of development residents have experienced. You should also understand that experiences or issues at any earlier stage can influence how a resident behaves now. Your responsibility is to learn how to support the resident.

For example, as a resident reminisces, they may be working through the task of maturity: reflecting on their life. They need to feel that they have been successful. They need to sort through their good and bad experiences. They need to feel they have resolved past issues. This is often necessary as older people prepare for the end of their life. Your responsibility is to support the resident through this process.

You also need to recognize your own feelings about this process. If you are uncomfortable with it, talk with the charge nurse. Chapter 22, End of Life, discusses this stage in more detail.

Assertive – being confident

Generativity – ability to produce or create something

Gross motor skills – abilities in the larger physical skills (running, catching a ball, etc.) vs. fine motor skills (drawing a picture, writing, etc.)

Hierarchy – a specific organized order or ranking

Integrity – being whole or complete

Theory – a set of ideas or principles offered to explain something observed

TABLE 3-1 ERIKSON'S EIGHT STAGES OF PSYCHOSOCIAL DEVELOPMENT

AGE	SUCCESS/CONFLICT	TASK	WHAT THE NURSE ASSISTANT CAN DO
Infant	Trust vs. mistrust	The infant must form a loving, trusting relationship with the caregiver.	In this phase the nurse assistant should hold the infant and be consistent and reliable to encourage trust. Feeding is the primary means to achieve success. Holding the infant during feeding supports this development.
Toddler	Autonomy vs. shame/doubt	The child develops physical skills, including walking, grasping, and bowel and bladder control. The child learns control at this stage.	The nurse assistant must support the toddler's physical development in walking and independent eating. Playing ball and other games is critical to develop gross motor skills. Helping with toilet training is critical for success. Praising the child and never scolding will help support their development.
Preschool child	Initiative vs. guilt	The child continues to become more assertive and independent, and starts to take more initiative.	The nurse assistant must support the preschool child's need to develop independence. The child will use their imagination in play. The child needs to be encouraged in their game playing.
School-age child	Industry vs. inferiority	The school-age child deals with demands to learn new skills and knowledge.	Helping the child be successful in learning is critical in this stage. This child needs to feel they are productive and can succeed. The child should be praised for completing their tasks.
Adolescence	Identity vs. role confusion	A teenager must achieve a clear sense of identity in sex roles at home, at school, and at work.	Talking with teenagers about their goals and friends is critical at this stage. Supporting them in decision making or even teaching decision making is important as teenagers sort through who they are and what they will do.
Young adulthood	Intimacy vs. isolation	The young adult learns to develop intimate relationships.	The ability to make a commitment is critical for the young adult's success. Discussing the person's relationships and supporting their commitments will help the person achieve success.
Middle adulthood	Generativity vs. stagnation	Adults need to feel they have accomplished something or supported the next generation.	A resident in this stage needs to feel they have accomplished something good. They must feel they have shared a part of themselves with people who are close to them. Talking with the resident will help them identify their successes.
Maturity	Ego integrity vs. despair	An older adult must have a sense of feeling fulfilled, that they have lived successfully.	In this stage the resident has to accept both the good and bad of their life. Allowing and encouraging the resident to discuss issues will help them in this stage.

Maslow's Hierarchy of Needs

All human beings have the same basic needs. We need to keep our physical bodies safe and functioning well. We need to nourish our social, spiritual, and sexual selves. With our own life experiences, we each have developed our own ways to meet these needs. We all have the same needs, but how we feel about them and satisfy them is different. As a nurse assistant, you can identify and help meet each resident's needs while they are in your facility.

Abraham Maslow described the most basic human needs in a hierarchy (Fig. 3-1). This means that there is a natural priority for how you meet needs at any one time. For example, if you have a physical need, such as eating, you will be more concerned about meeting that need than meeting a social need.

Physical Needs.   Physical needs relate to things necessary for survival, such as food, water, oxygen, rest, and movement. Everyone wants to meet their own physical needs independently. Healthy people get out of bed on their own, prepare their own meals, and take care of their own personal hygiene. As we grow older, because of physical changes we may need the help of others to meet our physical needs (Fig. 3-2). We must meet our physical needs before we can focus on the next level of needs.

> ***Consider this:*** Have you as an adult ever had someone else take care of you? You might find it pleasant at first, but not being able to take care of yourself for a long time is very frustrating. It can sometimes lead to feelings of worthlessness and depression.

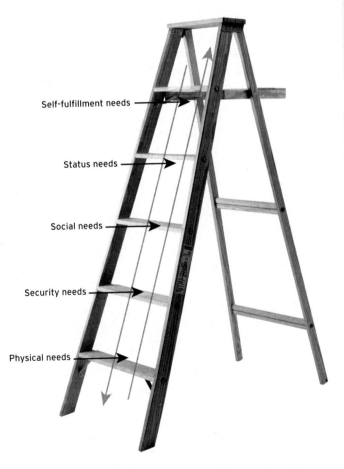

Self-fulfillment needs

Status needs

Social needs

Security needs

Physical needs

Fig. 3-1 — The ladder shows how Maslow prioritized human needs. Lower-level needs must be met before the resident can move up to higher ones.

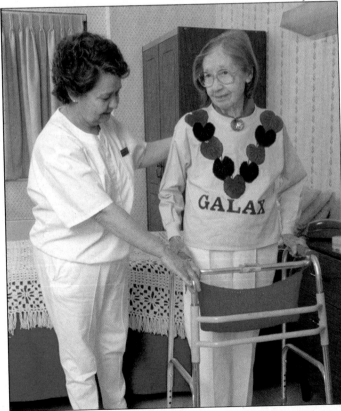

Fig. 3-2 — Nurse assistants help residents meet their physical needs.

When you help each resident meet their physical needs, such as eating, turning over in bed, and bathing, do it in a way that helps them be as independent as possible. Offer help as needed, but do not take over tasks that residents can do themselves. For example, you may need to open a milk carton for a resident and insert a straw, but let them hold the carton or glass while drinking. When turning or getting out of bed, a resident may move slowly but still can make the move with enough time and support. Be patient. Do not do something for residents simply because you think it "takes too long" for them to do it themselves. Remember that a resident has less independence if you do everything for them. Over time they may become more dependent and have less self-worth.

Safety and Security Needs. Safety and security needs are the second priority in Maslow's hierarchy. This includes physical safety, such as freedom from bodily harm. It also includes psychological safety, such as feeling secure. A person pays attention to safety and security needs only after meeting their physical needs. For example, if you were starving, you might risk your safety to get food. Once you meet your need for food, you behave more cautiously to protect yourself from danger.

Consider this: Infants and children depend on others to keep them safe. Children are very vulnerable to physical and emotional abuse or neglect because they depend on others to meet their needs. Society tries to protect children with laws and agencies that prevent abuse and neglect. As we become adults, we take care of ourselves, but laws still help protect our rights. As we grow older, our physical senses—sight, hearing, touch—may diminish, making us less independent. Then we again become vulnerable to injury and abuse. We may have to depend on others to help us stay safe. This is one reason elderly people become residents of long term facilities.

A resident may decide to move into a facility only after a long struggle to stay independent. For example, a person who has trouble seeing or maintaining their balance may fall or have an accident. Family members are then afraid for the person's safety and persuade them to move into the facility. A resident may have a serious medical problem that caused or resulted from the accident, but they still want independence. Sometimes you must balance your concern for a resident's safety with their need for inde-

pendence. Talk with the resident about safety. Make a plan together that gives them as much freedom as possible while also maintaining their safety needs (Fig. 3-3).

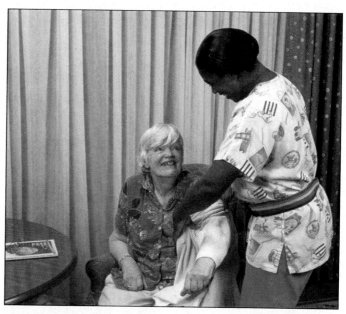

Fig. 3-3 – Residents should always be involved in the plan to meet their safety and security needs.

Social Needs. Social needs include a need for the approval and acceptance of others. When they are comfortable and safe in their surroundings, most people seek out friendships and group activities. Social needs include interaction with others, recognition, and a feeling of belonging.

Consider this: A key part of many people's personal identity comes from belonging to groups. These include family, church, and workplace groups. Interacting with others gives us a better sense of who we are. How we feel about ourselves depends a lot on how others react to us. When you wear a new outfit or a new hairstyle, how do you feel if family and friends do not notice? When you do a job well, you feel even better about it if someone else notices.

Recognition – to be acknowledged as important

Residents have the same needs for interaction and recognition. A new resident away from their usual support group may need your support for weeks or months after admission. A resident needs to establish new relationships but may not take the first step. Remember what it was like when you first came to a new school or job or your first training class? Most people are cautious in new situations, but everyone has their own way of dealing with new situations. Some people go right up to others, introduce themselves, and start talking. Other people wait before comfortably joining in. Most people will relate to others when they have something in common, but many have trouble taking the first step in new situations.

Special activities in the facility help residents get together and get to know each other (Fig. 3-4). You can also help bring residents together informally. You can do this at meals and when relaxing in common areas. You can bring together residents with similar interests. You may also help them attend community events.

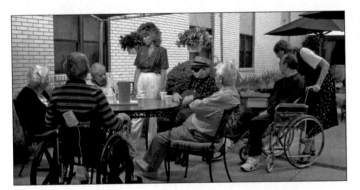

Fig. 3-4 – Social activities help residents develop new relationships.

Status Needs.   Status needs become important after one's social needs are met. Status involves respect from others. All people need to be treated with respect.

Consider this: Being rewarded for what you do is an important need. Respect and recognition can be shown in many ways: praise, a positive nod, a letter of acknowledgment. Have you ever really needed someone's approval or respect? As a child you looked to your parents for approval. As you grow older and have more life experiences, you need the respect of other people. School teachers, trainers, peers, bosses, co-workers, and spouses are just a few of the people whose respect we want. Each person fulfills your status needs in different ways, and the respect of each can have different meaning.

When you care for a resident, you can help fulfill their need for status. Show respect for each resident in every caregiving activity, in these ways:
- Call them by their proper name.
- Always ask their permission before acting.
- Explain the care you give.
- Knock on their door and wait for permission to enter.
- Respect their belongings.
- Recognize their achievements.
- Encourage them to get fully dressed and to use their personal belongings.

Self-fulfillment Needs.   Self-fulfillment needs are the highest level of needs. Self-fulfillment is a feeling that you are contributing and achieving your goals. You are satisfied with your life. Not everyone fully meets this need, and few people meet this need all the time. But most people want to make a contribution and feel that they have achieved something in their lives.

Consider this: Self-fulfillment involves achievement, independence, and being all you can be. This is the highest level people can reach. Think of Maslow's hierarchy of needs as a ladder. To reach the top, you must climb past all other needs. You go up and down the ladder of needs at different times to meet all your needs. The need for self-fulfillment is a lot like climbing the ladder. You have a goal, you plan how to reach it, and you take a few steps forward and maybe a few steps backward. Eventually you reach the top if you work at it.

Ask your residents what is important to them. This helps you understand where they are on the needs ladder and how you can help them reach their goals. Encourage residents to be as independent as possible. Any achievement can bring a feeling of self-fulfillment. For example, after a stroke a resident may feel that walking would be a great achievement. This resident may focus all their energy on that goal. Once they achieve it, they direct their energy to a new goal. Encourage residents to set new goals, and they will experience new achievements.

Status – position, rank, or prestige in relation to other people

Other Needs of Residents

Sexual Needs.   Sexual expression is both a physical and a social need. Sexual needs involve warm, loving, caring feelings shared between people. Sexuality may also involve feeling masculine or feminine. Sexual needs are not limited to sexual acts such as kissing, intercourse, or masturbation but can also be met through close physical contact. Unfortunately, our society often thinks of sexuality only for younger people. But it is a fact that the elderly often have sexual needs, too.

Many people have difficulty talking about sexuality. Yet people do not lose their need for close physical contact or their interest in sex just because they are over age 50 or 70 or any other age (Fig. 3-5). Studies of healthy adults show that most seniors are sexually active or interested in having sex into their 80s, 90s, and beyond. But many people treat older people as though they should not have sexual needs and feelings. Many seniors may accept this view. They may feel guilty about their feelings or may not seek meaningful sexual experiences.

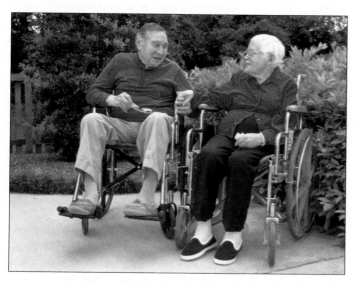

Fig. 3-5 – Sexual needs and feelings are normal at any age.

The physical changes of aging affect sexual activity. Men may take longer to have an erection and may have difficulty keeping it. Women often have vaginal dryness, which if ignored may make intercourse painful. Chronic illness or physical decline may make sexual activity uncomfortable or even unsafe. But older residents can make up for these changes if they know how.

The limited privacy in a facility often interferes with resi-

dents' sexual expression. Residents with roommates may have trouble arranging time alone with a spouse or intimate friend. You can help. Plan another activity for the roommate during such visits. Tell other staff not to enter the room until the resident or spouse requests them to.

Frail and very ill residents may have difficulty balancing sexual expression with their need for safety and supervision. Some staff may also be uncomfortable with residents having sex in the facility. If you feel uncomfortable about these matters, discuss your feelings with your charge nurse.

Many older people have difficulty meeting their sexual needs after losing their spouse to death or divorce. Since women usually live longer than men, single women far outnumber single men in older age groups. Yet sometimes a resident develops close, loving relationships with another resident. As long as both partners consent and there are no safety concerns, they have the right to privacy together. If family members or staff find this embarrassing or undesirable, help everyone to be more accepting. Encourage residents, family, and staff to talk about their feelings. Encourage residents to say how they want to be treated.

Masturbation is a normal outlet for meeting sexual needs, but some people are uncomfortable even thinking about it. Most people do not talk about it openly. Some older people grew up thinking that it is wrong. If you know that a resident masturbates, respect the person's needs and provide privacy.

Because of confusion or other factors, a resident may express their sexuality inappropriately around others. For example, a resident may masturbate or expose themselves in a group setting. This behavior usually makes other residents uncomfortable, and you must preserve all residents' privacy and dignity. You may need to move this resident to a private place or distract them with some other activity. Every long term care facility has a policy regarding matters of sexual expression. Make sure you read and understand the policy where you work.

Spiritual Needs.   Spirituality involves much more than religion, although many people meet their spiritual needs through religion. Spirituality can help a person meet their security, social, and self-fulfillment needs. Spirituality involves a meaning of life and feeling related to something greater than ourselves. A person may express spirituality through prayer, meditation, reading, and religious rituals.

Like anyone else, residents express their spirituality in different ways. Respect each resident's ways, do not judge them, and never impose your beliefs on a resident. As people grow older, they often look to their spiritual or inner selves for meaning in their lives. They benefit from reflecting on their life, remembering life events, and working through their losses, guilt, and regrets. They are not just "living in the past."

Following is an example of how you might work with a resident as they reflect on their life spiritually. Encourage the resident to talk about their past while you listen attentively. You can also help residents work through their feelings. The resident may say, "I wish I could have done more with my wife before she died." You can say, "Tell me what you and your wife did." Then you might add, "It sounds to me like you did a lot together and you were always there for her." This can help this resident reflect positively about experiences he had with his wife. Maybe he will resolve his regrets. This is part of the resident's search to find meaning in his life. You can play a major role by supporting this process.

Religious practices often give people spiritual comfort. This is especially true when residents are coping with major life changes like the loss of a loved one or their own approaching death. Rabbis, priests, and ministers can help residents with the question, "What has my life meant?" You can help residents attend the facility's place of worship (Fig. 3-6). If a resident requests a visit, notify their spiritual counselor. Provide privacy when the spiritual counselor is visiting. Residents or family members may ask you to pray with them. If you are comfortable with this, join in the prayer. If you are not comfortable, you can stay quietly with the resident or ask another nurse assistant to join them.

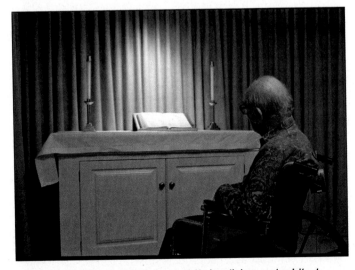

Fig. 3-6 – Assisting residents to meet their religious and spiritual needs can help them cope with life changes.

Many religious and ethnic groups observe special religious holidays. Often these involve ceremonies and traditional foods. Find out what special days your residents observe and help them experience their important rituals. You might also ask them to teach others about their rituals and to share religious ceremonies. Facilities often plan special activities for religious holidays such as Christmas, Easter, Rosh Hashana, and Yom Kippur. Also respect the rights of residents who do not observe these holidays. Give them privacy, if that is what they want.

Cultural and Values Differences

How a resident meets all their needs depends on many factors. Chapter 2 discusses values and culture. These factors affect how the resident meets their needs, along with the resident's family structure, where they lived, their education, and their financial status. Try to understand how the resident met their needs in the past and how they want to meet them now.

Some ways will be obvious to you. Some will be very different from how you meet your own needs. Do not pass judgment about different ways. Instead, learn about the resident. You can learn much about the resident's value system and culture. With this knowledge you can give the resident better care.

Meeting Different Needs

As we have seen, human needs occur on several different levels. As a person's needs change, they often move up and down these levels of need. For example, you probably get hungry several times a day. When you are hungry (or tired or ill), you focus on getting food (or rest or medical treatment). At that time you pay less attention to other needs. When you meet your physical needs, then you can again address safety and social needs.

Often one activity meets more than one need. For example, many social interactions involve food, such as family reunions, recognition banquets, and funerals. In one activity you meet a basic need for food at the same time you meet social needs and status needs.

Everyone meets their different levels of needs differently. For example, for some residents, being with people (social needs) is very important to their sense of well-being. For others, time alone to read or reflect on life (spiritual needs) is more important for their emotional stability.

As you work with residents, remember that their needs change often. What is important for a resident who is feeling well is different from what is important to them when they are in a lot of pain. This is why you must get to know the residents in your care (Fig. 3-7). You can see their changing needs and adjust your care accordingly.

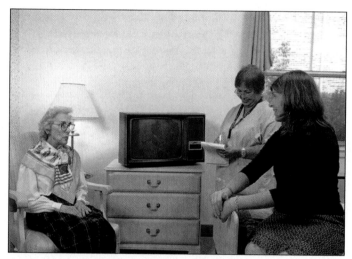

Fig. 3-7 – Asking residents and family members questions will help you get to know the resident better.

UNDERSTANDING A RESIDENT'S HISTORY

Always remember that each resident had a life with many experiences and relationships before coming to your facility. To successfully care for a resident, you must understand their history. Learn how the resident became who they are. As you read the following descriptions of residents, think about what each needs. Think about how you might approach their care.

Mrs. Thomas is a 70-year-old widow. Her three children live in different states a long way away. She has been active in her church and has enjoyed volunteer work since her retirement five years ago. She has lived alone since her husband's death two years ago. Her diabetes is controlled by diet and oral medication. Her vision is impaired by cataracts. Two months ago she fell and broke her hip. After recuperating from surgery in an acute care hospital, she entered a long term care facility for physical rehabilitation. She expects to return home and then have help from a home health agency.

Mr. Morton is an 82-year-old bachelor. He is a retired carpenter and has lived alone all of his adult life. Neighbors noticed a gradual decline in his functioning, and one of them called adult protective services to check on him. The caseworker found him confused and saw that his home was very dirty and cluttered. After he was hospitalized for treatment of high blood pressure and malnutrition, he was admitted to a long term care facility. He is diagnosed as having Alzheimer's disease. He is very confused and often wanders (Fig. 3-8).

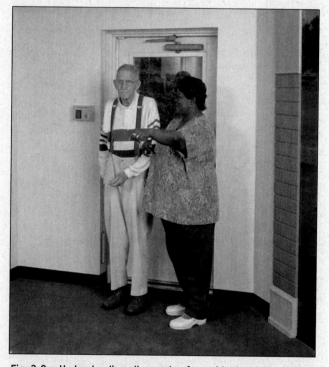

Fig. 3-8 – Understanding all aspects of a resident's history helps you understand and meet their needs.

Mr. Everett is a 72-year-old man who has lived with his wife for 54 years in their own home. He is a retired engineer and enjoys his garden and home workshop. After he retired 10 years ago, he and his wife enjoyed traveling to visit their children and friends. He had no serious health problems until he suffered a stroke three months ago. Now he is paralyzed on his left side. He is depressed and easily frustrated that he cannot communicate well or walk on his own. His wife comes to the facility every day and stays with him most of the day (Fig. 3-9, next page).

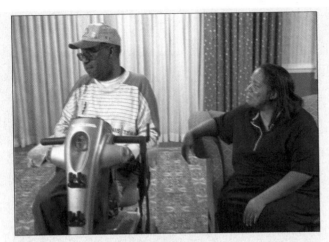

Fig. 3-9 – A loss of ability can cause problems for residents and their families that you need to understand.

Mrs. Cortez is a 68-year-old housewife who lived with her husband for 45 years. Four of their seven children live only a few blocks away. Mrs. Cortez worked all her life taking care of her family and her home. She was admitted to a nursing facility two weeks ago with terminal breast cancer that has spread to other organs. Several family members are with her most of the time. They want the facility to do everything to keep their mother alive as long as possible. Mrs. Cortez told facility staff that she is "ready to go" and wishes her family would let her die (Fig. 3-10).

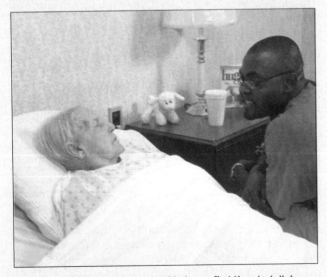

Fig. 3-10 – Nurse assistants should always find time to talk to residents about their thoughts and feelings.

Mrs. Lewis is an 85-year-old widow who lived with her son's family for the last 20 years. She kept house and cooked for the family until 2 years ago when she had a mild stroke that left her with left-side weakness. Her granddaughter then cared for her. She has had a gradual physical and mental decline and now experiences incontinence and is often confused. She entered the facility after her family became "just worn out" caring for her. Family members have a hard time dealing with their feelings about placing Mrs. Lewis in the facility. They do not visit very often or for very long (Fig. 3-11).

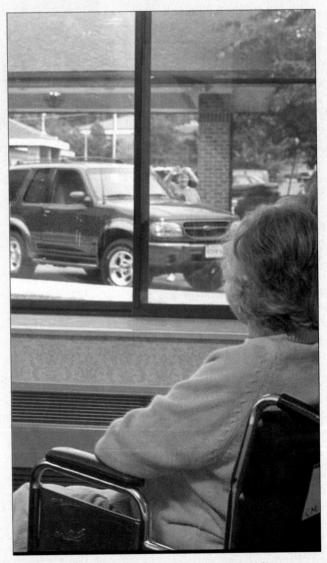

Fig. 3-11 – Residents often feel lonely after family visits.

Although these residents are different in many ways, they have some things in common. Moving into the facility was a big change in lifestyle for all of them. They each had to adjust to the changes of leaving their home and living in a different environment.

Moving into a long term care facility is often only one of many changes a resident has to cope with. As you learned in Chapter 1, people enter a facility because they need help with care. Depending on someone else to meet their basic needs is often the hardest part of aging for a resident. A resident loses the ability to control their life. Moving into the facility also involves giving up many personal possessions and familiar routines and people. Living in a group situation involves losing privacy. A resident also has to make adjustments because of other people's needs and demands.

You may not know all the changes or losses a resident experienced before they came to the facility or as a result of coming there. Some losses may not seem much to you, such as having to miss a weekly card game. For the resident, however, this may be a loss of a valuable support group and recognition. Only the person experiencing a loss knows its true meaning.

Remember that everyone has their own way of dealing with change. Residents react in many different ways.

Your interactions with residents influence how they adjust and react to their new life. Let residents know you care. Spend time with them, listen to them, and assure their privacy when giving care. Encourage residents to make their own decisions as much as possible. Even simple things like deciding when to take a bath and what to wear help residents feel in control. Encourage their independence by letting them do as much as they can for themselves. For example, even though it sometimes takes longer, let residents feed and dress themselves if they can. Encourage them to be with other residents in activities like meals, games, parties, and discussion groups. Give residents time alone when they want it.

IN THIS CHAPTER YOU LEARNED:
- How to get to know a resident
- Erikson's eight stages of psychosocial development
- Maslow's hierarchy of needs
- Ways to meet residents' needs
- How residents' basic needs are similar to your own
- How knowing a resident's history will help you to understand them better

SUMMARY
This chapter is about getting to know residents' needs. You learned two theories about psychosocial needs and development. Residents' sexual and spiritual needs are also important. A resident's culture and values influence how they behave. Remember the psychosocial changes that occur with aging.

The five scenarios you just read show how residents have the same basic needs even if they seem very different people. From these examples you can see the value of understanding why residents feel the way they do and how their life experiences affect who they are now.

PULLING IT ALL TOGETHER
Your own behavior patterns are similar at work, at home, and with friends. Be aware of how you relate to others and what situations make you uncomfortable. Are you uncomfortable with someone who is crying? Someone who is angry? You will encounter residents who behave like this in your job, and you still need to give them thoughtful care. If a situation is hard for you, ask for help from other nurse assistants or the charge nurse.

It is important always to be interested in who a resident is. You cannot just walk into a resident's room thinking that how you see them today is enough for you to give them the best care possible. As you read the following poem written by a resident, think about your responsibility to get to know all your residents.

ANONYMOUS POEM

What do you see, nurse, what do you see?
What are you thinking when you look at me?
A crabby old woman, not very wise,
Uncertain of habit with faraway eyes,
Who dribbles her food and makes no reply
When you say in a loud voice — "I do wish you'd try."
Who seems not to notice the things that you do
And forever is losing stockings or shoes,
Who, resisting or not, lets you do as you will
With bathing and feeding, the long day to fill.
Is that what you're thinking, is that what you see?
Then open your eyes, nurse. You're not looking at me.
I'll tell you who I am as I sit here still.
As I move at your bidding, eat at your will,
I'm a small child of ten with a father and mother,
Brothers and sisters who love one another;
A young girl of sixteen with wings on her feet.
Dreaming that soon now a lover she'll meet;
A bride now at twenty, my heart gives a leap,
Remembering the vows that I promised to keep;
At twenty-five now I have young of my own
Who need me to build a secure, happy home.
A woman at thirty, my young now grow fast,
Bound to each other with ties that should last.
At forty, my young sons have grown up and gone,
But my man's beside me to see I don't mourn.
At fifty once more babies play round my knee,
Again we know children, my loved one and me.
Dark days are upon me, my husband is dead,
I look at the future, I shudder with dread,
For my young are all rearing young of their own
And I think of the years and the love that I've known.
I'm an old woman now and nature is cruel
'Tis her jest to make old age look like a fool,
The body it crumbles, grace and vigor depart
There is a stone where I once had a heart.
But inside this old carcass a young girl still dwells,
And now and again my battered heart swells.
I remember the joys, I remember the pain,
And I'm loving and living life over again.
I think of the years, all too few, gone too fast
And accept the stark fact that nothing can last.
So open your eyes, nurse, open and see
Not a crabby old woman. Look closer, see me.

(From Regional Education Center: Geriatric Nurse Assistant
Manual, City College, Seattle, Washington, 1978.)

CHECK WHAT YOU'VE LEARNED

1. **You show your respect for a resident when you:**
   A. Get to know them as a human being.
   B. Give them a friendly nickname like "sweetie."
   C. Watch them from an open doorway as they get dressed.
   D. Surprise them by walking into their room without knocking first.

2. **What is an effective way to get to know a resident?**
   A. Discuss the resident with housekeeping staff.
   B. Read the resident's mail and personal papers.
   C. Ask the resident about their needs and preferences.
   D. Check with the resident's roommate for information.

3. **A person's psychosocial self usually involves their:**
   A. Medical history.
   B. Personality.
   C. Fluid balance.
   D. Temporary physical comfort.

4. **How can you help a resident be independent?**
   A. Select their clothing for them each day.
   B. Encourage the resident to do what they can.
   C. Insist on helping them with bathing.
   D. Leave them alone to take care of themselves.

5. **What is the task for the older adult in Erickson's theory of psychosocial development?**
   A. They must feel fulfilled with their life.
   B. They must learn to develop intimate relationships.
   C. They must learn to be assertive and to take the initiative.
   D. They must achieve a clear sense of identity in sex roles.

6. **What is our highest level of need in to Maslow's hierarchy?**
   A. Social needs.
   B. Sexual needs.
   C. Self-fulfillment needs.
   D. Safety and security needs.

7. **Mr. Humphrey wants to be alone with his wife during her visits. How should the staff react to his apparent need for sexual intimacy?**
   A. Give Mr. Humphrey and his wife privacy.
   B. Suggest that they play bingo instead.
   C. Tell Mr. Humphrey he's too old to behave sexually.
   D. Tell the charge nurse Mr. Humphrey is behaving inappropriately.

8. **Which of these statements about residents' spirituality needs is true?**
   A. Nurse assistants should never discuss religion with residents.
   B. Like all people, residents express their spirituality in different ways.
   C. If a resident doesn't talk about religion, they must not believe in God.
   D. Only family members and clergy can help residents meet their spiritual needs.

9. **What do all residents have in common?**
   A. They all enjoy playing bingo and watching TV.
   B. They all like to have a cup of coffee in the morning.
   C. Moving into a facility was a big lifestyle change for them.
   D. They feel completely abandoned by their families and friends.

10. **How can you help a new resident deal with change?**
    A. Leave them alone in their room until they are adjusted.
    B. Make all of their decisions for them.
    C. Suggest that they should not have moved into the facility.
    D. Encourage them to talk about their feelings.

(Answers to "Check What You've Learned" are in the Instructor's Manual.)

Chapter 4

UNDERSTANDING PEOPLE'S RIGHTS

Rights are things a person is entitled to. Always remember that residents are individuals who have the same rights as you. They have a right to be treated with respect and dignity, to pursue a meaningful life, to be free from fear. They also have the same legal rights as any other U.S. citizen. These rights include the right to vote and not be discriminated against because of their age, sex, race, religion, ethnic group, or disability.

All residents have the right to high-quality care. It does not matter how their care is paid for. Residents whose care is funded by Medicaid have the same right to good care as residents who pay for care themselves. The facility and all staff must protect and promote each resident's rights. Violating a resident's rights is breaking the law and can be punished by being fired and being fined or sent to jail.

In 1987, the nursing home reform law, the Omnibus Budget Reconciliation Act (commonly called OBRA 87), was passed. This law guarantees the rights of residents in long term care facilities. This law was needed because in the past, the rights of all residents were not being protected in all places.

In this chapter you will learn about residents' rights. You will learn your responsibility to help protect these rights. You will also learn what happens if a resident's right is violated or a resident has a complaint.

OBJECTIVES
- Define rights
- List the rights in the Residents' Bill of Rights
- Define terms used for abuse
- List what is required in an abuse program
- Define the role of the ombudsman

MEDICAL TERMS
- **Chemical restraint –** medication used to sedate a resident or slow their muscle activity
- **Circulation –** flow of blood throughout the body
- **Physical restraint –** any mechanical device that restricts a resident's movement or access to their body
- **Sedate –** to calm with drugs

"I depend on you to keep me safe, to respect me, and preserve my rights and freedoms."

ave you ever noticed how your environment affects how you behave? For example, in your own house you can play music loudly, dance all night, or turn up the television. But what if you moved to an apartment with neighbors nearby or had a roommate who does things differently? You would have to change some things because of common courtesy for others, but would you have to give up everything? Some things, like playing loud music, are not protected by law. But you would still have the same legal rights to voice your opinion, receive your mail without it being opened, vote in elections, and practice your religion.

When residents move into a long term care facility, they have to adjust to their new environment. They may have to change some behaviors out of courtesy for others. But they do not have to give up their rights.

LEGAL RIGHTS

In the early 1980s a study was done of what residents need to feel protected in long term care facilities. The led to the passing of OBRA 87, the nursing home reform bill. This reform defined residents' rights. These rights are found in the Code of Federal Regulations, Subpart B, "Requirements for Long Term Care Facilities," and are described in this chapter. These regulations state:

1. The resident has a right to a dignified existence, self-determination, and communication with and access to persons and services inside and outside the facility. A facility must protect and promote the rights of each resident.
2. A facility must care for its residents in a manner and in an environment that promotes maintenance or enhancement of each resident's quality of life.
3. The facility must promote care for residents in a manner and in an environment that maintains or enhances each resident's dignity and respect, in full recognition of their individuality.

Residents have many specific rights, listed in the Residents' Bill of Rights (Fig. 4-1). This chapter groups rights under the following headings to make it easier to remember them.
1. Right to exercise one's rights
2. Right to privacy and confidentiality
3. Right to information
4. Right to choose
5. Right to notification of change
6. Protection of residents' personal funds
7. Grievance rights

8. Admission, transfer, and discharge rights
9. Right to be free from restraint and abuse

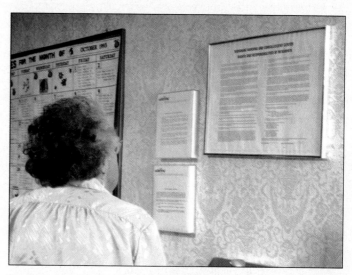

Fig. 4-1 – The Residents' Bill of Rights should be displayed where every resident can see it.

RIGHT TO EXERCISE ONE'S RIGHTS
- Each resident has the right to exercise the rights they have as a resident of the facility and as a citizen or resident of the United States.
- Each resident has the right to be free of interference, coercion, discrimination, and reprisal from the facility when they exercise any of their rights.
- If a resident is judged incompetent under the laws of a state, the person appointed by the state to act on their behalf exercises their rights.

Coercion – making someone do something against their will, often by a threat
Discrimination – a prejudiced or unfair action because of some characteristic of the person
Interference – act of obstruction; preventing a person from doing something
Reprisal – retaliation against or punishment of a person for doing something
Right – something one has a just or legal claim to
Self-determination – freedom to make your own choices and choose your own actions

How To Assist Residents To Exercise Their Rights

All residents must be able to exercise their rights. A person's rights do not change just because they enter a long term care facility. You may find that residents will ask you permission to do something like use the phone. Always tell the resident that of course they can use the phone. Remind them that in fact they can do all things they did at home here in their new home, the long term care facility.

You should encourage residents to exercise their rights. Give them choices and help them exercise their rights. For example, you can help them vote using an absentee ballot if they cannot go to a regular voting (sometimes called polling) place. If they are not mentally competent to make decisions, a person appointed by a judge acts on their behalf. Cooperate with residents to let them exercise their rights.

Consider this example of a resident exercising their rights:

> Mrs. Masucci tells you that at home she had tea everyday at 3:15 p.m. You tell her the kitchen is closed from 3 to 4 p.m., so she can only have her tea after 4 p.m. But the kitchen in fact does *not* close, and you told her this because your shift ends at 3:30 p.m., and from 3 to 3:30 you are busy reporting to the charge nurse and finishing documentation. You did not want to do anything for residents during that time. You were more interested in finishing your paperwork so you could go home. Did you violate this resident's rights?

RIGHT TO PRIVACY AND CONFIDENTIALITY

- Each resident has the right to confidentiality of their personal and medical records. They may decide whether anyone outside the facility may see their personal and clinical records. An exception occurs when a resident transfers to another facility. Then, the law requires release of their records to the other facility.
- Residents also have the right to privacy in their rooms. This includes privacy in written and telephone communications, during medical treatment and personal care, and when meeting with visitors or family members.

Confidentiality – keeping information private

Note: *In September 2013, updates were made to the Health Insurance Portability and Accountability Act (HIPAA) of 1996. These regulations determine how confidential health information should be handled and communicated. You need to be familiar with your facility's policies concerning this federal regulation.*

How To Protect Residents' Right to Privacy

Do not discuss residents' personal or medical information with anyone unless they have a legitimate need to know it. Do not talk about residents' personal information with other residents, with a resident's relatives or friends, with visitors, with the news media, or with your own friends. Even with other staff, share only the information they need to care for the resident. Give this information in private. Do not gossip.

When you care for a resident, always provide privacy. Knock on their door and give them enough time to say, "Come in." Then introduce yourself and ask if this is a good time. When giving care, pull the curtain and close the door. When giving personal care, drape their body correctly. You may have to ask visitors or other residents to leave the room when you give care.

If asked, you may help a resident read or write letters. But you must never open their mail unless they ask you to. If there is not a private telephone in each room, allow residents to have private phone conversations inside a phone booth or other area (Fig. 4-2).

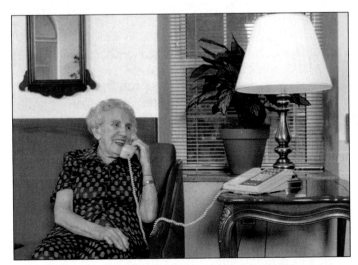

Fig. 4-2 – Residents should have privacy while using the phone.

Give residents time alone with visitors. Help them find a private place for visits, especially visits with spouses or significant others. If needed, involve their roommate in some activity outside the room to give the resident privacy.

Encourage residents and family members to join groups like a resident council or family support group. Staff often go to these meetings to answer questions and help solve problems. However, groups of residents have the right to meet without staff present.

Consider this example of a resident's privacy rights:

It is a warm day and you have been working hard at the facility all day. You feel very warm. When you go to care for Mr. Semino, his room feels hot to you. You open the window and do not close the curtain, so that you can cool off while you give care. Did you violate this resident's rights?

RIGHT TO INFORMATION

- The facility must inform each resident about their rights both orally and in writing.
- Each resident has the right to see their personal and medical records within 24 hours after asking. If they ask for a written copy of their records, they must receive it within two working days.
- Residents have the right to be fully informed, in words they can understand, about their total health status. They also have a right to know the rules and regulations governing resident conduct and responsibilities during their stay in the facility. If needed, a translator or interpreter must be present when giving information.
- Residents must be informed about services they cannot be charged for. This information must be given before or at the time of admission and periodically during their stay. They must be informed about all other services and the fees for them. Residents must be informed about any change in services. Residents have a right to see their financial records and to have everything explained to them.
- Residents must be given a written description of their rights. This should include their eligibility status for Medicaid benefits.
- The facility must post in an obvious place the names and addresses of resident advocacy groups and the ombudsman program (Fig. 4-3). You will learn more about the ombudsman program later in this chapter.
- Residents have the right to read the facility's most recent survey report written by federal or state

surveyors. They also have the right to read the facility's required plan for correcting any problems noted in the surveyors' report.

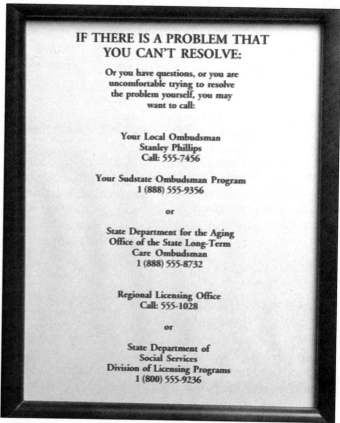

IF THERE IS A PROBLEM THAT YOU CAN'T RESOLVE:

Or you have questions, or you are uncomfortable trying to resolve the problem yourself, you may want to call:

Your Local Ombudsman
Stanley Phillips
Call: 555-7456

Your Sudstate Ombudsman Program
1 (888) 555-9356

or

State Department for the Aging
Office of the State Long-Term
Care Ombudsman
1 (888) 555-8732

Regional Licensing Office
Call: 555-1028

or

State Department of
Social Services
Division of Licensing Programs
1 (800) 555-9236

Fig. 4-3 – The Ombudsman's number must be posted where all residents and family members can see it.

Your Responsibilities for Providing Information

Much of the information listed above is given to residents and their families when the resident comes to live at the facility. This is a lot for anyone to remember, and a resident or family may later ask you about their rights. You should know where to find this information. If a resident asks to see their records, tell the charge nurse right away.

Ombudsman – person required by law to investigate complaints by residents or other violations of rights

Status – state, situation

A resident may see procedure manuals that contain the facility's policies to protect information rights. The Residents' Bill of Rights and instructions for contacting the ombudsman and other advocacy groups must be posted where residents and their families will see them. Usually these are in lounge areas or dining rooms.

If a resident asks you questions, help them find answers. Read the written residents' rights statement with them, or to them if needed. Go with them to read the posted information. If they express concerns about their medical condition or treatment plan, ask the charge nurse or physician to talk with them.

Consider this example of a resident's right to information:

> Mr. Connors' son calls while he is in the bathroom. He asks you to tell his dad to call him back. You want Mr. Connors to take his shower now, because you are behind in your work, so you decide to tell him about his son's call later on. Did you violate this resident's rights?

RIGHT TO CHOOSE

Residents have the right to choices about their living arrangements and medical care, as long as their choices do not interfere with other residents' rights.

- Each resident has the right to refuse a treatment and to refuse to participate in research.
- Each resident has the right to choose their personal physician and to help plan their own care. They must be informed in advance about changes in care or treatments that may affect their well-being.
- Each resident has the right to do voluntary or paid work in the facility. However, residents cannot be required to work.
- Each resident has the right to keep and use their own things as long as there is room and it is safe (they do not endanger themselves or others) (Fig. 4-4).
- Each resident has the right to share a room with their spouse, if both live in the facility and both consent.
- Each resident has the right to take their medications by themselves if the treatment team thinks it is safe (they are able to take the right medicine at the right time).
- Each resident has the right to choose their own activities, schedules, and health care based on their own interests and needs.
- Each resident has the right to interact with members of the community both inside and outside the facility.
- Each resident has the right to meet with others. The

facility must provide space and support staff for such meetings.
- Each resident has the right to have the facility reasonably meet their individual needs and preferences. For example, if a resident wants to have an annual family gathering, if space allows, the facility could help host the event (Fig. 4-5).

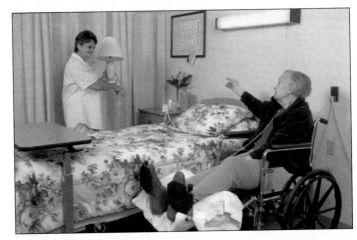

Fig. 4-4 – Encouraging residents to make decisions about their environment promotes their right to choose.

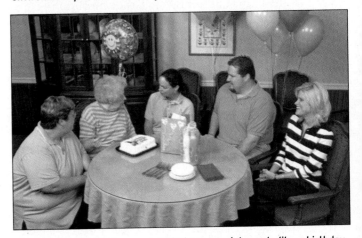

Fig. 4-5 – Residents have a right to have special events like a birthday party in the facility.

How To Help Residents Exercise Their Right To Choose

Make sure residents are aware of their choices. Tell them about activities in the facility. Learn their interests, and help them keep doing what they enjoy. Some residents may want to help with things like watering plants and making their own beds. They may also want to help other residents, such as assisting at mealtimes, but they are not allowed to feed other residents. No resident has to do such tasks, but some feel more useful and have more self-worth if they do things for themselves and help others. Future chapters will discuss other ways you can encourage and protect residents' choices about their care and their environment.

If residents want to stay active in their community, encourage their involvement with activities that interest them. They can attend meetings and events if their health allows. Think of ways to make life more enriching for residents. Do not arrange your routine just for your own convenience. Encourage residents to set up their own routines as much as possible.

A resident's choices may have to be limited if they interfere with other residents' rights. To prevent such problems, facilities have rules for the fair treatment of all residents.

Consider this example of a resident exercising their right to choose:

Mrs. Cain would like to wear her new pink dress that went to the laundry over a week ago. On your break, you saw that her dress has been ironed and is hanging in the laundry room, but you didn't feel like taking it to her just then. So you tell Mrs. Cain that you called the laundry and they said the dress is still not ready. Did you violate this resident's rights?

RIGHT TO NOTIFICATION OF CHANGE

- Each resident, family member, and physician must be told of any change in a resident's physical, mental, or psychosocial status and any accident that causes an injury.
- If treatment must change because of the resident's condition or resources, the resident must be told.
- Each resident must be told in advance of a planned change in their room or roommate.
- Every resident must be told about any changes in residents' rights.
- The facility must keep and update addresses and phone numbers of each resident's legal representative and interested family members.

When To Notify Residents of Change

If you must change a resident's care, such as changing a treatment time, tell the resident in advance. Try to give them a choice of times to schedule the treatment.

If you see an accident that injures a resident, tell the charge nurse so that the physician and family are informed. If a family member gives you a new address or phone number, note it in the resident's record.

Even with simple things like a meal delay, tell residents what time they will eat. Residents should be involved in a decision to move them to another room or assign them a different roommate. Help the resident become comfortable with the decision.

Consider this example of a change in a resident's condition:

The charge nurse tells you to call her when a resident's family member arrives for their daily visit. The charge nurse wants to report to them the fact that you accidentally scratched the resident when giving personal care. When they arrive, you do not tell the charge nurse. Did you violate this resident's rights?

PROTECTION OF RESIDENTS' PERSONAL FUNDS

- Residents have the right to keep and manage their own funds or have someone else do it for them. If a resident wants the facility to manage their funds, the facility must safeguard these funds. The facility must provide quarterly statements when the resident or legal representative asks. Funds over $50 must be maintained in an interest-bearing account. Funds under $50 can be maintained in a petty cash account.

Your Responsibility Regarding Residents' Funds

All staff must help safeguard residents' belongings. If you know a resident has a lot of money or is not managing their money appropriately, immediately tell the charge nurse, family, or legal representative so that they can protect the resident's funds. The facility must try to prevent theft of residents' belongings and money.

Consider this example about a resident's rights and money:

Mr. Belcher continually offers you money. He tells you that you are the best nurse assistant in the facility. You always say no. One day he offers you what he calls lunch money and says, "I have so much money, I wish you would take it." So you do. Have you violated this resident's rights?

GRIEVANCE RIGHTS

• Each resident has the right to make complaints without fear of retaliation or discrimination.
• The facility must act promptly on resident complaints.
• Federal law requires each state to have an ombudsman program. The ombudsman investigates complaints from residents and family members. The ombudsman then acts as their advocate to resolve complaints (Fig. 4-6). The facility must tell residents and their families about this program.

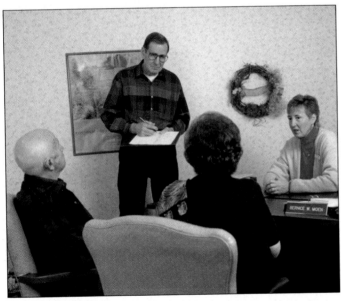

Fig. 4-6 – All residents have the right to voice their concerns to the facility's administration and/or the ombudsman.

Your Responsibility Regarding Residents' Grievances

Encourage residents to join resident councils. Offer written information to residents about the procedure for making a grievance. If a resident complains to you, tell the charge nurse or administrator as soon as you can. Never ignore a resident's complaint.

Do not let the complaint affect how you care for the resident. For example, if a resident complains that you have been rude, do not argue with them about what you said. Care for them with respect. Always make your best effort. Be sure to address their concern and explain to them how you will change their care to better meet their needs.

The facility must investigate any complaint of any kind. If a resident complains about you, the charge nurse must investigate. This does not mean that the people you work with will think you did something wrong. The investigation will determine what happened. This is for your own protection as well as the resident's.

If a resident or family member complains some more or says the facility is not fixing a problem, refer the family to the charge nurse or social worker.

If a resident complains to you about another staff member, tell the charge nurse or another supervisor. The facility will investigate. If you think the facility is not addressing a resident's complaint, you may contact the ombudsman yourself. Be sure to address these situations in a professional and neutral way, without becoming emotional or angry.

Consider this example of a resident with a complaint:

A resident complains to you that you never answer their call light on time. She says, "Please ask the charge nurse to come see me." You say, "I'm doing the best job I can," and you do not tell the charge nurse about the resident's complaint. Have you violated this resident's rights?

Grievance – a formal complaint
Retaliation – the act of getting revenge or punishing a person for doing something

ADMISSION, TRANSFER, AND DISCHARGE RIGHTS

Transfer and discharge involve moving a resident. A resident must be told about a transfer or discharge at least 30 days in advance. A resident can be transferred or discharged against their will only if enough advance notice is given that another place can be found, and only in one of these situations:

- The situation threatens their life or others.
- The resident no longer needs the services of the facility.
- The resident has failed to pay for services after reasonable notice.
- The facility ceases to operate.

Enough advance notice must be given to ensure the process is safe and orderly. If the resident plans to return to the same room, such as after hospitalization or therapeutic leave, the same bed may be held for the resident, depending on the facility's policy.

Your Role in Transfers and Discharges

If a resident is unhappy or frightened about a move, listen to their concerns. Do not discount their feelings by saying, "Don't worry about it. Everything will be all right." Help them understand why the change is needed. Make sure they have time to adjust.

Consider this example of a resident being transferred:

> Mrs. Helleberg's Alzheimer's disease is getting worse. She requires more skilled nursing care and is being transferred to the second floor this morning. The charge nurse asks you if you have prepared the resident for the change as requested. You did not prepare her, because you thought she wouldn't understand you. This morning you go into her room to pack her belongings. Mrs. Helleberg is extremely upset and surprised by having to move. Did you violate this resident's rights?

RIGHT TO BE FREE FROM RESTRAINT AND ABUSE

- Each resident has the right to be free from any physical or chemical restraints used either to discipline them or for the convenience of staff.
- Each resident has the right to be free from any verbal, sexual, physical, or mental abuse and from corporal punishment or involuntary seclusion.
- The facility must follow written policies to prevent mistreatment, neglect, or abuse of residents or their property.
- If a resident or family member complains of a violation of these rights, this complaint must be reported to the administration and other officials as required by state law. The facility must fully investigate these complaints and report the findings.

The Centers for Medicare and Medicaid Services (CMS) requires every facility to have a seven-part abuse-prevention program that includes staff education. Box 4-1 outlines the seven components. When you start work at a facility, you will learn more about its program. You are required to participate in your facility's program and follow its guidelines in your caregiving. The following section describes your role in preventing abuse and neglect.

ELDER JUSTICE ACT OF 2010

In March 2010, the federal government passed guidelines regarding reporting requirements for any suspicion of a crime committed against an older adult. The guidelines state: If an individual such as a health care worker has a reasonable suspicion that a crime has occurred involving a resident or person receiving care at the facility, that individual has the responsibility to report the suspicion directly to both local law enforcement and the state survey agency without fear of retaliation. The Elder Justice Act also provides very specific timelines and definitions regarding serious bodily injuries that are required to be reported within two hours. Any other suspicion of abuse is required to be reported within 24 hours. It is important to know your facility's specific policies, guidelines, and definitions regarding elder abuse.

Corporal punishment – physical punishment

Chemical restraint – medication used to sedate a resident or slow their muscle activity

Involuntary seclusion – isolation of a resident against their will

Neglect – failure to do something that should have been done

Physical restraint – any mechanical device that restricts a resident's movement or access to their body

Sedate – to calm with drugs

Transfer – move to another room in the facility

BOX 4-1.
SEVEN COMPONENTS OF ABUSE PROHIBITION PROGRAMS

SCREENING POLICIES FOR POTENTIAL HIRES:
- Interview applicants, keeping in mind desirable employee behaviors.
- Do criminal background checks.
- Check references.
- Conduct a screening for drug use.
- Check licensing or certification boards to be sure employees are in good standing.
- Start all employees with a probationary period.
- Screen all employees for past and present alcohol and substance abuse.

TRAINING OF EMPLOYEES THAT INCLUDES:
- definitions of abuse
- how to handle a difficult resident
- stress and burnout
- residents' rights
- regulations and responsibilities
- missing items, theft

FACILITIES MUST HAVE PREVENTION POLICIES AND PROCEDURES THAT:
- identify residents at risk
- define roles during the probationary period
- set up an ongoing education plan
- recommend staffing levels
- establish a plan for reporting incidents
- describe the investigation of missing items and theft

PROCEDURES FOR INVESTIGATING INCIDENTS AND ALLEGATIONS THAT INCLUDE:
- identifying when the suspected abuse may have occurred
- identifying all staff and residents who may have had access to the resident
- interviewing staff and residents in person
- obtaining written statements from both staff and residents about what happened, including:
  - the resident's behavior
  - staff members' response to the resident's behavior
  - unusual occurrences
  - observations
  - communications
  - everyone's immediate response to the situation

PROCEDURES FOR IDENTIFYING POSSIBLE INCIDENTS OR ALLEGATIONS THAT INCLUDE:
- what to do about complaints
- observations of what happened
- how to investigate injuries of unknown cause

PROCEDURES FOR PROTECTING RESIDENTS DURING INVESTIGATION THAT INCLUDE:
- securing the environment
- assessing the resident for harm and threats
- reassuring the resident

PROCEDURES FOR RESPONDING AND REPORTING THAT INCLUDE:
- reports to required agencies
- corrective actions
- analysis of the problem and solutions

Allegation – a person's statement or intended legal action
At risk – has a probability of having some type of medical incident (for example, falls, seizures, allergies, asthma, heart condition)
Incident – something happens that is unusual; it could be medical or behavioral
Securing – making something safe

What You Can Do To Prevent Resident Abuse

Abuse is willfully injuring a resident; unreasonably confining a resident; intimidating or punishing a resident; or causing physical harm, pain, or mental anguish. These terms are related to abuse:

- **Physical restraints** are any devices that limit a resident's movement or access to their body. Restraints may include bed rails, vest restraints that keep a resident in bed or in a chair, limb restraints that limit a resident's use of their arms or legs, tables that lock over a resident in a chair, or lap pillows that keep a resident from standing or walking. The resident must be able to remove any device or equipment used. Otherwise it is considered a restraint.
- **Chemical restraints** are medications used to sedate a resident, slow their muscle activity, or change their behavior.
- **Verbal abuse** includes using profanity, calling a resident names, yelling at a resident in anger, making oral or written threats, or teasing a resident in an unkind manner.
- **Physical abuse** is any action that causes actual physical harm. This includes handling a resident too roughly; giving a wrong treatment to a resident; or hitting, pushing, pinching, or kicking a resident.
- **Neglect** is failing to do something you should have done. Neglect includes not giving proper hygiene care, not turning a resident over in bed to improve their circulation, not giving food and water regularly, or not taking the resident to the bathroom when they ask. Neglect may also be considered physical abuse.
- **Negligence** is failing to act in the same way that a reasonable person with the same training would act in the same situation. Gross negligence is any action that shows no concern for the resident's well-being.
- **Sexual abuse** includes sexual acts between a resident and a staff member. It may also include touching residents in an intimate or suggestive manner, making sexual comments, or allowing another resident to engage in unwanted sexual acts with a resident.
- **Mental abuse** includes any action that makes a resident fearful, such as threatening them with harm or threatening to tell others something they do not want them to know. It includes actions that belittle or make fun of a resident.
- **Corporal punishment** is physical punishment, such as spanking or slapping.
- **Involuntary seclusion** is the isolation of a resident against their will, such as locking them alone in a room.

- **Theft** (or stealing) of a resident's belongings is another form of abuse.

When you understand these meanings of abuse, you will recognize abuse when you see it. In addition to direct abuse, such as hitting someone, abuse can be indirect, such as talking to another nurse assistant while ignoring a resident. It also includes saying negative things about a resident outside their room, whether or not the resident is likely to hear it.

Other examples of direct and indirect abuse are:
Direct abuse:
- calling a resident a disrespectful name
- screaming at a resident for being incontinent

Indirect abuse:
- making an indecent finger gesture behind a resident's door just because they need your help again
- ignoring a resident's call light when you're about to go on break

Help prevent theft of residents' belongings by marking them with the resident's name. List all belongings on the inventory record. Help residents keep their belongings in a safe place. You may suggest that family members take home expensive items. Also protect their items that have sentimental value to them.

Using a Restraint. A restraint may be used temporarily to help give a resident a medical treatment. For example, a resident may be placed in a limb restraint if they pull out tubes needed for medical treatment, even though the resident must already have agreed to the treatment. The limb restraint is used to restrict the resident's ability to move their arm and pull out the tube.

A restraint may also be used in an emergency if needed for a life-saving treatment. For example, an infection can cause a resident to become confused or delirious, and if they are not treated, they could die. A resident who is

---

Belittle – to make a person seem smaller or less important
Circulation – flow of blood throughout the body
Sentimental value – the value of the object comes not from the money it could be sold for, but because of the associations and memories it has for the owner—perhaps it was a present from a parent, child, or spouse

uncooperative or combative cannot be evaluated properly, so there may be a need to restrain them so that the nurse or physician can draw blood and do the proper assessment. The restraint would then be removed.

If a restraint is needed, the charge nurse will tell you which type of restraint to use and the proper procedure for using it. However, a physician's order is needed to use the restraint. The charge nurse must document the reasons for using the restraint according to the facility's policies.

When a resident is restrained, check that the restraint is used properly. Check the resident often to make sure the restraint does not cause a circulatory problem. Release the restraint frequently (without actually removing it), following your facility's policy. During your orientation, you will learn your facility's policies for restraints.

A resident who is sleeping much of the time or is suddenly slurring their speech may be receiving too much medication. Tell the charge nurse about any situation like this. Make sure it is documented in the resident's chart. This situation may be considered a chemical restraint.

Sometimes stress leads to abuse. Recognize your own stress and the stress of others around you. Join a stress management program offered in your facility and take breaks with co-workers (Fig. 4-7).

Report any signs of abuse to the charge nurse and the administrator. If you know about abuse and do not report it, you are just as responsible as if you did it.

The law requires the facility to have procedures to protect residents, and it severely punishes anyone who abuses residents. This can include fines and imprisonment of anyone convicted of abuse. Staff can be charged with assault for threatening to harm a resident. Anyone who actually causes physical harm can be charged with battery. You must protect vulnerable residents from abuse by other residents or others outside the facility.

📖

Battery – in law, the unlawful beating or use of force–or even touching someone without their consent

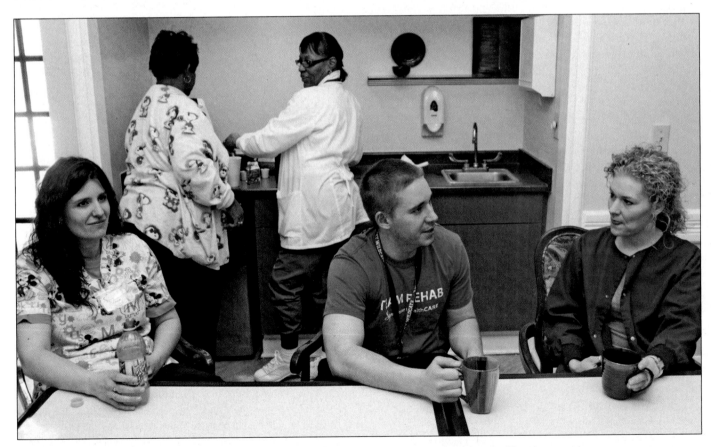

Fig. 4-7 – Being a nurse assistant can be stressful at times. Find time in your busy day to enjoy a break with your co-workers.

Whenever the resident or family alleges abuse, the facility must investigate and report its findings to state agencies. During the investigation, you may be asked about any actions you took. This does not mean that you have done anything wrong, but the facility must be able to document that it tried to protect its residents.

If a charge is brought against you, you have a right to a **hearing**. You may want to hire a lawyer. You may not be at fault even if you are charged. Like any other U.S. resident, you are innocent until proven guilty.

A nurse assistant who is found guilty of resident abuse loses their job and is reported to the state registry. Facilities refer to the state registry when hiring because they are not allowed to hire anyone who has been found guilty of neglecting, abusing, or mistreating residents or taking their property.

Consider this example of a resident's rights:

> You hear a resident swearing at another nurse assistant. The nurse assistant then tells the resident, "No dinner for you." Later, you serve that resident their dinner but do not report the other nurse assistant's behavior. Did you violate this resident's rights?

OMBUDSMAN PROGRAM

The Long Term Care Ombudsman Program was established because of growing concern about poor care in nursing facilities. This program was designed to protect the interests of residents. The law is part of the Older Americans Act. The facility must tell residents how to contact the local ombudsman program.

The law requires an ombudsman program to protect residents' rights. Each state must have an **advocate**, called the ombudsman. This person investigates complaints by residents or others about violations of rights. The law gives the ombudsman these responsibilities:

- identify, investigate, and resolve complaints made by or on behalf of residents
- provide information to residents about long term care services
- represent the interests of residents before government agencies, and seek administrative, legal, and other remedies to protect residents
- analyze, comment on, and recommend changes in laws and regulations concerning the health, safety, welfare, and rights of residents
- educate and inform consumers and the general public

about issues and concerns about long term care, and facilitate public comment on laws, regulations, policies, and actions
- promote the development of citizen organizations to participate in the program
- provide technical support for the development of resident and family councils to protect the well-being and rights of residents
- advocate for changes to improve residents' quality of life and care

(Source: U.S. Department of Health and Human Services, Administration on Aging, 330 Independence Ave. SW, Washington, DC 20201.)

The state ombudsman has authority to solve problems for a resident. If the ombudsman cannot resolve the problem, they may represent a resident, negotiate a solution, or file a lawsuit.

Ombudsmen also monitor state regulations and help strengthen laws that protect residents' rights. Ombudsmen help educate the public and train volunteers to help residents and their families. Since 1995, the National Ombudsman Reporting System (NORS) has collected information about complaints that ombudsmen investigate. This information is helping families, facilities, and government agencies improve the quality of long term care.

A facility must also post information about all relevant state client advocacy groups, including:
- the state's survey and certification agency
- the state's licensure office
- the state's ombudsman program
- the protection and advocacy network
- the Medicaid fraud control unit

📖
Advocate – someone who takes the side of another person and speaks for them

Hearing – initial examination in a criminal procedure

IN THIS CHAPTER YOU LEARNED:

• What rights are
• The specific rights in the Residents' Bill of Rights
• What abuse is and what terms are used for abuse
• What is required in an abuse prevention program
• The role of the ombudsman

SUMMARY

This chapter focuses on residents' rights. You are responsible for helping to protect residents in your long term care facility. Residents have many rights, and you can take many positive actions to protect and promote their rights. Although all of a resident's rights are important, the right of residents to be free from restraints and abuse is especially critical. Abuse can occur either directly or indirectly. You have a responsibility to report abuse. Every state has an ombudsman program to resolve complaints of violations of residents' rights.

PULLING IT ALL TOGETHER

The legal penalties for violating a resident's rights are severe. They show how important your role is to promote residents' health and well-being. Many residents are vulnerable because of their physical and psychological frailties. You must keep the facility environment safe for them. Treating them with dignity and genuine respect as unique individuals helps protect their rights. If you do your job in a caring way, you do not have to worry about violating residents' rights.

CHECK WHAT YOU'VE LEARNED

1. **What is a right?**
   A. A fact that we all know to be true.
   B. A promise one person makes to another.
   C. Something we have a just or legal claim to.
   D. Something we feel we deserve because of our past actions.

2. **If you suspect that someone has caused a serious bodily injury to an older adult resident, how soon must the incident be reported?**
   A. Before your shift ends.
   B. By the end of the week..
   C. Never; it's not your job.
   D. Within two hours

3. **Where can you find a written copy of the Residents' Bill of Rights in most long term care facilities?**
   A. In the staff lunchroom.
   B. In the clean supply room.
   C. In the maintenance engineer's office.
   D. On a wall where everyone can see it.

4. **The Residents' Bill of Rights includes:**
   A. The right to have a private room.
   B. The right to be happy all the time.
   C. The right to privacy and confidentiality.
   D. The right to receive all services free of charge.

5. **Which of these do residents have a right to choose?**
   A. Their personal physician.
   B. The wallpaper design for their room.
   C. Which nurse assistant cares for them.
   D. Whether to bring pets to live with them in the facility.

6. **When is it OK to use a restraint?**
   A. If a resident has frequent nightmares.
   B. When a resident frequently bothers staff at the nurse's station.
   C. When the doctor makes a written order for the restraint.
   D. If a resident repeatedly wanders into other residents' rooms.

7. **Which of these is an example of negligence?**
   A. Teasing a resident in an unkind manner.
   B. Threatening a resident with physical harm.
   C. Locking a resident in their room against their will.
   D. Not taking a resident to the bathroom when they ask.

8. **Mrs. Watson is refusing her bath. Making which of these statements would make you guilty of coercion?**
   A. "Either take your bath now, Mrs. Watson, or you won't get breakfast."
   B. "You can take your bath later, but then you won't be dressed in time for bingo."
   C. "Your friends are already bathed and dressed, and they're sitting on the patio."
   D. "Wouldn't you like to feel clean and refreshed when your daughter visits later?"

9. **If you see another staff member abuse a resident, what should you do?**
   A. Don't say anything unless someone asks you about it.
   B. Warn all your residents to keep away from that staff member.
   C. Report to the charge nurse exactly what you saw.
   D. Confront the staff member about what you think they did wrong.

10. **What rights does a resident have?**
    A. A resident's diagnosis must be kept private.
    B. Information cannot be shared with unauthorized family members.
    C. Pictures of a resident's wound cannot be posted on Facebook.
    D. All of the above.

(Answers to "Check What You've Learned" are in the Instructor's Manual.)

Chapter 5

YOUR ROLE IN ENSURING QUALITY OF LIFE

What do you want your residents to say when they are asked, "What it is like to live in this long term care facility?" How do you want your residents to answer this question? Do you want them to say that they feel they are well cared for, that they are treated with respect, and that their permission is always asked before something is done to them? Do you want them to say they feel well informed about what is happening in the facility? That the staff are familiar and pleasant to them and truly doing the best they can (Fig. 5-1)?

Chapter 1 asked you to think about what makes life worth living. What each resident thinks may be different from what you think. In Chapter 2, you learned you have to get to know the resident in order to give quality care. In Chapter 3, you learned about residents' needs and how their past affects how they behave. Chapter 4 described the rights of residents in long term care. Think about those chapters. What things would you want someone to consider when caring for you, your child, your relative, or your parent? If you were a resident, what would you want your family to say when asked, "What is it like to live in this long term care facility?"

In this chapter you will learn how to ensure that the resident's quality of life is the best it can be. You will learn what it means to treat a resident with dignity and respect. You will learn about customer service. You will also learn the importance of activities for residents and alternative forms of long term care.

OBJECTIVES
- Describe why treating a resident with dignity is important
- Describe what a customer service focus means for a nurse assistant
- Explain the importance of activities for residents
- Describe the principles of the Eden Alternative

MEDICAL TERMS
- **Bladder training** – a care plan to help a resident regain voluntary control of urination

"I've lived for a long time, and I look to you every day to help me continue my journey."

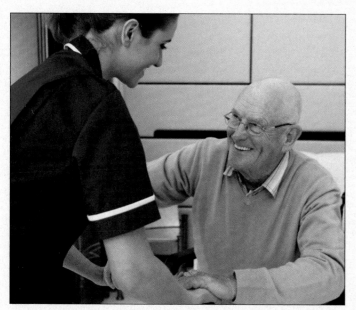

Fig. 5-1 – Residents have had many experiences. You will enjoy getting to know them.

When you consider a resident's quality of life, you should think about dignity, respect, and positive relationships. Dignity is a word you will see and hear often in your nurse assistant career. You will see the word when you read about residents' rights. You will hear your supervisor say, "Be sure to treat the resident with dignity when giving care." Always try to promote residents' dignity as you perform your daily tasks.

But what does dignity really mean? Why is it important to promote a resident's dignity, and how can you ensure it? All nurse assistants should ask themselves these questions, and you must find the answers as you work with each resident. Understanding what dignity is and how to promote each resident's dignity helps you give quality care and respect all residents. Treating residents with dignity and respect means that you are meeting their needs and supporting their quality of life. In addition, you enhance residents' quality of life when you support their existing relationships and help them create new ones both inside the facility and outside it.

WHAT IS DIGNITY?

What does dignity mean to you? If you asked residents what dignity means to them, what would they say? No one is born with a feeling of dignity. It must be learned. Our parents and teachers show us that we are valuable and that we deserve to be respected and treated with dignity. Our sense of self-worth must be reinforced throughout our lives, particularly if we become impaired or vulnerable in other ways. If you ask different people what dignity means to them, you will get many different answers. Nursing facility residents might say that a staff member treats them with dignity when a staff member

- shows respect
- gives individualized care and considers the resident's likes, dislikes, and preferences
- keeps them covered during personal care and maintains privacy (Fig. 5-2)

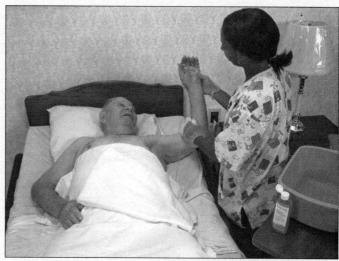

Fig. 5-2 – Keeping a resident covered when giving personal care shows respect for them.

- gives care in a pleasant and comfortable manner
- asks permission before giving care
- calls them by their preferred name
- shows them and other residents that they are important
- is sensitive to them and careful with their belongings
- is considerate of their needs, wants, and rights
- treats them the way they want to be treated

Dignity – a feeling pride and self-respect

All of these answers are part of dignity. Think about the last answer: "Treats them how they want to be treated." How do you know how people want to be treated? What clues do you get from residents?

The first thing to consider is your perception of residents. Is your mental image of a resident an accurate picture of who that person really is? **Perceptions** are impressions that you think are true, even if they are not actually true.

What do you see when you look at a resident? The following example shows how perception can work:

While she was on vacation, Sue noticed a man at the next table in a restaurant. She thought, "I know that man, but I can't remember where I met him." A few days later, Sue saw the same man picking up his son at school. Now she remembered him. His name was Mike, and his son Tommy was a friend of Sue's son. Sue saw Mike at least once a week, always at the school, but she didn't recognize him in another setting. Has something like this ever happened to you?

Sue didn't recognize Mike because she thought of him only as Tommy's dad. His face was in one category in Sue's mind—the father of her son's friend. That's why she had difficulty picturing him in another role. She didn't know that he liked to vacation in the same places she liked. She didn't know that he liked the ocean, that he read a lot, or that he was a firefighter (Fig. 5-3).

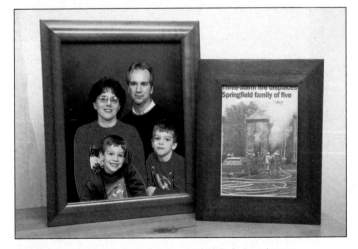

Fig. 5-3 – Everyone has many roles. Residents in long term care facilities have also had many roles.

When you have a **single-minded** image of someone, you miss opportunities to truly know them.

Close your eyes and imagine yourself walking through the halls of your facility, looking at residents as you pass them. What do you see when you look at each resident? Would you describe some of them as old, confused, noisy, incontinent, sick, or wrinkled? This is all that some people see. It is common to label a person—to form an image of them based only on what you see initially. Unfortunately, this keeps you from discovering other things about the person. You must learn to look beyond your initial impressions and truly get to know the resident.

Imagine meeting Mr. Roberts, who is being admitted to your facility for the first time. He is a 92-year-old man with Alzheimer's disease. He is confused and combative, and he appears angry. He has episodes of incontinence and is confined to a wheelchair. He cannot answer questions.

How would you describe Mr. Roberts? Would you say he is an angry old man with little mental and physical capacity left? That may be what you perceive when you see him for the first time, but is that who he really is? How can you see more to him than what is in front of your eyes? And how can you promote Mr. Roberts' dignity when you do not know much about him?

Having a single-minded image of Mr. Roberts as an angry man who cannot do much for himself can keep you from giving him quality care. If you think of him this way and talk about him in this way with co-workers, you set a pattern that is difficult to break. Labeling Mr. Roberts because of your first impression does not give you a chance to find out whether something caused him to behave as he did. Perhaps he does not usually act that way. Perhaps he acted that way only because:
• He was angry and scared of being admitted to a nursing facility.
• His disease affects how he expresses himself.
• The new surroundings are unfamiliar to him, and his sense of security is threatened.
• No one told him he was being taken to your facility.

Perception – a mental image of something
Single-minded – an attitude of seeing someone in only one way

Can you imagine leaving your home and moving to a facility where everyone is a stranger? Wouldn't you be angry and scared? It is very important not to label residents with a single-minded image. If you do, in most cases they will not receive the quality care they need and deserve. Once you label a resident, you will never know who they truly are.

How Perception Influences Dignity

How you perceive and label residents influences how you give them care and treat them in general. You may think you know how they want to be treated, but that may not be what they really want. In the example above, you might think that Mr. Roberts would be happier if people stayed away from him. You might think he is combative because he is angry. But your perceptions may be wrong.

Many factors influence perception. Exploring these factors helps you learn how the resident wants to be treated. These factors include your own:
• values
• morals
• culture
• religion (Fig. 5-4)
• environment
• life experiences
• likes and dislikes

For example, you may come from a culture in which people value keeping their emotions inside. If so, you may think that residents should not show feelings like sadness and anger in front of others. But a resident from a different background may feel that showing their emotions is natural and healthy. Respecting others—even when their behavior does not seem appropriate to you—is part of caregiving. It also is needed to treat others with dignity.

Once you discover that your first impression of Mr. Roberts may not be accurate, try to learn who he really is. Then it will be easier to treat him with dignity.

For example, you learn that Mr. Roberts has four sons, three of whom are married with children. All four of them live close by and plan to visit every weekend. Mr. Roberts was a truck driver for a local bakery. He loves boxing and football, and he played both sports when he was younger. As a football coach Mr. Roberts was well liked by the boys on the team. His team won the state championship three years in a row.

You now begin to see there is much more to Mr. Roberts than what you saw on the day he was admitted. To care for Mr. Roberts and give him the respect and dignity he deserves, you need to find out who he is.

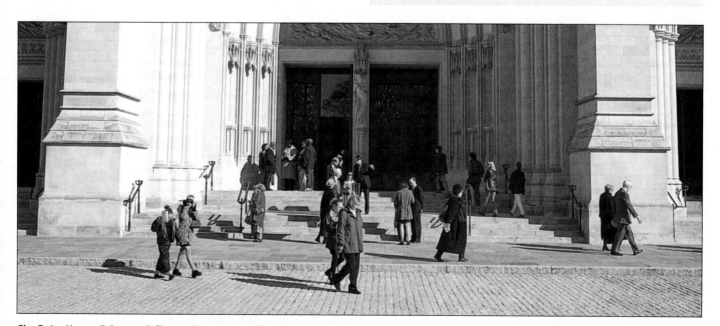

Fig. 5-4 – Your religion can influence how you perceive others.

Changing a Resident's Self-Perception

Residents, too, may have a single-minded image of themselves. Consider this example:

Mrs. Adams sees herself only as a wife. When her husband died, she felt a loss of self-worth and dignity because she no longer was a wife. She is now depressed, withdrawn, and uninterested in life. She moves slowly, does not join in activities, and does not want to eat. Her self-image—her identity as a wife—is gone.

Many residents have experienced loss. The loss of a spouse, a home, friends, or health can affect a resident's feelings of dignity. How can you help Mrs. Adams see that she is much more than a wife? What could you talk to her about to help her break out of this single-minded image? You could ask questions like "What things did you like to do? Did you enjoy cooking, reading, sewing, gardening, or painting? Tell me about your friends and neighbors. Did you work or do volunteer work? Where did you grow up? Do you have any sisters or brothers?"

In this way you will learn more about Mrs. Adams. Then you can help her to see that she is much more than just a wife. If you are successful, her self-esteem and self-worth will improve. By showing an interest in Mrs. Adams, you can influence her perception of herself and promote her dignity.

HONORING A RESIDENT'S LIFE

The following is a true story written by Anna Mae Halgrim Seaver, a resident who lived in a nursing facility. As you read this, think about Mrs. Seaver, what she likes, and how you could promote her dignity.

My World Now
Life in a Nursing Home, From the Inside*

This is my world now. It's all I have left. You see, I'm old. And I'm not as healthy as I used to be. I'm not necessarily happy with it but I accept it. Occasionally, a member of my family will stop in to see me. They will bring some flowers or a little present, maybe a set of slippers—I've got eight pair. We'll visit for awhile and then they return to the outside world and I'll be alone again.

Oh, there are other people here in the nursing home. Residents, we're called. The majority are about my age. I'm 84. Many are in wheelchairs. The lucky ones are passing through. A broken hip, a diseased heart, something has brought them here for rehabilitation. When they're well they'll be going home.

Most of us are aware of our plight—some are not. Varying stages of Alzheimer's have robbed several of their mental capacities. We listen to endlessly repeated stories and questions. We meet them anew daily, hourly or more often. We smile and nod gracefully each time we hear a retelling. They seldom listen to my stories so I've stopped trying.

The help here is basically pretty good, although there's a large turnover. Just when I get comfortable with someone they move onto another job. I understand that. This is not the best job to have.

I don't much like some of the physical things that happen to us. I don't care much for a diaper. I seem to have lost control acquired so diligently as a child. The difference is that I'm aware and embarrassed but I can't do anything about it. I've had three children and know it isn't pleasant to clean another's diaper. My husband used to wear a gas mask when he changed the kids. I wish I had one now.

Why do you think the staff insists on talking baby talk when speaking to me? I understand English. I have a degree in music and am a certified teacher. Now I hear a lot of words that end in "y." Is this how my kids felt? My hearing aid works fine. There is little need for anyone to position their face directly in front of mine and raise their voice with those "y" words. Sometimes it takes longer for a meaning to sink in; sometimes my mind wanders when I am bored. But there's no need to shout.

I tried once or twice to make my feelings known. I even shouted once. That gained me a reputation of being "crotchety." Imagine me, crotchety. My children never heard me raise my voice. I surprised myself. After I've asked for help more than a dozen times and received nothing more than a dozen conde-scending smiles and a "Yes, deary, I'm working on it," something begins to break. That time I wanted to be taken to the bathroom.

I'd love to go out for a meal, to travel again. I'd love to go to my own church, sing with my own choir. I'd love to visit my friends. Most of them are gone now or else they are in different "homes" of their children's choosing. I'd love to play a good game of bridge but no one here seems to concentrate very well.

My children put me here for my own good. They said they would be able to visit me frequently. But they have their own lives to lead. That sounds nor-mal. I don't want to be a burden. They know that. But I would like to see them more. One of them is here in town. He visits me as much as he can.

Something else I've learned to accept is loss of pri-vacy. Quite often I'll close my door when my room-mate—imagine having a roommate at my age—is in the TV room. I do appreciate some time to myself and believe that I have earned at least that courtesy. As I sit thinking or writing, one of the aides invariably opens the door unannounced and walks in as if I'm not there. Sometimes she even opens my drawers and begins rummaging around. Am I invisible? Have I lost the right to respect and dignity? What would happen if the roles were reversed? I am still a human being. I would like to be treated like one.

The meals are not what I would choose for myself. We get a variety but we don't get a choice. I am one of the fortunate ones who can still handle utensils. I remember eating off such cheap utensils in the Great Depression. I worked hard so I would never have to use them again. But here I am.

Did you ever sit in a wheelchair over an extended period of time? It's not comfortable. The seat squeezes you in the middle and applies constant pressure on your hips. The armrests are too narrow and my arms slip off. I am luckier than some. Others are strapped into their chairs and abandoned in front of the TV. Captive prisoners of daytime television; soap operas, talk shows and commercials…

…A typical day. Awakened by the woman in the next bed wheezing—a former chain smoker with asthma. Call an aide to wash me and place me in my wheelchair to wait for breakfast. Only 67 minutes until breakfast. I'll wait. Breakfast in the dining area. Most of the residents are in wheelchairs. Others use canes and walkers. Some sit and wonder what they are waiting for. First meal of the day. Only 3 hours and 26 minutes until lunch. Maybe I'll sit around and wait for it. What is today? One day blends into the next until day and date mean nothing…

…Back to my semiprivate room for a little semipri-vacy or a nap. I do need my beauty rest, company may come today. What is today, again? The afternoon drags into early evening. This used to be my favorite time of day. Things would wind down. I would kick off my shoes. Put my feet up on the coffee table. Pop open a bottle of Chablis and enjoy the fruits of my day's labor with my husband. He's gone. So is my health. This is my world.

* "My World Now: Life in the Nursing Home From the Inside" with permis-sion from her son, Richard H. Seaver, Sr., reprinted from *Newsweek*, June 27, 1994, p.11.

Who Is Anna Mae Halgrim Seaver?

How can you understand who a resident is? Ask the resident or the resident's family or friends what the person likes and dislikes. Ask about their past experiences and spiritual beliefs. Ask about where they grew up, what traditions they practice, their job experiences, and what they like to do to relax. You also can find out about residents from facility staff such as nurses, therapists, and social workers.

Who is Anna Mae Halgrim Seaver? Is she an old frail woman, incontinent and helpless? Or is she:

- a mother and wife
- compassionate and understanding
- independent
- proud of her accomplishments
- a teacher
- educated, with a degree in music (Fig. 5-5)

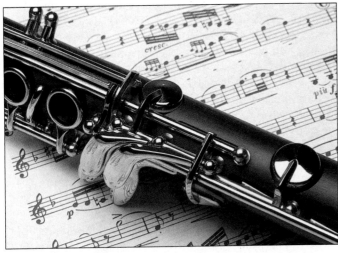

Fig. 5-5 – When you get to know a resident, you will learn many interesting things about them.

- able to hear very well with a hearing aid
- even tempered
- a woman who liked to travel, eat at restaurants, sing, play bridge, and visit friends
- a churchgoer
- active
- a human being

What does Anna Mae Halgrim Seaver like? Is she happy being called "y" names, like "deary," "sweety," or "honey"? Does she enjoy sitting in her wheelchair waiting to eat and being diapered to prevent her from wetting her bed? Or does Mrs. Seaver like:

- being with her family
- her home
- telling her own stories
- having one person care for her
- conversations on her level (not baby talk)
- activities (singing, playing cards, going on outings)
- private moments
- choices
- independence
- getting out of her wheelchair for exercise
- being treated as a person

To Mrs. Seaver, dignity means respecting her, maintaining her privacy and independence, treating her as an important person, and being sensitive to her and careful with her belongings. This is true for all residents.

Remember that your perceptions about residents are not always accurate. Learning about residents—about their values, morals, culture, religion, home environment, living experiences, and likes and dislikes—will help you promote their dignity.

In this example, Mrs. Seaver's dignity could have been maintained if the nurse assistant and others on the health care team:

1. Promoted, not blocked, communication with her by:
- asking Mrs. Seaver to share her life experiences and stories
- listening to her feelings
- talking to her as an adult, using an adult tone of voice
- asking her if she can hear, rather than shouting at her
- using touch appropriately, if she is comfortable with it

2. Promoted her independence by:
- asking Mrs. Seaver what she likes and dislikes
- offering her choices
- encouraging her to spend more time out of her wheelchair, for exercise and to participate in activities
- asking her what she would like to do between meals
- helping her regain continence through bladder training

Bladder training – a care plan to help a resident regain voluntary control of urination

3. Maintained her privacy by:

* knocking on Mrs. Seaver's door and asking for permission to come in before entering her room (Fig. 5-6)

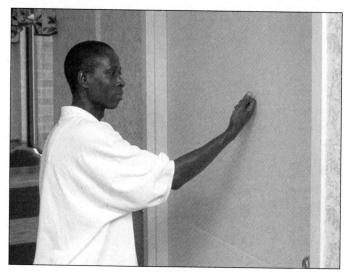

Fig. 5-6 – Knocking on the resident's door and waiting for permission to enter shows respect.

* not touching her personal belongings unless she gives permission
* honoring her likes and dislikes, culture, living experiences, and health when choosing a new roommate for her

4. Guaranteed her respect by:

* calling Mrs. Seaver by the name she prefers
* decreasing her need for incontinence products by maintaining bowel and bladder training
* positively reinforcing her functional abilities
* answering the call light promptly
* helping Mrs. Seaver stay clean and dry
* avoiding using labels to describe her
* acknowledging her intelligence
* treating Mrs. Seaver as a person. As she said, "I am still a human being. I would like to be treated as one."

HELPING RESIDENTS TO REDEFINE THEIR LIVES

Always try to understand who the residents are when they enter your long term facility. But it is just as important to help them understand that their new lives in the facility will likely involve a new view of life. You need to help the residents transition from their past lives to what their new lives will be in the facility. A good way to help them is to encourage them to bring their personal things to their rooms. Encourage them to talk about their pasts while getting used to their present situation. For example, talk to them about their past habits and preferences for how they lived, and help them find new ways to do the same things now. Maybe a resident always liked to curl up with a warm blanket and a book on a cold, rainy afternoon? If so, there is no reason why they can't do that now when the weather turns cold and rainy. Although the setting may be different, they need to know that their quality of life can still be good.

WHAT DIFFERENCE DOES PROMOTING DIGNITY MAKE?

Can you imagine living without positive communication, without choices, without privacy, and without respect? Would you feel like talking to others, eating, exercising, or improving your health? Probably not.

Think again about the earlier example of Mr. Roberts. How would you treat him if all you knew about him was that he looked old, acted angry and uncooperative, and could not do much for himself? Would you be slow to go to his room to give care? Would you feel frustrated if he did not cooperate? It is important to see Mr. Roberts as a person who has lived an active, productive, caring life—not as he happens to look and act at one time. Even if his mental capacities are limited today, he still deserves to be treated with dignity.

You can promote the dignity of residents by getting to know them and treating them as the important people they are. When residents have dignity, they feel better about themselves. When their self-esteem improves, they play a more active role in their own care. Their health may improve, and they may regain physical capacities they seemed to have lost. They engage in more social activities. They eat and sleep better and reach their optimum level of wellness.

ACTIVITIES

Activities are an important part of residents' lives in long term care facilities. Activities help the residents maintain their independence, feel important, and feel that they are a contributing member of society.

The facility's activity program is a critical part of the resident's care plan. Activities must be meaningful to the resident. If you know about a resident, you and the interdisciplinary team will have a better idea of what activities to offer them (Fig. 5-7). You can help the activities director by sharing your knowledge of the residents. Think about:

- what they did for a living
- their hobbies
- their role in their family
- their likes and dislikes

Be careful not to impose your own point of view on the resident, because their own values and culture are more important than yours. For example, a resident who has always thought that watching television is a waste of time is not likely to begin watching it for hours at a time. What a resident may really want is to spend some time outside or sit alone and read while other residents are at bingo. You may think this seems lonely, but it may have great meaning to a resident. If a resident does not want to participate in an activity, take the time to learn what they do want to do.

Encourage residents to select activities that give them positive experiences (Fig. 5-8). Try not to involve them in an activity that involves skills they may not have. For example, it's not a good idea to ask a resident with vision problems to attend a reading circle, where each resident reads aloud from a book. But this same resident may enjoy it when the activities director reads to the group.

The facility will offer both structured group activities, like a weekly bingo game, and unstructured activities, such as one resident visiting with another to discuss the daily news. The goal of both types of activities is to help residents become actively engaged—not sitting passively in

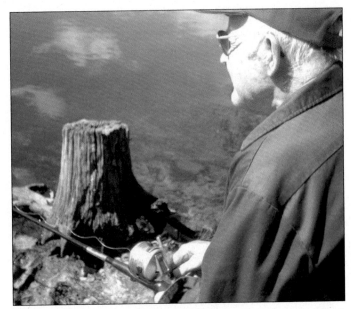

Fig. 5-8 – It is important that residents be able to continue activities that they enjoy even after they enter long term care.

front of the television or napping. Activities should not be childish. They should stimulate residents and help them feel involved. Most facilities post a schedule of events (Fig. 5-9). Talk with residents about events on the calendar so that they can choose which to attend. If a resident says that none of the activities interests them, tell the activities director and talk with the resident about what they would like to do.

As the person who spends the most time with the resident, you can give the charge nurse and the rest of the care team useful information about how the resident responds to activities. Then adjustments can be made to the resident's care plan. Just remember that not all residents like to do the same thing.

QUALITY OF LIFE

The Centers for Medicare and Medicaid Services (CMS) requires facilities to care for residents in a manner and environment that promote enhancement of every resident's quality of life. This includes:

- Treat the resident with dignity and recognize their individuality.
- Encourage self-determination and participation. Give residents choices about activities, schedules, and health care. Encourage them to interact with others both inside and outside the facility. Encourage them to make choices about all aspects of their life in the facility.

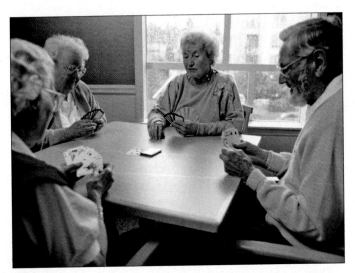

Fig. 5-7 – Activities are an important part of residents' lives in long term care facilities.

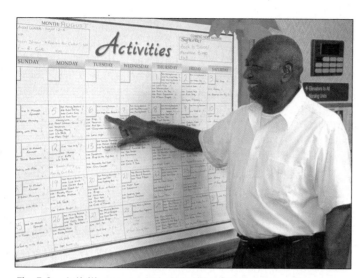

Fig. 5-9 – Activities are posted where all residents can see them.

- Encourage the organization of, and participation in, resident and family groups.
- Encourage participation in social, religious, and community activities as long as they do not interfere with the rights of other residents.
- Provide for an accommodation of the individual's needs and preferences within reason.
- Provide activities. The facility must have ongoing activities to meet the resident's interests and promote their physical, mental, and psychosocial well-being.

A DIFFERENT WAY TO PROVIDE CARE

All of us working in long term care want each resident to feel their life is still worth living. Based on this, Dr. William Thomas created a different type of long term care environment known today as the Eden Alternative.

To use this approach, staff in long term care facilities must understand three basic principles of care:

1. Every resident can grow as a person.
2. A resident's needs and capabilities must determine how we care for them.
3. Care must be continuous and long lasting, unlike treatment, which typically is intermittent and brief.

The idea behind the Eden Alternative is that to make life worth living, you must help prevent loneliness, helplessness, and boredom. Dr. Thomas says we must learn how to care, not just how to treat. When we treat residents, we manage only their disease. But when we care, we help the resident to grow.

Using the idea of the Eden Alternative, a long term care facility is transformed from an institution that treats residents into a home—one that meets residents' needs for companionship, their need to care for others, and their need for variety. Dr. Thomas says the facility should be a habitat with plants, gardens, and animals present. Residents then have the opportunity to care for the plants and animals, plant gardens, and even enjoy meals made with vegetables they grow (Fig 5-10).

Long term care facilities that implement the Eden Alternative include pets and flower and vegetable gardens in the environment. Some Eden programs include children. Day-care centers and after-school programs may be built into the facility, and children interact with the residents. In such an environment, residents grow and feel they are contributing to life. The Eden Alternative is not another activity program. It is a process that transforms the entire facility, the staff, and the residents.

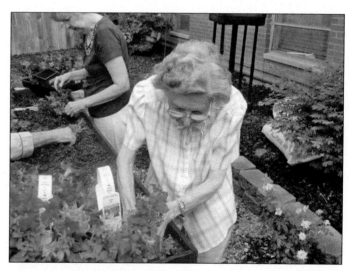

Fig. 5-10 – The Eden Alternative program encourages residents to plant their own flower and vegetable gardens.

Since the early 1990s, many long term care facilities have adopted similar approaches to caregiving. Generally these approaches are referred to as resident-centered approaches. So far the Eden Alternative has been the most popular of these.

Alternative – a choice, a different possibility
Habitat – a place where plants and animals are found growing naturally

IN THIS CHAPTER YOU LEARNED:

- Why treating the resident with dignity is important
- What a customer service focus means for a nurse assistant
- The importance of activities for residents
- The principles of the Eden Alternative

SUMMARY

This chapter explains how important it is for you to consider residents' quality of life when giving care. Treating residents with dignity and respect is the basis of quality. Your customer service focus will show residents you feel they are important. Activities are also a vital part of the resident's care plan. Promote activities that show residents you consider their likes and dislikes. The principles of the Eden alternative also help create an environment that transforms the long term care facility from an institution that treats diseases to a home that makes life worth living.

PULLING IT ALL TOGETHER

Imagine your first day at work in a long term care facility. Do you believe everyone is just there to die? What do you think a resident should expect from staff in the facility? Is it all about following your rules and routines? Think through these issues and your feelings about residents. You cannot improve or help maintain a resident's quality of life if you do not believe the resident has value.

Understanding the resident is the key to forming a successful relationship. What you learn about a resident will help you treat them with dignity and respect. Talk about this with other staff who have worked at the facility longer than you, and talk with the resident and the resident's family to learn more about the resident. They can help you discover who a resident really is.

CHECK WHAT YOU'VE LEARNED

1. **It is important for a nurse assistant to:**
   A. Order food and other dietary supplies.
   B. Treat residents with dignity and respect.
   C. Help with monthly pest control measures.
   D. Update a resident's billing records as needed.

2. **How can you promote a resident's dignity?**
   A. Tell them secrets about other residents.
   B. Tell them when you think their hair looks messy.
   C. Rearrange their belongings the way you think looks best.
   D. Be considerate of their wants, needs, and rights.

3. **Which of these statements about our perceptions is true?**
   A. Our perceptions about residents are always accurate.
   B. We should always believe that what we perceive is true, regardless of whether it may be right or wrong.
   C. Our perceptions influence how we behave toward others.
   D. Single-minded perceptions of residents help us get to know them better.

4. **How can you make a resident feel important?**
   A. Tell them what you don't like about them.
   B. Make decisions for them.
   C. Ask them to tell you about their life.
   D. Plan their day for them.

5. **How can you make a new resident feel that they belong?**
   A. Call them by the nickname "honey."
   B. Encourage them to participate in activities.
   C. Ask if you can borrow some of their jewelry.
   D. Leave them alone to adjust to the facility on their own.

6. **Which of these behaviors protects a resident's right to privacy?**
   A. Encouraging them to tell you their family secrets
   B. Telling them which other residents and staff members you think are nosey.
   C. Knocking on their door and announcing yourself before entering the room.
   D. Inviting a staff member in for a chat as you give the resident a bed bath.

7. **In order to avoid labeling a resident, you should:**
   A. Choose a nickname for them that suits their personality.
   B. Get to know them as an individual with their own feelings and needs.
   C. Always try to remember your first impression of them.
   D. Ask a family member to write the resident's name in each item of clothing.

8. **How can you honor a resident?**
   A. Give them a funny hat to wear on their birthday.
   B. Tease them about their appearance when they first wake up.
   C. Get to know their preferences and needs.
   D. Ask them why their family doesn't visit very often.

9. **You can add customer service to caregiving by:**
   A. Humming or singing as you do your job.
   B. Telling residents to talk to the charge nurse instead of you whenever they have a complaint.
   C. Doing all you can to solve residents' problems.
   D. Wearing a fresh flower above your name badge.

10. **Mrs. Marquez, a new resident, has shown no interest in any of the activities in the facility. What should you do?**
    A. Ask her what she is interested in and talk to the activity director about it.
    B. Leave her alone until she decides what she wants to do.
    C. Ask other residents to tell her how much they enjoy their bingo games and pressure her to join them.
    D. Tell her the rules say that she must attend at least one of the facility's organized activities.

(Answers to "Check What You've Learned" are in the Instructor's Manual.)

Chapter 6

THE ROLE OF THE FAMILY

Have you ever realized that your first impression of someone or something was not true? Maybe you realized that you did not have all the facts. Maybe you had misinterpreted what was going on. Sometimes, even when you have the facts, you do not let go of your first impression. This may be true even when the impression makes you uncomfortable.

Think about a family member walking into your facility and overhearing you talking to a resident who is resisting care. Think about how it might sound to the family member if you are trying to encourage the resident to get out of bed and take a walk. Are your conversations and actions always professional, kind, and considerate?

It is important to have a positive relationship with residents' family members, friends, and significant others. They are members of the health care team. Often they know the resident best. They can give you valuable information and guidance for your caregiving.

This chapter discusses the important role of residents' family members. They can affect the quality of your caregiving. Moving into a long term care facility has a big impact on the resident's family and friends, too. Like residents, they must make adjustments. You can do much to assist friends and family members in helping residents, too.

OBJECTIVES
- Define family
- State why family is important
- Define the family's adjustment process
- Describe how to make the resident's family feel like a valuable part of the health care team
- Explain how to develop a relationship with the family

"You are now a part of my family. Nurture your relationships with my children and loved ones."

ave you ever heard the saying, "You can attract more flies with honey than with vinegar"? Being kind and positive is more effective than being rude or negative. Think about how you interact with many people every day. Your experiences with others are affected much by the quality of your relationships with them. Think about how you like others to treat you. Don't you respond more favorably to someone who is kind and considerate? How do you react when someone is demanding or rude or ignores you?

In the same way, you need to work well with a resident's family members and friends. How you relate to them reflects on both your caregiving and the facility. Being friendly, caring, genuinely pleasant, and professional helps you form a positive relationship with them and gain their trust (Fig. 6-1). Then you can work more effectively with them. Being defensive or cold, on the other hand, hurts the relationship. Treating a resident's family well shows your respect not only for the family but for the resident, too.

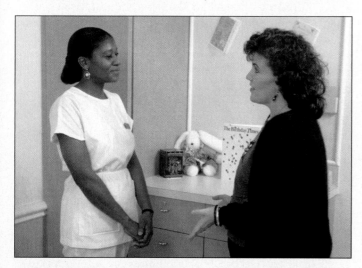

Fig. 6-1 – Being friendly with family members helps create a positive relationship with them.

WHAT IS FAMILY?

People are an important part of our lives. Think about the special people who matter the most to you: your family and friends. These are your significant others. They are important to you, and you care about them. Think about why they are so important to you. Can you imagine what life would be like without them? Family members affect us emotionally because of their personalities and actions. They influence us in many ways. They help bring meaning into our lives as we share experiences (Fig. 6-2).

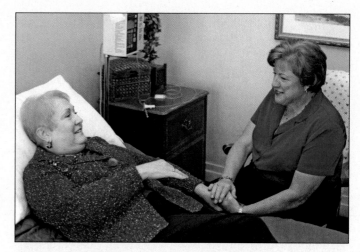

Fig. 6-2 – The resident's relationship with family members is an important part of the resident's life.

Residents may have a few or many significant others in their lives. Their family may include a spouse, brothers and sisters, nieces and nephews, children and grandchildren. Their significant others may include friends, a special person of the opposite or same sex, neighbors, and former co-workers. Because of their special bond with residents, family and significant others are very important. Since family and significant others are the same in this respect, this book will use the one word "family" for all significant others.

The Family as the Customer

Residents usually enter a long term care facility because family members and their health care provider have determined that the resident needs more support and care than they can receive at home or in the community. Family members often choose the facility. Most try to find a facility located close by.

In Chapter 5 you learned that the resident is your customer. The resident's family is also your customer. How you greet family members, how you talk with them about the resident, and how you address their concerns all affect how they think their loved one is cared for.

📖

Family – a group of persons of common ancestry or associated by marriage; includes significant others, or persons important to the resident

Consider the family in the same way as the resident. Keep an attitude that the family is your partner. With a partner you share common goals and decision making. Family members who are well informed will support the resident's goals for care. Keep them informed, treat them with respect, and they will support your efforts.

WHY IS FAMILY IMPORTANT?

Think of family members as an extension of the resident. Residents identify with family members because of their shared experiences and special memories. Usually these relationships are very personal and have lasted many years. Family members usually know a resident better than anyone else. In addition:
- Family members are familiar to residents when everything else in the facility is at first unfamiliar.
- Family can bring comfort to a resident.
- Family can share their knowledge about a resident.
- Family can help care for a resident.
- Family may provide financial support.

To give good care to the resident, consider who is important to them and how they value their relationships. Residents who have been close to family all of their lives want to keep these relationships. Think about how you feel when you are away from someone close to you. Do you sometimes feel hurt, angry, or sad?

Not all families are the same. Each resident has a unique relationship with their family. Some have strong family relationships. Others are more distanced. Some have difficult or stressful relationships. Be careful not to impose your own family values. Support each resident and their family whatever their relationship may be, even if you don't agree with it or find it hard to understand.

WHAT HAPPENS TO FAMILIES WHEN RESIDENTS ARE ADMITTED?

Think about how you live now. What might it be like to care for a dependent family member in your home? How would you manage? Could you find time for everything you needed to do? Would it be stressful for you? Maybe you are already caring for someone in your home and know how stressful it is.

When a resident is admitted to a facility, it is usually stressful for their family, too, because many changes happen at once (Fig. 6-3). The resident is physically and emotionally affected by this move, and these changes also affect the family.

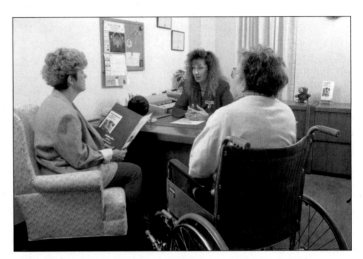

Fig. 6-3 – Admission of a family member to a facility is often a stressful time for the whole family.

Family members may have a range of feelings when their loved one enters the facility. Many find it hard to accept that they can no longer care for their loved one or that the person is no longer independent. They may have difficulty accepting that the resident may never come home.

Redefining the Family's Functioning

As discussed in Chapter 5, you need to help the resident redefine their life when they leave their home and enter the facility. Your assistance will also help the resident's family.

Most likely, for the first time, sons and daughters are in the uncomfortable position of having to make major decisions for their parents. These role changes and the change in their loved one's living arrangements dramatically affect families. Often they were comfortable with the way things used to be. Now they must make new decisions. This process begins when family members start looking for the right facility. Often they have to take a more active role in their loved one's financial and property matters. Now they are turning the day-to-day caregiving responsibility over to you and other facility team members who are strangers to them. They may now feel they have only a secondary role because you are their loved one's primary caregiver.

Stress – physical or emotional reaction that causes mental tension

With all these changes and stresses, family members may disagree or argue about some things. Unpleasantness may occur among family members, and possibly with the resident too. This may change their relationships and cause stress.

It is often stressful for families to care for elderly or ill relatives at home. In many families, every adult works outside the home, and no one can stay home to give care. Caring for one's parents is especially challenging for adults whose children also live at home. They may feel torn between the needs of their children and the needs of their parents.

Even so, most families try to care for elderly family members at home for as long as they can. They will place their loved one in a facility only as the last choice. Often this happens only when they are exhausted from caregiving responsibilities and when the community services that might support the family's care simply are not enough. By this time, the family often suffers from chronic stress. Families can feel burned out—physically and mentally exhausted—after caring for their loved one for a long time. In your work as a nurse assistant, you will encounter many families suffering from this type of chronic stress.

Understanding and talking with family members can help them cope with this stress. Sometimes it helps just to tell the family that you understand the changes must be hard for them. If you see that they need to talk about this, ask the charge nurse to arrange for the social worker to talk with them.

The Adjustment Process

Like residents, families must adjust before they can feel comfortable that their loved one is living in a long term care facility. It also takes time for the family to develop a trusting relationship with you (Fig. 6-4). The family may need six months or more to adjust to the facility.

During this time family members may have many different reactions. Watch for and try to understand their feelings. Even though their feelings are a normal part of the adjustment process, these feelings will certainly affect how they behave toward both you and their loved one. Accept that this adjustment period lasts until everyone is comfortable and a trusting relationship develops.

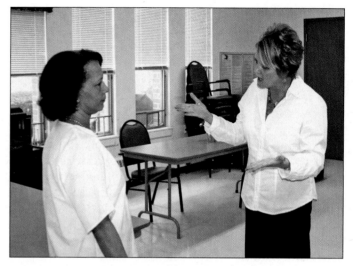

Fig. 6-4 – Family members can often be angry with staff.

Guilt.   Often family members feel **guilt** when they place their loved one in a facility. Some feel they are abandoning the person, no matter how difficult it would be to keep caring for them at home. Sometimes families had promised their loved one that they would always care for them at home. Then they had to break their promise because of a change in the person's health. They may feel very guilty. They may try to make up for it by visiting often and becoming very involved in care and decision making.

You can build trust by helping them stay involved and feel useful. Their attention often helps their loved one and makes the transition to the facility easier for everyone. You can help families get over their guilt. For example, you can say, "You made the right decision. Your mother will get the best care possible." Giving the very best care then helps the family resolve their guilt.

Anger and Resentment.   Some family members may be angry when they lose control of the care of their loved one. They may be the most challenging family members for you. They may resent staff, including you, because they think that all of you are replacing them. Their resentment may increase if they think the facility gives better care than they did.

Guilt – negative feelings experienced by someone who has committed an offense or believes they have done something wrong to another person

They may also be angry because of family disagreements about placing the loved one in a facility. This is especially true if a crisis forced them to make a quick decision. Angry family members may be critical and demanding of you or other staff. Sometimes a social worker or other staff member can help you and the family work together to resolve negative feelings.

Uncertainty.   Some families feel uncertain, nervous, or tense about their decision. They are not sure what to expect from the facility. They may worry whether they made the right decision. The facility is unfamiliar to them. They may be afraid for the future of their loved one in the facility because they want them to get the very best care. These families can be very emotional when they visit the resident. They may seem overly watchful as they try to make sure that their loved one is being cared for the way they want. By acting both professionally and compassionately, you can help them feel confident that you do care about their relative and are doing your best.

Sadness.   Some family members are very sad. They may have a hard time coping with being separated from their loved one if they have lived together or cared for them. They may grieve over the person's dependency or declining health during this period. Even though they visit the resident, they may feel a tremendous sense of loss.

These family members may seem upset or cry often when visiting. They may visit less often or stop coming because the situation upsets them so much. Let them express their feelings and help them talk about their distress (Fig. 6-5). Sometimes you can find a way to lighten the situation with a little laughter together, after the tears.

Loss of Control.   Many family members who cared for their loved ones for a long time feel a loss of control or responsibility when you and other staff take over the caregiving. Sometimes a family member's main role in life was to care for the loved one. Now they feel they have nothing to do. They may try to keep some control by becoming involved in care and decision making for their loved one.

Relief.   Some family members feel relieved when their loved one enters a facility. Taking care of the person at home may have been stressful and exhausting. This is especially so when the family members have other responsibilities. These families are relieved by the respite, or rest, from caring for their loved one.

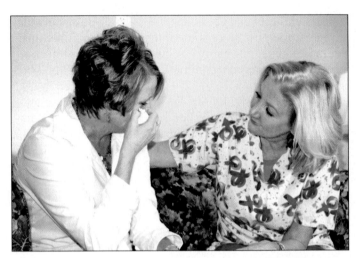

Fig. 6-5 – Support the resident's family members as they go through the adjustment process.

In this adjustment process, family members often move back and forth through different emotional stages. The key is to help them recognize what is happening and to support them through the stages. Once they feel comfortable with you and other staff members, they will come to rely on you.

YOUR RELATIONSHIP WITH THE FAMILY

From the moment you meet them, consider the resident's family part of the caregiving team. Family members can share information about the resident, interact with them, and help with their care. You can help families feel comfortable in this role.

When a resident is admitted, take the opportunity to get to know their family. Help make them comfortable by welcoming them and introducing yourself. Explain how you as a nurse assistant will help with their loved one's care. Get to know them by name. Take the time to understand their relationship with the resident.

If the family has not yet seen the facility or unit, let the charge nurse know so that they can have a tour of the facility. This helps them to become comfortable with an unfamiliar place that suddenly has become very important in their lives. Also, introduce them to other members of the health care team. Help them meet the families of other residents, too. Other families can give much support to each other and can become strong allies for your care team.

Families are interested in their loved one's activities. Let them know about upcoming events. Show them the calendar of events, and explain the activities that are available for residents. Your facility may have special events that involve families. Encourage family members to participate in any of these activities.

Find out what their family member's daily routines were at home, and consider how you can include these in the resident's care plan. Let them know when the resident will have meals, therapy sessions, and recreational activities. (This may also be a good time to let the family know about special policies at the facility.) Encourage visits and family participation.

Family members need to feel important and useful. Help them decide if they want to be involved in their loved one's care. If so, what would they like to do? If not, make sure they know that is OK, too. Encourage interested family members to bring in the resident's favorite things or foods, after they have checked with the charge nurse for any food restrictions or policies about bringing in food. Family members can help motivate a resident who seems depressed or is upset by illness or therapy. Family members are often the best cheerleaders (Fig. 6-6).

family members, understand their feelings, and help them adjust to their loved one's new circumstances.

INVOLVING THE FAMILY IN CARE

Some family members want to help care for their loved one. They may have cared for the person already, perhaps for years, and still need to feel useful. Family members may still want to help the resident, but often they are unsure how they can help. They may not want to seem pushy or to interfere with your caregiving. Try to find out what role they want to play. Don't wait for them to offer to help.

Family members can participate in the resident's care in many ways. They can do all or part of the resident's personal grooming at bath time. They may want to help their loved one eat and drink (Fig. 6-7). They can be good companions during physical therapy sessions. They may want to join them for a special activity such as crafts, music, or games. The family can also participate by shopping for clothes or special items for the resident. In addition,

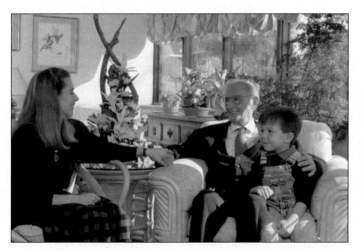

Fig. 6-6 — Family members can help motivate and cheer up a resident.

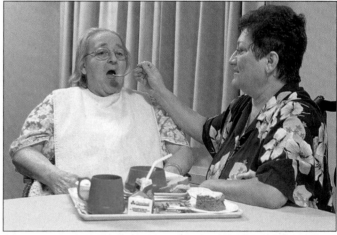

Fig. 6-7 — Family members can play an important role in caregiving, such as helping feed a resident.

You will work with the family as long as you care for their loved one. Stay involved with the families of residents who have lived in the facility a long time as well as new families. How the family feels about the care being given their loved one affects their attitude toward you and other staff. If the family feels their loved one is receiving good care, they will have positive feelings for you and other staff. They will trust you. But if they feel their loved one is unhappy or not well cared for, they will react negatively and have a hard time adjusting. Because you spend so much time with each resident, you can get to know their

encourage family members to participate in resident care conferences (Fig. 6-8, next page). Their knowledge of the resident is valuable. Family members can become involved in the family council and help shape the facility's policies for the benefit of all residents. Both care conferences and family councils are good opportunities for families to participate and feel satisfied with their involvement and contributions.

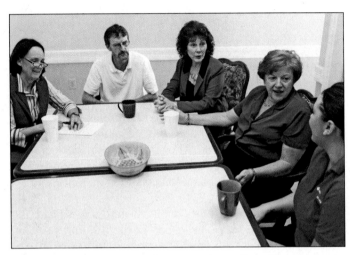
Fig. 6-8 – Residents' care conferences and council meetings are great times for family members to get involved.

You, too, may find it very helpful when families are involved in their loved one's care. Acknowledge their contributions with positive feedback and thanks. Just as you like to know that you are appreciated for doing a good job, families need to know this, too. Positive feedback helps keep families motivated to stay involved. But don't take advantage of their help or take it for granted. Some families may try to give all the care because it makes them feel more comfortable or useful. You can help them feel OK by making them confident of your care.

However, sometimes you may be uncomfortable when family members help care for a resident. You may be used to giving the resident care in a certain way, and the family member may do it differently. Or you may feel the family member is looking over your shoulder or trying to do your job. Family members may sometimes tell you how to care for the person. Always listen to what they are saying and never argue. They may know that the resident prefers care in a certain way, so let them know you will consider their suggestions. If you are uncomfortable with their suggestions or actions, discuss the situation with the charge nurse.

Communicating Effectively With Family Members

Be comfortable talking with the family about a resident openly and supportively. Family members can tell you much about a resident. They can share their medical history, habits, and likes and dislikes. They can share stories about the resident's life before they entered the facility. This information helps you and other staff understand the resident

better and give better care (Fig. 6-9). Let the family know that by helping you, they are helping their loved one.

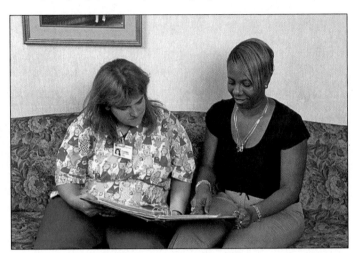
Fig. 6-9 – Family members are good sources of information about the resident.

To work well with the family, you need to communicate well with them. Use the skills described in Chapter 7, Communication. Good communication begins when the family knows you and you know them. Be available to talk with the family during their visits or on the telephone. Let them see how you interact with their loved one.

Often family members will ask you about a resident's condition, their progress, and how they have been feeling or acting. You should feel comfortable answering their questions (but refer questions about medical treatments, etc. to the charge nurse). You can also ask them for advice when their loved one behaves in certain ways. Remember that the family cares about the resident's well-being. They look to you for support and guidance.

Show your support by really listening to what the family says. Don't let other things distract you when you are with them, or the family member may feel you are not really listening (Fig. 6-10, next page). If a family member asks to speak to you when you are busy, try to agree on another time in the near future when you will have time to focus on them. Find a quiet spot so you can both relax and talk. This helps develop a positive relationship.

Be careful not to judge what family members say or do. Stay objective. Do not agree or disagree with their opinions,

📖
Feedback – information received that is corrective or evaluative

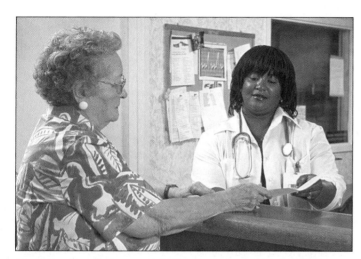
Fig. 6-10 – Always give your full attention when sharing information with a resident's family member.

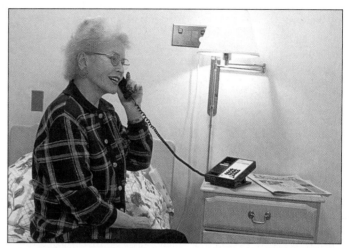
Fig. 6-11 – Talking on the phone is an important way for residents to stay in touch with family members.

especially if they are angry or frustrated. If family members disagree with each other or with their loved one, do not take sides. That would only cause more problems.

When you are talking with family members, repeat back to them the feelings, questions, and concerns they have expressed to you. This helps explain exactly what they are saying. When you let them know you understand their feelings, they are reassured that you have been listening to them.

Never try to hide a problem from the family. If you are uncomfortable discussing something with them, or if they ask questions you cannot answer, ask them to talk to the charge nurse or the social worker. The charge nurse is the one who should report any change in a resident's condition to the family right away. This way, they will not be surprised by any change that they notice during a visit.

Family members need to feel they are not cut off from their loved one. If you become aware of any barriers to communication, work to remove them. Be sure residents have access to the telephone and writing paper so that they can contact family members. By encouraging family members to visit, making their visits comfortable, and involving them in care, you enhance a resident's relationship with their family.

FAMILY VISITS

Most families try to keep a close relationship with their loved one in the facility. They stay in contact through visits, telephone calls, cards and letters, and outings outside the facility (Fig. 6-11). Most residents look forward to these interactions with their families. You should encourage interactions as much as possible.

During family visits, residents can talk about old times and share their feelings and experiences with the people who matter the most to them. This is a personal time. Make sure residents have privacy with their visitors and few if any interruptions. Family members may bring in photos, special foods, or gifts for their loved one (Fig. 6-12). They may take the resident to the chapel or for a walk outside. They may simply sit and hold hands.

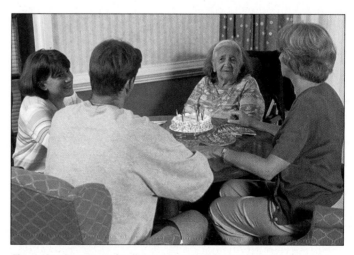
Fig. 6-12 – Encourage family members to be involved in events and activities that are important to the resident.

Some family members visit regularly and often. A husband may come every day at lunchtime to eat with his wife. A daughter may bring her children to visit their grandmother every Saturday. Family members may come in pairs or groups. Some may come alone. Most visits are unannounced. When the resident knows a family member is coming to visit, help prepare the resident in any way they wish so they can look and feel their best.

If a resident cannot communicate with family members or is in failing health, visits can be difficult for the family. Always continue to support the family.

Managing Family Members' Expectations

Different family members often have different expectations for how their loved one should be cared for. For example, one family member may have given most of the care at home. But now that the resident has come to your facility, other family members may become more involved. They may have a different opinion about caregiving. It is uncomfortable for staff when family members have differing opinions about their loved one's care.

If you encounter a situation involving conflict like this, try to carefully address each family member's concerns as if it is the most important thing you can do for the resident. Do not blame other family members or say anything negative about their opinions. Do not make excuses about how care is given in the facility. Be sure to tell the charge nurse about the family member's concerns. The nurse can hold a family meeting to help prevent future conflicts and try to help them reach agreement about the care. Otherwise, conflicts among family members can become a burden for staff. If the issues are not resolved, you may end up trying to make different family members happy but not satisfy anyone.

When Families Express Distress

Sometimes family members express their distress in ways that make you uncomfortable. This usually happens when they are emotional and have not yet adjusted to their loved one being in the facility. But they may have other stresses in their life, too. These may cause them to be demanding, critical, or hostile to you and other staff. They may even expect that you and other staff can somehow make their loved one better. Do not take their comments personally. Be supportive. Try not to judge the situation, but report it to the charge nurse.

Sometimes a family member has a justified criticism. Listen carefully. In this case staff must recognize the problem and work harder to meet the resident's needs. Remember the tips in Chapter 5 about managing customer issues. Do not ignore a problem or make excuses for it. If

you cannot correct it on your own, tell the charge nurse about it.

Some family members may not visit or call very often. They may live far away or be busy with their jobs, family, or other responsibilities. Some may seem to have little interest in a resident. They may be upset when they do have contact with them, perhaps because it is hard to accept changes in the resident's physical or mental state.

A resident who is aware of this lack of attention may make these family members feel even more guilty when they do visit. You can help by warmly greeting these visitors by name and telling them you are glad they came. Offer them something to drink and sit with them for a few minutes. Encourage the resident to tell their loved one what they have been doing. If a resident cannot communicate with them, you should do so. If a resident has memory loss, you may need to remind them of the names of family members. Reinforce the family's positive feelings about the visit by thanking them for coming.

A family support group or family council can be a great help to family members who are feeling distressed. They will get emotional support from others who feel the same way about their own loved ones living in the facility. Encourage the family's participation. Tell them when these groups meet and who in the facility can give them more information. Sometimes the social worker can help family members work through their feelings (Fig. 6-13). Families need to know about these resources and where to find them. You are a necessary and important link.

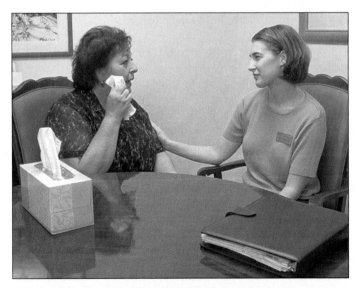

Fig. 6-13 – When a resident's health changes, family members may become upset. The social worker can lend support to the family.

WHEN YOU BECOME LIKE A FAMILY MEMBER

You may have more contact with some residents than their own family members do. Some residents may rely on you more and even trust you more than their own family. You may be the most consistent and caring person they see every day. For all of these reasons, a close, caring relationship may develop between you and a resident. You may come to feel like their family member yourself. Enjoy this special relationship and appreciate their trust. But don't let your feelings interfere with your caregiving for them and for other residents. Even though you may prefer to be with some residents more than others, give equal attention to all the residents you work with.

Because you are the resident's primary caregiver, you are a tremendous resource and support for families. Many family members will openly appreciate your efforts and thank you. In some cases, you may become attached to a resident's family. This often happens when a resident cannot communicate and you do most of the communication with the family.

IN THIS CHAPTER YOU LEARNED:

- What family means
- Why family is important
- How the family adjusts to the resident's new living arrangement
- How to help the family feel like a valuable part of the health care team
- How to develop a relationship with the family

SUMMARY

This chapter describes the important role of the resident's family. Consider the family as anyone—not just a relative—who is important to the resident. The resident's family has valuable information about the resident. The family also must undergo an adjustment process, which may cause them to react negatively to you from time to time.

Be sure to treat the resident's family as a customer. Always deal with their concerns in a manner that is open, and do not be defensive. Create an environment that supports their visits. This is an important part of the service you provide as a nurse assistant. It also shows the family how you welcome their active support of your caregiving.

PULLING IT ALL TOGETHER

You are taking care of Mrs. Connors, an 87-year-old resident with congestive heart failure and arthritis. She complains about how difficult it is for her to walk. She has three daughters and one son. Her daughter-in-law often comes to visit and has a great relationship with the staff.

One Sunday, Mrs. Connors' daughter visits and complains to you about what her mother is wearing. She also complains because you are encouraging her mother to take a walk. But you know that Mrs. Connors' daughter-in-law bought the outfit and agrees with you about the importance of daily walks. How should you handle the situation?

Talking with the daughter about why it is important for her mother to take walks will help her to understand why you encourage it. It will also help if you ask the daughter if she wants you to change her mother's clothes. The key is to be responsive to the needs of the resident's daughter. Do not promote conflict by telling Mrs. Connors' daughter that her sister-in-law, like you, wants her mother to walk.

It is important to make the charge nurse aware of this family conflict while it is still manageable. It may seem a small concern now but can become a major conflict later on. The charge nurse may choose to set up a family meeting. That way, everyone can have the same information and the family can reach an agreement about who should be informed when issues arise later on.

1. **Who is considered part of a resident's family?**
   A. All significant others.
   B. Only relatives of common ancestry.
   C. Only people related to the resident by blood or marriage.
   D. Everyone the resident knows.

2. **Families are important because:**
   A. They may bring food or gifts for staff.
   B. They can bring comfort to the resident.
   C. You can always count on them to help with bathing and dressing the resident.
   D. You can take a break from your duties whenever they are visiting.

3. **What is guilt?**
   A. A feeling that something bad is going to happen.
   B. Making someone do something against their will.
   C. A feeling that you've done something bad.
   D. A black mark written on your employment file when you make a mistake.

4. **When a resident is admitted to a long term care facility, their family at first is likely to feel:**
   A. A loss of control.
   B. Total confidence in your caregiving.
   C. Happiness and joy.
   D. No reaction at all.

5. **How can you help a family get over their guilt when a resident is admitted into a long-term care facility?**
   A. Encourage them to question their decision to admit their family member.
   B. Give their family member the best care you can.
   C. Tell them they are in charge of bathing and dressing their family member whenever they visit.
   D. Just nod and smile whenever they make suggestions about their loved one's care.

6. **How can you help to make a family visit pleasant?**
   A. Always take part in their visit with the resident.
   B. Include the resident's roommate in conversations.
   C. Tell them all the problems you are having.
   D. Give the family privacy and time to visit their loved one.

7. **Mr. Carey's son thinks staff does too much for Mr. Carey, while his daughter thinks they don't do enough. As his caregiver, what should you do?**
   A. Tell them you are just following orders.
   B. Tell each of them in private that you think they are right and the other one is wrong.
   C. Tell them they should both file written complaints.
   D. Explain why residents are encouraged to do all that they can for themselves.

8. **When a family member is angry or critical, you should:**
   A. Take their comments personally.
   B. Explain that the facility is understaffed and there's nothing anyone can do.
   C. Be supportive and report the situation to the charge nurse.
   D. Pretend you agree that the facility is not very good.

9. **How can you support family members who are never happy with their relative's care?**
   A. Tell them they should not expect so much from the staff.
   B. Encourage them to move their relative to another facility.
   C. Tell them about a family support group or family council offered at the facility.
   D. Suggest that they ask their physician for medication to help them stop worrying so much.

10. **A resident might think of you as a family member because:**
    A. You look like their favorite cousin.
    B. You share their interest in antique dolls.
    C. You are paid to pretend you are a family member.
    D. They know you care for them and respect them.

(Answers to "Check What You've Learned" are in the Instructor's Manual.)

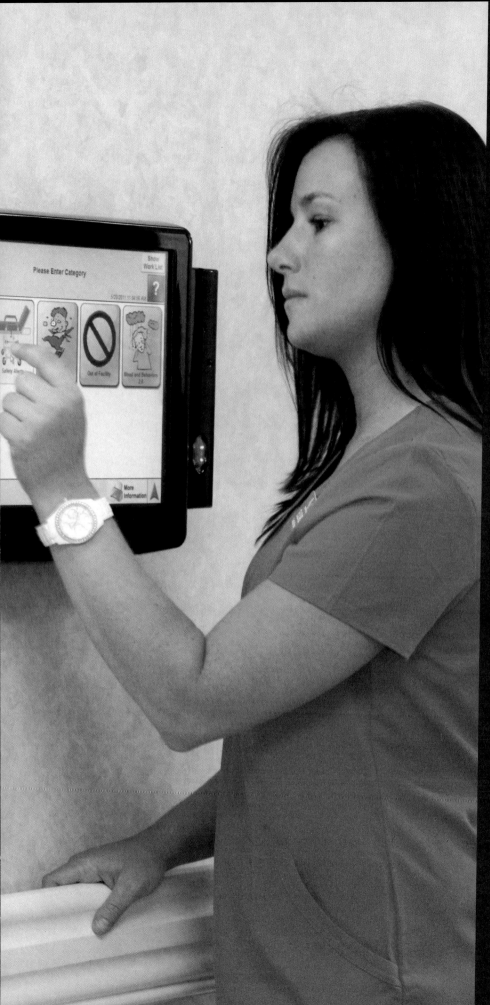

You Are Responsible For Quality Care

Chapter 7

COMMUNICATION

All people need to feel they are being heard. Moving into a long term facility often makes residents feel isolated and lonely. They are surrounded by strangers whom they depend on to help them meet their most basic needs. Talking to someone helps reduce their feelings of loneliness and isolation.

When you show a resident that you understand their feelings, they begin to trust you. Residents who feel you understand them are more likely to share their feelings and needs. A trusting relationship can develop when they feel cared for and know what to expect. Effective communication is the key to creating a trusting relationship. Effective communication is important because:

- It helps you understand each resident's needs.
- It promotes a trusting relationship.
- It makes your job easier and more enjoyable.
- It improves residents' quality of life.
- It helps you gain residents' cooperation.
- It adds to the resident's satisfaction, the family's, and your own.
- It helps staff know what changes you have observed about residents.
- It helps the health care team plan individualized care for each resident.

This chapter describes the skills you need for effective communication. You will learn how to communicate in different ways to meet the resident's special needs. You will also learn how to use your communication skills to resolve conflicts.

OBJECTIVES
- List ways to make verbal communication effective
- Explain the importance of nonverbal communication, touch, and listening
- List general guidelines for good communication and active listening
- Explain ways to communicate with residents who have special communication needs
- Describe ways to handle residents' inappropriate behavior or aggression
- Describe how to resolve conflicts
- Explain when it is OK to talk about yourself with residents
- Demonstrate proper telephone courtesy

MEDICAL TERMS
- **Aphasia** – condition in which a person has difficulty putting thoughts into words

"I trust you because you always take the time to listen and understand."

A big part of your job as a nurse assistant involves communicating with residents. Our culture emphasizes words in many forms: newspapers, magazines, books, radio, television, movies, lectures, and conversation. But communication is more than just words. Communication also occurs through symbols, such as traffic lights and road signs. When you were very young, you learned that a red traffic light means to stop and a green one means to go. You make another symbol for stop when you hold your hand up with the palm out. Words and symbols help give our lives structure, safety, and comfort. This is true in long term care facilities as well (Fig. 7-1).

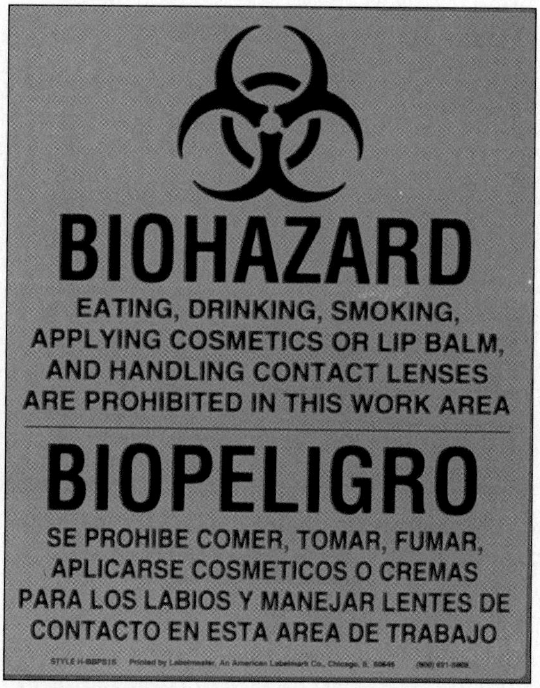

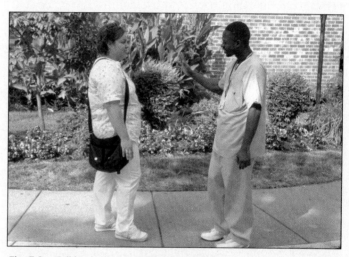
Fig. 7-2 – Talking is one way of communicating.

(verbal communication) (Fig. 7-2), through our body language (nonverbal communication) (Fig. 7-3), through touch, and through listening. Think of communication as a thread woven through a piece of cloth. If the thread is pulled or cut away, the cloth is damaged: A hole may form, or a hem in a pant leg can fall. Like cloth, a relationship needs the thread of communication to hold it together. Effective communication can improve the quality of your relationships and caregiving.

BIOHAZARD

EATING, DRINKING, SMOKING, APPLYING COSMETICS OR LIP BALM, AND HANDLING CONTACT LENSES ARE PROHIBITED IN THIS WORK AREA

BIOPELIGRO

SE PROHIBE COMER, TOMAR, FUMAR, APLICARSE COSMETICOS O CREMAS PARA LOS LABIOS Y MANEJAR LENTES DE CONTACTO EN ESTA AREA DE TRABAJO

STYLE H-BBPS15   Printed by Labelmaster, An American Labelmark Co., Chicago, IL 60646   (800) 621-5808.

Fig. 7-1 – Symbols and signs communicate information, such as this biohazard warning sign.

Body language is also a form of communication. When we are very young we learn to "read" the body language of others. Remember your mother's look when you tracked mud on the floor? She may have used words too, but they probably weren't as powerful as the look on her face that told you she was angry.

All of these aspects of communication are very important in your role as a nurse assistant. Communication is at the core of all relationships.

Communication involves both sending and receiving messages. We send and receive messages through words

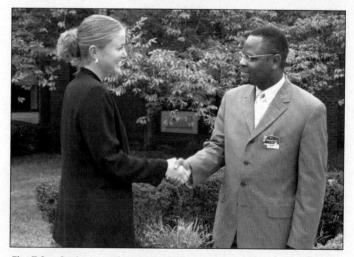
Fig. 7-3 – Gestures such as handshaking and nonverbal cues such as smiling are other ways we communicate.

Communication – Sending and receiving messages verbally and nonverbally

HOW WE COMMUNICATE

Verbal Communication

Verbal communication involves spoken or written words. That sounds simple enough, doesn't it? But words can have many different meanings, depending on one's background, culture, and education. Take the word "frequently," for example. To a health care worker it may have a very specific meaning related to a health condition. A physician who hears that a resident is frequently thirsty may consider this a symptom of a health problem. But a resident who says he is frequently thirsty may simply be telling you that the hot weather is causing him to drink a little more than usual today.

You cannot always automatically know exactly what someone means, even when they use familiar words. You have to understand the context of their words. As a nurse assistant, you must communicate in a manner that the resident understands. You must make sure the resident understands you, and you must pay attention to clues that show you when they do not.

We all learn to use words in particular ways by listening to our friends, family, and others. In the same way, you can learn the meaning of residents' words by really listening to them.

Your tone of voice, the speed at which you speak, and the clarity of your speaking often tell the listener much more than just what the words mean. You can make it easier for others to understand what you are saying if you follow the do's and don'ts listed in Box 7-1.

If you do not speak a resident's primary language, you must find someone to translate for you, such as a family member or staff member. But you also show that you really care if you try to learn some words in the resident's language. You can post these words in the resident's room to help other caregivers communicate with the person.

If your own primary language is not English, and a resident you care for speaks only English, remember to speak only English with them and around them. Staff who speak to each other in a language that residents do not understand are indirectly violating these residents' rights. Residents often feel that staff are talking about them and feel intimidated or threatened (Fig. 7-4). This is particularly

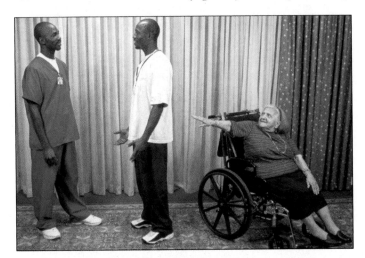

Fig. 7-4 — Speaking in a different language in front of a resident indirectly violates the resident's rights.

📖

Context – the whole situation, background, or environment that gives meaning to someone's words

---

BOX 7-1.
THE DO'S AND DON'TS OF COMMUNICATION

DO
- Use words that you know are familiar to the resident to be sure they understand.
- Speak clearly and slowly.
- Look directly at the person you are talking to.
- Try to be at the person's eye level.
- Use a pleasant tone.
- Reduce or eliminate other sounds such as radio, TV, and housekeeping equipment. Turn down the volume or close the door to the room.

DON'T
- Don't use medical terms or slang, which many residents do not understand.
- Don't put your hands near your mouth while speaking.
- Don't talk with food or chewing gum in your mouth.

true with a confused resident who may already be having difficulty understanding what is going on around them. By speaking in another language, you may also give them the impression that you do not want them to understand what you are saying.

Avoid using medical terms, or else explain their meaning if they are routinely used in the facility. For example, instead of saying, "I need to check your vital signs," say, "I need to check your temperature, pulse, breathing rate, and blood pressure." When a resident is NPO ("nothing by mouth"), explain that this means they temporarily cannot eat or drink anything. Then explain why and for how long.

Nonverbal Communication (Body Language)

Nonverbal communication, also called body language, is communicating without words. Body language includes how you hold your head, arms, hands, and whole body, as well as your expression and movement. Here are some examples:
- Standing with your hands on your hips or with your arms crossed over your chest conveys anger.
- Friendly eye contact conveys attention and caring.
- Moving quickly communicates that you are in a hurry.
- Sitting down to talk with someone says that you are interested in them and care enough to take the time to talk.

Your facial expressions can convey many feelings, including happiness, humor, concern, pain, or sadness. If you feel anger or frustration, your face will usually show it.

Consider this interaction:

> Cheryl and Kate are talking about an experience Cheryl had earlier in the day.
> Cheryl: Gosh, Mrs. Peacock was mad when I told her I had to take the salt from her tray.
> Kate: What did she say?
> Cheryl: Oh, she didn't say anything. She just slammed her fork on the table and glared at me.

We often watch other people's facial expressions to see if they received the message we meant to communicate. For example, if you explain something to someone and you see them wrinkle their eyebrows, you may guess they did not understand you.

Often we are unaware of the nonverbal messages our own body language or expressions are sending to others.

Even if you didn't mean to communicate a feeling, the message may be sent nonverbally. Although someone may try to use words to hide their feelings, their body language often conveys their true feelings. That is why most people pay attention to the nonverbal messages others give them: to get the real message.

Think about a task you should do but don't really have time for. For example, a resident with very long hair asks you to help wash and braid her hair. It is a busy day for you, but her family is coming to visit in the evening and she wants to look good. You know that helping her will take as much as an hour of your time.

You may say, "Yes, I'll be glad to help you." But did you take a deep breath before you answered? Did you look at your watch and cringe? Did you hurry to towel-dry her hair and accidentally pull it? The resident may not say anything. She may even be quieter than usual. But think of the messages she received from your nonverbal behavior. How might this affect your future relationship with her?

Pay close attention to messages you send residents with both verbal and nonverbal communication. When a resident asks you to do something you cannot easily do now, instead of saying yes and frowning, try discussing alternatives with them. Together you can create a plan that is good for both of you.

Residents, too, may send different messages with nonverbal and verbal communication. For example, a resident may say they are not in pain, but you see an expression of pain on their face. When you are caring for a resident, watch for their nonverbal messages as you listen to their verbal communication. Some examples of body language to avoid are:
- rolling your eyes
- sighing
- smirking
- turning your back on the resident
- folding your arms across your chest
- putting your hands on your hips

Touch. Touch is an important form of nonverbal communication. Some people often use their hands when talking and just naturally touch others. Others are not

---

Nonverbal communication – sending and receiving messages without the use of words

Smirking – smiling in a way that gives the impression you are superior to another person

comfortable being touched—to them touch is an invasion of personal space. For many people, hugs are a common way of saying hello to friends or family members or communicating congratulations or **condolences** (Fig. 7-5). But others give hugs only in intimate relationships.

Learn about each resident's comfort level for touching. Be aware how you yourself feel about touching others or being touched. Some find it easier to touch someone than to accept being touched by them.

The old saying, "A picture is worth a thousand words," is true also of nonverbal communication. What a person sees is often much more important than what they hear.

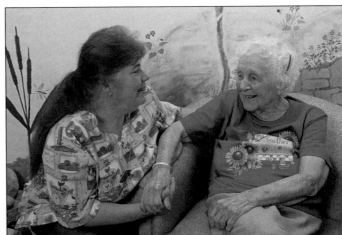

Fig. 7-6 – Sitting down and looking at the resident shows you are listening when they are talking.

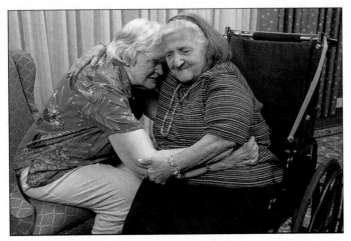

Fig. 7-5 – Hugging can communicate different messages such as welcome, congratulations, or condolences.

Listening

The more you know about another person, the better you can communicate with them. You have many chances to learn about residents through your daily contact. The skill you need most is listening (Fig. 7-6). Listening means hearing the other person's words, observing their body language, and experiencing the feelings behind their words.

Listening takes time, but you can listen while you care for residents. You can learn much about their likes and dislikes, what activities they participated in before entering the facility, and their family relationships. But also take time to sit and talk with them about whatever is on their mind. This shows that you are interested in them and that they matter to you.

Being relaxed and unhurried when you talk with residents helps put them at ease. Show your interest by making eye contact, leaning toward them, and nodding as they talk. Whenever you can, keep your face at the same height as theirs by sitting, squatting, or kneeling close to their bed or chair. Let silences happen when residents talk; do not try to hurry them.

If you do not understand something a resident says, ask them to repeat it. If you still do not understand, ask someone else for help. Do not pretend to understand, because a trusting relationship depends on honesty and understanding. Residents need to trust you if they are to communicate their real feelings and needs to you.

To show your interest and confirm you understand what a resident is saying, you can ask, "Is this what you mean?" and then say what you think they meant. This technique is called reflection. You re-state in your own words what the other person said. You also can use this technique to encourage a resident to continue talking. You might say something like, "It sounds like you have difficulty talking to your grandchildren about your feelings." If your interpretation is correct, this shows you understand the person's feelings. If your interpretation is not correct, this gives the person a chance to **clarify** what they were saying.

Be aware of your body language when you are listening. If you say you want to listen but your attention is on your task, you are not communicating real interest in what the person is saying. Have an open posture, with your arms

Clarify – make sure something is clearly understood
Condolences – expressions of sympathy or sorrow

comfortable at your sides or in your lap. Do not cross them in front of you or put them on your hips. Touch the resident from time to time on the shoulder or arm if you and the resident are both comfortable with that. Sit close enough for them to see you clearly but not so close that you threaten their sense of personal space. Box 7-2 outlines good listening skills.

BOX 7-2.
GOOD LISTENING SKILLS

• Stop what you are doing.
• Make eye contact.
• Sit down and stay at the person's eye level.
• Prevent distractions such as personal pagers and cell phones.
• Keep your body language positive.
• Validate what you hear the other person saying.

Validating Communication

How do you know if a resident receives exactly the same message you meant to send? You need to **validate**, or check out, whether the other person understands your intended message. If you are giving instructions, for example, you can ask the other person to repeat what you said or to do the activity. To be sure you have successfully communicated an idea or feeling, you might ask, "What did you hear me say?" Sometimes you know the communication was effective because the person does what you requested. Watching the person's body language closely also provides strong clues about their understanding. Body language like nodding or shaking the head, an open or puzzled facial expression, and posture can communicate a lot (Fig. 7-7).

PROMOTING EFFECTIVE COMMUNICATION
Many of the methods you have already learned for protecting residents' rights also promote effective communication. The following are guidelines for promoting effective communication:

• Show respect for residents by calling them by their title and **surname** (Mrs. Jones) unless they request otherwise. Do not use **nicknames** such as "sugar" or "honey."
• Always ask residents first if it is OK to do something. Explain new procedures before you do them. Plan activities with them, and always keep your word (Fig. 7-8). If

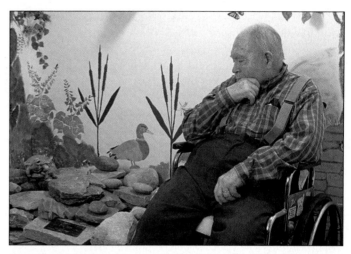

Fig. 7-7 – Facial expressions and body language give you information about how a resident feels.

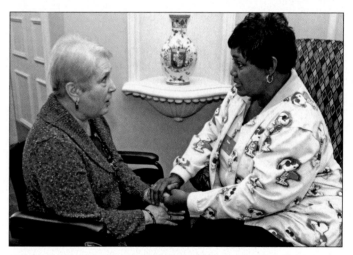

Fig. 7-8 – Telling the resident when you will be back and keeping your word promotes effective communication.

you cannot do something you promised, explain why.
• Respect a resident's feelings. If a resident says they feel sad, use a reflective response, such as "Do you feel discouraged right now?" Do not disrespect their feelings by saying things such as "Things aren't all that bad" or "Don't talk like that. It's going to be fine."

📖

Nickname – a familiar name that family and friends use
Surname – last name or family name
Validate – prove to be valid, sound, or effective

Give hope, but not false reassurances. Instead of saying, "You'll feel better tomorrow," say, 'I know you're having a tough time. But I think you'll be more comfortable if we....." Always assume that a resident can hear you. Even if the person seems unresponsive, continue to explain who you are and what you are doing.

- Offer residents choices in all their daily activities. Look for ways to encourage residents to keep control over their lives. Ask them what they want to wear, when they want to take a bath, and when they want care. When possible, teach residents or family members how to do some of the resident's grooming, if they wish.
- Ask open-ended questions that encourage residents to talk, rather than asking questions with yes or no answers. Say, "How do you feel about this?" or "Tell me about that."
- Respect residents' privacy by not sharing personal information about them except with staff who need to know. If a resident asks something personal about another resident, give only general information. For example, you can say the person is fine and ask if they would like to visit with the person. Or you can say that the person went to the hospital, but do not share the medical reason why.

ENDING A CONVERSATION

Communication is important, but so is getting your work done. How do you end a conversation when you must leave to do something else? Try to end the conversation so that the resident feels good. You can simply say, "I've really enjoyed talking to you. Can we continue this conversation after dinner? I have to check on some other residents now." When you start a conversation, you can say, "I have about 10 minutes before I have to do something else. Could we talk for a few minutes?" When the time is up, you can say, "I have to go now, but I'd like to talk more later." Set a time for this if you can, and be sure you come back. Never make a promise you cannot keep.

PROBLEMS OF INEFFECTIVE COMMUNICATION

What happens if you are not communicating effectively with a resident? You may not be able to meet their needs because you do not completely understand them. A resident may not tell you about a change in their condition that could indicate a serious medical problem. They may not report a complaint, and then the larger problem may not be corrected.

A resident or family member who is not comfortable talking with you may take a problem to an outside agency, although your facility could have solved it more easily. A resident may withdraw, feel that no one is interested in them, and miss opportunities for relationships with other residents. You can become frustrated and discouraged in your work if you feel you do not have a helping relationship with the residents you care for.

SPECIAL COMMUNICATION NEEDS

Some residents may develop a childlike dependence on staff and family after entering the facility. They may demand that you do everything for them. Their family may also expect you to give all their care, so that the resident does nothing. In such cases, use your communication skills to explain the importance of independence.

Other residents have physical problems that make communication difficult, such as a hearing or vision loss. They may have difficulty speaking clearly because they have an illness or stroke, or because their dentures do not fit properly. Residents who are depressed or who have memory loss have other special communication needs. All these special communication needs are discussed in the following sections.

Communicating With Demanding Residents

Sometimes residents feel that because they are paying for care, they should receive whatever they want whenever they want it. The family may encourage them to feel this way. They may say, "If my mother could bathe herself, she'd still be at home." The reasons for reactions like these can be complicated. Family members may be going through the adjustment process you learned about in Chapter 6. Or residents may be afraid to do things for themselves.

Some residents or their family members may also be perfectionists. That means they set rigid standards for themselves and others and have difficulty being flexible in different situations. They may insist you do everything in a certain way and the same way every time. Or they may demand that the resident's things stay in exactly the same place at all times.

People often learn these behaviors in childhood. Then, in stressful situations, such as when they move into a facility—an unfamiliar environment—they may act this way to cope with their loss of control. In these situations, follow these guidelines:

- Remember that these behaviors are efforts to cope with stress. Try to respond in a nonthreatening manner.

- Do not take their behavior personally.
- Encourage residents and family members to have as much control as possible, within the rules of the facility. For example, tell them how much time you have now and ask what they would like you to do in that time.

Try to recognize, rather than ignore, the family's and resident's reaction. Listen to the resident's concerns, using the listening skills and effective communication guidelines you learned about earlier. If the resident or family member is still unhappy, offer to call the charge nurse. Remember, never make excuses or be defensive. Work together with the charge nurse, family, and resident to resolve any problems.

It is natural to react personally to things that happen on the job with residents or family members. You may become angry if a resident or family member criticizes the care you give. It is normal to feel defensive when criticized, but make sure you do not express negative feelings to residents or family members. Talk to someone else when you have negative feelings. A co-worker or supervisor may have had similar experiences and can suggest how to deal with your feelings.

Sometimes just talking about the incident is enough. If needed, move away from the situation to cool off after you make sure a co-worker or supervisor knows where you are and will care for residents during this time.

Communicating With Residents Who Need Encouragement

Encourage residents to do all they can for themselves. Physical activity helps maintain good muscle tone and joint flexibility. Being independent also helps you feel better about yourself. If residents ask you to do something for them that they can do themselves, you can suggest, "You do as much as you can, and I'll help you with what you can't do." (Fig. 7-9).

The caregiving team should use a consistent approach for a resident who needs more encouragement. For example, if a resident goes from one staff member to another asking for help, the team may pick one person to answer all their requests. When a resident starts taking responsibility for their care, give encouragement and praise. Say things like:
- "You did a good job. You should be proud of your accomplishment."
- "I'm glad to see you out of your room. I hope we'll see you out more."
- "I'm glad you tried that. Tomorrow maybe you can do a little bit more."

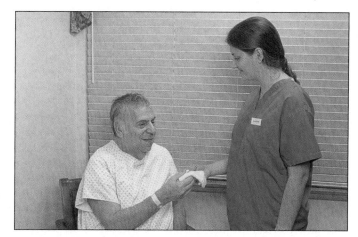

Fig. 7-9 – Encouraging residents to do as much as possible for themselves helps maintain their independence.

Communicating With Residents Who Have a Visual Impairment

With a resident who is blind or has impaired vision, follow these guidelines for more effective communication:
- Be sure the room is well lighted, and sit where the person can best see and hear you. If a resident has glasses, make sure they are wearing them and that the glasses are clean.
- If a resident has another vision aid, such as a magnifying glass, encourage its use (Fig. 7-10).

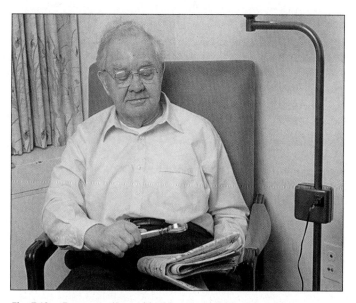

Fig. 7-10 – Encourage the resident to use available vision aids.

- Be sure you always introduce yourself when you start talking to the resident. Keep talking so they know what you are doing and where you are.
- When appropriate, touch a resident to let them know where you are. Encourage the resident to use touch to find things in their environment. Try to keep things in the same place (a place the resident prefers), so that the resident becomes familiar with their location. This helps residents be more independent in self-care.
- If a resident asks you to read their mail or personal documents to them, of course do so—but only when asked.
- Describe things the resident will be using, including their location. For example, describe the food on the resident's plate using the "clock" description on p. 205.

Communicating With Residents Who Have a Hearing Impairment

Follow these guidelines for more effective communication with a resident with a hearing impairment:
- Eliminate or reduce background noise.
- Face the resident when you are talking so they can see your lips. This helps residents understand what you are saying. Speak clearly, using your lips to emphasize sounds.
- Use gestures or point to objects as you are speaking. Speak to the person's stronger side, if one ear is better.
- You may touch a resident to get their attention.
- Encourage the resident to use their hands to point to things they want.
- If a resident with a hearing impairment neglects to use their hearing aid, encourage its use. Be sure the hearing aid is clean and working properly.
- Repeat what you said if a resident asks you to. If necessary, say it again using different words.
- Be sure you have the person's attention, and maintain eye contact.
- In some cases you may need to write down on paper what you are saying (Fig. 7-11).
- Always be patient.

Communicating With Residents Who Are Depressed

Some residents become depressed and withdrawn when they are having trouble adjusting to the facility. They may already have experienced many losses. With these residents, use the communication techniques described earlier. Most important, be patient, understanding, and consistent. The following tips promote communication with a

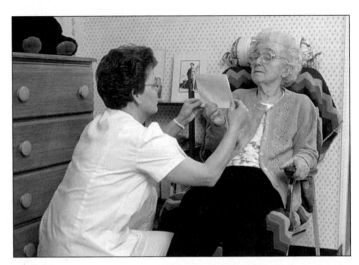

Fig. 7-11 – If a resident has difficulty hearing you, write down what you want to say.

depressed resident:
- Spend extra time just sitting with this resident, even if they are not talking to you.
- Invite them to participate in their own care as well as in social activities in the facility. You might say, "I'll get a basin of water. While I'm doing that, why don't you get out your shaving cream and razor?"
- Set goals for the resident. Make suggestions like, "Today we'll walk just to the nurses' station and back. Tomorrow I'd like you to walk with me to the dining room."
- Ask family members and friends about the resident's interests in the past. Then try to engage them in conversation about these interests.
- In all your efforts, keep trying. When you show you care, the resident may finally respond.

Communicating With Residents Who Have Cognitive Impairment

Some residents may be cognitively impaired and have much memory loss. Many residents cannot remember recent events but clearly remember things from their childhood. Encourage them to talk about things they

---

📖

Cognitive impairment – condition in which memory, thinking, or problem-solving skills have changed or been damaged

remember. Follow these guidelines for communicating with those who have difficulty remembering things in the present:

- Keep your questions and your directions short and simple. Repeat information if needed.
- Try to understand the resident's feelings and their perceptions of the world, and use words appropriate for them.
- Use helpful visual reminders, such as referring to calendars and clocks throughout the facility (Fig. 7-12). A wall chart in the room can help a resident remember daily routines, such as the steps in getting dressed or the times that meals are served.

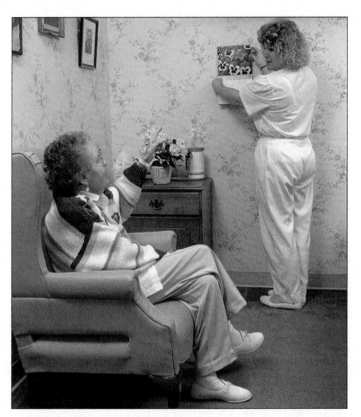

Fig. 7-12 — Wall charts, calendars, and clocks can serve as visual reminders to residents with cognitive impairment.

- Because of their memory loss, some things a resident says may not make sense to you, even though they are trying hard to fill in gaps in their memory. Never laugh at or make fun of anything they say.

Communicating With Residents Who Have a Speech Impairment

Strokes and other brain injuries often cause aphasia. Residents with aphasia may have difficulty expressing themselves or understanding what you are asking them. Some residents cannot speak but can read. Others may not be able to read or speak. The resident's specific limitation depends on the underlying reason for their loss of speech. Talk with the charge nurse to learn more about a resident's aphasia. The nurse can guide you in how best to communicate with the resident.

Residents who have difficulty being understood may give up and become depressed. They may become withdrawn and no longer try to communicate. With these residents, too, your time and patience can make a big difference. Try these ways to promote communication:

- Encourage the resident to use their hands to point things out or touch things to help communicate their message.
- Ask questions they can answer with a yes or no.
- Since it is frustrating for these residents to make themselves understood, let them express their anger and frustration. If needed, sit quietly with them and let them cry. Keep trying to understand what they are saying.
- When you understand what a resident's particular sounds or symbols mean, tell other staff, too, so they can communicate better with the resident. You can put a chart on the resident's wall to tell others what the symbols mean. You can also post a list of common phrases a resident might use so that they can simply point to what they need.

COMMUNICATION AND INAPPROPRIATE BEHAVIOR

Special communication needs arise with residents whose behavior makes you uncomfortable. Some residents may make sexual advances or be physically abusive to you.

Responding to Sexual Advances

Sometimes a resident's or family member's behavior may make you uncomfortable. They may make sexual advances or comments. In such cases you need to communicate

---

📖

Aphasia — condition in which a person has difficulty putting thoughts into words

that you do not like the behavior without being negative about the person. You might say, "That makes me very uncomfortable. Please don't do it again."

Some residents, however, cannot control their behavior. Sometimes the best thing you can do is to distract them with another topic or activity.

Some residents' behaviors, like sexual advances, may make other residents uncomfortable. A resident who is not mentally competent must be protected from unwanted sexual advances. Other residents often will tell you if they see someone making another person uncomfortable. Watch vulnerable residents closely. You must also protect others from unwanted sexual advances by a mentally incompetent resident. At times you may have to move them into a different area to keep them from annoying or threatening other residents. Try to spend time alone with them and look for activities they might enjoy. This may help replace their inappropriate behavior with positive social contact.

Responding to Physical Abuse

Some residents may verbally or physically abuse you or other residents. You must protect others from harm, but you also must protect the rights of the abusing resident. In a case of verbal abuse, you can say, "You must feel very angry—can I help?" Often the person is saying angry things just to feel better, as we all do sometimes.

In cases of physical abuse, you must act to prevent harm to others. For example, you may have to step between two residents or take away an object a resident may try to use to hurt another. You may have to move the residents to separate areas for a cooling-off period. Other residents who see such a conflict may become anxious and need your extra support and reassurance that staff will keep them safe.

In extreme cases, an aggressive resident may try to injure another resident or staff member. A resident may express their distress by yelling or cursing, hitting, kicking, head-butting, biting, spitting, or throwing things. The best way to prevent aggression and possible injury is to know residents very well—what they are feeling and thinking and why they act as they do. Constantly monitor their moods, which can change without any reason you can see. To prevent aggressive behavior, try to understand what they are feeling, and fit your words and actions to meet their needs. Understanding aggressive residents is not always easy, especially if they are on medication, depressed, ill, very tired, or in pain. Something that makes

sense to a resident may not make sense to you. Still, you can learn what they are feeling by talking to them, watching their facial expressions for changes, and paying attention to what the shift before yours reports about their actions. Avoid these things:

- Never surprise the resident or let them surprise you.
- Never walk up behind a resident and touch, startle, or surprise them.
- Never give a resident orders as if you are their boss.

Whenever you approach the resident, smile and talk in a soft, friendly voice. Use short sentences and ask simple yes-or-no questions. When appropriate and when it will not surprise the resident, gently touch them. This can be reassuring and help to let the resident know that you care.

Remember two things when helping a potentially aggressive resident:

- Don't rush. Find out if the resident is willing to listen to you and then allow plenty of time for them to hear and understand you. Give instructions that have simple steps. When needed, repeat instructions using exactly the same words. Sometimes, because of your own frustration or a resident's, it may be better to try again later. Give the resident a hug or change the subject. If the conversation between the two of you becomes very tense, you may need to leave the room.
- Even if an upset resident is looking at you when they begin an aggressive behavior, do not take their actions personally or consider yourself to be the cause. An aggressive resident may have a brain disease and not mean to hurt or annoy you. They are struggling with

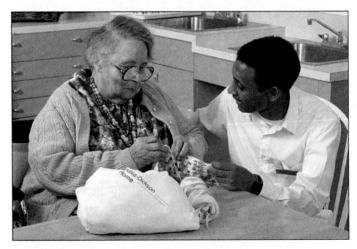

Fig. 7-13 — Always be calm and patient with residents, and reassure them that you care.

feelings or pain that is difficult to understand, and you just happen to be there when they could not cope any longer. Never argue with any resident, no matter what they say to upset you. Always stay calm and patient (Fig. 7-13).

In situations involving an aggressive resident, be patient and understanding. Evaluate the situation as unemotionally as you can. Try to communicate with the resident. If you consistently use this approach, both you and the resident will become more aware of what is going on and can avoid surprises and injuries resulting from aggression. Many abusive residents are mentally impaired and cannot be held responsible for their behavior. Try to distract them with another topic or activity.

CONFLICT RESOLUTION

Resolving conflicts can be a very rewarding growth experience. **Conflict resolution** also helps you to maintain residents' dignity and rights, as well as positive employee relations when you are working with other facility staff members.

Have you been in a situation where someone criticized how you did something? Perhaps you forgot to use your turn signal while driving, and the driver behind you yelled at you or blew their horn. When something like this happens, do you feel angry or defensive afterwards? Do you feel you're being attacked without having a chance to defend yourself. How do you react in the following situations when:
• someone raises their voice when speaking to you?
• someone questions your ideas or your words?
• someone ignores you?

Do these things make you uncomfortable or uneasy? Many people feel physically sick in conflict situations. They may have an upset stomach, feel shaky inside, or have flushed skin. Understanding the causes of conflict and how people react is very important. With this understanding you can learn to resolve conflicts in a productive, successful, and rewarding way.

What is conflict? Some people define conflict as a:
• situation in which one side or person tries to gain something at the expense of another
• situation in which people have incompatible or seemingly incompatible ideas, interests, or values
• disagreement
• situation in which people are trying to meet a goal in different ways

Dictionary definitions of conflict include "things that clash or are in opposition, competing or opposing actions, and opposing desires or tensions." How would you define conflict? Conflict is often a very personal thing. What you perceive as a conflict may not be viewed that way by someone else. The opposite may also be true: someone else perceives a conflict, but you do not.

Do you know the saying, "Perception is reality"? This means that if someone believes that a situation or threat is real, it is real to them—whether or not it is a true situation or threat. You cannot simply change their belief. For example, a person who is afraid of dogs feels threatened every time a dog is nearby. Even if the dog is very friendly, they feel afraid because they believe every dog is dangerous. Perceptions of conflict also differ: Some people feel arguments are part of daily life, even fun. Others feel uncomfortable whenever someone disagrees with them or raises their voice.

Understanding Yourself

Before you can practice the steps of conflict resolution, you should recognize your own reaction to conflict. When you find yourself in a situation that causes you conflict, step back and look at your own motives. Try to understand your emotional response and judge whether it is appropriate. This process of self-discovery helps you channel your emotional energy so you can find a more productive solution.

Following are the keys to understanding yourself when dealing with conflict:
• **Recognize the energy that arises from an emotional reaction to a conflict.** Ask yourself, "What is going on? Why am I so upset?"
• **Channel this energy and step back to observe the situation and yourself.** Take some time to understand what is going on. Ask yourself, "Am I reacting to this situation or to something else?"
• **Consider how effective communication can help.** The communication tips in the next section can help you resolve the conflict.

Conflict resolution – use of effective communication to resolve problems

Reactions to Conflict

People react to conflict in different ways. Typical reactions to conflict include the following:

- **Avoidance.** Avoidance is trying to escape from, rather than deal with, an issue. With this approach, the conflict is not dealt with at all and usually continues.
- **Competition.** Competition is the opposite of avoidance. One of the parties in the conflict takes action against the other person in an attempt to "beat" that person, as if the conflict involves a competition. The action taken may not have anything to do with the original conflict.
- **Accommodation.** When you "give in," or accommodate, the other person, your own needs are not being met. In this case, you are doing what the other person wants you to do against your better judgment.
- **Compromise.** Compromising means that both people give up something that they want in order to resolve the problem. Neither wins or is completely satisfied. Usually, both sides have to settle for something less than or different from what they wanted. In this situation no one is happy even though both parties agree at the moment to let the issue go.
- **Collaboration.** This is the best reaction to conflict. When both sides collaborate to resolve a problem, they work together to come up with a reasonable solution. Often both parties feel they win when they collaborate. To collaborate, each party must understand the other's position and work together on the solution.

Nondefensive Communication

People react defensively when they feel another person is attacking their integrity. Did you ever feel that someone was questioning your competence, your ethics, or your values? When this happens and you become defensive, it is very difficult to resolve the conflict. There are four common defensive reactions to conflict. Have you ever reacted in any of the following ways?

1. **Taking things personally**

    If you take things personally, you may say something like "Why are they doing this to me?" or "I'm always the one who gets yelled at." When you feel this way, you need to realize that other people may have a different point of view when they disagree with you about how you have handled something. But if someone disagrees with you, it does not necessarily mean they are attacking you personally.

2. **Running for cover**

    Have you ever had a disagreement with a supervisor about how to do something and the supervisor said only, "This is how we do things here. You have to follow our rules." Some people call this "running for cover." In this case the supervisor is not really communicating what they believe but is "hiding behind" the facility's policies and procedures. Sometimes only a simple explanation is needed to resolve a conflict.

3. **Creating a diversion**

    Someone who brings up past events during a disagreement about a present issue is creating a diversion. The conflict cannot be resolved unless both parties stay focused on the same issue.

4. **Attacking the other person**

    Some people use words to attack others when a conflict arises. They may feel they are being attacked personally and make a counterattack. They may try to deflect their anger or frustration onto the other person. Attacks—even when they are only verbal and not physical—usually result in someone being hurt.

None of the four reactions outlined above is helpful. Each of them can make it more difficult to resolve the conflict. The following guidelines can help you to communicate openly and avoid acting defensively:

1. **Remove yourself from the situation.** Stop and ask yourself, "What is the issue here?"
2. **Put yourself in the other person's place.** Try to imagine how they feel. If the problem does not need to be addressed right this moment, you also can try acting it out, or role-playing. Ask a friend to play your part while you play the part of the other person involved in the conflict.
3. **Ask the other person questions that help clarify the issues.** Clear up any misconceptions. Be sure you are both talking about the same thing.
4. **Communicate directly and honestly.** Use "I" statements, such as "I feel," instead of "you" statements, such as "You always.…"
5. **Try not to take the situation personally,** even though that can be very difficult. At work remind yourself, "This is a business situation. It is not about me or my friendship with co-workers."

Some of these guidelines may already be familiar to you. Practicing these skills will help you in your work every day.

📖

Diversion – anything that distracts a person's attention

Effective Communication When Conflict Occurs

Understanding other people can be very challenging for all of us. Has anyone ever said to you, "You're not listening to me" or "You just don't get it"? When people say things like this, they usually mean that you do not understand what they are saying. Misunderstandings happen because you may be experiencing the same event or situation differently.

Communication sometimes breaks down when people are defensive and view conflict as a personal attack. But defensiveness is a barrier to effective communication. A barrier is a block, something that gets in the way. Many things can be barriers. Some people have trouble handling their feelings, so they do not let others know how they feel. You often cannot tell how strongly someone feels about something. Have you ever been surprised at how angry another person became over what you thought was a minor problem? Maybe you, too, have surprised others with your own strong reaction to something they thought was "nothing."

Feeling helpless is another barrier to communication. If you feel powerless in a situation, you may not even bother to let anyone else know how you feel.

Understanding these barriers will help make you a better communicator. Follow these general guidelines for effective communication and conflict resolution:

1. **Understand your role in the conflict and the barriers to communications**. Try writing down what things upset you and how people react to you when you are upset. Then review what you have written and see if it helps you see a pattern in your behavior.
2. **Consider the timing of your communication**. When conflict occurs, step back and think about the situation. Relax, take deep breaths, or take a walk before you discuss the problem.
3. **Always address the issue, not the person, to prevent them from becoming defensive**. Talk about the way you see the situation, not the way the other person behaved.
4. **Use "I" statements, not "you" statements**. With "I" statements you take responsibility for your feelings. For example, say "I feel uncomfortable when you walk away from me. It makes me feel as if you don't care about me," not "You make me feel uncomfortable when you walk away from me."
5. **Watch your nonverbal communication**. If you are trying to be open to what the other person is saying, for example, do not fold your arms across your chest.
6. **Be understanding, open, and honest**. Do not make people guess what you are thinking or feeling. Have you

ever waited for someone to figure out why you were angry? Did you get angrier as you waited?
7. **Consider where you will talk about the conflict**. Try to talk in a private place (Fig. 7-14). Never discuss personal issues in front of others, especially residents.

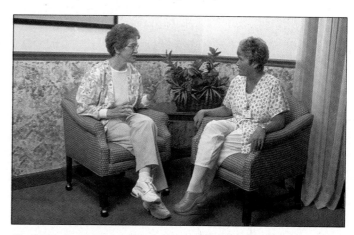

Fig. 7-14 – Resolving conflicts is an important part of your job.

8. **Be sure the other person understands your point and that you understand theirs**.

By practicing these techniques, you can improve your communication skills. But remember that developing new skills takes time. Try focusing on one skill at a time. It can be difficult at first to adopt a new behavior, try a new technique, or develop a new style. But it will be worth the effort as you learn how to resolve conflicts successfully.

Conflict resolution is a process in which people understand the problem and then agree to a solution. Learning to resolve conflicts is an important part of your job training because an unsolved problem can affect your caregiving. When you feel angry or resentful, you may be impatient with residents or co-workers. You may not even realize that you have hurt someone's feelings or that the quality of your work has suffered. Over time, small problems that would be easy to fix, but aren't fixed, can turn into major issues.

Steps for Conflict Resolution

Even when you communicate effectively, you may have a conflict at work or at home. When conflict occurs, resolve it so that it does not become a larger problem. Following are steps to resolve conflict that will work in almost all situations. These steps can also help to prevent conflict from occurring in the first place.

Step 1. Try to understand the other person's position or feelings.

The best way to do this is to ask how the other person sees the problem. This will show you that you have an open mind and want to know how important the problem is for the other person. This also helps prevent an embarrassing situation if your perception of the other person's position or feelings is incorrect.

When considering the other person's viewpoint, you should:

- Agree that you both are interested in understanding each other's position before resolving the problem. You agree to listen to each other.
- Try to learn the other person's thoughts and feelings. This shows you are open and willing to listen.
- Ask the other person for help to understand their position. Ask specific questions so that you are clear about their point of view.
- Use your own words to re-state the other person's message. By using your own words, you show that you understand the message.
- Ask for clarification. Be sure that you truly understand the other person's point of view.

Step 2. Explain what you mean.

You also need to let the other person know exactly what you mean. Choose your words carefully and state your position clearly to prevent any misunderstanding. As you speak:

- Ask the other person to listen carefully to you, as you listened to them.
- Explain what you feel about the other person's viewpoint. Explain your emotions.
- State your case using "I" statements. Tell how you feel and how the situation affects you.
- Ask the person to repeat what you just said. Be sure the other person clearly understands your concerns as you do theirs.

Listening carefully and then explaining your position are necessary to understand the problem as each of you sees it. This also helps calm strong emotions because each person gets a chance to be heard. Sometimes Steps 1 and 2 by themselves lead to resolution of the conflict. But when they do not, use the third step.

Step 3. Collaborate.

- Agree that you both understand each other's position. You each must at least acknowledge each other's position.
- Agree to work together on a solution. Both parties must agree to try to solve the problem.

- List all possible solutions. You both should think of a complete list of possibilities before you go back and consider each idea.
- Together, choose the best solution you can both agree to. If you cannot agree, at least agree to continue to try to understand and respect each other.

The steps for conflict resolution should be used in this order, to ensure that both parties have an opportunity to be heard. Each person needs the opportunity to vent their emotions and clear up any misconceptions. If you do not follow these steps in order, you cannot know for sure if a solution is agreeable to both parties.

COMMUNICATING ABOUT YOURSELF

As you talk to residents about their personal lives and families, you can share things from your own life. This sharing often promotes communication. However, stay focused on the resident and do not make the conversation all about you. For example, you may share an amusing family story similar to a story the resident told you. This can be a good way also to engage a depressed or withdrawn resident in conversation (Fig. 7-15).

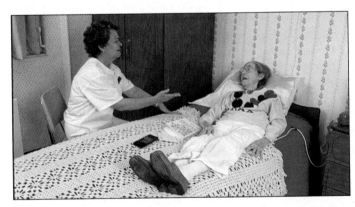

Fig. 7-15 – You can help a withdrawn resident join in a conversation by sharing an experience of your own.

Like everyone else, you will have bad days. But telling the resident your problems may make them feel they cannot tell you theirs. Focus on residents' feelings rather than your own. Talk with your supervisor if you can't focus on your work because of a personal problem. If you notice that a co-worker seems to have a personal problem, find a private moment and ask if you can help. Help may be as simple as listening for a few minutes or letting a supervisor know that another employee needs some extra attention.

A resident may ask you about your family or children in a way that shows they want a two-way conversation about each other's problems. With their wisdom and years of experience, residents can often help you solve you own problems. Use your good judgment. Talk to the charge nurse or social worker if you are unsure if you should be talking with a resident about your problems.

TELEPHONE COURTESY

Courtesy is very important in your job. You have a great opportunity to give a good impression of your facility to others. Telephone courtesy is just as important as courtesy in person. Always think how you would feel if you were treated rudely on the phone. Although at times you may be rushed in your work and you might feel the telephone is an irritation, remember that rudeness or **curtness** is never appropriate. You are a representative of the facility you work for.

Whenever you answer the phone you should:
- State the facility's name, the unit, and your name.
- Find out why the caller is phoning by asking how you can help.
- Try to meet the caller's request. You might bring a resident to the phone or find the appropriate staff person to answer a question. Never yell or call out for someone, but instead go to get them.
- Never put a caller on hold for more than 2 to 3 minutes.
- If you cannot meet the caller's request, take their telephone number and say you will give the message to the right person so they can call back.
- Thank the caller for calling.

Be sure you follow through on anything you say you will do.

Curtness – being so short or brief that you are not polite; brusque

IN THIS CHAPTER YOU LEARNED:
- Ways to make verbal communication effective
- The importance of nonverbal communication, touch, and listening
- General guidelines for good communication and active listening
- Ways to communicate with residents with special communication needs
- Ways to handle inappropriate resident behavior or aggression
- How to resolve conflict
- When it is OK to talk about yourself with residents
- Proper telephone courtesy

SUMMARY

This chapter is about communicating effectively. Successful verbal and nonverbal communication and listening are the keys to establishing positive relationships. Communication skills are also used to resolve conflicts. Both general communication guidelines and specific techniques will help you communicate with residents with special needs. As you develop relationships with residents, you will also develop a sense of what is appropriate to share with them about yourself. As the person that spends the most time with the resident, you may find that you want to talk about your own life with them. Sharing information is a good way for you and the resident to get to know one another. But remember the main focus should always be on the resident. Residents should not feel burdened by your problems.

PULLING IT ALL TOGETHER

You are scheduled for the first time to care for Mrs. Taylor, a 90-year-old woman who is depressed. She is scheduled to have a psychiatric evaluation soon. Her three daughters come often to the facility. Staff have had many meetings with the daughters in order to understand Mrs. Taylor's likes and dislikes.

Her daughters are perfectionists. They consider themselves to be perfectly groomed and expect Mrs. Taylor to be that way, too, although they themselves never help with her care. They have not accepted the fact that their mother is depressed. Mrs. Taylor tells everyone on staff that she does not want to be "fussed over." But her daughters are constantly criticizing the staff, and staff members are starting to avoid them.

After reading this chapter, how do you think you could communicate effectively with Mrs. Taylor and her daughters?

When you enter her room, you find that two of her daughters are visiting. You introduce yourself to them. You tell them that you will be caring for their mother today. What can you do now to engage them in her care? Using your communication skills, you can begin to develop a relationship with them by explaining what needs to be done, then asking them for tips or advice on how they would like things done. You could even encourage them to assist you so that they can show you how they want things done. At the same time they will feel more involved. If you sit down with them, ask them their advice, validate what you are doing right and what they want done, you will be using effective communication skills to build a relationship with the family and the resident that will contribute to the quality of Mrs. Taylor's life.

Tact is the art of saying the right thing politely at the right time. Few people are tactful all the time, but you can get better with practice. Take the time to get to know residents. If you listen and watch for clues in their body language, you will be able to respond in ways that show you understand their needs and concerns. In addition, the more aware you are of your own needs and ways of relating, the more empathy and tact you will have for others.

CHECK WHAT YOU'VE LEARNED

1. **Effective communication helps you:**
   A. Convince residents' family members not to interfere by offering to help care for their loved one.
   B. Make residents do what you want them to do.
   C. Develop a trusting relationship with the resident.
   D. Hide any mistakes you happen to make when giving care.

2. **Others will understand you better if you:**
   A. Talk very softly.
   B. Speak clearly and slowly.
   C. Talk very loudly.
   D. Use correct medical terms whenever possible.

3. **Which of these nonverbal behaviors helps develop a positive relationship with a resident?**
   A. Smiling warmly.
   B. Always keeping your facial expressions neutral.
   C. Looking over the resident's shoulder when you speak to them.
   D. Folding your arms across your chest.

4. **If the resident you are caring for speaks only English, what language should you use to communicate with a co-worker whenever you both are with the resident?**
   A. Your native language.
   B. Your co-worker's native language.
   C. Sign language.
   D. English.

5. **As you give care, what can you do to promote good communication with a resident with a visual impairment?**
   A. As you give care, talk very loudly.
   B. Encourage the resident to point to things they want.
   C. Write down on paper what you are saying.
   D. Let them know where you are and what you're doing.

6. **Mrs. Ford, who is recovering from a stroke, has difficulty putting her thoughts into words. The term for this problem is:**
   A. Ataxia.
   B. Anoxia.
   C. Aphasia.
   D. Anemia.

7. **How can you support a resident who is trying to tell you something but has difficulty talking?**
   A. Tell her you'll come back after she sees a speech therapist.
   B. Tell her to call you later when she's able to talk.
   C. Ask her to point at what she needs or write it down.
   D. Just stare at her until she decides what she wants to say.

8. **To communicate with a resident who cannot hear well, you should:**
   A. Cup your hands around your mouth and yell.
   B. Give the resident a small chalkboard and a box of chalk.
   C. Face the resident when you talk so they can see your lips.
   D. Use background music to reduce the resident's stress level.

9. **Mr. Laramie, a resident in your care, has just yelled at another resident. What should you say to him?**
   A. "OK, what did I miss?"
   B. "I can tell you're angry. Can I help?"
   C. "Mr. Laramie, what are you going on about now?"
   D. "Calm down this minute. There's no excuse for this type of language."

10. **You're involved in an argument with a co-worker. In order to resolve the conflict, you should:**
    A. Tell the co-worker what's wrong with their point of view.
    B. Bring up past conflicts you've had with the co-worker.
    C. Take time to understand the other person's point of view.
    D. Calm things down by joking about their point of view.

(Answers to "Check What You've Learned" are in the Instructor's Manual.)

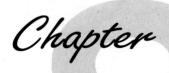

Chapter 8

DOCUMENTATION PRINCIPLES AND PROCEDURES

From your first minute on the job as a nurse assistant, you are flooded with information. People talk to you and give you things to read. They show you things and encourage you to ask questions (Fig. 8-1). This is two-way communication. You are listening, observing, and reading but also talking, being observed, and writing things down. Giving residents the best care depends on clear, thorough, accurate information. Other health care team members, including residents, depend on the information you communicate.

You have a responsibility to accurately document information. Centers for Medicare and Medicaid Services (CMS) guidelines require that facilities collect standard data for every resident using an instrument called the Minimum Data Set (MDS). The interdisciplinary team uses the MDS to develop the resident's care plan. The MDS is also used by state and regulatory officials to evaluate the facility. It is also used for the facility to obtain Medicare or Medicaid reimbursement. Like other health care staff, you will be asked to give information about residents. Your information becomes part of the resident's medical record.

This chapter focuses on the communication skills you will use as you observe, report, and document activities and gather information about residents to help develop their care plans.

OBJECTIVES
- Name all the locations where resident information can be found
- Explain the difference between objective and subjective information
- Explain your role in the care-planning process
- Explain when and how to report and document information
- Identify medical terminology and abbreviations

"It is such a comfort to know that you are ever watchful of how I'm doing."

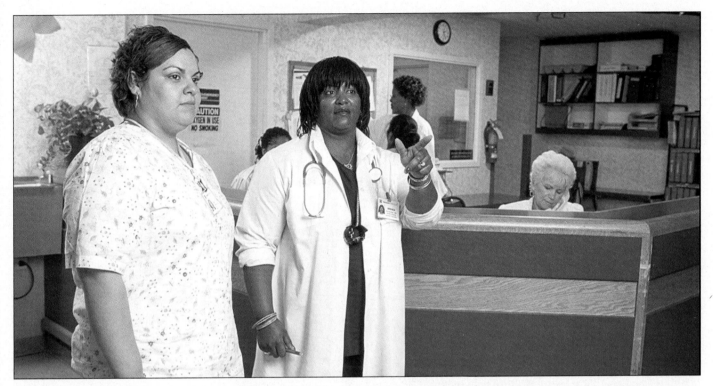

Fig. 8-1 – When you start your job as a nurse assistant, you will be provided with a lot of information. With time you will learn everything you need to know.

Think back to a special event you experienced months ago, like a birthday or holiday. Try to remember the event in detail. What were people wearing? What did they talk about? What did they eat and how much? What was their mood? What time did each person come and go? You have probably forgotten many of these facts. It's only human to forget details like these.

Because of memory limits, we often have to write things down. For example, insurance companies expect us to write down the facts and details after a car accident. Then we can read our notes months or even years later to remember the specifics. If we didn't write down the details, the only known "facts" would be what we happened to remember. Much information would then be lost. We might not know at the time how important some details could be later on, and therefore we might not pay enough attention to them to remember them. The documentation you do on the job has the same purpose. The health care team uses what you write down to care for residents. Some written notes may be used months or years later. You and others in the facility can later state facts with certainty because you wrote them down.

GATHERING INFORMATION ABOUT RESIDENTS AND THEIR CARE ACTIVITIES

In earlier chapters you learned that to give the best care possible, you must get to know the resident. Gathering information about residents is also a job responsibility required by regulations. As you give care, you will receive much information from residents and others. This information will be used to create the resident's care plan. The care plan provides an interdisciplinary approach for each resident's care.

There are many sources of information about residents. The next sections describe the most common ones.

Care plan – a written, interdisciplinary document developed for each resident, listing the resident's needs and goals as well as the actions and approaches that staff will take to help the resident to meet their goals

Documentation – written reports that the facility maintains

Residents

Residents are the main source of information about themselves. A resident can give you valuable information about their care preferences and needs. Be sure to verify this information with the charge nurse. Some residents might be confused or tell you something that they wish were true. For example, a resident may tell you that they are going home tomorrow. You must verify this with the charge nurse before starting to prepare them for discharge. It is especially important to listen to and report or document residents' feelings and preferences. Then other members of the health care team can understand the residents better and give more personalized care.

The Resident's Chart

A resident's health record is also called the medical record or the chart. It is the main communication tool used by the interdisciplinary team (Fig. 8-2). It is also a legal record of a resident's stay in the facility.

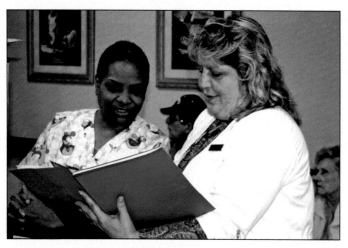

Fig. 8-2 – The resident's medical record is the main communication tool used by the interdisciplinary team.

As the basic tool for planning, recording, and evaluating a resident and their care, the chart helps organize all the information gathered about a resident. The chart is confidential and belongs to the facility. Because it is a record of each resident's condition and care, it must be complete and accurate.

There is a common saying: "If it isn't in the record, it didn't happen." In other words, if there is information, but it's not in the chart to be communicated to the interdiscipli-

nary team, it might as well not exist at all. Weeks or years later, no one will clearly remember facts not written down. Then it will be as if the situation never happened. The purpose of the resident's chart is to provide accurate, permanent information about the resident that can be used by the facility, the staff, and the resident.

A typical chart has many different pieces of paper, including the resident's medical history (past conditions and events), current records, and care plans (Fig. 8-3). All team members record information in the chart. Most charts include the following types of information:

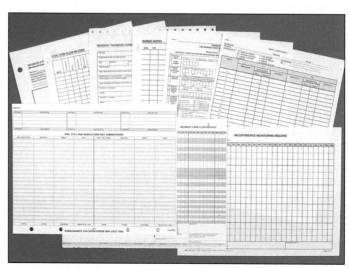

Fig. 8-3 – The resident's chart includes information such as the resident's medical history and care plan.

- the resident's identifying information (name, medical record number, birth date, etc.), often on a form called the face sheet
- the resident's admission papers outlining the reason for admission
- permission forms signed by the resident or representative, such as a "consent for treatment" form, and instruction forms, such as a "no cardiopulmonary resuscitation" order
- sections of documentation from individual disciplines, such as a section for the physician's orders that may include orders and notes from a clinical nurse practitioner, physician's assistant, and other consulting physicians
- progress notes from other health care team members, such as the dietician, respiratory therapist, and physical therapist
- test results such as lab tests, X-rays, and hearing tests
- graphs or flow sheets used for recording nursing activities,

such as vital signs, weights, bowel movements, activities of daily living (ADLs), and intake and output (I & O) of food and fluids—each added to the record as completed

Nurse assistants often document information on flow sheets. A flow sheet records objective facts. Objective means what you can see, hear, smell, or touch. Each flow sheet is used for only one type of information, such as the vital signs record, the intake and output record, and the weight chart. Flow sheets make it easier to see changes in residents over time.

You can evaluate your observations by comparing them with previous findings. For example, at first it may not seem important that a resident did not have a bowel movement today. But as you record this on the flow sheet, you discover this is the fourth day in a row that they have not had a bowel movement. As you record facts about residents, you can monitor their progress and notice changes that could become problems if not taken care of (Fig. 8-4).

Other departments also document information in the medical record. This information can be important to you, too. For example, if you care for a resident whose speech is unclear, you need to know if there are other ways to communicate with them. You can read the speech therapist's notes, which might say the resident should use an alphabet board to spell out words. You may also learn this information from the resident's care plan. This part of the chart describes how the team is working together to help a resident reach their goals. For example, the care plan may contain the recommendation for using an alphabet board.

In some facilities, the chart is kept all together in a holder like a notebook. In others, different sections of the chart are kept in different places. For example, the weight charts for all residents may be stored in one notebook near the weight scales to make it easier to record weights. The weight sheet is still a part of the resident's health record even if it is kept in a different place. It is still a legal record.

In some cases the information on worksheets later becomes part of the chart. For example, staff may use an intake and output worksheet form throughout the day for a particular resident. At the end of the day the numbers are added up, and the total intake and output are recorded in that resident's chart. In your orientation, you will learn your facility's requirements for documentation.

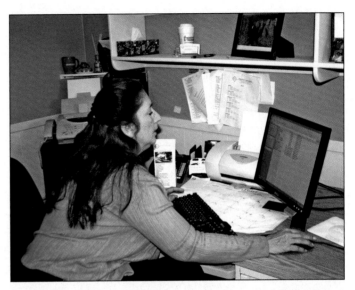

Fig. 8-4 – Accurate documentation on a computer helps you monitor a resident's progress and notice changes that need to be reported.

Other Communication Devices and Systems

Other communication devices give you additional information about residents. Different facilities use different systems. You will learn about these in your orientation. For example, a resident's wristband has their name on it and may include other information. Some facilities identify residents with diabetes or other diseases or conditions by different colors of wristbands. To identify a resident accurately, you must check their wristband, ask another staff member, or check a photo of the resident in their chart. If you do not know a resident, always check their wristband (Fig. 8-5, next page). Do not just ask them their name. Sometimes residents forget their names or respond to any name they are called.

Words and symbols on residents' door cards may communicate other information. A door card is the name sign on or beside the door to a resident's room. In some facilities colored dots on door cards identify blind or deaf residents who would need special help in an emergency. Other signs with words or symbols by the resident's bed may provide more information. Be sure you understand all this information so that you can provide safe, effective care for each resident.

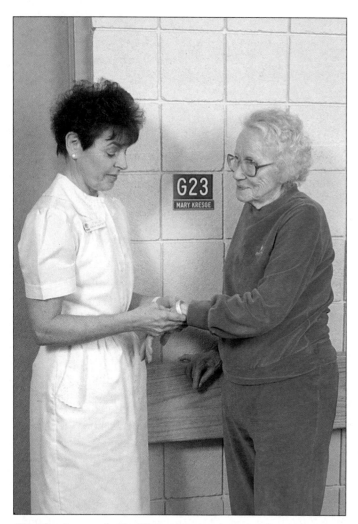

Fig. 8-5 – One way to identify a resident accurately is to check their wristband.

Other People

Others with whom you work will tell you about residents. Staff in other departments who have worked with a resident often have much information. Other nurse assistants also have information you can use to give individualized care.

Family members and visitors can also tell you much about residents. Be careful to verify their information because they may not always know the full situation. Information from the family is often useful. For example, a family member may tell you that a resident always took a nap after lunch at home. When you check with the charge nurse, you learn the resident has a physical therapy appointment scheduled after lunch. Because you commu-

nicated this information to the charge nurse, the nurse can talk to the therapist and make future appointments that let the resident take their afternoon nap.

Facility Policies and Procedures

Facility policies and procedures are rules for how to do things in the facility. Policies and procedures tells you how and why things are done. For example, a procedure called "Completing the Personal Possession Record" describes how to document items that a resident brings from home.

Policies and procedures help you care for residents in specific situations. For instance, if the "Policy and Procedure for Residents Leaving the Facility" states that residents should sign out in the "leave notebook," this may remind you to ask a resident if they will be returning in time for the next meal. Always follow facility policies and procedures to ensure your actions are correct.

There is so much information in the chart and other places in the facility, in policies and procedures, and from other staff, residents, and visitors that you may find it a challenge to keep it all straight. But once you know all these sources, gathering information will become easy for you.

If you are unsure of anything when talking with members of the team, the resident, or family members, just ask. Don't assume anything you're not sure of. Asking questions and clarifying information are important forms of communication for the whole team.

In addition you will learn about the Health Insurance Portability and Accountability Act, known as HIPAA. This law covers privacy issues related to the resident's health care, including who has access to information. During your orientation, your facility will give you guidelines to follow.

THE DIFFERENCE BETWEEN OBJECTIVE AND SUBJECTIVE INFORMATION

Your observation of a resident is an excellent source of information. Objective information is factual information. You observe objective information by looking, listening, smelling, and touching. For example, the statements "This resident weighs 127 pounds" and "That resident's skin is warm and dry" are objective data (Fig 8-6, next page).

Objective – information that can be observed; factual; not subjective

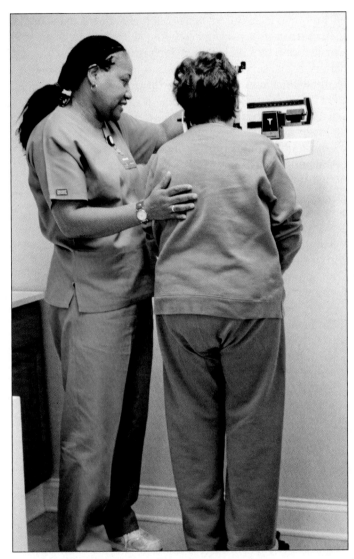

Fig. 8-6 – Weighing a resident gives you factual, objective information. Always weigh a resident without their shoes.

Subjective information is your guess or hunch about what you observe. It is also what the resident feels inside and tells you about. If you see that a resident did not drink any milk at lunch, you might guess what that means. You might think that they do not like milk. This guess is subjective. It might be right or wrong because it is not a fact. Maybe the resident does like milk but did not drink it this time for some other reason.

Subjective information can be very helpful as long as you identify it as resident's feeling or yours. Another example is telling the charge nurse that you noticed that a resident just seems different today. After the nurse assesses the

resident, the resident is discovered to have an infection. Your report of this subjective information allowed for early treatment of the infection.

Imagine a situation in which you hear a loud crash and a resident yelling, "Help me! I fell." When you run into the room, you see the resident lying on the floor and the tray table tipped over. You guess that they fell down. You report to the nurse, "I heard a loud crash, then I heard him call, 'Help me! I fell.' When I walked into the room, I saw him lying on the floor with the tray table on the floor beside him. I think he fell." In this way you clearly identify which information is objective and factual (what you heard and what you saw) and which information is your subjective guess ("I think he fell"), and your report is clear and accurate.

Now imagine that something else actually happened in that situation. Maybe the resident carefully lay down on the floor, pushed his tray table over, and then called, "Help me! I fell." Maybe he wants his family to think that he fell so that they will come to visit after the nurse calls them to report the "fall." The objective data that you reported is still correct, but your guess was wrong. You were correct to identify it as a guess (as subjective information) and not as a fact (objective information). Your report would be inaccurate if you stated subjective information ("I think the resident fell") as though it were an objective fact ("The resident fell"). Because you did not observe what actually happened, you cannot state "The resident fell" as a fact.

Accurate observations and reports collect both subjective and objective information. It is always key to use language that clearly identifies what is a fact and what is a guess.

Good observations focus on detail. You will know more about the situation if you use all your senses. For example, danger signs in a resident with diabetes are heavy sweating, a red face, "fruity" smelling breath, and the person saying, "I don't feel right." If you suspect this, quickly gather as much information as you can to give the nurse a full report. For example, is the room very warm or is the resident covered with heavy blankets, which might account for the sweating and red face? Do you smell a particular odor in the room? Ask the resident for more detail: "What do you mean, you don't feel right?" Then report all this information to the charge nurse so that the right actions can be taken. Your accurate observations and reports improve the resident's care.

Subjective – guess or hunch about what you observe, or something a resident feels inside and tells you about; not objective

RESIDENT ASSESSMENT

If your television won't turn on, you look for the problem. Maybe it isn't plugged in, or maybe the batteries in the remote control are dead. You assess its condition by looking at all relevant factors. Health care includes many **assessments** of a resident and their condition. The first step in assessment is to gather data. This includes objective information. As a nurse assistant, you are a key part of this process, especially gathering data, because you spend so much time with residents. All other departments use and depend on your observations of residents.

The most important assessment tool used for all residents in a Medicaid or Medicare facility is the **Resident Assessment Instrument (RAI)** The RAI has five parts (Fig. 8-7):

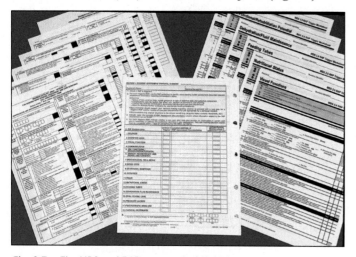

Fig. 8-7 – The MDS and RAPs are part of the RAI.

- the Minimum Data Set (MDS)
- Resident Assessment Protocols (RAPs)
- care plan development
- care plan implementation
- evaluation and outcome

You will often hear the nurse talk about this assessment process. Often this is called completing the MDS, but in fact it involves all five components.

The RAI is first completed for a resident on admission. A new assessment is done at least yearly and whenever a resident's condition changes. A partial assessment (called a quarterly review) is done more often. You may be asked for information about the resident each time an assessment is done for the RAI or MDS. If a resident enters the facility under Medicare, the RAI may be performed more often.

The nurse uses the MDS to collect information about the resident. It has several different sections. These are usually done by staff in other departments, such as the dietary, social services, activities, and nursing departments. Most facilities have an MDS coordinator who ensures that the MDS is completed on time.

Each section of the MDS includes observations by many different staff members, including you. The resident's memory, communication abilities, hearing, vision, emotional and social behavior, activity patterns, nutrition, and dental status are all assessed. Two areas on the MDS are especially important to the nursing department. One assesses the resident's physical functioning, including the activities of daily living: bathing, dressing, transferring, toileting, and eating. The other assesses resident's bowel and bladder continence.

Although you will not write on the MDS form yourself, the nurse will ask for your information for it. As with all reports, you must clearly identify objective information ("Mr. Brown puts on his own shirt, but he doesn't button the buttons himself") and subjective information ("I think that he could button his shirt himself if he had bigger buttons").

Some MDS items may have meanings different from the usual ones in your facility. For example, the term "bed mobility" on the MDS includes not only how a resident turns from side to side in the bed but also how they sit up and lie back down. Be certain that you understand items you are asked about so that you give accurate, full information.

As the person who spends the most time with residents, you are often first to observe a change in a resident's condition. Everyone will see a big change caused by a serious illness, but nurse assistants are often the first to see small or gradual changes. Imagine, for example, a resident who has been able to dress themselves and take care of their own personal hygiene after you help them sit up. Over the last few days, you observe and report that they need a little more help. You and other staff then observe these changes more closely.

📖

Assessment – an evaluation of a patient or condition

Minimum Data Set (MDS) – resident information on the RAI, including levels of physical functioning and bowel and bladder continence

Resident Assessment Instrument (RAI) – an assessment tool used in long term care facilities to document key information about residents including their care plans and outcomes

Resident Assessment Protocols (RAPs) – section of the RAI that includes a more detailed assessment of problem areas

A new MDS is done when a resident improves or declines. This is called a "significant change in status assessment." Without your observations and report, subtle changes might be missed. Individualized care starts with a thorough and accurate assessment based on information from nurse assistants and other staff who know a resident well and who communicate their observations clearly.

After the MDS is done, a resident is assessed in more detail in possible problem areas. This is done using the Resident Assessment Protocols (RAPs). For example, a resident may have a mobility problem. You provide information about the resident so the staff can decide whether the care plan should address this as a problem. The RAPs give the staff additional information or "protocols" to determine if this is a problem.

All facilities manage MDS information on a computer. The data collected on the MDS is centrally located. The system tracks certain kinds of resident data. It can automatically inform staff when the RAPs should be used to determine if the resident has a problem that should be on the care plan. The computer system allows staff to document, save, retrieve, and track information. If you will use the computer in your facility, you will learn about it in your orientation.

Quality Indicators

Quality indicators are another type of information from the MDS. A quality indicator summary report can tell staff, for example, how many residents have pressure ulcers or incontinence. State surveyors use this information when assessing the quality of care the facility provides. Such reports do not necessarily mean that care is poor but help staff know what areas may need improvement.

You will learn about the quality indicators used in your facility. All facilities that receive Medicare and Medicaid reimbursement use indicators based on CMS standards. Some other facilities have their own indicators based on their own goals and objectives.

RESIDENT CARE PLAN

A care plan is an interdisciplinary document that lists a resident's needs and goals as well as the actions and approaches the team will use to help the resident to meet their goals. Many health professionals in the facility have input into the plan. All staff use the care plan to ensure consistent care. The care plan is usually kept at the nurses' station, where all staff have access to it. It may be kept in a loose-leaf notebook (Fig. 8-8).

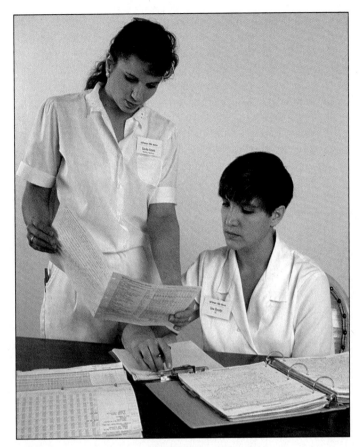

Fig. 8-8 – The care plan is used by every member of the interdisciplinary care team so everyone knows what the resident needs.

The care plan is based on assessments of the resident on admission. It is fully developed within 7 days after the RAI. The care plan is never considered "done," however, because it must change as the resident changes. Change means either improvement or decline in any area. It also changes because of information that you and other staff gather about the resident's needs, preferences, strengths, weaknesses, and goals.

The care plan lists each resident's medical, nursing, and psychosocial needs, often listed as problems. For each problem, an objective or goal is written. For example, a problem statement is: "Resident is having difficulty walking

---

📖

Quality indicators – outcomes or a summary of the entire facility's MDS information, which indicates the quality of care provided by a facility

since injuring left hip." A possible goal may be: "Resident will walk to the bathroom (10-15 feet) independently within 45 days." The care plan also lists the actions that staff will take, called approaches, to help the resident meet the goal. Following are some example approaches:

- "Nurse assistant takes resident to physical therapy every morning at 9 a.m."
- "Physical therapist stands resident at parallel bars for two minutes three times a day."
- "All staff encourage resident to use their walker."
- "Nurse assistant gives range-of-motion exercises to both legs, five times per leg at bedtime."

To help the care plan team evaluate a resident's progress, a time frame (sometimes called a goal date) is set. Table 8-1 gives an example of a problem, goal, time frame, approaches, and staff involved.

Your observations and experience with a resident are especially important for developing the care plan and keeping it up to date. From observing the resident, you can report whether the care plan is working. In the example in Table 8-1, you might discover that this resident also likes peanut butter sandwiches at bedtime. You report this information so that it can be included in the care plan. Then the staff who work with this resident will know that even if the protein drink and ice cream are refused, this alternative might appeal to this resident.

Your Role in the Care-Plan Meeting

The interdisciplinary team, including the resident and family, reviews and revises the care plan. This is done as needed, or at least every 90 days. Some team members may write their information for this review. Most sit down with the resident and family to discuss the care plan and their progress toward meeting the goals. This is sometimes called a care conference (Fig. 8-9). Problem solving

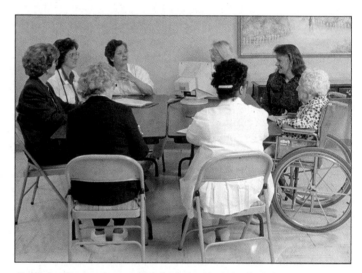

Fig. 8-9 – A care-plan meeting includes the interdisciplinary team, the resident, and family members.

TABLE 8-1
SECTION OF A RESIDENT'S CARE PLAN

PROBLEM	GOAL	APPROACHES	STAFF
• Poor appetite and weight loss since beginning chemotherapy	• Resident will gain 2 pounds within three weeks	• Dietary and physician consult • Weigh every Friday a.m. • High-calorie diet • Monitor tray and record intake • High protein drink at 10 a.m. and/or bedtime • Resident likes ice cream, so offer ice cream if they refuse to drink high-protein drink • Offer snacks at bingo • Son will eat with resident at noon. Serve tray in A wing lounge.	• Nurse • Nurse assistant • Dietary • Nurse assistant • Nurse assistant and dietary • Nurse assistant • Activities department • Nurse assistant

is an important part of this meeting, with everyone sharing ideas, observations, and information.

Good communication skills are needed in care-plan meetings because many people are sharing a lot of information. Sometimes the group struggles with difficult situations. Your role is to come well prepared and to be knowledgeable about the resident. You should be open to new ideas and approaches and ready to share information. Since some areas of any resident's care and progress may be sensitive, being tactful is especially important. It can be exciting for a resident to participate in this meeting, but it also might be stressful. You should give professional and caring support to every resident in these meetings.

HOW TO REPORT INFORMATION

You report different information in different ways. Usually you report to the charge nurse, but sometimes you need to report to other facility staff. Since all staff maintain the confidentiality of information about a resident, you can safely report to other members of the interdisciplinary team. However, use a private place to give an oral report so others will not overhear you (Fig. 8-10).

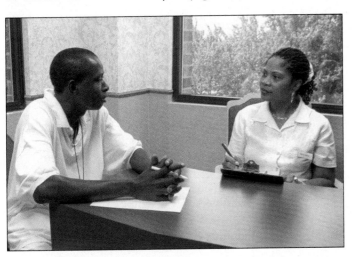

Fig. 8-10 – Information about a resident should be reported in private.

Because information about residents is confidential, be careful when talking with family members and visitors. Even information that is routine to you may not seem that way to others. For example, you might tell a resident's husband that his wife slept two hours that afternoon. He be-comes alarmed and says, "She never sleeps that long. She must be sick!" Always check with the charge nurse first before making reports to residents or family members.

Most of your reports are directly to another person, giving information face to face. Sometimes you report things in writing with a note or a form. For example, you might write a request to the maintenance department to tighten a faucet handle.

Routine Reporting

At the end of your shift, always report to the charge nurse about the residents you cared for. This is called routine reporting. Report objective and subjective information that can wait until the end of the shift. This is information that was not immediately important when you first observed or learned it. With routine reporting, you share information about the care you gave during your shift. Before you report, ask yourself, "What did I see, hear, smell, or touch when caring for each resident? Was anything new or changed? Did I meet each resident's needs?"

You can wait until the end of your shift to report much general information. For example: "Mrs. Jones is continuing to walk without limping" and "Mr. Smith wants us to tell the night shift to wake him up at 7 a.m. because his son is telephoning him at 7:15." You can make general reports at any time convenient for you and the person you are reporting to.

Immediate Reporting

Some observations must be reported immediately. You must report right away any dangerous situation, such as the following:

- A frayed electrical cord
- Any unusual incident, such as a resident's fall (Fig. 8-11, next page)
- Any suspicion of resident abuse
- Any resident's complaint of ill health, such as a complaint of pain or dizziness
- Any unusual observations, such as a resident's temperature of 103° F or confusion and agitation in a normally alert resident

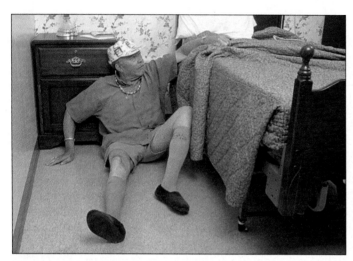

Fig. 8-11 – Some information must be reported immediately, such as a resident's fall.

"By a Certain Time" Reporting

A third type of reporting is called "by a certain time" reporting. This involves information needed by a set time. For example, the nurse may need a resident's temperature before the physician calls. If you are unsure when to report something, ask the charge nurse.

INCIDENT REPORTS

Incident reports document an accident or an injury. They provide information about what happened. These reports also protect residents, you, the facility, and others involved. An incident report documents the incident and all related facts (Fig. 8-12). Because an incident may be involved in a future legal action, the incident report is an important document. You may give objective information (what you heard, saw, smelled, and touched) to someone else who fills out the report, or you may write it yourself. The guidelines for documenting an incident are the same as for documenting other information in the chart.

YOUR ROLE IN DOCUMENTATION

The facility maintains many kinds of written information and reports. In addition to residents' charts, you will also document information on worksheets and facility records such as incident reports. Most written records communicate information to other staff. But your documentation may be used in other ways too, such as by an insurance company or in a court case. You follow the same guidelines for documentation as all other health professionals.

CONFIDENTIAL AND PRIVILEGED
PERFORMANCE IMPROVEMENT INFORMATION
PREPARED FOR ADVICE BY COUNSEL IN ANTICIPATION OF LITIGATION

INCIDENT EVENT REPORT (Connecticut and Texas)
(Resident/Visitor)

Facility #:____ Name:____ City:____ St.:____
Resident/Visitor Name:____ Date of Admission:____ Age:__ Sex: ☐ M ☐ F
Current Diagnosis:____ Room #:____ Bed #:____
Date/Time of Occurrence:____ Location of Occurrence:____
Nature/Summary of Occurrence:____
____ Med. Rec'd. #:____

ACTION TAKEN:
Immediately:____
Vitals: BP:____ P:____ RESP:____ TEMP:____
Within 24 hours:____
Follow-up/Summary:____

DISPOSITION:
D1 ☐ Remained in Facility D2 ☐ Seen in Facility by MD
D3 ☐ ER Visit D4 ☐ Hospital Admittance
D5 ☐ Returned to Facility - Date/Time:____

NOTIFICATION: **TIME/BY WHOM**
☐ Family:____
☐ Guardian:____
☐ Physician:____
Address:____

WITNESS INFORMATION (to be recorded by staff) **FOR EACH WITNESS:**
Name:____ Phone #:____
Address:____
Reason for Presence in Building: ☐ Visit ☐ Volunteer ☐ Resident ☐ Employee ☐ Vendor or Delivery ☐ Other (Explain)
If Employee: ☐ Regular ☐ *Per diem* ☐ Agency____
Were Statements Made or Given to Staff:____

REVIEWED BY:
Director of Nursing:____ Date:____
Administrator:____ Date:____
Medical Director:____ Date:____

SIGNATURE OF EMPLOYEE PREPARING REPORT:
Name:____ Date:____

CONNECTICUT ONLY
____ - A__ B__ C__ D__ E__ - __ __ - ____
Facility Lic. # *Classification* *Year* *Sequential # of Report*
CCNH__ RHNS__ No. of Beds____
Condition before occurrence (mental and physical):____
Condition after occurrence (mental and physical):____

SEE INSTRUCTIONS ON REVERSE

N-RM F 6.3 A CT-TX (8/99)

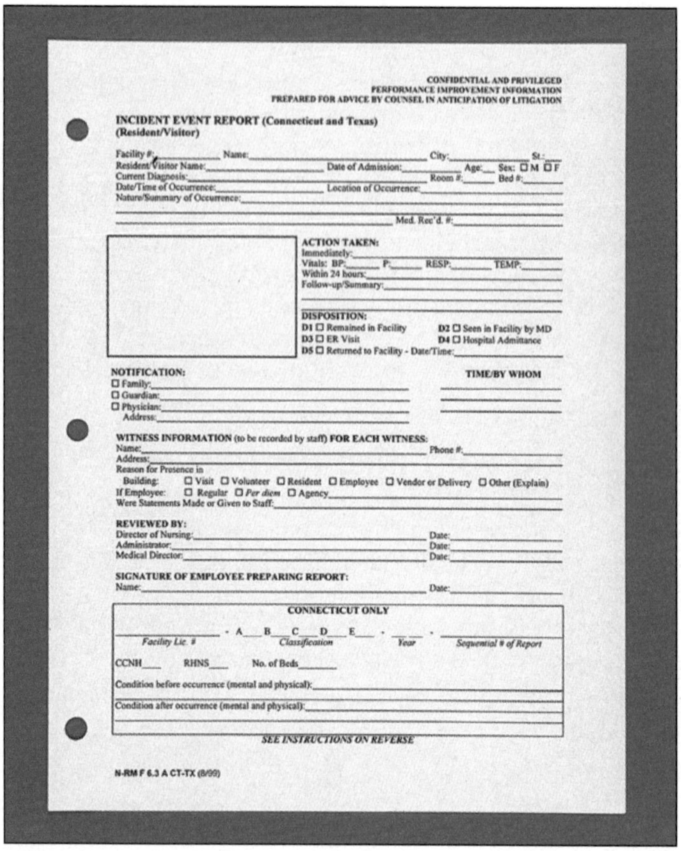

Fig. 8-12 – Incident reports must be completed after an accident or injury.

Even documentation that seems routine is important. For example, you take a resident's blood pressure and write it on the vital sign sheet. Her pressure is 150/86, which is not especially high for an elderly woman. But when you compare it with her usual blood pressure readings, which are around 100/60, you see that it is quite high. You should immediately report this possibly serious change.

When you are documenting, you may discover something that also needs to be reported. For example, as you record a resident's weight, you notice that they have lost weight since the last recorded weight. You report this information to the nurse in addition to documenting it.

Documentation involves watching for trends as well as changes. For example, when writing in a food intake record, you discover a resident often does not eat their vegetables. Since the dietitian needs this information to better plan meals, you report it to the dietitian in addition to writing it down.

Be sure you understand your facility's policies and procedures for your documentation. Different facilities have different policies. In some facilities nurse assistants write progress notes. These are notes about a resident and the care you give. This information is listed by date. It may include the following:

- general statements of care given
- the resident's appointments and activities
- any complaints from the resident
- general statements about the resident's psychological well-being
- visitors, including physician's visits

Some facilities use check-off sheets that require only your initials and simple documentation, such as an "L" to note a large bowel movement. You may record intake and output numbers directly in the chart or on worksheets that the unit clerk or charge nurse later adds up and records in the chart.

Your facility may use a combination of different charting methods. For example, your assignment sheet may need your initials on one side but have a few lines on the other side for progress notes.

Electronic Documentation

As the world of health care advances, additional changes will occur in the methods and systems you will use for your documentation. Facilities will increasingly be using an electronic documentation system to record the care given to your residents. It will be important to understand the specifics of your facility's system. Timely and precise reporting of residents' condition is one of your priorities. When using an electronic documentation system, accuracy becomes even more important. It can be difficult to correct a mistake within an electronic system and may require the assistance of your charge nurse. If you are uncertain what to do or how to use the system, check with your supervisor for guidance.

Guidelines for Documentation

Common-sense rules help ensure that chart documentation is clear and easy to read. Follow the documentation guidelines listed in Box 8-1 to prevent misunderstandings. These rules also help prevent any inappropriate changes of the record. The rules maintain the chart as a legal record. If

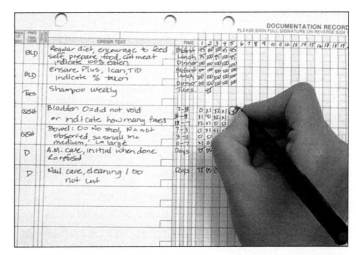

Fig. 8-13 – Neat handwriting is important so everyone can read entries in the resident's record.

BOX 8-1.
GENERAL GUIDELINES FOR DOCUMENTATION

- The resident's name should be on every page of the chart. It is written on each new page before anything else is written.
- Write all entries in permanent blue or black ink, not pencil or felt-tip markers that may smear when wet.
- Write each entry so that it is easy to read. Pay attention to your penmanship (handwriting). Use neat printing instead if it is easier for others to read.
- Charting is continuous. Do not leave spaces or skip lines between entries.
- Document only your own actions and observations.

- Do not tamper with or change entries made into the chart unless you make an error. If you make an error, correct it immediately and properly.
- Use standard medical terminology and standard abbreviations (see Appendices A and B).
- Write down the date and the time of each entry as required.
- Sign each entry and include your title after your name. In some cases you may initial the entry when your signature is somewhere else on the form.

entries in the chart cannot be read or seem wrong or changed, it would be very difficult to be certain of the facts.

Always use neat handwriting or printing when writing in the record (Fig. 8-13). An entry that cannot be read might as well not be there at all. Never skip lines or leave open spaces in the record because someone could later write something in that space. (See "Correcting a Mistake in Documentation," below.) If there is a space in the chart for you to write your initials after doing a task, for example, follow your facility's rules for filling in that space even if you did not complete the task. Leaving that space empty would enable someone to change the record later. In addition, chart only your own actions and observations. It is illegal to chart for someone else. All staff are responsible for their own work.

Correcting a Mistake in Documentation

The resident's chart and most forms on which you document information are legal records. People who look at

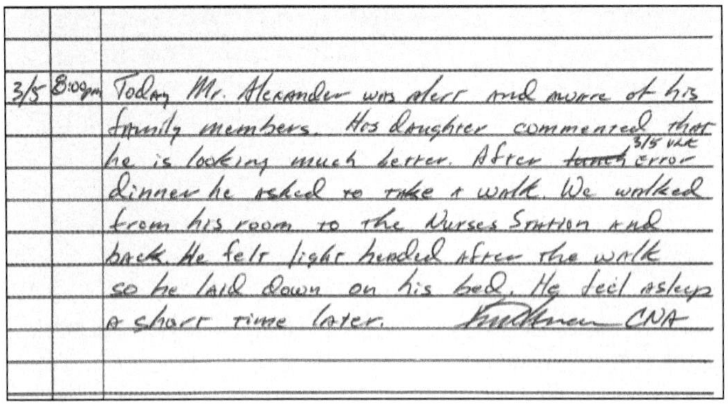

Fig. 8-14 – Always follow the proper procedure for correcting an error.

records for legal purposes examine alterations closely. Lawyers, state surveyors and other inspectors, and insurance company officials may carefully inspect residents' records. To prevent problems and misunderstandings, all health professionals use a standard method for correcting mistakes in documentation.

If you make a mistake, you must correct it so that the information is accurate for other members of the health care team. For example, if you misspell a word in the health record, you must correct it to prevent a possible misunderstanding. Follow these steps to correct it:
1. Draw a single line through the word.
2. Print "error" above or beside the word.
3. Add your initials and the date above it.

BOX 8-2.
GUIDELINES FOR CORRECTING DOCUMENTATION ERRORS

- Draw a single line through the error. Do not completely cover the error with X's, scribbles, or correction fluid (White Out). Do not erase entries. What you wrote should remain readable.
- Print the word "error," your initials, and the date above or beside the error.
- To correct a charting mistake in a small box or area, circle the mistake and write the correction, the date, and your initials on the reverse side of the sheet or in the margin (Fig. 8-15).

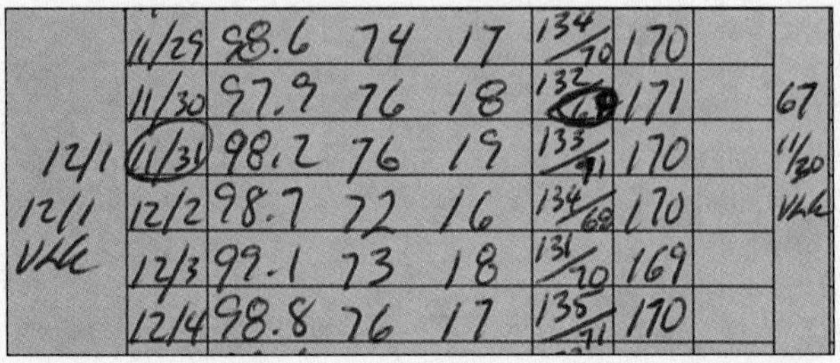

Fig. 8-15 – For mistakes in flow charts, circle the mistake and write in the correction, date, and your initials on the back of the sheet or in the margin.

- To correct a large amount of charting, indicate the reason why in the margin (for example, "wrong resident" or "charted entry twice"). This is not necessary for correcting short entries.
- Ask the nurse or medical records department for help if you cannot figure out how to clearly correct a documentation mistake.

4. Then write the correct word before continuing (Fig. 8-14).

Do not try to cover an error with X's or scribble all over it, because readers then could not tell what was originally written. A person could later claim that you had originally written something very different, and you would not be able to prove that their claim was wrong. Box 8-2 summarizes the guidelines for correcting errors.

If you have to correct a large amount of writing, be sure to write the reason you are making the correction. Many health professionals have written a detailed progress note only to discover they were writing on the wrong resident's chart! If that happens to you, draw one large X through the note or single lines through each line of charting, and write "wrong resident" in the margin, along with your initials or signature.

Sometimes it is difficult to correct a documentation mistake. When you have to write your initials or numbers in a little box, there may not be enough room to correct a mistake in that place. In this case draw a circle around the entry and write a note on the back of the sheet, or in the margin if there is not room on the reverse, to describe what happened. Include the date, your initials, and the correct information.

In some situations it can be very difficult to correct a mistake. Maybe there is not enough room on the form to correct an error. Maybe you realize days or weeks later that you made a mistake. In these unusual cases, talk to the charge nurse or the medical records department about how to make the correction. Your responsible attitude and desire to have only accurate information in the record are signs of your good intentions.

COMMON MEDICAL TERMS AND ABBREVIATIONS

Imagine meeting with a banker to discuss a loan. You are already a little nervous, and then the banker starts using financial and banking terms you never heard before. You feel lost, as if the banker is speaking a foreign language! This is a common feeling for residents and family members in health care settings. Medical terms like "perineum" are used instead of words the general public commonly uses, such as "crotch" or "privates." Medical terms and abbreviations are also used throughout the medical record.

As you gain more experience in health care, medical terms and abbreviations will become familiar to you. Although abbreviations are used less commonly now, the Joint Commission for Accreditation of Healthcare Organizations (JCAHO) has asked health care providers to carefully consider the use of abbreviations in their health care settings and not use any that may increase the risk of medication errors. JCAHO has a "Do Not Use" list of abbreviations, acronyms, and symbols and another list of those that may be added in the future. Be sure you know the "do not use list" in your facility.

Remember that the medical terms you use may not be understandable to everyone, especially residents, visitors, new staff, or staff in other departments. Medical terminology can be very confusing to people new to health care. For example, a nurse assistant once asked a new resident if he needed to urinate. He replied, "No, I don't have to do

that—I've just got to pee."

That example may be humorous and generally harmless, but misunderstandings can also be dangerous. For example, a nurse assistant might want to ask a resident about their chest pain. If the nurse assistant asks, "Are you experiencing angina?" the resident might answer no even if they do have chest pain. Maybe they do not know what "angina" means. This could be a potentially dangerous situation for a resident who is having real chest pain.

Generally, try to communicate with residents in simple, nonmedical terms. For example, say "I'm going to wash between your legs now" instead of "I'm going to wash your perineum now." Define terms a resident might not understand. For example, you might say, "I'm going to take your axillary temperature now. That means I'm going to put the thermometer in your armpit."

Because you must do much documentation, you will often use standard medical terminology and abbreviations in records. Most facilities use many of the same standard terms and abbreviations. Some facilities use their own terms and abbreviations, however. Never be embarrassed to ask what something means. It is much worse not to ask and guess wrong. For example, a physician was confused because he read in the record that a resident was walking with SBA (standby assistance) and thought that SBA must be a new kind of leg brace.

Appendices A and B define common medical terms and abbreviations. You may use some of these in your facility. But it is more important to document information clearly than to use complicated medical terms. Sometimes health professionals think that they must use an "official" medical term when they could have used a simpler term that communicated the information more clearly. For example, someone might write, "The resident ambulated on their own BID today" instead of simply saying "The resident walked by himself two times today."

IN THIS CHAPTER YOU LEARNED:
- Different places where resident information can be found
- The difference between objective and subjective information
- Your role in care planning
- When and how to report and document information
- When and how to use medical terminology

SUMMARY
In this chapter you learned the importance of communicating information about the resident through clear, accurate documentation. Much information is available to help you do your job successfully. You have a very important role in gathering information about the residents you care for. Others on the team count on you for information for the RAI and the care plan. You also have a major role in the resident's care planning process. Finally, you learned the importance of reporting information both accurately and on time.

PULLING IT ALL TOGETHER
Mr. Smith is a quiet, gentle resident in your care. He usually gets up early in the morning and walks around the facility's grounds. He tells you that in his younger years he was a runner. This morning you notice he doesn't seem himself. While taking his routine weekly vital signs, you note an increase in his oral temperature to 100.6°. You put a note about this in your pocket and tell yourself not to forget to record his vital signs and report the temperature increase to the charge nurse later on.

A week later Mr. Smith is admitted to the hospital for pneumonia. During a care planning meeting the charge nurse asks you to get Mr. Smith's medical record for her to review. She notes that Mr. Smith's vitals signs were not recorded last week. This concerns the charge nurse, because the care plan states to take weekly vital signs to monitor his cardiac condition. The charge nurse asks you why you didn't take his vital signs last week. You suddenly realize that a week ago you forgot to document his vital signs. You also forgot to report that his temperature was elevated and that he seemed quieter than normal.

What do you think might have happened if you had documented and reported his changes a week ago? Could his hospitalization have been prevented with early treatment? As the person who spends the most time with residents, you have information that other staff need. Others count on you to communicate information about residents so that the best care possible can be given.

1. **The interdisciplinary care team uses the minimum data set (MDS) to:**
   A. Make roommate assignments.
   B. Develop a resident's care plan.
   C. Keep a record of monthly expenses.
   D. Teach nurse assistants correct medical terminology.

2. **Who is the primary source of information about a resident?**
   A. The resident.
   B. The charge nurse.
   C. The social worker.
   D. The resident's physician.

3. **A medical record is used to maintain:**
   A. The facility's financial information.
   B. The facility's equipment maintenance record.
   C. Lab results and reports by all care staff.
   D. Correspondence between the resident and their family.

4. **Mr. Houston's weight is checked each day. Before the end of your shift, you would record this information on:**
   A. A wall calendar.
   B. A flow sheet.
   C. The Quarterly Review form.
   D. The Resident Assessment Protocols.

5. **You have just taken Mrs. Cotton's temperature. It is 98.4°. This is a type of:**
   A. Objective information.
   B. Subjective information.
   C. Resident Assessment Protocol.
   D. Quality indicator.

6. **The minimum data set (MDS) is one part of the:**
   A. Quality indicators.
   B. Resident's care plan.
   C. Resident Assessment Instrument (RAI).
   D. Resident Assessment Protocols (RAPs).

7. **A resident's care plan is used as a tool to:**
   A. Determine whether the resident qualifies for Medicaid payments.
   B. Invite family members to facility parties.
   C. Plan for new building improvements.
   D. Coordinate all treatments and services for the resident.

8. **Your role in the care plan meeting includes:**
   A. Sharing information about the resident.
   B. Serving coffee and doughnuts to the interdisciplinary team.
   C. Deciding which doctors and nurses should attend.
   D. Diagnosing the resident's medical condition.

9. **Routine information about residents is usually shared with the charge nurse:**
   A. On your lunch break.
   B. At the end of your shift.
   C. During weekly personnel meetings.
   D. Immediately.

10. **When you write in a resident's chart, you should:**
    A. Erase any mistakes and then write in the correct information.
    B. Get the doctor's permission before you write anything.
    C. Write neatly and legibly.
    D. Correct any mistakes you see that were made by others.

(Answers to "Check What You've Learned" are in the Instructor's Manual.)

Chapter 9

PREVENTION AND CONTROL OF INFECTION

People die every day from infections. They may come into a health care setting with an infection or acquire one there. Today residents are at risk of exposure to bacteria that have become resistant to antibiotics. Many infections can be prevented. The challenge in a long term care facility is to provide a healthy environment for both residents and staff. Infections spread because of careless infection control practices. Simple handwashing and common sense cleaning practices can often prevent these tragedies.

How do you define a challenge? Most of us think of a challenge as something that is difficult to achieve but important. We feel satisfied when we meet a challenge. Infection control procedures can sometimes be a challenge. It is a challenge to care for residents with an infection. It is also a challenge to prevent the spread of infection to other residents and to maintain a clean environment (Fig. 9-1). Residents who are elderly, frail, or already weakened by another illness can be more seriously affected by infection than younger or healthier adults. This makes it even more of a challenge.

You have a very important role in preventing and controlling infections in residents. You can do many things to prevent the transmission of microorganisms.

In this chapter you will learn how microorganisms are transmitted and what you can do to prevent the spread of infection. As a nurse assistant you are responsible for practicing proper infection control procedures.

OBJECTIVES
- State how microorganisms are transmitted
- Demonstrate the skill of handwashing
- Demonstrate the proper way to put on and remove gowns, aprons, gloves, masks, and eye protection
- Explain your facility's policies and procedures related to isolation precautions
- State your role in cleaning objects and disposing of soiled items in the resident's environment

MEDICAL TERMS
- **Antibiotics** – drugs that reduce or kill microorganisms
- **Bacteria** – one-celled microorganisms that may cause infection (bacterium is the singular form)
- **Chicken pox** – contagious disease caused by a virus; one early symptom is a low-grade fever
- **Diarrhea** – very frequent and liquid stools
- **Emesis** – related to vomiting, as in an emesis basin
- **Fungus** – a type of microorganism like yeast and mold (fungi is the plural form)
- **Gonorrhea** – contagious bacterial venereal infection that is sexually transmitted
- **Human immunodeficiency virus (HIV)** – viral infection transmitted by contact with blood and other body fluids such as semen and vaginal secretions
- **Immunization** – administration of a vaccine to make the person immune (not susceptible) to a specific infection
- **Infection** – condition produced when an infective agent becomes established in or on a suitable host; infections usually have signs and symptoms
- **Influenza (flu)** – contagious viral disease which has a sudden onset, fever, and severe aches and pains
- **Intestines** – part of the digestive tract through which food passes after leaving the stomach that helps digest food and eliminates waste
- **Measles** – contagious disease caused by a virus, which produces red spots on the skin
- **Microorganisms** – viruses, bacteria, or fungi that cannot be seen with the naked eye; also called germs
- **Nonpathogenic** – microorganisms that do not cause infection
- **Outbreak** – sudden, dramatic increase in cases of a particular disease or harmful organisms
- **Pathogenic** – microorganisms or substances that can produce disease
- **Pathological** – caused by disease
- **Secretions** – substances such as saliva, mucus, perspiration, tears, etc. that come out of the body

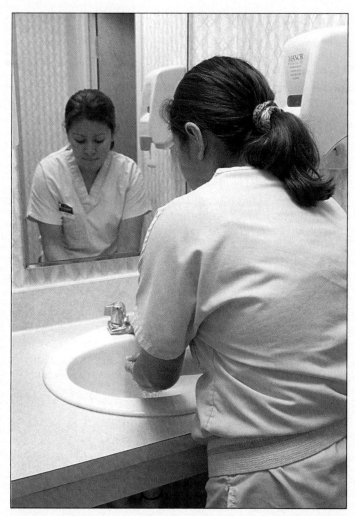

Fig. 9-1 – Infection control practices such as handwashing can reduce the spread of infection.

"It seems so easy for me to get sick these days, but I don't need to worry because you do everything you can to keep me healthy."

Did you ever wonder why colds and **flu** are more common in the winter? People used to think that being cold made it easier to catch a cold, but that theory has been proven wrong. Colds are more common in the winter because people stay inside more often. They are in closer contact with each other. Anyone can catch a cold at any time, but cold germs, or **microorganisms**, spread more easily among people in close contact. They spread easily when someone coughs or sneezes. Someone in a weakened condition is more likely to get a cold, because the body's natural defenses are less able to resist, or fight off, the **infection**.

Fortunately, not all microorganisms are **transmitted** as easily as the ones that cause colds. But infections can be serious for residents in a long term care facility. You and other staff in the facility face the challenge to work together to control and prevent the spread of microorganisms.

- **Shingles** – viral inflammation that affects the nerves in the skull and spine
- **Syphilis** – a chronic, contagious venereal infection that is sexually transmitted
- **Tuberculosis (TB)** – infectious, bacterial, communicable disease that primarily affects the lungs
- **Virus** – a type of microorganism that survives only in living things

📖

Infection – condition produced when an infective agent becomes established in or on a suitable host; infections usually have signs and symptoms

Influenza (flu) – contagious viral disease which has a sudden onset, fever, and severe aches and pains

Microorganisms – viruses, bacteria, or fungi that cannot be seen with the naked eye; also called germs

Transmit – transfer an infectious agent from one person or place to another

HOW MICROORGANISMS CAUSE INFECTIONS

Microorganisms are so small they can be seen only with a microscope. The most common types are **viruses**, **bacteria**, and **fungi**. People often call these microorganisms "germs."

Many microorganisms live naturally on the skin. They also live in the **intestines**, vagina, mouth, and other parts of the body. These bacteria are called natural flora. In a healthy person, these bacteria are in balance and do not cause problems. However, if the natural balance is destroyed because of illness, poor nutrition, stress, fatigue, or certain drugs, these microorganisms may cause infection. Microorganisms that live in one part of the body without causing problems can cause a serious infection if they reach another part. For example, some *Escherichia coli* bacteria (*E. coli*) normally live in the gastrointestinal tract. They can cause a urinary tract infection if they get into the bladder. You commonly hear about *E. coli* contamination of food caused either by improper food handling or by contaminated water.

HOW MICROORGANISMS ARE TRANSMITTED: THE CHAIN OF TRANSMISSION

Microorganisms are transmitted from one person to another in a process involving six steps or conditions. You can think of this as a chain with six links (Fig. 9-2). Each link must be present to make the chain complete in order for the infection to be transmitted. These links are:

1. the microorganism that can cause infection
2. the **reservoir** (person, animal, or environment where the microorganism lives)
3. a **portal of exit** (route) from the reservoir
4. a mode of transmission from the reservoir to a susceptible host
5. a **portal of entry** (route) into the susceptible host
6. the **susceptible host** (person with little resistance to an infectious disease)

As you read the next sections about these links, think about what you need to do to break the chain. Breaking a link prevents infection. Think about who or what can be the source of the infection, who is at risk, and how the infection spreads.

The Microorganism

The first link in the chain is the microorganism that causes the infection. Many types of viruses, bacteria, and fungi cause infections. Microorganisms that cause infections are called **pathogens**; those that do not are called **nonpathogenic**. Without a pathogenic microorganism, there can be no infection.

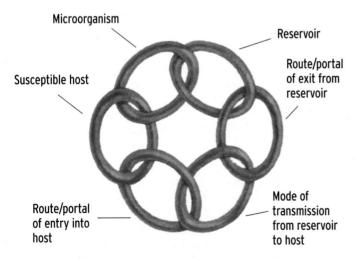

Fig. 9-2 – Transmission of microorganism involves six steps or links. All six must be present for the microorganism to be transmitted.

Bacteria – one-celled microorganisms that may cause infection (bacterium is the singular form)

Fungus – a type of microorganism like yeast and mold (fungi is the plural form)

Intestines – part of the digestive tract through which food passes after leaving the stomach that helps digest food and eliminates waste

Nonpathogenic – microorganisms that do not cause infection

Pathogenic – microorganisms or substances that can produce disease

Portal of entry – natural openings in the body where microorganisms can enter

Portal of exit – a route taken by microorganisms leaving the body, such as blood and the natural openings of the body

Reservoir – a person, animal, or environment in which an infectious agent lives

Susceptible host – a person who is not resistant to infection by a microorganism

Virus – a type of microorganism that survives only in living things

The Reservoir

The second link is called the reservoir. This is where the microorganisms live. The human body is a reservoir for many different types of microorganisms. They also live in animals, plants, soil, food, and water as well as on surfaces in the environment.

Portal of Exit From the Reservoir

The third link in the chain is the portal of exit, or route, from the reservoir. The microorganisms must exit from the infected person or other reservoir to be transmitted to another person. Portals of exit include all natural body openings. They include breaks in the skin such as tears and wounds (also called broken skin or nonintact skin). They also include openings made during medical procedures such as surgery. For example, microorganisms in the lungs can exit the body when a person coughs or sneezes. Microorganisms in the bladder exit in urine. Microorganisms in the intestinal tract exit in stool.

Modes of Transmission From the Reservoir

In the fourth link, organisms are transmitted from the reservoir to the portal of entry of a susceptible person. This can happen by several pathways, or modes. They include direct, indirect, and airborne transmission. These are described in the next sections.

Direct Transmission (Person-to-Person).   Direct transmission of microorganisms from one person's portal of exit (such as the mouth or genitalia) to another person's portal of entry can occur by touch. This includes activities such as kissing and sexual intercourse (Fig. 9-3). Direct transfer also occurs when small drops of mucus from coughing or sneezing come in contact with another person's eyes, nose, or mouth. This is most common when people are within three feet of each other. Direct transmission easily spreads microorganisms. For example, droplet-transmitted diseases such as **chicken pox** and **measles** spread quickly among children. Direct transmission may also occur if one person's blood or other body fluids with pathogenic organisms come in direct contact with another person's broken skin or mucous membranes.

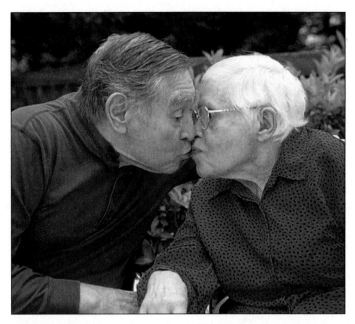

Fig. 9-3 — Kissing is an example of how microorganisms spread by direct transmission.

Indirect Transmission (Person-to-Intermediate Object-to-Person).   Indirect transmission occurs from an intermediate object between the portal of exit and the portal of entry of another person. Intermediate objects include the hands, soiled linen or dressings, and **contaminated** surfaces, water, and food.

In long term care facilities, hands are the most common intermediate objects involved in indirect transmission of microorganisms from one resident to another (Fig. 9-4, next page).

Chicken pox — contagious disease caused by a virus; one early symptom is a low-grade fever

Contaminated — impure or unclean

Direct transmission — direct transfer of microorganisms from one person to another

Indirect transmission — transmission of infection by an intermediate object, such as food, water, medical equipment, or a person's hands, into the portal of entry of a susceptible host

Measles — contagious disease caused by a virus, which produces red spots on the skin

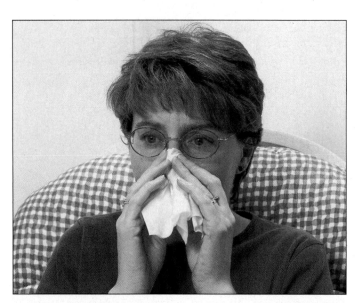

Fig. 9-4 – Your hands are considered an intermediate object in the transmission of germs.

Consider this example:

You are caring for Ms. Swenson and Ms. Ritter, who are bedridden and are roommates in a two-bed room. As you deliver lunch trays to both residents, you discover that Ms. Swenson has been incontinent of urine. You give Ms. Ritter her lunch tray but put Ms. Swen-son's tray aside until you can clean her and her bed.

Just as you finish cleaning Ms. Swenson, Ms. Ritter asks you to help her open a plastic wrapping on a cookie. If you fail to wash your hands, your hands may have microorganisms from Ms. Swenson's urine on them. Your contaminated hands touch the cookie, to which some of these microorganisms are transferred. When Ms. Ritter eats the cookie, she takes in some of these microorganisms. This is an example of indirect transmission.

Airborne Transmission. Airborne transmission of microorganisms occurs when the person (reservoir) coughs microorganisms into the air and a susceptible host breathes them into their lungs. Only a few microorganisms are transmitted by this mode, including the bacteria that cause **tuberculosis (TB)**. TB microorganisms can live in the air, but airborne transmission can be prevented if the facility has appropriate ventilation and air exchange.

Portal of Entry Into Susceptible Host

The fifth link is the portal of entry. Most commonly the portal of entry is a natural opening in the body. For example, a susceptible host may breathe in microorganisms through their nose and mouth from another person's cough or sneeze. Microorganisms that cause **diarrhea** may enter the susceptible host in food the person eats, if someone preparing or handling the food did not wash their hands after using the bathroom. Sexually transmitted disease microorganisms enter through the vagina or penis. The portal of entry may also be an open wound. This includes skin tears and pressure ulcers.

Susceptible Host

The sixth and final link in the chain is the susceptible host. All people are susceptible to infections caused by viruses, bacteria, and fungi. A resident can become more susceptible to infection because of various other diseases or conditions. A person may also be more susceptible because of treatments with steroids or chemotherapeutic agents that weaken the immune system, breaks in the skin, use of equipment like catheters, an unclean environment, or simply old age.

STRATEGIES FOR BREAKING THE CHAIN OF TRANSMISSION

If even one link in the chain is broken, infection cannot be transmitted. Many different infection prevention and control measures can be used to break different links in the chain. The next sections describe these infection prevention and control techniques. Remember, breaking even one link breaks the chain of transmission of infection (Fig. 9-5, next page). Use the following strategies when you are providing care.

Airborne transmission – route of infection that occurs when the reservoir coughs microorganisms into the air and a susceptible host breathes them into the lungs
Diarrhea – very frequent and liquid stools
Tuberculosis (TB) – infectious, bacterial, communicable disease that primarily affects the lungs

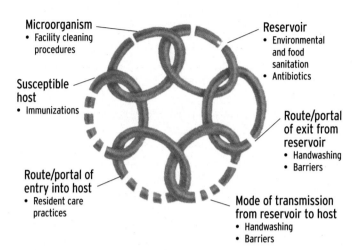

Microorganism
• Facility cleaning procedures

Susceptible host
• Immunizations

Route/portal of entry into host
• Resident care practices

Reservoir
• Environmental and food sanitation
• Antibiotics

Route/portal of exit from reservoir
• Handwashing
• Barriers

Mode of transmission from reservoir to host
• Handwashing
• Barriers

Fig. 9-5 – The chain of transmission can be broken by using proper infection control procedures.

Breaking the Chain With Handwashing and Other Strategies

Barriers and many different care practices break the chain at the portal of entry. Handwashing and the use of barriers like gloves, gown, mask, and goggles can break the chain at the portal of exit and at the mode of transmission. Environmental sanitation and disinfection measures will reduce or eliminate environmental reservoirs.

Breaking the Chain at the Reservoir Link

When a person has signs and symptoms of an infection and is diagnosed with one, antibiotics are often used in the treatment. This treatment reduces the number of bacteria and severity of the infection and allows the person to get well. Then the person no longer is a reservoir.

Food sanitary practices prevent food from becoming a reservoir for microorganisms. This includes using clean equipment for preparation, adequate refrigeration for storage, and proper handwashing, especially after using the bathroom, coughing, or sneezing. If food sanitation is not maintained, many people can become ill from eating contaminated food.

Antibiotics – drugs that reduce or kill microorganisms
Barrier – something that protects, or separates, a person from an infectious microorganism

Breaking the Chain at the Mode of Transmission Link

Diseases such as gonorrhea, syphilis, and human immunodeficiency virus (HIV) infection are transmitted by direct contact during sexual activity. HIV can also be transmitted through direct contact with the blood of an infected person. There are no vaccines for these diseases. Using barriers such as condoms are one way to break the chain of transmission of sexually transmitted diseases.

Another microorganism transmitted by direct contact is the virus that causes fever blisters or cold sores (herpes simplex virus). For example, you may have a fever blister on your lip. A resident may have chapped lips, with a slight break in the skin. You happen to touch your fever blister with your finger and then give the resident mouth care without putting on gloves. The virus from your fever blister can enter the resident's body through the opening in their skin. Wearing gloves when giving mouth care is one way to break the chain. Another way is using a mouth care sponge with a handle, so that you do not touch the resident's mouth with your fingers.

Airborne transmission can be reduced when the facility has appropriate ventilation and air exchange. Staff also need to recognize when a resident's cough is a symptom of infection and to report this or other symptoms to the nurse. Recognizing and treating airborne diseases at an early stage helps to prevent transmission. These include tuberculosis, measles, and shingles. Masks can be effective if worn properly when a resident or staff member has an infection that may spread by airborne transmission. Later in this chapter you will learn the proper way to wear a mask.

Condom – a thin, flexible covering commonly made of latex rubber, worn over the penis to reduce the risk of pregnancy and susceptibility to or transmission of sexually transmitted diseases
Gonorrhea – contagious bacterial venereal infection that is sexually transmitted
Human immunodeficiency virus (HIV) – viral infection transmitted by contact with blood and other body fluids such as semen and vaginal secretions
Mask – protective covering for the face
Sanitation – the promotion of hygiene and prevention of disease by maintaining clean conditions
Shingles – viral inflammation that affects the nerves in the skull and spine
Syphilis – a chronic, contagious venereal infection that is sexually transmitted

Breaking the Chain at the Susceptible Host Link

People become immune to some microorganisms after one infection. For example, after having chicken pox only once, you have lifetime immunity to this virus. However, other microorganisms can cause infections again and again in the same person because immunity does not occur. This is true for many gastrointestinal diseases.

Breaking the chain at the susceptible host link depends on the microorganisms and the individuals. If a vaccine is available, the best way to protect susceptible hosts is to vaccinate them. **Immunizations** against many diseases can keep you and residents from being susceptible hosts. Vaccinations are commonly used to prevent infection and the spread of infection. Annual flu shots should be given to residents and staff if not contraindicated. CMS currently recommends that all eligible residents be offered an influenza immunization every year and and a pneumococcal immunization every five years.

The best way to protect residents who are susceptible hosts from becoming sick with microorganisms that are already in their bodies is to help them maintain their nutritional status and mobility.

The best ways to protect yourself from infectious diseases are to be immunized against those diseases for which there are vaccines, stay as healthy as you can, use barriers appropriately, and wash your hands often and well.

Table 9-1 summarizes the chain of transmission and ways it can be broken. As you can see, using common sense often breaks the chain of transmission. Many procedures for preventing or controlling infection are not your responsibility alone. All staff must work together to control and prevent infection. Note that handwashing helps break the chain at every link. Handwashing is the single most important thing you can do to prevent or control infection.

Use your common sense and be mindful. Never let infection control activities become routine. Ask yourself these questions if you suspect an infection is present:

1. **Who or what may be infected?** What or who is the source of the infection? The source may be a resident, a staff member, a visitor, or something in the environment. It may include the equipment in the resident's room or a food source.
2. **Who is at risk?** A resident may be more susceptible to infection due to old age or underlying disease. Risk is also increased by treatments with steroids or chemotherapeutic agents, breaks in the skin, and the use of **invasive** devices such as urinary catheters, intravenous catheters, and G-tubes.

TABLE 9-1   BREAKING LINKS IN THE CHAIN OF INFECTION

LINK	HOW THE CHAIN IS BROKEN
Microorganism	Facility cleaning procedures Handwashing
Reservoir	Environmental sanitation Identification and treatment of infections with antibiotics Food sanitation procedures such as cleaning equipment and adequate refrigeration Handwashing
Portal of Exit	Use of barriers like gloves and masks Handwashing
Mode of Transmission	Use of barriers like gloves and masks Handwashing
Portal of Entry	Use of barriers such as gloves, masks, and goggles Proper equipment disinfection Handwashing
Susceptible Host	Immunizations against disease Use of barriers such as gloves and masks Handwashing

3. **How can the microorganism be transmitted?** Microorganisms can be transmitted through all routes. The most common routes in a facility are direct and indirect contact, droplet, and airborne transmission.
4. **What do I need to do to protect residents and myself?** Use barriers, wash your hands between residents and procedures, and change your gloves often. Change gloves between residents and whenever they are contaminated. Promote good nutrition and exercise. Encourage annual influenza and pneumococcal vaccinations.

Immunization – administration of a vaccine to make the person immune (not susceptible) to a specific infection
Invasive – something that enters the body

Handwashing

Note: *Check the sink, soap dispenser, and towel dispenser before beginning. Ask yourself: "Will I contaminate my hands touching these items after I wash my hands?" If your answer is yes, prepare these before you begin.*

1. Remove your watch and roll up your sleeves.

Note: *Minimize the amount of jewelry worn on your fingers and around your wrist.*

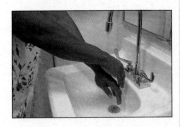

2. Turn on the water to a comfortable temperature. Wet your hands and wrists.

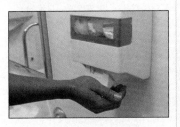

3. Apply soap to your hands.

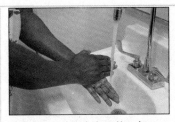

4. Rub your hands together in a circular motion with friction for a minimum of 20 seconds.

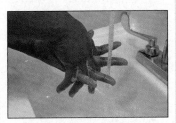

Lace your fingers together to wash in between them). Clean under your fingernails: Use a nail brush or orange stick, or rub your nails briskly in your palm to clean them.

Note: *Because acrylic or silk-wrap (artificial) nails are difficult to clean under and may harbor bacteria, they should not be worn.*

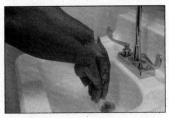

5. Rinse your hands with warm water, keeping them downward, allowing the water to run from the wrist to the fingers.

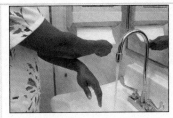

6. Get paper towels from the dispenser.

Note: *If you have to touch the dispenser to remove the towel, you must have the towel ready before you start so you do not contaminate your hands.*

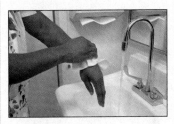

7. Dry your hands with paper towels. Start at the top of the fingers and work downward toward the wrists.

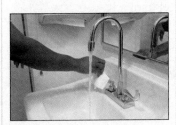

8. Turn off the faucets with a paper towel.

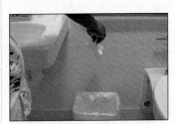

9. Discard paper towels in appropriate receptacle.

Note: *You should use a moisturizing lotion on your hands if they are dry. This will prevent them from cracking.*

No procedure is more important than washing your hands to prevent the transmission of disease and infection. Practice the procedure carefully and consistently.

CLEAN VERSUS DIRTY

To practice infection control, you must also understand the concept of clean versus dirty. If something is considered clean, it remains clean until it is contaminated with something considered dirty. For example, if you wash your hands properly before preparing supplies for bathing a resident, your hands are considered clean. But if you answer a phone call, open the door for someone, or blow your nose, your hands are now considered dirty until you wash them again. The safest approach is to always assume that everything is dirty and needs to be cleaned. This includes a table, a glass, and your hands. Keep the concept of clean versus dirty in mind at all times. This awareness will help decrease the spread of germs that could be harmful both to you and residents.

TREATMENT-RESISTANT MICRO-ORGANISMS

Antibiotic-resistant microorganisms are among the most serious threats in any health care facility. These resistant microorganisms cause infections that cannot be managed with usual forms of treatment. These infections are very serious especially in older or medically compromised residents.

Following are some of the most common threats to long term care residents:

1. Clostridium difficile (C. diff): This bacteria causes a form of diarrhea in patients after antibiotic use. It is classified by the Center for Disease Control (CDC) as a severe threat due to the number of people who are affected and the severity of the symptoms.

2. Methicillin-resistant Staphylococcus aureus (MRSA): This bacteria causes a range of illnesses from skin and wound infections to pneumonia and bloodstream infections that can cause sepsis and even death.

3. Vacomycin-resistant Enterococcus (VRE): This bacteria can cause a range of illnesses, usually among patients in health care facilities. The illnesses include bloodstream infections, surgical site infections, and urinary tract infections.

These infections are hard to treat and can be fatal. As a nurse assistant, you must make sure that you follow all isolation and protection policies within your facility. The CDC issues guidelines for long term care facilities to follow to prevent and control the spread of each type of treatment-resistant infection.

Of the many treatment-resistant microorganisms, the examples above are the most common in long term care settings. You are likely to encounter many such infections in your career. Prevention is always the best way to control the spread of infection. Daily use of proper infection control practices is the best defense for both you and your residents.

HANDWASHING

Every facility has readily accessible handwashing areas. Wash your hands with soap and lukewarm running water immediately before and after all care procedures. Proper handwashing is needed to cleanse the skin of contamination by potentially infectious microorganisms.

When soap and water are not available for washing your hands or other body areas, use an alcohol-based hand cleanser and rub your hands thoroughly until they are dry.

Wash your hands before putting on gloves and immediately after removing gloves or other personal protective equipment. If you come in contact with blood or other potentially infectious materials, immediately wash your hands and the affected skin areas with soap and water. If your mucous membranes (such as your eyes or inside your nose or mouth) are splashed with blood or fluid, flush the area with water immediately. Such contact may occur from the splattering of fluids, such as when you are emptying a urinary drainage bag or rinsing a bedpan.

Note: *Recent studies have shown that more bacteria are present under longer fingernails. The Centers for Disease Control and Prevention (CDC) recommends nails should be no longer than one fourth of an inch. Acrylic and silk nails harbor more bacteria and should not be worn. Chipped nail polish also allows more bacteria than freshly painted nails. All of these situations are more likely to transmit germs to residents.*

It is also recommended to reduce the amount of jewelry you wear on your fingers and around your wrist.

Almost anytime is a good time to wash your hands at work. But at certain times we must all wash our hands:

- before and after each shift worked
- before and after every resident contact
- between different care activities (after helping the resident toilet and before helping with the bath)
- after using the bathroom
- before and after handling food
- after handling anything you think is contaminated (dirty)
- after contact with blood or body fluids
- before and after cleaning an area
- before and after handling body fluids collected for testing

PUTTING ON AND REMOVING GLOVES

Putting on Gloves

1. Wash your hands.

2. Slip gloves on, covering your entire hand and wrist.

Note: *If you are putting on gloves along with a gown and mask, put the gown on first, then the mask, and then the gloves. Pull the gloves up over the gown's cuffs.*

Remove the gloves after you complete the task. Remove them as described below if you are right-handed. If you are left-handed, use the opposite hand from the one described in each of these steps.

Removing Gloves

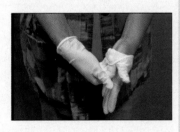

1. Using your right hand, grasp the glove on the left hand at the inside of the wrist, turning the glove inside out as you pull it down over your left hand.

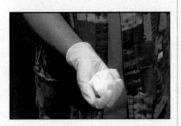

2. Hold the used left glove in a ball in your gloved right hand.

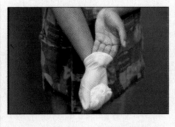

3. Grasp the inside of the right glove at the top of the wrist with your left hand.

Note: *If you are wearing fitted, sterile gloves, you will not be able to grasp the inside of the top of the right glove, so you must cuff (fold over) the top of the right glove before you begin to remove the glove.*

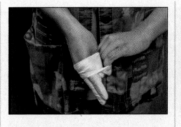

4. Pull the right glove down over your right hand and over the used glove held in that hand. The right glove is now inside out, with the left glove enclosed in it.

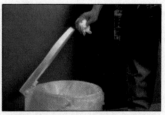

5. Dispose of the gloves in the trashcan. Follow your facility's infection control policies to dispose of soiled waste.

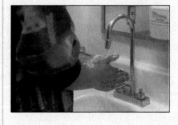

6. Wash your hands.

- after smoking a cigarette
- before putting on gloves
- after removing gloves
- after covering a cough or sneeze
- after blowing your nose

USING BARRIERS

Barriers include gloves, gowns or plastic aprons, masks, and eye protection. Barriers do not replace handwashing but should be used along with handwashing. Barriers protect your hands, skin, clothing, eyes, and mucous membranes from microorganisms that may be in a resident's secretions or excretions. They also protect residents from microorganisms that may be on your hands, skin, or clothing.

Gloves

Putting On and Removing Gloves. If you are using gloves without any other barrier, put them on immediately

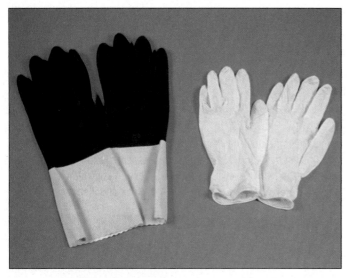

Fig. 9-6 – When cleaning, heavy utility gloves should be worn rather than single-use gloves.

before your hands come into contact with broken skin or mucous membranes. Put on gloves anytime you need a barrier between you and a resident's secretions or excretions. Follow these steps for putting on gloves:

You usually use single-use disposable gloves. Gloves are made from different materials. Most gloves are made of latex, but vinyl or other non-latex gloves are available for people who are allergic to latex. These gloves are pack-

aged as clean, not sterile.

Some types of gloves fit better than others. Your facility will have various sizes of gloves. Good-fitting gloves are needed for fine motor skills. Most of the time, you do not need sterile gloves or tight-fitting gloves.

Change your gloves and wash your hands before caring for each resident. Change your gloves and wash your hands anytime the gloves become visibly contaminated.

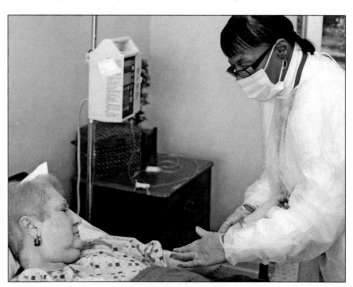

Fig. 9-7 – A plastic apron helps protect the front of your clothing from contamination.

Wash your hands after removing gloves because they may become contaminated from small defects in the gloves, from tears in the gloves during use, or from when removing the gloves. This helps prevent carrying potentially infectious microorganisms from one resident to another or contaminating the resident's environment, such as the call light or bed rail. You must also change your gloves when moving from a contaminated body site to a clean one. For example if you remove the resident from a bedpan and then give them a bath, you must change your gloves.

When you clean equipment or surfaces like a bedside table, you should wear heavy utility gloves rather than single-use clean disposable gloves (Fig. 9-6). The chemicals in cleaning solutions may irritate your hands, and heavy utili-

📖

Secretions – substances such as saliva, mucus, perspiration, tears, etc. that come out of the body

ty gloves protect you better. You can reuse utility gloves for cleaning unless they are cracked or worn out, just as you reuse similar gloves at home.

Whenever you are about to care for a resident, ask yourself, "Will my hands touch something wet or moist?" If the answer is yes, then you need to wear gloves. You may also wear other protective equipment, especially if there is a risk of a spill or splash. Always discuss the situation with the charge nurse if you are not sure what to do. Wash your hands whenever you touch something moist and after you remove your gloves.

Gowns and Plastic Aprons

A gown is a barrier covering your skin and clothing. Gowns are made of cloth, paper, or plastic. Follow your facility's policy for when to wear a gown. In individual situations you may have to judge yourself when you need a gown to protect your skin and clothing from a resident's secretions or excretions. Plastic aprons are barriers that cover the front of your clothing (Fig. 9-7).

They are particularly useful if your clothing may get wet, such as when you are helping a resident to bathe. Plastic aprons are also useful when changing soiled linen that cannot easily be folded on itself to contain the soilage.

Microorganisms are not easily transmitted by clothing. Nurse assistants do not "carry germs home" to their family on their clothing. No one likes to wear soiled or dirty clothing, however, and gowns and aprons help to keep your clothing clean.

Gowns. If you are using gloves and a gown, put on the gown first. Then put on gloves as described earlier. Remove the gown after completing your task with the resident.

Disposable Plastic Aprons. Disposable plastic aprons usually have a neck strap and ties at the waist. They do not protect your arms. To put on a plastic apron, slip the strap over your head and tie the waist ties. The apron keeps the front of your clothes clean and dry.

Remove a plastic apron by first untying the waist ties and pulling the neck strap over your head. Then roll the apron into a ball with the contaminated surface on the inside, similar to removing a gown. Discard a disposable apron in the trash. Wash your hands.

If you are wearing both gloves and a plastic apron, put on the apron first, then the gloves. Remove the gloves first, then the apron. Wash your hands.

Putting on a Gown

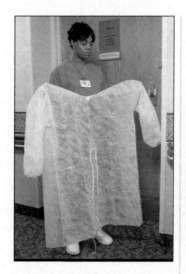

1. Open the gown.

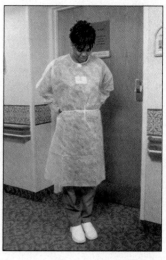

3. Tie the gown at your neck and waist.

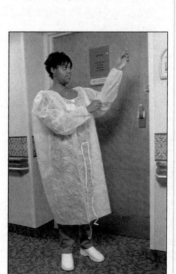

2. Put your arms in the gown's sleeves, with the opening in the back.

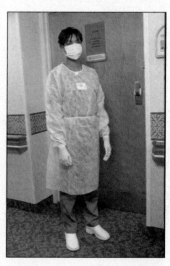

4. Then put on your gloves and pull the gloves up over the gown's cuffs.

Removing a Gown

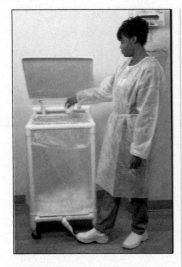

1. Remove your gloves first and dispose of them properly.

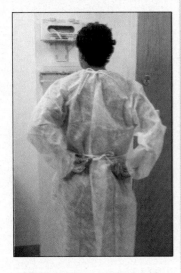

2. Untie the gown at your neck and waist.

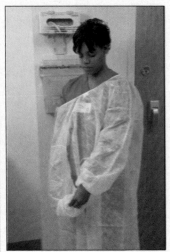

3. Grasp the cuff of one of the sleeves and pull the sleeve down over that hand.

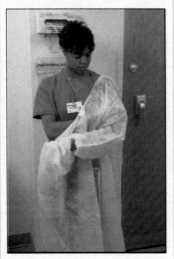

4. Pull the other sleeve off with your covered hand.

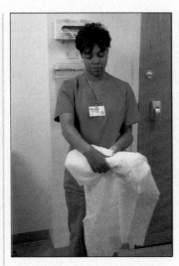

5. Carefully roll the gown up, keeping the soiled surface inside.

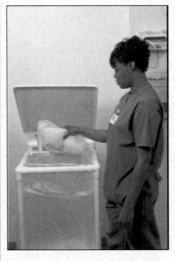

Note: *With a cloth gown that will be laundered, put it in the appropriate linen hamper. Put a disposable paper gown in the trashcan, following your facility's policy. In most states, gowns are thrown out as regular waste.*

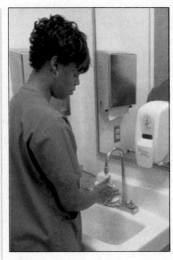

6. Wash your hands.

Masks

Masks protect the mucous membranes of the mouth and nose from splashes. Masks are an effective barrier to splashes or splatters (Fig. 9-8). You do few tasks, however, that might result in the splashing or splattering of your face, nose, and mouth.

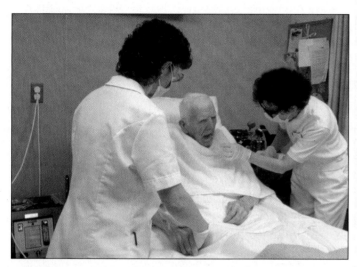

Fig. 9-8 – Masks can protect the mouth and nose from splashes.

A mask also protects against inhaling droplets in the air. The mask must fit tightly so that you do not inhale air easily around the sides of the mask. If you will be spending a long time with the resident, change your mask every 20 minutes. Change it sooner if it becomes moist.

Masks are used in the operating room to protect surgical patients from microorganisms in the staffs' respiratory secretions. Very few situations in long term care facilities require wearing a mask to protect residents from you. Although some people believe you should wear a mask if you have a cold, cold viruses are actually transmitted more often by the hands. Wear a mask to protect residents from droplets if you have a cold with a cough. Handwashing is the best way to prevent spreading the common cold.

Although there are different kinds of masks, all have a metal bar on the bridge of the nose and ties, straps, or elastic to secure the mask. Follow the correct steps for putting on the mask.

If you are wearing a mask, gloves, and a gown or apron, put on the gown or apron first. Then put on the mask, and put on the gloves last. Remove the gloves first, then the gown or apron, and then the mask. Wash your hands after you have removed all these barriers.

Putting on a Mask

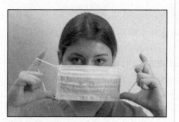

1. Put the mask over your nose and mouth.

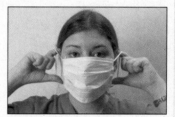

2. Tie or secure the straps around your ears or the back of your head so that the mask fits tightly.

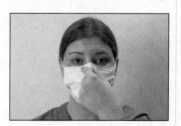

3. Pinch the metal piece on the bridge of the nose to make a tight seal.

Removing a Mask

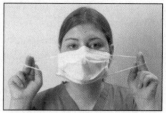

1. Remove the mask by untying the ties or pulling the straps over your ears or head.

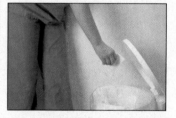

2. Fold the outside edges of the mask together, keeping the soiled sides together. Dispose of the mask in the trash, following your facility's policy.

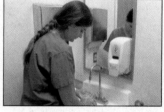

3. Wash your hands.

Eye Protection

Goggles or glasses with side shields protect the eyes from splashes and splatters. As you will learn in Chapter 10, the OSHA Bloodborne Pathogens Standard requires using a mask and eye protection together if splashing or splattering of the face is likely (Fig. 9-9). Very rarely will you be in situations requiring this protection.

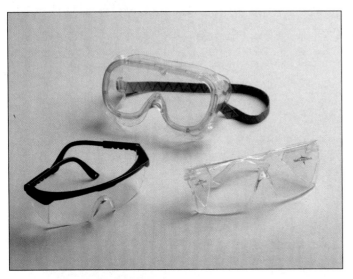

Fig. 9-9 – Goggles protect the eyes from splashes or splatters.

If you wear eyeglasses and want to use them for splash protection, they must have side shields to protect against splashing from the side. Side shields are devices that add to your glasses. Then you do not have to remove your glasses or wear goggles over them when doing a task where splashing is likely. The infection control practitioner in your facility can help you find the correct side shields for your glasses.

If you do not wear glasses and need eye protection for a task, use goggles or a face shield. Goggles can be washed, dried, and reused. Most face shields can also be washed, dried, and reused. Some manufacturers make a single-use combination mask and eye protection shield. These shields can be worn over corrective eyeglasses and protect against splashes from the front and sides.

If you are using eye protection and a mask along with a gown or plastic apron and gloves, put on the eye protection when you put on the mask. Remove it when you remove the mask. As always, wash your hands after you remove all barriers.

Wastes Requiring Special Handling

Different terms are used to designate wastes that require special handling. These include regulated waste, infectious or infective waste, biohazardous waste, and special waste. All states have regulations about wastes contaminated with blood or secretions and excretions.

Waste regulations differ from state to state and from city to city. Your infection control practitioner will tell you about your facility's procedures for waste.

ISOLATION PRECAUTIONS

Isolation precautions are things a facility does to keep microorganisms from spreading from one resident to others. Isolation precautions involve many different practices in long term care facilities. These are usually described in the facility's infection control manual or isolation manual (Fig. 9-10). The infection control practitioner will teach you how to use the facility's isolation precautions system.

The CDC has specific recommendations for isolation precautions. In addition to the standard precautions described in Chapter 10, the CDC recommends using transmission-based precautions for residents who are known (or suspected) to be infected with highly transmissible pathogens.

📖

Biohazardous – anything that is harmful or potentially harmful to humans or the environment; contaminated material

Isolation – set apart from others

Transmission-Based Precautions

Transmission-based precautions are used along with standard precautions. There are three types:
- airborne precautions
- droplet precautions
- contact precautions

Airborne Precautions.   In addition to using standard precautions, use airborne precautions for residents who are known (or suspected) to be infected with microorganisms transmitted by airborne droplets that remain suspended in the air and that can be dispersed (spread) by air currents. For example, this precaution is used for a resident with active tuberculosis (Fig. 9-11). This is the suggested procedure:

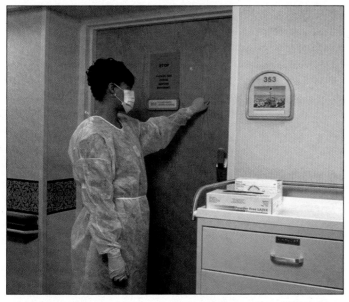

Fig. 9-10 – Use proper infection control procedures when caring for an infectious resident.

1. Place the resident in a private room with a special ventilation system. Keep the room door closed.
2. Wear a special mask, which has been fit-tested for you, as respiratory protection when entering the room. The charge nurse will explain these precautions to you.
3. Limit the number of times that the resident is taken into and out of the room. Place a mask on the resident when they are taken out of the room.

Droplet Precautions.   In addition to standard precautions, use droplet precautions for residents who are known (or suspected) to be infected with microorganisms transmitted by droplets produced by coughing, sneezing, talking, or performing procedures. For example, this precaution would be used if there was a flu outbreak. This is the suggested procedure:
1. Place the resident in a private room.

Note: *When a private room is not available, the infected resident should be separated by at least three feet from other residents and visitors. Special ventilation and air exchange are not necessary.*

2. The door may remain open.
3. Wear a mask when you are working within three feet of the resident.
4. Transport the resident from the room only for essential purposes. Place a mask on the resident when they are transported from the room.

Contact Precautions.   In addition to standard precautions, use contact precautions for residents known (or suspected) to be infected with microorganisms that can be transmitted by direct or indirect contact. Transmission can occur when you perform care activities involving hand or skin contact. Transmission can also occur by indirect contact. This includes touching environmental surfaces or items in the resident's room that have been contaminated. For example, use this precaution with a resident with a draining wound. This is the suggested procedure:
1. Place the resident in a private room if possible. If a private room is not available, the infected resident should be separated from other residents and visitors by at least 3 feet. Special ventilation and air exchange are not necessary.
2. Put on gloves as soon as you enter the room. When giving care, change your gloves if they are visibly contaminated with infective material before you start another task with that resident. Remove the gloves before leaving the room. Wash your hands immediately with an antimicrobial agent or a waterless antiseptic agent. After handwashing, do not touch potentially contaminated environmental surfaces or items in the room.
3. Wear a gown when entering the room if your clothing may contact the resident, environmental surfaces, or

Outbreak – sudden, dramatic increase in cases of a particular disease or harmful organisms

items in the room. Also wear a gown if the resident is incontinent, has diarrhea, or has wound drainage that has not been contained by a dressing. Remove the gown before leaving the room. Then make sure that your clothing does not contact potentially contaminated environmental surfaces.

4. Move or transport the resident from the room only if needed. Do not share equipment between residents. If an item must be used elsewhere or for another resident, properly clean and disinfect it first.

Applying Isolation Precautions

You should be familiar with the isolation precautions used in your facility. Be consistent in using these precautions with resident care. Talk to the charge nurse about isolation precautions to be sure you understand the correct way to do things. Following is an example of how a facility would handle a certain infection.

Tuberculosis (TB) is caused by bacteria. When TB bacteria are coughed into the air by a person with pulmonary tuberculosis, some of them stay in the air in very tiny droplets. If you inhale these droplets, you can become infected with tuberculosis bacteria. Therefore, the facility would add airborne precautions to the standard precautions.

Residents with active pulmonary tuberculosis are usually transferred to acute care facilities for treatment. But a resident who is still infectious may return to the long term care facility if it can provide adequate care. However, this resident requires a private room with special ventilation.

If you are caring for a resident who is still infectious with tuberculosis, keep the door closed at all times. Wear respiratory protection whenever you enter the room. Teach the resident to cover their nose and mouth with a tissue when they cough, and to discard those tissues in the appropriate container.

Psychosocial Needs of Residents on Isolation Precautions

A resident on isolation precautions may have to be confined to their room but can still have visitors and social stimulation (Fig 9-12, next page). Residents who are not allowed to leave their rooms may feel they have done something wrong or are being punished. Help them understand how germs are spread. Explain that the situation is only temporary and when they are better they will no longer be in isolation, as in this example:

Mrs. Henderson developed an intestinal obstruction in the facility. She is transferred to an acute care hospital for abdominal surgery and develops a post-operative wound infection. The physician starts treatment with intravenous antibiotics in the hospital, and her wound begins to heal. As she improves, her treatment changes to oral antibiotics. She returns to the facility five days after surgery. Her abdominal wound is still draining so she is put on contact precautions.

Because of Mrs. Henderson's wound infection, she may need a private room. Caregivers wear gloves when caring for her wound and also a gown, if soiling of clothing is likely. They wash their hands before and after care and when they take off their gloves.

You are taking care of Mrs. Henderson. She has been on oral antibiotics for three days. Her wound is almost completely healed, and she is feeling much better. She would like to go to the dining room for dinner. Her healing wound is completely covered with a dressing that contains the drainage, and she wants to put on regular clothing. Is there any reason why Mrs. Henderson should not be permitted to go to the dining room?

You discuss the situation with the charge nurse, who must determine whether Mrs. Henderson presents a risk to anyone in the dining room. Because her wound drainage is completely contained in the dressing and there is no portal of exit for the microorganisms, the nurse decides that eating in the dining room will be beneficial for Mrs. Henderson. She can visit with other residents and will feel much better. You then help her get dressed and encourage her to eat a good dinner because good nutrition contributes to wound healing.

Only rarely are long term care facility residents confined to their rooms with restrictions on visitors. However, this may happen with pulmonary tuberculosis, as described earlier. Confinement can be very disorienting for an elderly person, particularly if they are cognitively impaired. Explain to the resident and family why the resident must stay in the room and for how long. Help them understand that it is not punishment. Provide as much mental stimulation as possible through activities the resident enjoys.

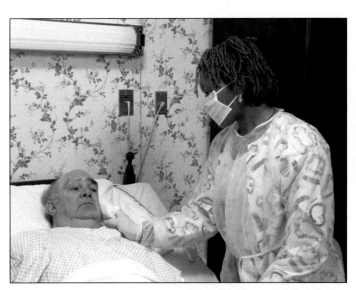

Fig. 9-11 – Spending time with a resident in isolation is important so they do not feel alone.

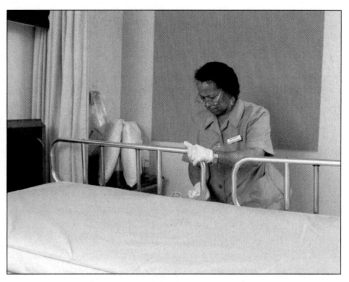

Fig. 9-12 – After a resident is discharged, the housekeeper will thoroughly clean the resident's room.

CLEANING, DISINFECTION, AND STERILIZATION

Cleaning

Cleaning is the removal of soil from objects. Water, detergent, and scrubbing are used to clean things. Cleaning helps control and prevent infection and keeps the environment pleasant and free of odors, dust, and dirt.

The facility's housekeepers regularly clean floors, carpets, walls, and large items. They also clean drapes, curtain dividers, and furniture as needed. When a resident is discharged, housekeepers may thoroughly clean the bed, chairs, overbed and bedside tables, and the entire room. Then the environment is clean and attractive for the next resident (Fig. 9-13).

In some facilities, nurse assistants clean the resident's immediate environment during daily care activities. Be sure you know which staff member is responsible for cleaning certain objects in residents' rooms. For example, know who cares for tabletop items and discards them after use.

Disinfection

Disinfection is a process that eliminates virtually all microorganisms on objects. Disinfection usually involves special chemicals, sometimes combined with a detergent. The detergent or disinfectant is used for general cleaning of objects such as overbed tables, side rails, and plastic-covered mattresses. When you use a disinfectant, wear gloves to protect your hands from being burned or damaged. If your skin comes in contact with any disinfectant, consult the **material safety data sheets (MSDS)** for what action to take (see Chapter 10, Personal Injury Prevention and Protection).

Sterilization

Sterilization is the complete elimination of all microorganisms from an object. Many items used for resident care come in a sterile condition or are disposable. This includes gauze pads, surgical supplies, urinary catheters, needles used to give injections, and bags of fluid used for intravascular (IV) therapy.

An autoclave is a machine used to sterilize things such as surgical instruments and operating room supplies with pressurized steam (Fig. 9-14, next page). Objects that cannot be steam heated are sterilized with ethylene oxide gas. Other chemicals may also be used to kill all microorganisms.

Material safety data sheets (MSDS) – written information sheets describing chemicals used in a facility

Sterilization – elimination or destruction of all microbial life

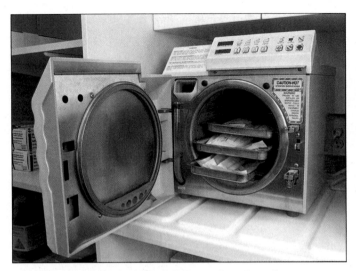

Fig. 9-13 – An autoclave sterilizes instruments and supplies.

Designated Clean and Dirty Areas of the Facility

Most facilities have designated clean and dirty utility rooms or other areas. These are used to separate clean and dirty supplies, equipment, and functions. Clean utility rooms are used to store supplies such as bandages and tape, dressings, urinary catheters and tubing, bed-saver pads, bottles of irrigation fluid, irrigation sets, feeding tubes and supplies, bedside kits (with wash basin, water pitcher, cup, and **emesis** basin), and other clean supplies (Fig. 9-15). Some supplies for a resident may also be stored in their room if there is enough space.

All objects and supplies that have been used by a resident or caregiver are considered dirty. Some used supplies, such as soiled dressings or bed-saver pads, are disposable. These may be discarded in an appropriate trashcan. Other supplies will be reused after being cleaned. Follow your facility's policy for cleaning reusable supplies. When you take a piece of dirty equipment (like a used bedpan) to the dirty utility room to be cleaned, always wear gloves (Fig. 9-16, next page). Most dirty utility rooms or areas have a deep flushing sink similar to a toilet. Liquid wastes can be poured into this sink and go directly into a sanitary sewer system. Then return the clean bedpan to the resident's bedside or bathroom. Many dirty utility areas also have waste receptacles for the disposal of sharps containers and other regulated wastes. This may be called "red-bagged trash." You must know the regulations for all of these types of wastes in your facility, because regulations vary from state to state.

Some cleaning functions can be done in the resident's bathroom. You may use the toilet to empty bedpans,

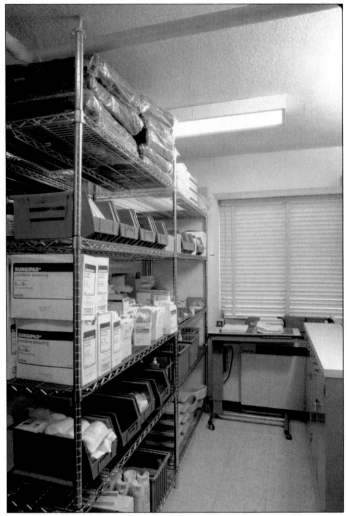

Fig. 9-14 – Clean utility rooms are used to store clean supplies.

urinals, and emesis basins. Bedpans can be rinsed in the bathroom if the toilet has a pull-down lever or spray cleaning device. Bedpans should not be washed in the same sink that you or the resident use for handwashing or brushing teeth. Stool from bedpans can contaminate the sink with microorganisms, which can then later contaminate your hands or other items that you or other people use. If these microorganisms from contaminated hands reach a person's mouth, they may cause gastrointestinal illness.

📖

Emesis – related to vomiting, as in an emesis basin

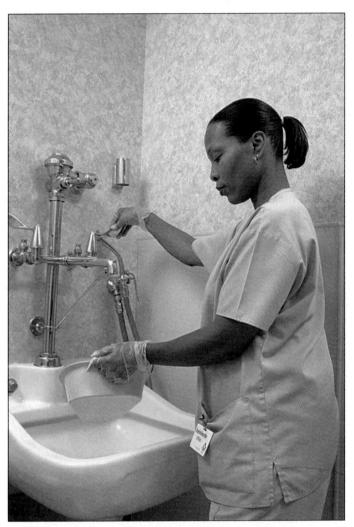

Fig. 9-15 — Always protect yourself when cleaning used items.

IN THIS CHAPTER YOU LEARNED:

- How microorganisms are transmitted
- How to wash your hands properly
- The proper way to put on and remove gowns, aprons, gloves, masks, and eye protection
- How to follow your facility's policies and procedures for isolation precautions
- Your role in cleaning objects and disposing of items in the resident's environment

SUMMARY

Your role role in preventing and controlling infection is very important. Knowing how microorganisms cause infection and are transmitted helps you prevent infection. Many methods are used to prevent and control infection. The single most effective method is handwashing. Other methods include barriers such as gowns, gloves, masks, and goggles. Isolation is sometimes important to protect the resident and others by helping reduce the spread of infection. You have a valuable role in supporting a resident in isolation. Finally, you must always work to maintain a clean environment.

PULLING IT ALL TOGETHER

A pandemic is a global disease outbreak. Today, with so many people traveling around the world, it is hard to keep outbreaks within a localized area. For example, you have probably heard of outbreaks of the Asian flu in the United States. The virus may have originated in Asia but was carried to the United States. Such an outbreak can spread like wildfire. The principles you have learned in this chapter will help you, your family, and your residents stay as healthy as possible. Use your common sense and the infection control principles, and you will be successful.

1. **In the chain of infection, a microorganism leaves an infected person through:**
    A. The reservoir.
    B. The portal of exit.
    C. The portal of entry.
    D. Direct transmission.

2. **You can help to break the chain of infection at each link by:**
    A. Sterilizing all bed linen every morning.
    B. Disinfecting all surfaces.
    C. Wearing a gown and protective eyewear at all times.
    D. Washing your hands before and after every contact with a resident.

3. **Which type of infection can be transmitted through the air?**
    A. Syphilis.
    B. Hepatitis.
    C. HIV.
    D. Tuberculosis.

4. **What is the minimum amount of time required to wash your hands?**
    A. 5 seconds.
    B. 10 seconds.
    C. 20 seconds.
    D. Until they appeat clean.

5. **If you are putting on gloves along with a gown and mask, in what order do you put them on?**
    A. Gloves, gown, mask.
    B. Gloves, mask, gown.
    C. Gown, mask, gloves.
    D. The order does not matter.

6. **When a resident with an infection is on contact precautions, you should:**
    A. Never allow any visitors under any circumstances.
    B. Request that the charge nurse provide all care.
    C. Wear gloves when providing care.
    D. Install a special air ventilation system.

7. **Disinfecting contaminated equipment results in:**
    A. Complete elimination of all microorganisms.
    B. Elimination of most microorganisms.
    C. Elimination of bacteria only.
    D. Elimination of viruses only.

8. **How should you dispose of a red bag that has a biohazard label?**
    A. Dispose of it with all other bags of trash.
    B. Leave it in the hallway outside the resident's room to be picked up later.
    C. Follow your facility's procedure.
    D. Dispose of it in the kitchen's trashcans.

9. **Which of the following items is stored in the facility's clean utility room?**
    A. Dirty laundry is stored there until the laundry service picks it up.
    B. Used bed pans are left there temporarily as long as they are on the floor.
    C. Used bed saver pads are stored there for use again with the same resident.
    D. Clean and sterile resident care equipment and supplies.

10. **What is a pandemic?**
    A. When many people call in sick.
    B. When many people in the facility get the flu.
    C. When many people in your family are sick.
    D. When many people in the world get sick.

(Answers to "Check What You've Learned" are in the Instructor's Manual.)

Chapter 10

PERSONAL PROTECTION AND INJURY PREVENTION

Nursing staff often have musculoskeletal problems caused by on-the-job injuries. These injuries result from caregiving tasks. The health care industry spends billions of dollars related to these injuries. But occupational injuries can be prevented if staff use common sense and follow guidelines for working safely with residents.

Being mindful about preventing injuries in the workplace will improve the quality of your work. This improves the quality of care you give residents. Although some staff members try to do everything by themselves, that may put them at risk for injury. All caregivers should ask themselves three questions before beginning any task. "Am I at risk for exposure to any bodily fluid?" "Is there a better way to do this?" and "What equipment do I need to do the task safely?"

This chapter begins by discussing how to protect yourself from bloodborne pathogens. This is a critical issue in all health care settings. You will also learn what you need to know to do your job safely—how to prevent injuries to yourself and residents. You will learn about ergonomics and common sense rules to follow to prevent injuries. You will learn how to prevent resident falls. Your role in facility injury prevention programs will be described. You will also learn about chemical and electrical hazards and how to be prepared for possible disasters.

OBJECTIVES
- Explain standard precautions
- Define the OSHA Bloodborne Pathogens Standard
- Define ergonomics
- List at least 10 common-sense rules for preventing injury
- Demonstrate good body mechanics
- Describe how to prevent resident falls
- Discuss your role in preventing injuries in the long term care environment
- Describe your role in disaster preparedness

MEDICAL TERMS
- **Antibody** – type of protein that the body produces to fight infection or illness
- **Biceps** – strong arm muscles used for lifting
- **Hepatitis** – infection or inflammation of the liver
- **Insulin** – hormone involved in breaking down carbohydrates in the body; it can be given as a shot to control diabetes
- **Standard precautions** – activities based on recommendations of CDC for facilities to use in handling blood, body fluids, secretions, excretions (except sweat), nonintact skin such as cuts and wounds, and mucous membranes to prevent infection

"I need your strength to help me. Please take good care of yourself and keep us both safe from injury."

earning something new does not automatically make a positive difference in your life. You have to apply the information. We all know the importance of seat belts, for example. But have you ever been in a hurry to get somewhere? Did you ever drive off without fastening your seat belt because you were going only a block or two? Often people take shortcuts and skip important safety steps. But what if someone hits your car that one time you're not using your seat belt?

We all know that we should wear seat belts, brush our teeth, look both ways before crossing the street, and limit the fats and sugar we eat (Fig. 10-1). But do we always follow these simple rules of healthy living? Sometimes we just think, "It won't happen to me." Ignoring common sense may not have immediate consequences. Having a second bowl of ice cream just once won't make you overweight. But some actions, like not wearing your seat belt, can lead to pain, suffering, and injury to yourself or others. Bad things won't happen because of every unwise or thoughtless choice, but when they do happen, all the wishing in the world cannot undo the bad results.

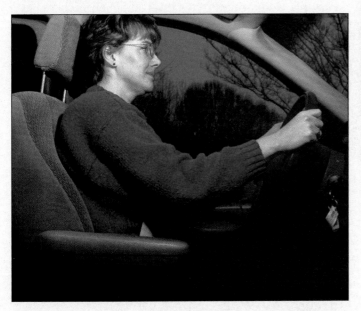

Fig. 10-1 – Using common sense rules for safety, such as wearing a seatbelt, can prevent or minimize injuries.

Ensuring safety for yourself and residents is your most important role as a nurse assistant. Usually only a little extra effort is needed to prevent accidents and injuries. Most of the time you need only be mindful in your actions, and use common sense and the right equipment to prevent injuries.

PROTECTING YOURSELF FROM BLOODBORNE INFECTIONS

Several different viruses can live in people's blood, even when the person does not appear to be sick. Health care providers are most concerned about the hepatitis B virus (HBV), the hepatitis C virus (HCV), and the human immunodeficiency virus (HIV).

Standard Precautions

To prevent transmission of these bloodborne viruses and other infectious diseases, the Centers for Disease Control and Prevention (CDC) developed standard precautions. All health care staff must use these whenever they will have possible contact with another person's body fluids (Fig.10-2). Body fluids include blood, secretions, excretions (except sweat), nonintact skin such as cuts and wounds, and the mucous membranes. Standard precautions are an approach to infection control and prevention.

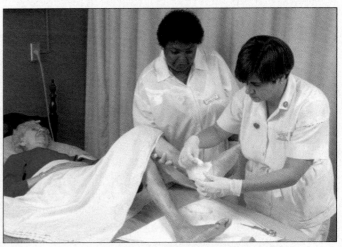

Fig. 10-2 – Wear gloves when changing a resident's dressing.

Hepatitis – infection or inflammation of the liver
Standard precautions – activities based on recommendations of CDC for facilities to use in handling blood, body fluids, secretions, excretions (except sweat), nonintact skin such as cuts and wounds, and mucous membranes to prevent infection

The goal of standard precautions is to reduce the risk of transmission of microorganisms from both recognized and unrecognized sources. This means that you use the same precautions around someone you think is healthy as you would use around someone who is known to have a bloodborne virus. You should assume that all human beings and their blood, body fluids, wounds, and mucous membranes may be infected. You cannot know for certain that any person does not carry a bloodborne virus.

Standard precautions include many work practices that minimize or eliminate your exposure to pathogens. Information you learned in Chapter 9 about preventing infection transmission is a part of standard precaution practices. This includes handwashing and the use of barriers. Standard precautions are summarized in the next sections.

Handwashing
- Wash your hands after touching blood, body fluids, secretions, excretions, and contaminated items.
- Wash your hands after removing gloves, between resident contacts, and between tasks if your hands become contaminated.
- Use plain soap and water to wash.
- Use an antimicrobial agent or a waterless antiseptic agent in certain situations as directed by the facility.

Gloves
- Wear gloves when touching blood, body fluids, secretions, excretions, or contaminated items.
- Wear gloves when touching mucous membranes or broken (nonintact) skin.
- Change gloves between tasks, before giving care to another resident, and before touching noncontaminated items and environmental surfaces.

Mask, Eye Protection, and Face Shield
- Wear a mask and eye protection or face shield to protect mucous membranes of your eyes, nose, and mouth during tasks and activities that are likely to involve splashes or sprays of blood, body fluids, secretions, or excretions. For example, use these when emptying a Foley catheter drainage bag or assisting a nurse with suctioning a resident.

Gown
- Wear a gown (a clean, nonsterile gown is adequate) to protect your skin and prevent soiling of your clothing while you are performing tasks and activities that may splash or spray you with blood, body fluids, secretions,

or excretions. For example, wear a gown when a resident has diarrhea, is vomiting, or has large amounts of drainage from a wound.
- Remove a soiled gown as soon as possible.

Resident Care Equipment
- Handle equipment that has been soiled with blood, body fluids, secretions, or excretions in a manner that prevents contact with your skin and mucous membranes or contamination of your clothing. At a minimum, wear gloves and gown.
- If splashing or splattering may occur, also wear a mask and eye protection when handling equipment.
- Ensure that reusable equipment is not used for the care of another resident until it has been cleaned and disinfected appropriately.
- Ensure that disposable (single-use) items are disposed of properly.

Environmental Control
- Know your facility's procedures for the routine care, cleaning, and disinfecting of environmental surfaces, beds, bedrails, bedside equipment, and other frequently touched surfaces.

Linen
- Handle used linen that has been soiled with blood, body fluids, secretions, or excretions in a manner that prevents exposure of your skin and mucous membranes or contamination of your clothing. At a minimum, wear gloves. Always carry linen by holding it away from your uniform, even if it is not visibly soiled.
- If the linen is very wet, also wear a gown (Fig. 10-3, next page).

Occupational Health and Bloodborne Pathogens
- Take care to prevent injuries from needles and other sharp instruments like razors. An injury may occur when handling sharp instruments after procedures, when cleaning used instruments, or when disposing of used needles.
- Never recap (put a cap back on) used needles (Fig. 10-4, next page).
- Use needles with attached safety devices.

Exposure – a condition of being in direct or indirect contact with an infectious microorganism

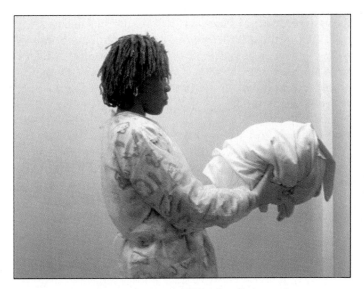

Fig. 10-3 – Wear gloves and a gown if linen is soiled or wet.

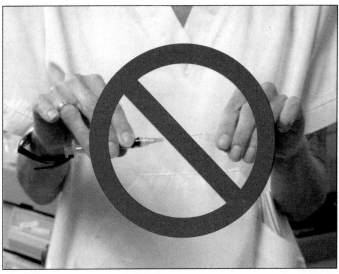

Fig. 10-4 – Never recap a needle.

- Place used disposable syringes and needles and other sharp items in appropriate puncture-resistant containers located near the area where the items are used (Fig. 10-5).
- Have mouthpieces or resuscitation bags available in areas where there is a likely need for resuscitation, so you can avoid giving mouth-to-mouth resuscitation. If mouth-to-mouth resuscitation must be given, use appropriate barrier protection.

Resident Placement
- If a resident frequently contaminates the environment or does not (or cannot) help maintain appropriate hygiene or environmental control, they should be placed in a private room.

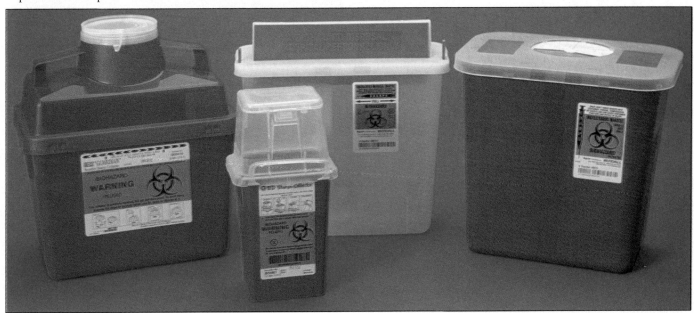

Fig. 10-5 – Discard needles and other sharps in a proper puncture-resistant container.

The OSHA Bloodborne Pathogens Standard

The Occupational Safety and Health Administration (OSHA) Bloodborne Pathogens Standard requires all health care agencies, including long term care facilities, to follow the CDC standard precautions for bloodborne pathogens. In addition, there are several other requirements, which are described in the following sections.

Prevention of Needlesticks. Microorganisms in the blood of one person can enter another person's body through an accidental needlestick injury. Consider this example:

The nurse has just given Ms. Anderson an **insulin** injection. Ms. Johnson, her roommate, faints and falls out of bed just as the nurse removes the needle from Ms. Anderson's skin. The nurse quickly puts the needle and syringe down by Ms. Anderson's pillow and rushes over to help Ms. Johnson.

You are in the hallway and hear Ms. Johnson fall. You come into the room to see if the nurse needs help. You notice Ms. Anderson is very concerned about her roommate's fall. You go over to comfort her. You do not see the needle and syringe by the pillow until you feel a prick in your arm as you adjust Ms. Anderson's pillow.

The needle is an intermediate object that can transfer the resident's blood to you through your skin. If Ms. Anderson has microorganisms in her blood, the needlestick could transfer them to you. If a needlestick ever happens, you must follow the facility's policy for evaluation and follow-up.

Of course, you and the nurse know that the nurse should have discarded the needle and syringe immediately in a needle disposal container. However, Ms. Johnson's fall distracted her, and Ms. Johnson needed immediate help. Before she helped Ms. Johnson, the nurse did not take the time to cover the needle with the attached safety device and carry the needle to the sharps disposal container on the medication cart or in the resident's room.

The nurse intended to return to Ms. Anderson's bed and discard the needle correctly as soon as she finished helping Ms. Johnson, but you came into the room before she could return. If you were the nurse, what would you have done?

Exposure Control Plan. OSHA requires all facilities to have a written exposure control plan to eliminate or minimize employees' exposure to blood and body fluids. Every department in the facility is covered by this plan. Every employee should be aware of the plan and be able to review it at any time.

Engineering and Work-practice Controls. Engineering controls use various devices to reduce hazards. For example, a needle disposal container is located near the place where needles and sharps are used so that sharps can be disposed of directly without being transported to another location. OSHA requires using only safety needles and syringes that have attached safety devices. For example, with one type, after using the needle, you press it against a hard surface and the needle retracts to a safe position out of the way. If you use any of these devices in your facility, know how to use them correctly.

Personal Protective Equipment. Personal protective equipment includes barriers to prevent contact between the reservoir and the susceptible host—for example, between a sick resident and a caregiving nurse assistant. Gloves, masks, eye protection, and gowns or aprons prevent you from contacting blood or other body fluids from residents (Fig. 10-6). The proper use of these barriers is described in Chapter 9.

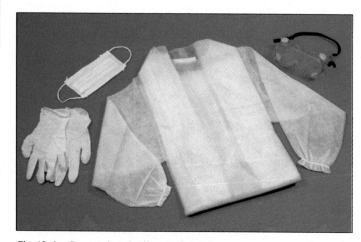

Fig. 10-6 – Personal protective equipment.

📖
Insulin – hormone involved in breaking down carbohydrates in the body; it can be given as a shot to control diabetes

Housekeeping. The facility's environment must be kept clean and sanitary. A written cleaning schedule is required for each facility. This includes the methods for decontaminating surfaces or equipment soiled with blood or body fluids. If you have questions about how the OSHA Bloodborne Pathogens Standard is followed in your facility, ask the infection control practitioner.

Hepatitis B Vaccination and Post-Exposure Evaluation and Follow-up. OSHA requires all facilities to provide the hepatitis B vaccine free of charge to all employees who may have occupational exposure to blood or other infectious materials (Fig. 10-7). OSHA also requires that facilities offer and encourage a free blood test one to two months after they have received the last shot in the hepatitis B vaccine series. This test determines if the vaccine will be effective for them. The facility cannot require employees to take the vaccine or blood test. If an exposure occurs, the facility must provide immediate post-exposure evaluation and follow-up either in the facility or elsewhere. The facility must pay for this.

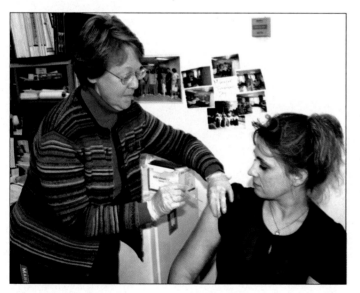

Fig. 10-7 – All facilities must provide the hepatitis B vaccine to all employees.

Information and Training Requirements. The OSHA Bloodborne Pathogens Standard requires facilities to give information and training to all employees during working hours. This training must include information about blood-borne pathogens, tasks that involve occupational exposure, and ways to reduce the risk of exposure.

Information About Bloodborne Pathogens The OSHA standard protects workers from all known and unknown diseases transmitted by blood. The three viruses of greatest concern at present are hepatitis B virus (HBV); hepatitis C virus (HCV); and the human immunodeficiency virus (HIV), which causes acquired immunodeficiency syndrome (AIDS).

HIV and AIDS The signs and symptoms of HIV infection vary greatly among different people. HIV infection can be detected with an HIV-antibody test within a few weeks or months after a person is infected. However, signs and symptoms of the infection may not occur for 10 years. During this time the person can transmit the infection to others.

HIV is transmitted through blood and other body fluids, such as semen and vaginal secretions. Transmission occurs through sexual contact, sharing drug needles, contaminated blood products (now rare because blood products are tested), and from an HIV-infected mother to her infant.

Occupational transmission between a health care professional and a patient has occurred from puncture injuries with HIV-blood-contaminated needles and sharps. It has also happened from blood contact with broken skin or mucous membranes. But you do not have to worry about caring for a resident with HIV as long as you follow the required standard precautions.

Hepatitis B and Hepatitis C Hepatitis B and hepatitis C are viruses that cause inflammation of the liver. There is a vaccine to prevent hepatitis B, but not one for hepatitis C. Hepatitis C is transmitted in the same ways as hepatitis B and HIV infections.

Hepatitis B is far more common than HIV. The hepatitis B virus (HBV) is present in high concentrations in the blood of an infected person. This means there is a greater chance of infection with HBV from an exposure than there is to HIV. People who have been vaccinated against hepatitis B will not become infected, however.

The most serious problem with hepatitis B and hepatitis C infections is that some people with these infections never get well. Their liver damage may be so serious that they eventually will need a liver transplant. Vaccination can prevent serious liver damage from hepatitis B. When contact with blood is likely, careful attention to sharps safety and the use of barriers helps protect you from hepatitis C infection.

📖

Antibody – type of protein that the body produces to fight infection or illness

Nurse Assistant Tasks Involving Exposure to Blood.
Because you provide most resident care, you may notice
blood in a resident's stool, urine, or vomitus or in drainage
from a wound. Always wear gloves to protect yourself
when handling any resident's body secretions and excretions (Fig.10-8).

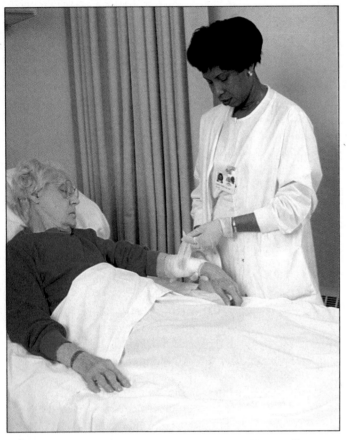

Fig. 10-8 — Gloves will protect you from resident's body secretions,
wound drainage, and excretions.

The risk of being splashed in the eyes, nose, or mouth
with any fluid containing blood can be minimized if you
follow standard precaution procedures. If you are at risk of
being splashed with any body fluids—even just a little—
always wear the appropriate eye, nose, and mouth barrier
protection.

You may sometimes clean up spills on the floor or in a
resident's bathroom. These spills may include blood or
other body fluids. Follow the facility's procedure for cleaning up spills, using the correct detergent and **disinfectant**.
Wear a gown or plastic apron if your skin or clothing may
be soiled when cleaning up the spill. Always wear gloves
when cleaning up any type of spill. The infection control
practitioner or head housekeeper can teach you the best
way to clean up spills.

SPECIAL EQUIPMENT AND SUPPLIES FOR INFECTION PREVENTION AND CONTROL

Sharps Safety Equipment

Nurse assistants do not usually perform tasks using needles or other sharps. Some nurse assistants may change
sharps disposal containers, however. Injury and exposure
could occur if needles are improperly disposed of, are
sticking out the top of the container, or have punctured
the side of the container. To prevent accidental injury,
examine the sharps disposal container carefully before you
touch it.

Punctures from needles and other sharps and cuts from
used scalpels put health care workers at risk for many
infections, including HIV, HBV, and HCV. All facilities have
policies and procedures for handling and disposing of
used sharps. Sharps disposal containers should be located
as close as possible to where they are used. Usually these
containers are on medication carts and in medication
rooms. Some facilities have sharps disposal containers on
the walls of residents' rooms. Know the location of all the
sharps containers in your facility.

Wastes Requiring Special Handling

Many wastes require special handling, including:
* pathological wastes
* lab cultures
* liquid waste
* human blood
* products of blood
* items saturated with blood or body fluids
* items contaminated with blood, such as used sharps

The OSHA Bloodborne Pathogens Standard defines regulated wastes and makes rules for waste handling, storage,
or shipping. Regulated wastes are discarded in red bags or
bags that have a special biohazard label (Fig. 10-9).

Disinfectant – an agent that inactivates microorganisms on inanimate
objects

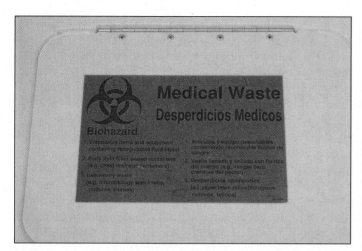

Fig. 10-9 – The biohazard label indicates waste that requires special handling.

INJURY PREVENTION

Ergonomics

Ergonomic studies have shown how job injuries can result from:
- repetitive body movements, which result in tired muscles
- awkward posture, which increases the force on body parts
- lifting residents or items that are too heavy, which puts a strain on the body
- using the wrong equipment, or using equipment incorrectly

Injuries from these actions can be prevented by a five-step approach to prevent injuries when caring for a resident:
1. Determine the resident's capabilities.
2. Determine the equipment you need.
3. Determine and communicate to other staff the steps needed for safe handling.
4. Follow the care plan.
5. Evaluate the success of tasks performed.

You are not responsible for implementing these steps alone. The interdisciplinary team helps determine the right steps for you and the resident.

Have you ever had a resident fall asleep with their arm in an awkward position. Did they wake up shaking their arm (Fig. 10-10)? Did they say their arm fell asleep? This happened because the blood supply was cut off because of the position. Imagine if you had to hold your body in that same awkward position all day, every day. What do you think would happen to your arm? Would your muscles get sore? Would you have aches and pains? Could you keep doing that task for any length of time?

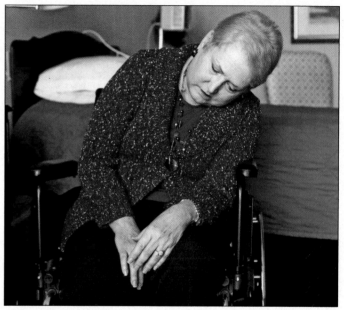

Fig. 10–10 – An awkward posture can lead to a muscle strain.

Many caregiving tasks place you in awkward positions for a long time. You also may have to lift or help someone in situations where the physical demands are beyond your capability. But if you practice good ergonomic principles, consider your capabilities and the resident's, and use equipment, you can make the task easier and safer. You will learn to plan to use this equipment before you begin the task.

Repetitive job motions such as bending, lifting, turning, and reaching put you at risk of injury. A resident's unpredictable actions also increase the risk. If you don't use the right equipment correctly or you misuse your body when performing your duties, you can seriously injure yourself and the resident.

Ergonomics – the study of relationships between workers' physical capabilities and their job tasks

Injuries result from not knowing how to do something safely or from practicing bad habits. Sooner or later, an injury will happen if you are not careful to prevent it. As you begin your job as a new nurse assistant, you have a perfect opportunity to develop safe habits. Good work habits based on ergonomic principles will lower your risk of being injured.

MINDFUL DECISION MAKING: INJURY PREVENTION

Mindful decision making begins with participating with the interdisciplinary team in the assessment of a resident's capabilities. Categorizing the resident's abilities helps you to know what you must do to move, transfer, or reposition them. You also learn how to help the resident with their daily care.

Box 10-1 presents an example of how residents can be categorized. In your training and orientation, you will learn your facility's system for communicating this information about residents. This communication must not violate the resident's right to privacy but should give staff the information they need to work safely with the resident.

Using the right equipment for each resident is an important part of ergonomics. Many kinds of equipment can help you move residents from bed to chair, chair to toilet, and chair to bed. Other equipment can help you position and reposition residents in their beds and chairs.

The key is to know what is available to you and to follow the manufacturer's directions for its use. Table 10-1 lists examples of equipment you can use to help move, transfer, or reposition a resident and help with the activities of daily living.

You should consider safety and injury prevention to be one of the most important parts of your job. Being mindful about safety means paying attention to details, always evaluating the situation, and being observant. You must also be willing to ask questions and to change your ways of doing things. Ask the charge nurse about any procedure, equipment, or anything else you are not completely sure about (Fig. 10-12). Never put yourself or your resident at risk. Ask the charge nurse to help you learn to evaluate situations. Remember, because every resident and every situation are different, your actions have to change to meet each resident's unique needs.

Ergonomic principles are the basis for the policies, equipment, and staff training needed to provide quality care.

BOX 10-1. ICON SELECTION MATRIX

CATEGORY	EQUIPMENT OPTIONS	ICON TO USE	DESCRIPTION OF THE RESIDENT'S ABILITIES
Limited Assistance	Gait Belt		Resident highly involved, setup help only OR one person physical assistance
	Slide Board		
	Sit-to-stand Lifter		
Total Dependence	Sling Lifter		Limited to nonweight bearing; full staff performance of activity

TABLE 10-1 EQUIPMENT USED TO HELP MOVE RESIDENTS

TYPE OF EQUIPMENT	USES
Mechanical lifts, including: • total body lifts (Fig. 10-11) • stand-assist lifts • ambulation lifts • bath/shower lifts	Move residents from one location to another, such as from the bed to a chair, from the chair to the toilet, or off the floor
Slide boards Transfer mats Slippery sheets (friction-reducing devices) Draw sheets Trapeze bars	Lateral transfers between two horizontal surfaces, such as when you move from the bed to a stretcher Positioning
Gait belt Transfer belt with handles Pivot discs Range-of-motion machines	Ambulation Repositioning Transfer from bed to chair Manipulation of a body part
Shower/toilet combination chairs Extension-hand tools Pelvic-lift devices	Help with activities of daily living (ADLs) (bathing, dressing, transferring, toileting, and eating)

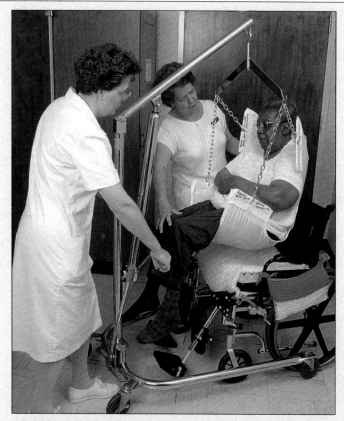

Fig. 10-11 — Mechanical lifts help move a resident from one place to another, such as from bed to chair.

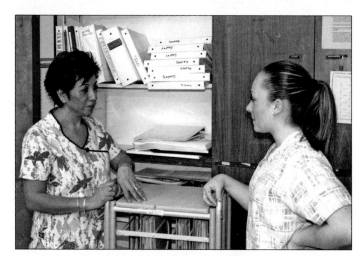

Fig. 10-12 — If you are unsure about how to move a resident safely or how to use a piece of equipment, talk to the charge nurse.

Common Sense Rules

Following are common sense rules that promote safety for both you and residents. These safety rules are grouped by how they affect residents, you, and the environment. Some safety rules involve all three. Consider each resident's own safety needs. For example, the needs of residents with visual impairments are different from those with hearing impairments. The key is to know your residents and their special needs, the equipment you can use, and other staff who can help. With this knowledge you can adjust the rules for each situation.

Residents
• Before walking with a resident, check their path for potential trip hazards, such as a bed crank.
• Encourage residents to use handrails and grip rails.
• When bathing residents, test the water temperature carefully to be sure it is not too hot (or too cold).

- Always turn off the hot-water faucet before the cold one, to prevent hot water from dripping on a resident's skin or yours.
- Encourage residents to always use their assistive and prosthetic devices, such as using their glasses or their walker when they get up at night to use the bathroom (Fig. 10-13).

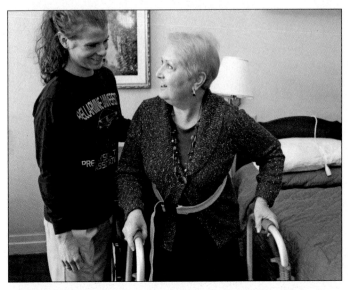

Fig. 10-13 — Encourage residents to always use their assistive and prosthetic devices.

- Always respond to call lights immediately. Be sure the call light button is close by each resident and that residents know how to use it.
- Familiarize residents with all furniture and equipment in their surroundings.
- Always keep each resident's bed in its lowest position when they are resting or not in bed.
- Frequently inspect residents' assistive devices, such as walkers and canes. Be sure that the rubber tips on the device are in place and the device fits the resident correctly.
- When moving a resident onto or off a piece of movable equipment, such as wheelchairs, shower chairs, beds, etc., always lock the wheels of the equipment first.

Nurse Assistants
- Wear nonskid shoes.
- Avoid jerky movements, such as fast, awkward turns. When you turn, move your feet so that your body can follow smoothly. Avoid twisting motions. Never reach

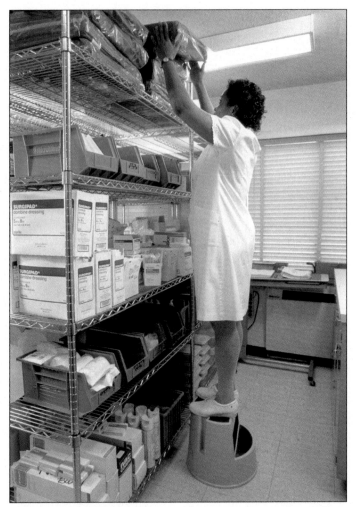

Fig. 10-14 — Always use a stool if you cannot reach something safely.

high overhead for something. Instead, use a stool (Fig. 10-14).
- Use equipment instead of using your body whenever handling a resident.
- Always ask for help.
- Always use good body mechanics.
- Never run down a hallway. Use caution when turning a corner, because someone may be there.
- Never use electrical equipment near water.
- Report any nonworking equipment.
- Keep yourself healthy.

Body mechanics – principles of using your body efficiently to do something

Environment
- Always clean up spills immediately.
- Keep residents' rooms and hallways free of clutter.
- Make sure hallways are well lit.
- Use night lights.
- Always store chemicals like cleaning solutions and medicines in their proper place.

Following these common-sense rules helps you protect residents and yourself from injury.

BODY MECHANICS

Body mechanics involve how you use your body to do something. If a resident must be manually lifted or moved, use the proper lifting aid to minimize the risk of injury to you and the resident. Safe lifting is an important part of your job. Regardless of whether you are using a mechanical lift or a lifting aid device, or are lifting the resident by yourself, always use proper body mechanics. Proper body mechanics help prevent injury to you and residents.

Proper body mechanics increase your efficiency and safety by using the body efficiently and minimizing stress. With good body mechanics, the body does less work in the task. With poor body mechanics, on the other hand, the back or other body areas can be injured. Even though injuries like strains and sprains may not seem serious, over time these smaller injuries build into a more serious injury. Unless you use good body mechanics every time you do something, you are at risk for injury.

Pay attention to protecting your back all day long. Before you lift something, take a moment to assess the situation. If you are about to lift a resident, for example, find out first if and how they can help you. Use equipment available to you. If you have any doubt about your ability to lift someone with or without equipment, get help before you try.

Principles of Body Mechanics

Think of the principles of body mechanics in three steps:
1. Consider the situation before beginning to lift, move, or position a resident.
2. Prepare yourself by considering your body mechanics.
3. Determine how to do the lift, move, or position.

Step 1: Things to Consider
- Adjust the height of the bed. Move it up to the height of your elbow when giving care, such as when giving a complete bed bath, and down when moving someone out of the bed. Changing the height reduces the amount

of bending you have to do (Fig. 10-15).

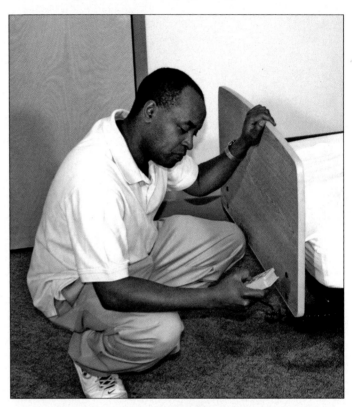

Fig. 10-15 – Adjust the height of the resident's bed to reduce the amount of bending you do when giving care.

- Never reach over things like bed rails, tables, or people. To avoid reaching injuries, bring what you need close to you.
- If you are moving a resident in bed, consider putting your knee up on the bed. This lets you get closer to residents without reaching. You may also want to use a friction-reducing device. Place a barrier such as a sheet or towel between your knee and the bed sheets (Fig. 10-16).

Step 2: Prepare Yourself
- Put your feet about shoulder-width apart for better support and strength.
- Put one foot slightly in front of the other for a stronger base of support.
- Tighten your abdominal muscles by pulling in your stomach. This gives support to your spine.
- Keep your back neutral.
- Bend your knees and lift the resident by using your leg and arm muscles, not your back. Leg and arm muscles have the greatest strength (Fig. 10-17, next page).

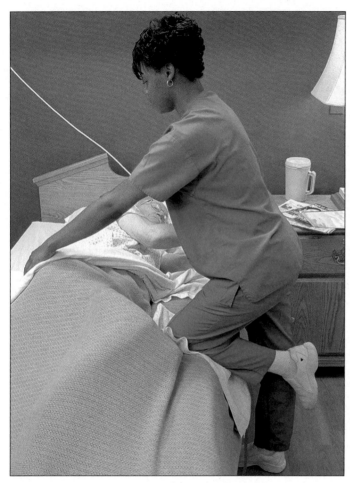

Fig. 10-16 – If necessary, put your knee on the bed to get as close to the resident as possible.

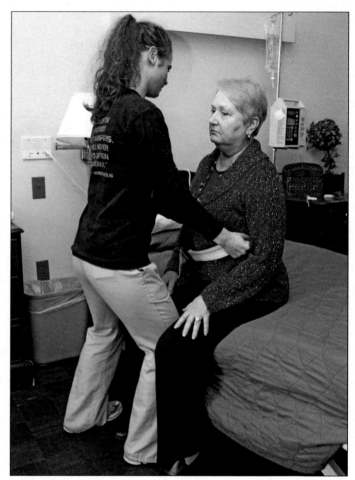

Fig. 10-17 – With your knees bent, lift using your arm and leg muscles.

Step 3: Determine How To Move

- Get as close as possible to what you are lifting or moving. The "hug" position is very supportive. Bring a resident or the item you are moving as close to you as possible. Use a gait or transfer belt with handles to get a good grip on the resident. Getting close also gives you more strength (Fig. 10-18). Compare how you feel when you carry something with your arms stretched out to the way you feel when you carry that same object with your arms close to you.
- Keep your palms up when lifting. Get under what you are lifting, and use your biceps.
- Breathe in deeply before you begin to lift, and breathe out while you lift. This helps pump blood and oxygen to your muscles.

- Rock to gain momentum for a lift or move. Rocking is moving your body very slightly in small motions, either back and forth or side to side. This shifts your weight toward and away from the object you are moving and increases your strength in the move. Always be careful not to move a resident too fast, which could potentially cause injury. When possible, use a sliding board as a bridge between the bed and chair and a friction-reducing device.

Use these principles as you learn the procedures of resident care. In Chapter 15, Learning to Position and Move Correctly, you will learn many different skills for helping a

---

📖

Biceps – strong arm muscles used for lifting

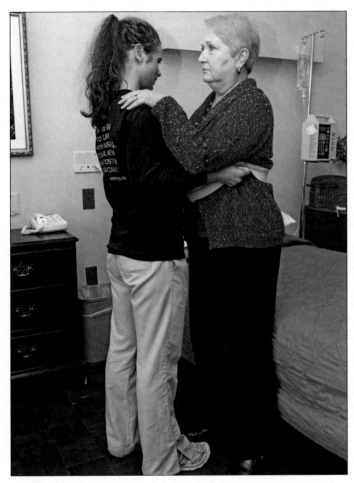

Fig. 10-18 – While moving the resident, bring them as close to you as possible.

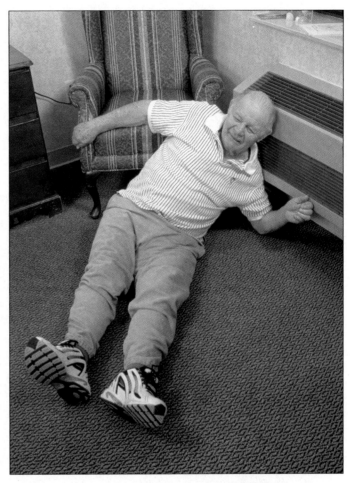

Fig. 10-19 – Falls can cause serious injuries. Prevention is the key.

resident move in bed and between bed and chair. You can injure your back in any procedure if you are careless about body mechanics. Be mindful about doing it the right way, and your body will thank you for it.

Using good body mechanics helps prevent injury. It is like deciding to wear your seat belt: No one but you can make the decision, but the right decision can prevent injury.

PREVENTING RESIDENT FALLS

Many long term care facilities have fall prevention programs. Falls can be a serious problem at any age. When an elderly person falls, it can be extremely dangerous (Fig. 10-19). Falls can cause injuries such as fractures or cuts and bruises. Even if an injury does not occur, a resident who has fallen may become fearful and less independent. Residents may stop walking by themselves or getting out

of bed to go to the bathroom. This loss of mobility can lead to number of other problems. In later chapters you will learn that maintaining the resident's independent mobility is important for their health and quality of life.

Why Residents Fall

Residents fall for a number of reasons. You will learn in Chapter 11, The Aging Process and Disease Management, about aging-related changes that everyone experiences. Changes in the musculoskeletal system, which maintains posture and balance, make falls more likely. Many residents in long term care are frail and have health conditions that affect their posture, balance, and mobility. Some medications also affect residents in ways that make them more likely to fall.

Falls are more likely in crowded or cluttered residents' rooms. Needing to go to the toilet more often, another aging-related change, also increases the risk of falling. In addition, a fall can occur if you are not using the ergonomic principles described earlier when moving, transferring, or walking a resident.

Preventing Falls

To prevent or minimize falls, consider all the factors involved. Work with the interdisciplinary team to prevent falls. Talk with other staff and share your ideas about things that need to be changed. For example, although you may not know what medications a resident is taking, you may have noticed that at night after they receive their evening medication, they have trouble keeping their balance.

You can also discuss the resident's routines with the team. For example, you might share the information that a resident drinks lots of fluids late in the day and goes to bed early, and then often gets up in the night to go the bathroom. If the night staff know about this, they can assist with toileting more often and thereby prevent a fall. You can also ensure that the resident's path to the bathroom is free from clutter and well lighted (Fig. 10-20)

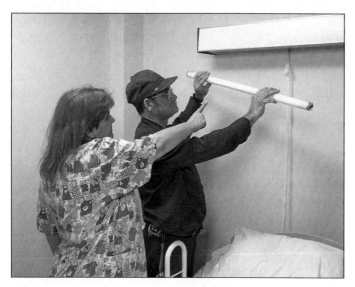

Fig. 10-20 – Keep the resident's path clear and well lighted to help prevent falls.

Make sure there are no obstacles in the pathway, such as chairs or equipment that is not being used. Ensuring that the bed is locked and in the lowest position is also your responsibility.

Box 10-2 lists other guidelines to help prevent resident falls. In Chapter 15 you will learn what to do if a resident does fall.

BOX 10-2. GUIDELINES FOR PREVENTING RESIDENT FALLS

- Report changes in a resident's behavior.
- Report broken equipment.
- Report any lighting problem.
- Keep paths clear and well lighted.
- Use mechanical devices for transfers.
- Eliminate clutter in the resident's room.
- Remove unnecessary items from the resident's room and bathroom.
- Keep the resident's personal items (like glasses) within their reach.

Devices and Equipment Used To Prevent Falls. An interdisciplinary approach is needed to help prevent residents from falling. You will participate in meetings to discuss residents who have a history of falls or who have fallen recently. You may be asked about how a resident sits in their wheelchair or chair. For example, does the resident slide forward or slouch in the chair, lean over onto one side, or lean forward?

Your knowledge about residents will help the team determine whether a piece of equipment or device can help prevent them from falling. For example, seating devices can support a resident's posture. Motion-detection devices are available that turn on lights or alarms when a resident approaches stairs or opens a door.

In addition, support handles can be installed in the resident's bathroom. A raised toilet seat makes it easier to get on and off the toilet. All theses devices can help prevent a resident from falling.

In Chapter 4, Understanding People's Rights, you learned that residents must not be restrained. Always keep this in mind, and never restrain a resident because you think that will prevent a fall. Residents must be able to move freely. Seat belts on residents' wheelchairs may be used to remind the resident to call the nurse when they want to get up from the chair. These straps usually fasten together with Velcro and may be used only if the resident can easily open the belt.

Side rails (or bed rails) may be used when they are part of the resident's care plan. Side rails can be useful in helping residents turn and reposition in bed. They can provide a handhold for getting into or out of bed. They give some residents a feeling of comfort and security. Follow your facility's policy for the use of side rails. Your facility may require a health care provider order for their use.

Note: *Side rails should never be raised automatically for any resident. In fact, some residents may become injured or even die if they become caught or entangled in the rails or between the mattress and rails. Residents can be seriously injured if they try to climb over the rails and fall. Residents who are frail or elderly, or those who are confused, in pain, or have uncontrolled body movements or other conditions, are at greater risk of injury when side rails are used. Remember to always follow your facility's policy for their use.*

ENVIRONMENTAL AWARENESS

In addition to being safe in your actions, you need to be aware of the environment in the long term care facility. The environment may involve hazards you can control to prevent injuries.

Wet Floor

Everyone is responsible for cleaning up spills. Whether you make a spill or only find one, you must ensure it is cleaned up immediately. Even if you are responding to a medical emergency at the time, you can call out so that someone else cleans up the spill before anyone slips and is seriously injured.

Floor cleanup is simple. First make sure that everyone is alerted to the danger with an easily seen "Wet Floor" sign (Fig. 10-21). For a large wet area, use more signs as needed. Don't leave the spill to get the sign, but ask another staff member to bring you the sign and cleanup equipment.

Dry the floor as much as possible. If the area is very large or is heavily used, ask the housekeeping department to dry the floor immediately. Remove the warning signs after the floor is dry so that people do not get in the habit of ignoring them.

Remember that it is everyone's job to clean up spills. The guidelines above apply not only to wet floors but also to anything on the floor that could cause a person to slip or trip. Keep an eye out for any hazards on the floor. These may include urine, water, broken floor tiles, soap, paper clips, bed cranks, and food (Fig. 10-22).

When working with water, such as when helping a resident with a shower, be extra careful. Never assume that everyone is on the lookout. You know about the increased chance for a slip or fall, but not everyone is as aware as you. Be careful to keep your work area clean and dry. Watch out for your co-workers.

Electrical Safety

Electrical safety also is everyone's concern. While working with or around electricity, follow these guidelines:
- Never use electrical devices near water.
- Always dry your hands before using electrical equipment.

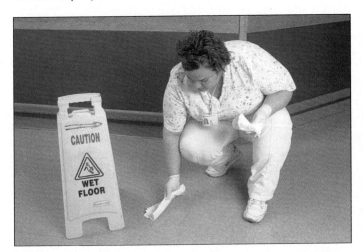

Fig. 10-21 – Everyone in the facility is responsible for wiping up spills.

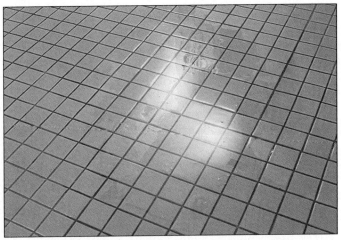

Fig. 10-22 – Pay attention to all potential hazards that can cause a person to trip or slip, such as water standing in a shower room.

- Never use extension cords or outlet expanders (devices with multiple outlets that plug into a single outlet). Laws prohibit their use in facilities.
- If you're not currently using the device, turn it off.
- Report any electrical shock from a device to your supervisor. The device should not be used again until it is repaired.
- Never try to repair an electrical device yourself.

Pay attention to electrical items that family members bring in. Things like electrical razors, televisions, fans, radios, and lamps should be examined by maintenance staff for potential electrical problems. Some facilities have a policy requiring an inspection before the item can be used. Supervise any resident's use of equipment.

Always watch to be sure every electrical device is in working order. Watch for frayed cords, sparks, excessive heat, missing safety guards, exposed wires, cracks, or any other signs that the device may not be in proper working order. Report any such conditions to your supervisor immediately.

Chemical Safety

By law, all employers and employees must know about any chemical hazards in the workplace and how to protect themselves. Employers must communicate this information to all employees through training programs. The most common chemicals in long term care facilities are disinfectants and cleaners. If you follow the manufacturer's directions for their use, you and your residents will be safe.

If you will use any hazardous chemicals in your facility, you will receive specialized training called hazard communication training, or "haz com." OSHA requires this training, which includes all safety information you need to know. All facilities must also make available a material safety data sheet for every chemical used in the facility.

Material Safety Data Sheets (MSDS). As part of your training about chemicals used in your facility, you will learn about material safety data sheets (MSDS). Each sheet lists the substance's chemical contents, fire and health hazards, use precautions, clean-up procedures, disposal requirements, necessary personal protective equipment, and first aid procedures. These sheets are kept in an accessible location such as the nurses' station (Fig. 10-23). If you are exposed to a chemical and have a reaction, go to the emergency room of the nearest hospital and take the MSDS with you.

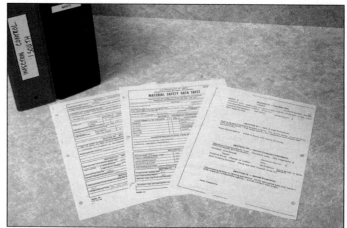

Fig. 10-23 – Every facility must have MSDS for all chemicals used in the facility.

Container Labeling. Your training will also include understanding container labels. You must get in the habit of reading and following the directions on labels. Labels contain most of the information you need to protect both you and your residents (Fig. 10-24, next page). If you find a container without a label, do not use it in any way or smell it to guess what it is. Instead, take it to the charge nurse immediately. The nurse can then contact the person responsible for getting the correct labeling directly from the manufacturer.

Emergency First Aid for Chemical Exposures. If you or someone else is exposed to a chemical, what to do depends on the kind of chemical. Following is the general emergency first aid related to chemicals:
- Follow the guidelines in the material safety data sheet for the chemical.
- See your supervisor immediately, who will contact the local Poison Control Center if needed to find out what emergency actions to take.
- If you or a resident inhales a chemical, get into fresh air as soon as possible.
- If you or a resident gets a chemical on your skin, rinse it off with lots of running water.
- If you or a resident swallows a chemical, do not induce vomiting. Rinse out your mouth or theirs.
- Follow the instructions from the Poison Control Center (Fig. 10-25, next page).

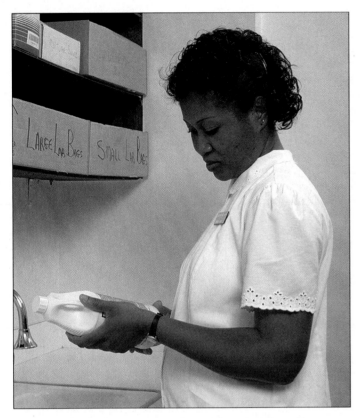

Fig. 10-24 — Always read the directions on the label before using any product.

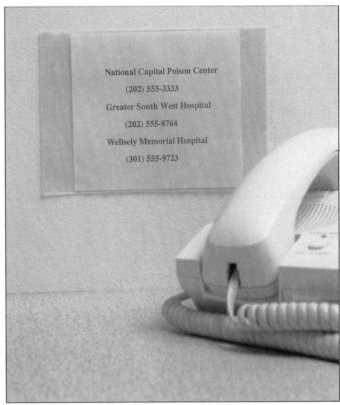

Fig. 10-25 — If you are exposed to a chemical, call the Poison Control Center.

For chemical spills or splashes in your eyes, follow these guidelines:
- Immediately flush your eyes with cool running water for at least five minutes. Remove contact lenses.
- Continue flushing for at least 15 minutes, holding the eyelids open to ensure the entire eye is rinsed.

The "Right to Know" Law. As an employee, you have a right to see certain kinds of personnel and safety records. In addition to your employment and medical histories and job description, you have the right to see documents affecting safety in the facility. You can request to see your department's chemical inventory list, material safety data sheets, and the OSHA publication "Access to Employee Exposure and Medical Records Standard." You may want to read these if you have questions about what chemicals you may be exposed to on the job or what to do in an emergency. Submit your request in writing to your supervisor. Include your full name, the date, a description of the information you want, and your signature.

Safety Around Oxygen

Oxygen (O_2) is an important gas in your facility. Because oxygen increases the risk of fire and explosion, you must remember certain important facts and follow precautions in areas where oxygen is being used.

Oxygen can come from several different sources. It may come from a valve in the wall, from various sizes of green tanks of compressed gas, or from a machine called an oxygen concentrator (Fig. 10-26, next page). Regardless of the source of the oxygen, certain precautions always apply:
- Oxygen is not flammable itself but makes other things easier to ignite and burn. Keep all flames and potential sources of sparks away. There must be no smoking when oxygen is in use.
- Always put a "No Smoking—Oxygen" sign on a door where oxygen is in use (Fig. 10-27, next page).
- *Never* put any kind of lubricant on hoses or fittings used with oxygen, because this could start a fire. If the pieces don't go together smoothly, tell the charge nurse. *Never try to force a fit.* The tank may be labeled incorrectly.

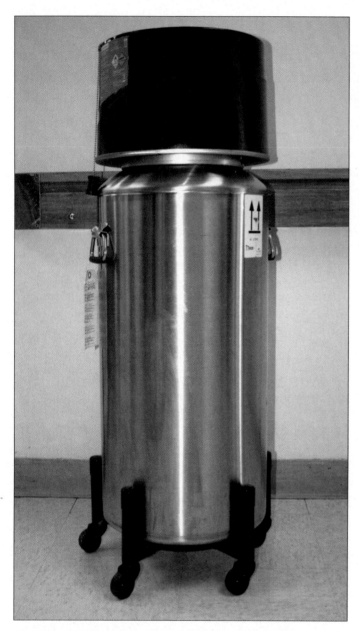
Fig. 10-26 – Oxygen may be administered from tanks like this.

You will learn more about oxygen in Chapter 11 and Chapter 24.

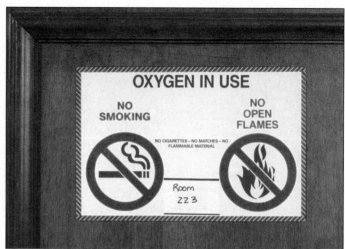
Fig. 10-27 – "No Smoking–Oxygen" signs should be posted in plain view.

DISASTER PREPAREDNESS

All facilities have written disaster plans in case of an emergency. These plans usually say that employees must first move residents to safety and then care for them. Regardless of problems caused by the disaster, you must still meet the needs of your residents.

Disaster plans do not assign tasks to people by name because different staff are on duty at different times. Emergency tasks are assigned by job description. You must be familiar with your facility's disaster plan and know the role of nurse assistants if a disaster strikes. Disasters include natural disasters such as dangerous weather conditions and fires.

Weather

Possible weather disasters depend on your area's climate. Emergencies can occur suddenly, as with a violent storm, or with advance warning, such as with a hurricane. The charge nurse will tell you when to evacuate residents following either the **internal evacuation** or the **external evacuation** plan.

External evacuation – moving residents out of the facility to another site for safety
Internal evacuation – moving residents to another section within the facility for safety

Evacuations follow the principle of "priority of movement." This is the order in which residents should be moved. The evacuation starts with residents who require the least amount of help. This frees staff members to help those who are dependent and unable to move themselves to the new location. Following is the usual order of evacuation:

1. ambulatory residents
2. residents who need wheelchairs and walkers
3. bedridden residents

To evacuate bedridden residents, you use emergency transfer methods that are quick, efficient, and safe. These are different from the transfer techniques you use normally. These emergency methods are described in Appendix D, Emergency Transfer Techniques (Fig. 10-28).

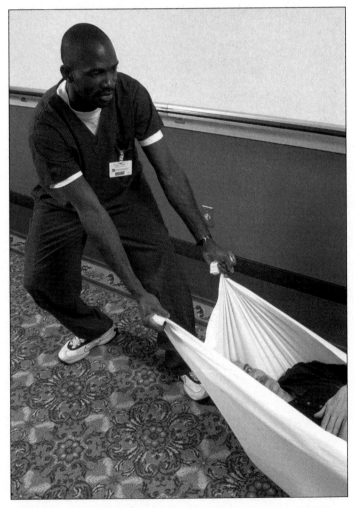

Fig. 10-28 – During a disaster use an emergency transfer method that is quick, efficient, and safe.

Fire

Fire safety and preparedness are a major responsibility for all employees. In your new employee orientation, you will learn your facility's fire plan. Fire procedures are posted in each department and at each nurses' station near the phone. Local emergency phone numbers should also be posted for the fire department, police or sheriff, ambulance, and Poison Control Center.

Fire drills are held at least every three months on each shift. You must participate fully in these drills to ensure that you and all staff are as prepared as possible.

To prevent fires, follow these guidelines:
- Report any unsafe condition so that corrective measures can be taken right away.
- Enforce no-smoking regulations. Safety ashtrays should be used and cigarettes must always be out when discarded.
- Never store anything within 18 inches of a water sprinkler head. Do not park linen hampers or food carts where they will block or hide a wall-mounted fire alarm "pull."
- Watch corridors and doors for safety. Keep corridors and exits free of equipment that cannot be wheeled out of the way.
- Exit doors should never be locked or blocked (Fig. 10-29). Smoke or fire doors also must not be blocked.

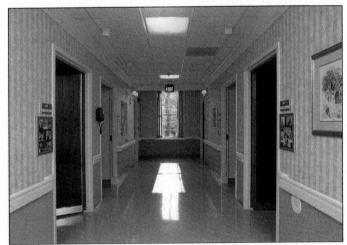

Fig. 10-29 – For fire safety, corridors and exit doors must never be blocked or locked.

- Doors to maintenance areas, elevators, equipment rooms, and boiler rooms should always be kept closed.

Your role in emergency preparedness is so important that you must always be alert for problems. Participate in all prevention activities to help everyone stay safe.

If You Are the First To Notice a Fire.   If you enter a room where there is a fire or are first to see a fire, do this:
1. Stop and quickly assess the situation.
2. Yell for help, and sound an alarm if one is present.
3. Immediately remove all residents from the area. Do this quickly because it is smoke inhalation that causes most deaths in fires, not the actual fire. If possible, turn off residents' oxygen.
4. Do not open the windows.
5. When everyone is out, close the door to the room. Most doors in health care facilities are fire doors. They help contain a fire for one to two hours.
6. Evacuate the residents from rooms on both sides of the room that is on fire.
7. Never open a closed door during a fire unless you have no other choice. If you must open a door, put your hand on it first to check if it is warm, and look for smoke coming from underneath it. If it is warm or you see smoke, do not open the door. If you did, oxygen would enter the room and cause the fire to explode, seriously injuring you and making the fire grow.
8. Move residents at immediate risk to the end of the wing farthest from the fire, or remove them from the wing or unit entirely if instructed to do so.
9. Fight a fire with a fire extinguisher only if it is very small and contained, such as in a wastebasket. Do not try to fight a larger fire because it can get out of control very quickly.

If a Fire Alarm Sounds on Another Wing or Unit.
1. Follow your facility's emergency plan and the charge nurse's instructions.
2. Clear residents out of hallways into their rooms and close the doors. Remember that these are fire doors.
3. If several residents are in a gathering area, close the doors to that room instead of moving them through fire doors to return them to their rooms. Act calmly and reassure the residents.
4. Make sure the halls are free from obstructions.

If an Evacuation Is Ordered.   Evacuate residents in this order:
1. those nearest the fire
2. ambulatory residents
3. ambulatory residents who need assistance

4. residents who use wheelchairs
5. residents who are bedridden
6. residents' charts and medication carts

The reason for this priority order is that if evacuation began with bedridden residents who take more time to be moved, the process would take longer and more residents are likely to be caught in the burning area. If ambulatory residents are moved first, more residents will be saved if the fire spreads quickly (Fig. 10-30).

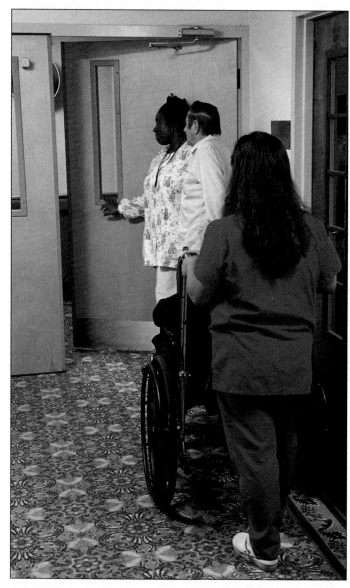

Fig. 10-30 – Follow the priority order for evacuating residents in case of a fire.

INCIDENT REPORTING

Sometimes, no matter how careful and mindful everyone is to prevent injuries, an accident does happen. As human beings, we're not perfect. Even if you follow the rules, a problem can occur. If an accident or injury does happen, you may need to complete an incident report.

This is called an incident report rather than an injury report because all incidents must be reported, not just injuries. An incident is anything that goes wrong that should not happen again. Regardless of whether the incident involved equipment, staff, or a procedure failure, tell your supervisor immediately. The sooner a problem is reported, the sooner it can be corrected. Chapter 8, Documentation Principles and Procedures, describes in more detail how to make an incident report.

IN THIS CHAPTER YOU LEARNED:
* How to protect yourself from bloodborne pathogens
* The principles of ergonomics
* Common-sense rules for preventing injury
* Good body mechanics
* What to do to prevent resident falls
* Your role in preventing injury in the long term care environment
* Your role in disaster preparedness

SUMMARY

This chapter introduced you to information you need to know to do your job safely and prevent injuries to yourself and residents. It is critical that you understand how to protect yourself from bloodborne pathogens. Know what to do if you are exposed. You must also understand the principles of ergonomics and good body mechanics to prevent injury. You learned about how to prevent resident falls. It is also important for you to know about chemical and electrical hazards in the facility as well as your role in disaster preparedness.

PULLING IT ALL TOGETHER

In Chapter 2 you learned what it means to be mindful. You learned never to let routines become automatic. Being mindful about safety principles is critical to ensure you and residents are not injured.

Consider the following:

You arrive to work on the day shift and learn that two other nurse assistants have called in sick. The charge nurse says not to worry, because one of the night staff will stay and another unit can spare a staff member. You get your assignment. Because you know these residents best, you are assigned to care for most of the residents who need total or partial assistance.

One of these residents, Mrs. Reynolds, is anxious to get up. The label above her bed states that she needs the mechanical lift to transfer to her wheelchair. You go to get it but find that it is in use elsewhere. Instead of checking when it will be available, you go back to Mrs. Reynolds and ask her if she can stand up to do the transfer. Mrs. Reynolds says she will try.

You now decide to do the transfer without the lift. You clear the pathway for the move, and position the wheelchair and lock it. You ask Mrs. Reynolds to sit up on the side of the bed, and you explain what you are going to do. You get into position and consider your body mechanics, and you feel ready.

You tell Mrs. Reynolds to stand up on the count of three and turn toward the chair. "Ready, 1, 2, 3." You help Mrs. Reynolds up to a standing position, and suddenly she is nervous that she will fall. She grabs onto you around the neck and you cannot move. You ask her to let go, but she only becomes more nervous. You can't hold her weight up any longer — you start to fall, and so does Mrs. Reynolds.

How could you have prevented this incident? If you had talked to the charge nurse about the problem of not being able to use the lift right away, maybe the two of you could have found another solution. The charge nurse would have told you that the lift is always used with Mrs. Reynolds because she is afraid of falling and feels safe only when the lift is used with two staff. The charge nurse could also have helped you communicate with Mrs. Reynolds, asking her to wait a little longer until the lift was available.

1. **Ergonomics is the study of the relationship between:**
   A. Nurse assistants and residents.
   B. Residents and their families.
   C. Workers' physical capabilities and their job tasks.
   D. Workers' attitudes and their job satisfaction.

2. **What is the purpose of ergonomics?**
   A. To help workers cope with stress.
   B. To design better care plans for residents.
   C. To help workers buy better health care insurance.
   D. To prevent injuries in the work place.

3. **What is the first step you take to prevent being injured when caring for a resident?**
   A. Weigh the resident.
   B. Ask family members to help you with all care tasks.
   C. Determine the resident's capabilities.
   D. Join a weight-lifting group to make your muscles stronger.

4. **To make sure a resident is safe during a bath, you should:**
   A. Close the tub room door.
   B. Undress the resident in the tub room.
   C. Check the water temperature.
   D. Remove all your jewelry.

5. **Which of these actions will help to prevent resident falls?**
   A. Be sure all residents eat all of their meals.
   B. Limit the number of times you move the resident.
   C. Move the resident's personal things, like eyeglasses, well out of the way.
   D. Eliminate clutter in the resident's room.

6. **Using good body mechanics will help you:**
   A. Get all your work done before your shift ends.
   B. Lose weight.
   C. Avoid injuries.
   D. Develop stronger muscles.

7. **Standard precautions are used whenever your work involves:**
   A. Touching a resident in any way.
   B. Preparing snacks for residents between meals.
   C. Meeting with unknown family members.
   D. Handling anything that may be contaminated with blood or other body fluids.

8. **The OSHA Bloodborne Pathogens Standard is intended to protect health care workers from:**
   A. All diseases.
   B. Colds and flu.
   C. HIV and hepatitis.
   D. Syphilis and gonorrhea.

9. **Which residents are usually evacuated first from the facility during a disaster?**
   A. Bedridden residents.
   B. Confused residents.
   C. Ambulatory residents.
   D. Residents who use walkers.

10. **In which of the following situations should an incident report be filed?**
    A. When a resident spills juice in the dining room.
    B. When a resident falls in the shower.
    C. When the nurse assistant replacing you on the next shift calls in sick.
    D. When a family member is late for a visit with a resident.

(Answers to "Check What You've Learned" are in the Instructor's Manual.)

Chapter 11

THE AGING PROCESS AND DISEASE MANAGEMENT

As the person who spends the most time with residents, you are in a unique position to influence the quality of their care. You can observe and report even a small change in a resident. Your observation and reporting can help ensure that early intervention begins as soon possible, reducing complications.

To give residents quality care, you must understand changes they experience. Some changes may be part of normal aging, but others may be more serious. A change may result from a disease that needs immediate treatment. You must recognize what is normal aging, what is normal for a resident, and what is a problem that should be reported.

In this chapter you will learn about each body system. For each, you will learn its anatomy (structure, or parts) and physiology (functions, or what it does) and the changes that happen with aging. You will learn signs of abnormal changes to watch for as you care for residents. You will also learn about common illnesses and problems that occur in different body systems. For each, you will learn its objective signs (what you can observe and collect) and subjective symptoms (what a resident experiences or feels and tells you), and how to care for these residents. The observations you report to the charge nurse can significantly improve the quality of a resident's care.

OBJECTIVES

- Identify four general characteristics of aging
- Define the terms "acute," "chronic," "observation," "signs," and "symptoms"
- Explain why no one should be labeled by their disease or condition
- Explain the importance of early detection of cancer
- Describe how the body responds to infection
- Identify the structure, function, and aging-related changes of the 10 body systems
- Give an example of each body system's changes as the body ages
- Give five examples of information that should be reported to the charge nurse
- Complete a resident's chart with a description of an illness, disease, or problem; signs and symptoms; your role in observation and intervention; the goals of care; and interventions or skills for care

MEDICAL TERMS

- **Acute** – problem that begins rapidly and typically lasts 7-10 days; then the person recovers
- **Adrenal gland** – located on top of the kidneys, this gland secretes hormones that regulate metabolism, increase blood sugar, control blood vessel constriction, and help us react in emergency situations
- **Alveoli** – air sacs in the lungs
- **Arteries** – blood vessels that carry oxygenated blood to all parts of the body
- **Arthritis** – joint inflammation that causes pain and limits movement in affected joints
- **Blister** – elevated area of epidermis containing watery liquid
- **Bronchi** – left and right airway passages to the lungs (bronchus is the singular)
- **Bronchioles** – branches of each bronchus
- **Capillaries** – tiny blood vessels that connect arteries and veins, where oxygen is exchanged for carbon dioxide inside organs
- **Cataract** – cloudy film that develops in the lens of the eye and reduces sight
- **Cerebral vascular accident (CVA)** – condition that occurs when blood flowing to the brain is interrupted (also called stroke)
- **Chemotherapy** – use of chemical agent to treat or control disease
- **Chronic obstructive pulmonary disease (COPD)** – chronic inflammatory disease of bronchial passages and lungs; three most common types of disease are bronchitis, emphysema, and asthma

- **Circulatory system** – body system that includes the heart and blood vessels that carry oxygen and nutrients to the body and remove carbon dioxide
- **Congestive heart failure (CHF)** – condition that occurs when the heart muscle weakens and the heart becomes ineffective in moving blood through the body
- **Constipation** – condition in which bowel movement is delayed and feces are difficult to expel from the rectum
- **Coronary artery disease (CAD)** – condition that results from reduced flow through the coronary arteries, which nourish the heart
- **Cyanosis** – bluish or purplish discoloration of the skin caused by not enough oxygenation of the blood
- **Dermatitis** – inflammation of the skin; contact dermatitis is a skin reaction resulting from coming in contact with something you are allergic to
- **Dermis** – second layer of the skin
- **Digestive system** – body system that provides the body with a continuous supply of nutrients and fluid and removes waste products
- **Edema** – swelling because of fluid gain, most commonly observed in the legs and ankles
- **Endocrine system** – body system made up of many glands that secrete hormones
- **Enema** – procedure that introduces fluid into the rectum to stimulate a bowel movement
- **Epidermis** – top or first layer of the skin

- **Fallopian tubes** – two tubes that carry egg cells from the ovaries to the uterus
- **Fecal impaction** – condition that may occur when constipation is not treated; hard feces are packed in the rectum
- **Fracture** – broken bone
- **Heimlich maneuver** – technique used to free a foreign object from the airway when a resident is choking
- **Hypodermis** – lining beneath the epidermis
- **Integumentary system** – body system made up of the skin, nails, and hair
- **Malignant** – refers to a tumor or condition that tends to spread abnormal cells
- **Mole** – a colored spot on the body
- **Multiple sclerosis** – progressive disabling disease that affects nerve fibers
- **Muscle atrophy** – muscle wasting
- **Musculoskeletal system** – body system made up of bones, muscles, tendons, ligaments, and joints
- **Nervous system** – body system made up of the brain, spinal cord, and nerves
- **Osteoarthritis** – joint inflammation caused by wear and tear of the joint
- **Osteoporosis** – condition in which bones become weak and brittle due to loss of minerals, especially calcium
- **Ovaries** – organs in the female's pelvic area that secrete hormones involved in sexual function and becoming pregnant

- **Pancreas** – digestive system organ located near the stomach; its cells secrete insulin
- **Parkinson's disease** – neurological disease that affects motor skills
- **Penis** – male organ of sexual intercourse and urination
- **Peripheral vascular disease (PVD)** – condition that causes diminished blood flow to the arms and legs
- **Pituitary gland** – gland located in the brain that secretes hormones and regulates other glands
- **Pneumonia** – lung infection
- **Pus** – a yellowish-white fluid formed when an infection is present
- **Radiation** – medical treatment using X-rays
- **Reproductive system** – body system that provides sexual pleasure and allows for human reproduction
- **Respiration** – exchange of oxygen and carbon dioxide in the lungs
- **Respiratory system** – body system that takes in oxygen (inhaling) and expels carbon dioxide (exhaling)
- **Rheumatoid arthritis** – inflammatory joint disease
- **Sacrum** – bottom part of the spine
- **Sebaceous glands** – glands that are located in the dermis and secrete oil
- **Sensory system** – body system of sense organs that gain information from the world outside the body

- **Sign** – body characteristic that can be observed objectively, such as a red rash or bruising
- **Subcutaneous** – under the skin
- **Surgery** – operation; procedure done to the body
- **Symptom** – any condition that accompanies or is caused by a disease or medical disorder; may be something observable or something reported by the patient
- **Testes (testicles)** – the two oval glands that manufacture sperm cells and the male sex hormone testosterone
- **Thyroid gland** – gland located in the neck that secretes hormones that help regulate metabolism
- **Urinary system** – body system that helps maintain fluid balance and eliminates liquid wastes
- **Uterus** – muscular reproductive organ in which the fetus develops during pregnancy; it sheds its lining during menstruation
- **Vagina** – muscular canal in the female leading from the uterus; involved in sexual intercourse, childbirth, and passage of menstrual flow
- **Veins** – blood vessels that carry deoxygenated blood from the body back to the heart and lungs
- **Vulva** – external structure of the female sex organs
- **Wart** – horny bump on the skin caused by a virus

[Some of the words in this chapter are defined in the text rather than in the footnotes.]

"I'm so lucky that you know what to watch for so that any problems are caught before they get worse."

The body is made up of different body systems. Each has different organs. Every organ has its own **structures** and **functions**. We can study each system separately to better understand it, but in the body all these systems work together to support life. For the body as a whole to be healthy, each part of each body system must work by itself, and each system must work with other systems.

Each system of the body ages. There is no one pattern of aging for everyone, and different body systems age in different ways. Still, aging causes general changes you should understand. Changes caused by aging:

• reduce the functioning of the system
• happen gradually
• happen naturally
• happen to everyone

Aging often scares people, but the aging process actually begins at birth. Aging is a natural process that happens to everyone. Many factors influence aging. How a person lives and their family history affect how they will age—but these do not change the fact that aging will occur eventually. For example, exposure to the sun influences how the skin ages (Fig. 11-1). Everyone's skin eventually wrinkles with age, but wrinkling occurs faster if you have spent more time in the sun.

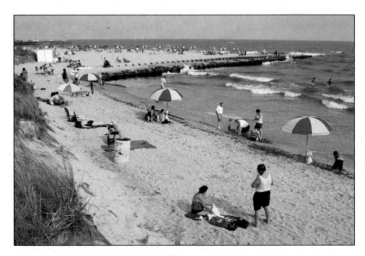

Fig. 11-1 – Exposure to the sun influences how the skin ages.

📖
Function – key action(s) of an organ or body system
Structure – a definite pattern of organization (like organs in a body)

LEARN HOW RESIDENTS FEEL ABOUT AGING

Some people try not to think about aging because they are afraid of growing old. If you ask a group of people what they fear the most about aging, you will hear different things. People are different in this way as in many other ways. To learn how a resident feels about aging, ask questions like:

- Do your limitations with walking cause problems for you?
- Does your stiffness in the morning prevent you from getting ready for the day?
- What do you do to start your day in a better way?

By asking questions, you can better understand the psychological effects of aging on the resident. You can also learn about any abnormal **signs** and **symptoms** they may have.

The residents you care for depend on you to notice any changes. Remember what you learned about reporting objective and subjective information in Chapter 8. In this chapter you will learn about the signs and symptoms of common illnesses, diseases, and problems. When describing a sign of a disease, you are reporting objective information. When describing a symptom, you are reporting subjective information. You must carefully observe those symptoms and recognize and report any changes to the charge nurse. Use all your senses to observe any abnormalities.

Think for a minute about someone you know well, such as a co-worker, your child, or a friend. How can you tell when they are sick or not feeling well? Don't you use all your senses? You may see that they are pale, hear that they sound hoarse, or feel that their skin is warm. The same is true as you get to know residents. When you observe something different about a resident, try to find the reason for the change. Look for other signs of a change. For example, a person who is flushed and sweaty might be ill, or maybe the person just finished exercising. You will learn to observe each resident carefully and report any changes.

AVOID LABELING

Have you ever known someone with a serious health problem? Maybe you know someone with a heart problem. Did you ever find yourself calling them "the man with the heart condition" instead of "my neighbor, Mr. Stein"? Doing this labels Mr. Stein by his problem. That label makes his illness his most important feature, and you tend to think of him as a condition instead of as a person just like you.

As a member of the interdisciplinary team, take care not to label residents that way. By referring to a resident as "the women with Alzheimer's in 3B" or "the blind man," you are thinking of these residents as diseases rather than people. When you focus on what is wrong, you don't see what is right or healthy about them. Residents with diseases and problems need the same general care as other residents. Their care may simply have a different emphasis. Having a disease does not mean that the person deserves less respect and dignity than everyone else.

Be careful also not to judge someone by how they look. If someone looks old, that doesn't mean that they don't think clearly or don't have feelings like you. Never confuse aging with poor health. No one should think that aging takes away their ability to live happily.

ACUTE VERSUS CHRONIC PROBLEMS

There are usually differences between **acute** and chronic health problems. Acute problems develop rapidly or suddenly. An acute problem usually lasts only a limited time and is predictable, then the person usually recovers. The common cold, for example, is an acute problem. It comes on quickly and lasts 7 to 10 days, and you recover completely.

Most infections are also acute problems. It is important to identify an acute problem as soon as possible so that it can be treated effectively. Watch for clues to such problems. Clues are signs you observe in your daily care of residents. Some clues, like a skin rash and fever, can be specific signs of infection even if the resident can't tell you where they hurt or how they feel. The sooner a problem is identified, the quicker the resident will be treated and recover.

Chronic problems, on the other hand, last a long time or recur often. Residents with chronic problems may experience signs and symptoms on some days, but not on others. Some residents, however, live with constant pain from chronic illness or disease. Chronic back pain and **arthritis** are two problems that involve constant, nagging pain.

Acute – problem that begins rapidly and typically lasts 7-10 days; then the person recovers

Arthritis – joint inflammation that causes pain and limits movement in affected joints

Sign – body characteristic that can be observed objectively, such as a red rash or bruising

Symptom – something subjectively felt but not observable by another, such as when a resident tells you they feel a sharp pain in their chest

Recognize a resident's efforts to focus on life, however, regardless of what chronic problems they may have.

At times a chronic condition can worsen and need medical treatment. For example, a resident with arthritis may wake up stiff on most days and need time to get "loosened up." But during a flare-up, this resident can have terrible pain. Some joints may be swollen, red, and hot to the touch. This is an example of a chronic problem in an acute phase. This is one reason you must monitor residents and identify and report any changes. If you give the charge nurse accurate information about a resident, treatment can start before the problem gets worse.

Many chronic illnesses, diseases, and problems have both acute and chronic phases. A chronic problem can also affect an acute problem. For example, residents with chronic lung disease have a greater risk of catching the flu (influenza). It also takes longer for them to recover from the flu because of their chronic illness.

CANCER

Cancer is a **malignant** growth of abnormal cells called a tumor. Most cancers grow locally, sometimes rapidly. First the cancer invades one organ or body system. Sometimes the cancer then spreads throughout the body. Health care professionals often talk about the primary site, which is the first system or organ affected by the cancer. For example, a resident's prostate gland (in the reproductive system) may be the primary site of a cancer that spreads to bones (the musculoskeletal system) or the lungs (respiratory system).

Because cancer can spread, early detection is important for treatment to begin. Report to the charge nurse any cancer warning signs you observe in a resident. Box 11-1 lists the cancer warning signs. Warning signs do not mean the resident has cancer. They are observations that need to be reported to the charge nurse. General signs and symptoms of cancer include fever, fatigue, pain, unintentional weight loss, and changes in the skin.

Cancer treatments include **surgery**, **radiation**, **chemotherapy**, or a combination. Surgery often removes the cancer. Often the original organ is removed along with surrounding tissue. Radiation uses X-rays to destroy cancer cells. Chemotherapy uses drugs that target tumor cells.

Unfortunately, radiation and chemotherapy kill not only cancer cells but also some normal cells. Residents receiving these treatments often experience nausea and vomiting, hair loss, and a risk for bleeding and infection. A resident may tell you that they felt better before they started the treatment. Listen to their concerns and help them through their very trying treatment program.

BOX 11-1.
CANCER WARNING SIGNS

1. change in bowel or bladder habits
2. a sore that does not heal (Fig. 11-2)
3. unusual bleeding or discharge from a body opening
4. a lump or thickening in the breast or elsewhere on the body
5. difficulty swallowing or indigestion, or weight loss
6. an obvious change in a wart or mole
7. nagging cough or hoarseness

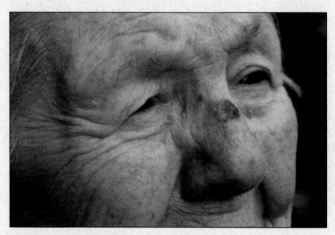

Fig. 11-2 – A change in a sore that does not heal is one of the warning signs of skin cancer.

Chemotherapy – use of chemical agent to treat or control disease
Malignant – refers to a tumor or condition that tends to spread abnormal cells
Mole – a colored spot on the body
Radiation – medical treatment using X-rays
Surgery – operation; procedure done to the body
Wart – horny bump on the skin caused by a virus

INFECTION

Like cancer, infection can begin in one place in the body and spread. The body may respond in many different ways. The response depends on the type of microorganism causing the infection and its severity. The three general types of responses are the localized, whole-body, and silent responses.

Localized Responses

You can see some kinds of infections by looking carefully at a resident's skin. For example, if a resident has a skin tear that becomes infected, the area around the tear becomes warm and red, and there may be yellowish pus in the wound. This is called a localized response because it affects only the one area on the skin.

Whole-Body Responses

Pneumonia is an example of an infection that affects the entire body. Body temperature rises due to fever. Other signs and symptoms may include respiratory distress, aches, pain, cough, sputum production, and sometimes a change in mental status—the whole body is affected. Fever can be a sign of infection. In older people fever is usually not as high as in children and younger adults. A temperature a little over 100 F in a person 80 years old may be as serious as a temperature of 102 F in a small child (Fig. 11-3).

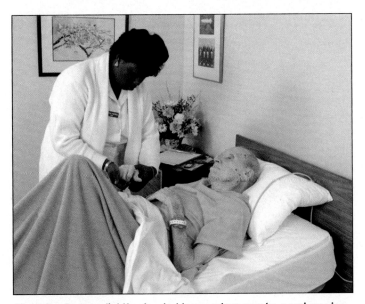

Fig. 11-3 – Even a slightly elevated temperature may be a serious sign of illness in an elderly person.

When a resident doesn't feel well, has a fever, and has a change in behavior such as lethargy, irritation, or agitation, these may be early clues that they are developing an infection. A resident's change in temperature should be reported to the charge nurse.

Silent Responses

Some infections are called silent because they cause no symptoms. They are found only with lab tests. For example, most people infected with the human immunodeficiency virus (HIV), the virus that eventually causes AIDS, have a silent infection that can be identified only with special blood tests.

Some microorganisms that cause infections in childhood can stay in the body silently for many years. An example is the chicken pox virus. As some people get older and their immune system weakens, the chicken pox virus "wakes up" and causes painful blisters called shingles. If you have never had chicken pox, you can catch this virus from a resident with shingles. You may then become ill with chicken pox.

To prevent transmission of the virus, wear gloves when caring for a resident with draining shingles. Wash your hands well. If you have already had chicken pox, however, you cannot catch it again.

IDENTIFYING SIGNS AND SYMPTOMS OF COMMON INFECTIONS

Because the body responds to infections in certain ways, you can often recognize the clues of common infections. A symptom of infection happens in the person's body when microorganisms cause disease. The infected individual feels certain symptoms and may describe them to you. For example, a fever blister on the lip causes a burning or tingling sensation of the skin before the fever blister breaks out. If a resident cannot describe this symptom, you cannot know that a fever blister is about to erupt.

A sign of infection, on the other hand, can be known to someone else. Some signs of infection are visible, such as redness and drainage caused by an eye infection. Other signs of infection can be identified by lab tests (Fig. 11-4, next page). For example, a complete blood count may indicate a high number of white cells in the blood, which

Blister – elevated area of epidermis containing watery liquid

Pus – a yellowish-white fluid formed when an infection is present

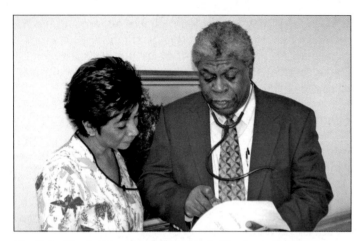

Fig. 11-4 – The doctor will order a complete blood count test that can indicate an infection if the white blood cells are elevated.

is a sign of infection. Other signs of infection can be measured with instruments. For example, a thermometer is used to measure elevated temperature, which is a sign of infection. An X-ray can identify signs of pneumonia in the chest.

Signs and symptoms of infection are clues that you can observe in your daily care of residents. Putting several clues together helps you form a picture of infection, even if residents can't tell you where they hurt or how they feel. When you put clues together well and report them to the nurse, you improve the quality of life for residents.

Clues to Infection in Older Adults

Clues to an infection are not as clear in older adults as they are in younger people. Also, a resident with cognitive impairment may not be able to tell you when they feel symptoms. You have to look for signs that indicate some change. Some clues to infection that you may observe when giving daily care include drainage from a wound, dark and smelly urine, or greenish thick sputum. Remember that even a small change, such as a change in their skin coloring, mood, or activity level, can be an important clue that something may be wrong.

You can also identify infection when it first appears. You are often the first person to notice a change in a resident's normal behavior or condition. The change may be a clue that a resident is developing an infection. Tell the charge nurse about any change you observe so that the resident can be evaluated promptly. Then treatment can begin before the infection becomes serious. Antibiotic treatment works much better early in an infection than after a resident becomes seriously ill.

Putting Together Clues to Infection

When you identify clues to a possible infection, you need to put them together in a meaningful way. You know residents better than anyone else in the facility. You know when a resident looks, acts, or sounds different than usual. These differences may be clues to infection, but you need to put them together and report your observations to the charge nurse so that action can be taken if needed (Fig. 11-5). Consider this example:

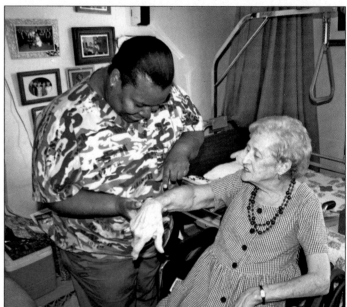

Fig. 11-5 – Report all your observations to the charge nurse.

Mr. Cavanaugh is usually eager to get out of bed and be active. But on Tuesday morning when you go in to get Mr. Cavanaugh ready for breakfast, he tells you he didn't sleep well and felt cold all night. He coughs, and you notice that his nose is running. He tells you he really doesn't feel like getting out of bed this morning. You might want to take Mr. Cavanaugh's temperature because fever is a sign of infection. If Mr. Cavanaugh just has a cold, however, he may not have a fever. His runny nose and cough are other clues you should report to the charge nurse so that he can be evaluated further.

It is important that you describe the signs and symptoms you have observed. Tell the charge nurse that Mr. Cavanaugh has a runny nose and cough and doesn't feel like getting out of bed, and that his temperature was only 98 F. This specific information helps the charge nurse evaluate Mr. Cavanaugh further and talk with the physician. The charge nurse should be pleased that you have already taken Mr. Cavanaugh's temperature. The physician may prescribe a cold medication to help Mr. Cavanaugh be more comfortable. For the next few days watch for changes in his condition because a simple cold can sometimes lead to pneumonia.

Putting different clues together may also help identify a possible urinary tract infection. For example, a common symptom of urinary tract infection is a burning sensation on urination. A resident who is cognitively impaired may not be able to describe this. But if you watch their facial expression and body language, you may notice that they feel pain during voiding. A pained facial expression during voiding may be a clue of a urinary tract infection, although there could some other reason for the pain. A specific clue is dark or smelly urine, or urinary incontinence in a resident who usually can control bladder function. If all three clues are present in a resident, they probably have a urinary tract infection. Report this information promptly to the charge nurse.

INTEGUMENTARY SYSTEM (SKIN)

Structures

The skin has two main layers (Fig. 11-6):
• The epidermis is the top layer you can see and feel.
• The dermis is the thicker layer beneath the epidermis.

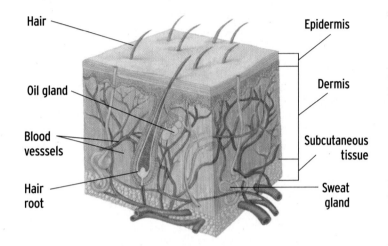

Fig. 11-6 — The skin and its components.

Beneath the two layers of skin is a cushion of subcutaneous tissue. This cushion of fatty tissue helps the skin look smooth. Five structures within the skin help the skin stay healthy and help protect the body:
• The oil glands, called sebaceous glands, help keep the skin moist.
• The sweat glands help the body get rid of heat and waste products.
• The hair roots and hair over parts of the body help protect the skin.
• Melanocytes are cells that give color to the skin.
• Blood vessels nourish the skin and help control body temperature.

Three other integumentary structures are extensions or outgrowths from the skin:
• hair
• fingernails and toenails
• mucous membranes lining the inside of the nose, mouth, and other body openings

Functions

The skin is very important to health because it covers the entire body and protects the body in two ways:
- It prevents germs in the environment from entering the body. This is the first line of defense against infection.
- It helps control body temperature. The skin sweats when it is hot, and the blood vessels to the skin dilate (expand) to let heat out. When it is cold, blood vessels constrict (narrow) to keep heat in.

Aging Changes

The skin often shows the signs of aging sooner than other body systems. This is especially true with lifelong exposure to sun, wind, cold air, and drying soaps. Table 11-1 lists the changes that occur in the skin and hair as a person ages.

TABLE 11-1
CHANGES IN THE INTEGUMENTARY SYSTEM WITH AGING

CHANGE	RESULT
Inability of skin to retain moisture	Dryness of skin and hair
Thinning of the dermis layer of the skin	Wrinkling of the skin
Decreased elasticity of the skin	Sagging skin
Shrinkage of the hypodermis layer of skin, due to loss of fatty tissue	Difficulty adjusting to heat loss, especially on the face and back of hands
Decreased production of melanin in hair bulbs	Graying hair
Decrease in rate of growth of hair follicles	Thinning hair

Abnormal Signs and Symptoms

- change in color or size of any skin growth such as a mole, freckle, wart, etc.
- bleeding
- rash (red bumps on skin)
- reddened areas
- open sores
- bruises
- cuts
- flaking skin
- complaints of itching or pain
- very hot skin
- cold, damp skin

Observations To Report

- What does this resident's skin normally look like?
- Is a growth new, has it changed, or has it always been there?
- Has the resident done something new, such as trying a new skin lotion or wearing new clothes, that might have caused a rash?
- Does the reddened area go away when you change the resident's position?
- What has the weather been like? Is a resident's skin dry and flaky because of the weather?
- Is the resident concerned about the appearance of their skin?
- Has the resident's attitude about personal hygiene changed?
- Does the resident have a history of allergies?

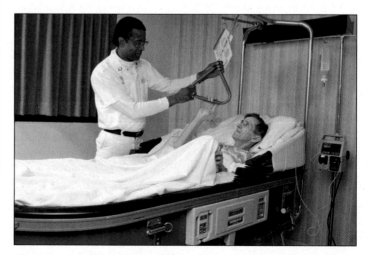

Fig. 11-7 – A special mattress can be used to help prevent pressure ulcers.

ypodermis – lining beneath the epidermis

Common Chronic Illnesses, Diseases, and Problems of the Integumentary System

One of the worst skin problems is the formation of a pressure ulcer. The prevention and treatment of pressure ulcers (Fig. 11-7, previous page) is described in Chapter 19, Maintaining Skin Integrity.

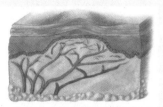
Stage 1 pressure ulcer

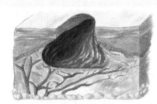
Stage 3 pressure ulcer

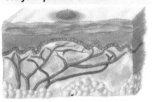
Stage 2 pressure ulcer

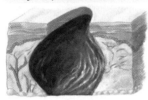
Stage 4 pressure ulcer

Dry Skin.   With aging and weather changes, skin dryness is a common problem. Dryness may also result from other factors such as irritating wool clothes or rough sheets or linens. Dry skin is annoying but can usually be handled easily.

Signs and Symptoms of Dry Skin
- flaky areas on skin
- reddened areas
- complaints of itchiness
- scratching

Nurse Assistant's Role in Observation and Intervention
- Pay attention to a resident's skin when giving care. You may find reddened areas, or the resident may tell you their skin feels itchy. The skin may be more itchy at night.
- Inspect the skin for flaking, redness, or scratch marks. These can be signs of a problem.
- Always report any complaints to the charge nurse.
- Keep the resident's skin well lubricated (moisturized).

Goals of Care
- Eliminate the dryness and itchiness.
- Help the person feel more comfortable.
- Prevent problems such as tears in the skin caused by scratching.

Interventions or Skills for Care
- Limit the amount of soap used on the skin.
- Use a moisturizing cream on the affected area. Massage the cream gently into the skin to enhance absorption. Let residents choose what cream they want used. If the resident does not have a preference, any moisturizing skin cream will work.
- Add bath oil to the bath if the resident prefers and the charge nurse says you may.
- Use a therapeutic bath solution if ordered by the physician (see Chapter 16, Personal Care).
- Encourage the resident to drink more fluids, especially water (unless they are on fluid restrictions).
- Keep the resident's nails trimmed and clean.

Contact Dermatitis.   Contact dermatitis is a skin reaction resulting from a resident contacting something they are allergic to.

Signs and Symptoms of Contact Dermatitis
- rash (red bumps on skin)
- complaints of itchiness

Nurse Assistant's Role in Observation and Intervention
- Identify and report to the charge nurse what changes occurred before the rash developed. For example:
  – new clothing
  – new detergent used in laundry
  – new food
  – new medication
  – new jewelry
- Report any rash to the charge nurse because it may indicate an infection or an allergic reaction.

Goals of Care
- Identify the source of the allergic reaction.
- Relieve the itchiness.
- Prevent problems such as skin tears caused by scratching.

Interventions or Skills for Care
  Help the charge nurse with the following:
- Use over-the-counter topical ointments as the physician recommends. Most of these ointments contain hydrocortisone to relieve the itching.
- Cover the area with a dry dressing if the physician orders.
- Use therapeutic bath solutions if the physician orders.

MUSCULOSKELETAL SYSTEM

Structures

The **musculoskeletal system** is made up of bones, muscles, tendons, ligaments, and joints (Fig. 11-8):

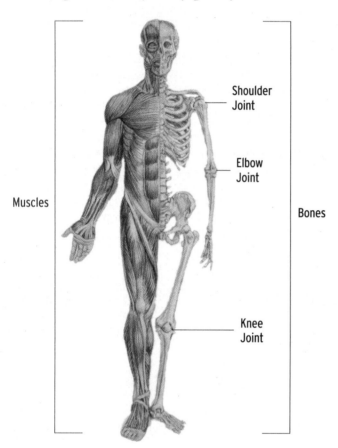

Shoulder Joint

Elbow Joint

Muscles

Bones

Knee Joint

Fig. 11-8 – The musculoskeletal system and its components.

* Bones are the frame for the body.
* Muscles allow the body to move.
* Tendons attach muscles to bones.
* Ligaments attach bones to other bones.
* Joints are where two or more bones come together.

Functions

The musculoskeletal system helps give the body its shape and enables it to move. Movement is important for good health.

Aging Changes

Table 11-2 lists the changes that occur in the musculoskeletal system as a person ages.

TABLE 11-2
CHANGES IN THE MUSCULOSKELETAL SYSTEM WITH AGING

CHANGE	RESULT
A shortening of the spinal column due to compression of vertebrae and changes in posture	Loss of height
Loss of minerals from bones	Greater risk of broken bones
Loss of muscle mass	Loss of strength
Loss of elasticity	Muscle stiffness

Abnormal Signs and Symptoms

* swollen, reddened joints
* bumps or bruises on arms and legs
* complaints of increased stiffness, inability to move, or pain

Observations To Report

* Does a resident favor a certain position?
* Is the resident's position changed often?
* Does the resident get up and move or walk enough? Do they need help?
* Does the resident have problems moving in the morning or after sitting awhile?
* Does the resident favor one arm or leg over the other?
* Do the resident's shoes and assistive devices fit properly?
* Can you do anything to promote and support the resident's ability to move (offer your arm, move things out of the way)?

Common Chronic Illnesses, Diseases, and Problems of the Musculoskeletal System

Arthritis. Arthritis is a common joint problem that causes pain and limits movement in joints affected by it. The two most common types are osteoarthritis and rheumatoid arthritis. Osteoarthritis is more common. It is caused by age and a lifetime of wear and tear on the joint. The cartilage in joints between bones thins and breaks down, resulting in less shock absorbency. Because of this, the body produces bony protuberances (swellings, bumps) at the sides of the joints (Fig. 11-9). Rheumatoid arthritis is an inflammatory disease of the joints. Because of the inflammation the joints become swollen, warm, and painful.

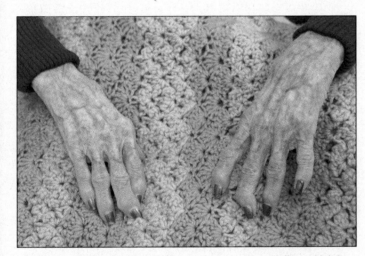

Fig. 11-9 – A resident with arthritis can have swollen, disfigured joints.

Signs and Symptoms of Arthritis
* stiffness
* painful joints
* in rheumatoid arthritis, red, swollen, and hot joints

Nurse Assistant's Role in Observation and Intervention
* Promote the resident's capabilities and encourage them to do whatever they can.
* Plan care around scheduled pain management.
* Encourage independence. Recognize the resident may need more time to complete an activity .
* Help the resident maintain as much mobility as possible.
* Encourage the resident to use adaptive equipment.

Note: *Residents may resist movement due to pain, but it is important for the joints to move as much as possible to prevent problems. When a resident does not use a joint, disfigurement may occur caused by an abnormal position of the joint, known as a contracture.*

Goals of Care
* Minimize pain.
* Prevent injury.
* Promote mobility.
* Keep joints movable (by providing range of motion (ROM) exercise).

Interventions or Skills for Care
When caring for someone with joint pain, you should:
* Let the resident know you care, understand, and want to help, since residents in constant pain can feel hopeless and depressed.
* Plan your schedule for care and other activities such as ROM exercises to enable residents to receive their pain medication first. Talk to the charge nurse about this.
* Help the resident with ROM exercises to prevent deformities. But never move a joint that is very painful, red, or swollen (Fig. 11-10).
* Properly position a resident in bed or a wheelchair. Encourage good posture.
* Help a resident put on splints or braces.

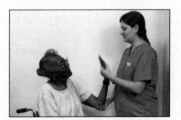

Fig. 11-10 – Range of motion exercise can prevent deformities. Never move a joint that is painful, red, or swollen.

* Plan your schedule to help the person back to bed for rest periods as needed. Don't push a resident to be active when they are tired, because this can damage joints.
* Report any joint problems to the charge nurse.
* Encourage a resident to do as much as possible to help maintain their independence.

Osteoporosis. Osteoporosis is caused by a gradual loss of minerals, especially calcium, from bones. Bones become weak and brittle. Osteoporosis is most common in women after menopause. Often this condition is not diagnosed until a resident is injured. Many postmenopausal women have a bone density screening as part of their physical examination. Calcium supplements and prescription drugs help minimize the mineral loss from bones. Residents with osteoporosis have a higher risk for fractures. Use the information you learned in Chapter 10, Personal Protection and Injury Prevention, to prevent falls.

Signs and Symptoms of Osteoporosis
- loss of height
- falling
- fractures

Nurse Assistant's Role in Observation and Intervention
- Monitor residents who are frail or have a history of falling and previous fractures.
- Anticipate problems when residents move, and use safety measures.
- Encourage weight-bearing activities.

Goals of Care
- Promote safety.
- Encourage good nutrition and exercise as tolerated.

Interventions or Skills for Care
- Always use assistive devices, like a gait belt, when moving a resident from bed to chair or chair to bed and when helping them walk.
- Encourage residents to use a cane for support or a weight-bearing walker, especially when they start to move.
- Be sure a resident has a clear path to leave the bed to walk, to prevent injury from bumping into things.
- If a resident starts to fall when you are with them, try to guide them to the floor.
- If you find a resident on the floor, call the charge nurse immediately and follow their instructions.
- Encourage residents to eat healthy, balanced meals, especially those rich in calcium.

Fracture. A fracture is a break in a bone, caused most commonly by a fall (Fig. 11-11). The most common fracture in elderly residents is a fractured hip.

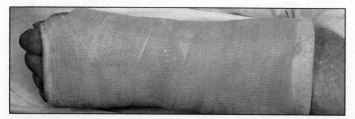

Fig. 11-11 – A resident who breaks a bone needs a cast to assist in the healing process.

Signs and Symptoms of Fractures
- swollen, black and blue area at the break site
- complaints of pain or altered sensation
- inability to put weight on leg or to use arm
- abnormal shape of arm or leg, including possible shortening of the limb

Nurse Assistant's Role in Observation and Intervention
- Report any abnormality you see in a resident's arms or legs.
- Report any pain.
- Provide a safe environment. Keep the call light within the resident's reach.
- Promote activities that enhance healing and mobility. Follow the recommendations of the nurse and physical therapist.

Goals of Care
- Prevent complications from the fracture, such as muscle weakness and joint abnormalities.
- Help the resident regain their former level of mobility.

Interventions or Skills for Care
- Assist the resident with mobility according to their care plan.
- Do ROM exercises to keep other joints and muscles working, as directed on their care plan.
- Use proper transfer techniques to avoid harmful movement at the fracture site.
- Encourage the resident's independence.
- Support a resident going to physical or occupational therapy for rehabilitation. Help them to use the toilet. Encourage and assist them to dress in comfortable clothing.
- Follow the physical therapist's guidelines for movement, such as walking with a walker.
- Recognize that a resident may fear falling and fracturing the bone again and therefore may avoid some activities. Be supportive and offer help until the person feels secure.
- Follow the instructions of the charge nurse and physical therapist about positioning the resident properly in bed and in a chair. Improper positioning can slow the healing of a fracture.

Fracture – broken bone

RESPIRATORY SYSTEM

Structures

The main structures of the respiratory system
(Fig. 11-12) are:
- The nasopharynx is the nasal passage.
- The oropharynx is the mouth and oral passage.
- The trachea connects the mouth and nose to the bronchi.
- The right and left bronchi enter the lungs like tree trunks.
- The bronchioles are branches from each bronchus. These air passages inside each lung look like an upside-down tree.
- The lungs take air in, move oxygen into the blood, and remove carbon dioxide from the blood.
- The alveoli (air sacs) look like hundreds of blossoms on the bronchioles.

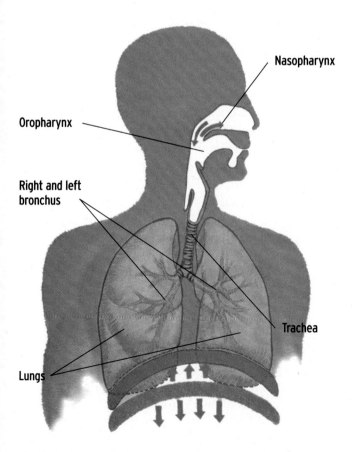

Nasopharynx

Oropharynx

Right and left
bronchus

Lungs

Trachea

Fig. 11-12 — The respiratory system and its components.

Function

Breathing (respiration) is the exchange of oxygen and carbon dioxide in the lungs. This is one of the most basic and important body functions.

The respiratory system takes in oxygen through the nose or mouth as we breathe in (inhale or inspire) air. The air passes through the bronchi and bronchioles and into the alveoli.

The oxygen then passes into the blood vessels and is carried by the blood to all body parts. The blood exchanges oxygen for carbon dioxide. The air that we breathe out (exhale or expire) gets rid of the carbon dioxide from the body. The heart and lungs work together to oxygenate the blood.

Aging Changes

Table 11-3 lists the changes that occur in the respiratory system as a person ages.

TABLE 11-3 CHANGES IN THE RESPIRATORY SYSTEM WITH AGING	
CHANGE	**RESULT**
The chest wall and lung structures become more rigid. Respiratory muscle strength decreases.	There is not as much room for air in the lungs, and it is more difficult to take deep breaths.
A decreased amount of air is exchanged with each breath.	During exercise, illness, or stress, a person has to breathe faster to get enough oxygen in and carbon dioxide out.

Abnormal Signs and Symptoms

- cyanosis
- gasping for breath or labored breathing
- rattling or gurgling noise when breathing
- foul-smelling breath
- very fast or very slow chest movements
- very cold or very hot skin
- sweating
- needing to sit up to breathe
- pain with breathing
- shortness of breath, unusual color sputum, or funny taste in their mouth.

Observations To Report

- Has the resident's breathing changed?
- What do the resident's lips, nail beds, and skin usually look like? Are they different now?
- Is the resident sitting upright? Is it difficult for the resident to lie flat?
- Does the resident's breathing sound strange?
- Does the resident take frequent rest periods?
- Does the resident complain of shortness of breath, difficulty breathing, or decreased ability to do things?
- Has the resident coughed up unusual sputum (lung secretions)?

Common Chronic Illnesses, Diseases, and Problems

Cold and Flu. The common cold is an upper respiratory infection caused by a virus. Colds sometime accompany the flu. Flu causes more symptoms. A resident with the flu will have cold symptoms along with fever, body aches, and headache. The flu can be a major problem for residents. Today most residents receive an annual flu shot.

Signs and Symptoms of a Cold and Flu
Cold:
- runny nose
- cough
- watery eyes
- stuffiness or a sense of fullness in the face, called sinus pressure

Flu:
- all the cold symptoms listed above plus
- aching muscles and joints
- possible fever
- headache
- weakness

Nurse Assistant's Role in Observation and Intervention
- Report symptoms early to prevent further illness.
- Provide care to relieve symptoms.
- Practice infection control procedures, especially proper handwashing, to keep the infection from spreading to other residents and yourself.

Goals of Care
- Help the resident to be comfortable.
- Monitor their symptoms.
- Prevent spread of infection to yourself and others with proper handwashing.

Interventions or Skills for Care
- Encourage the resident to drink plenty of fluids (unless they are on fluid restrictions).
- Encourage them to rest.
- Encourage the resident to get out of bed for short periods. If they cannot get out of bed, be sure they change position often. Keep the head of the bed elevated to limit their respiratory distress.
- Remind the resident to breathe deeply and cough often to prevent mucous secretions from building up in the lungs.

Cyanosis – bluish or purplish discoloration of the skin caused by not enough oxygenation of the blood

- Keep tissues handy. Use gloves when handling tissues with secretions. Dispose of tissues in proper containers.
- Provide comfort by fluffing pillows, giving back rubs, etc.
- Measure the resident's vital signs as directed and report any changes.
- Observe their symptoms and report even a small change to the charge nurse.
- Wash your hands before and after contact with a resident.
- The doctor may order a sputum specimen and other tests to be sent to the lab.

Sputum Specimens

Sputum is a substance often present in a person's mouth after coughing. It contains saliva, mucus, and at times purulent (infected) secretions or drainage. Usually it is thicker than saliva. Sputum comes from further down in the airway or lungs. A sputum specimen can be helpful in diagnosing a disease or condition affecting the respiratory system. Procedure 11-1 describes how to collect a sputum specimen.

Pneumonia. Pneumonia is a lung infection caused by a virus or bacteria. It may follow a cold or bronchitis (an infection in the bronchial tubes).

Signs and Symptoms of Pneumonia
- difficulty breathing
- cough, sometimes with increased sputum
- shortness of breath
- complaint of painful breathing
- possible elevated temperature
- possible lethargy or weakness

Nurse Assistant's Role in Observation and Intervention
- Report symptoms to the charge nurse.
- Give care to relieve symptoms and provide comfort.

Goals of Care
- Keep resident comfortable and promote rest.
- Relieve symptoms.

Interventions or Skills for Care
- Encourage the resident to drink plenty of fluids (unless they are on fluid restrictions).
- Encourage good nutrition to aid in the healing process.
- Encourage the resident to rest.

PROCEDURE 11-1.
COLLECTING A SPUTUM SPECIMEN

 REMEMBER: BE AWARE

Items Needed
- specimen container and label
- gloves
- biohazardous bag

Note: *Make sure a resident who chews tobacco has not done so before you collect the specimen. If the resident has just eaten, ask them to rinse out their mouth. Try to collect the specimen in the morning. Often large amounts of sputum are coughed up first thing in the morning.*

1. Give the resident the sputum collection container or hold it yourself. Take care not to touch its inside surface, or lining.

2. Ask the resident to take deep breaths and cough deeply from the chest. They may need to cough several times to get enough sputum for the sample. Ask them to try not to spit only saliva into the container.

3. Place the lid securely on the specimen bottle. Label it with the resident's name, room number, and the date and time of the collection. Place the specimen in a biohazardous bag.

4. Report the color, amount, and consistency of the specimen to the charge nurse.

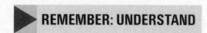 **REMEMBER: UNDERSTAND**

- Encourage the resident to get out of bed for short periods. If they cannot get out of bed, be sure they change position often. Keep the head of the bed elevated to reduce their respiratory distress (Fig. 11-13).

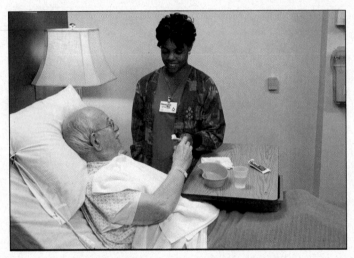

Fig. 11-13 – Keeping the head of the bed elevated will reduce a resident's respiratory distress.

- Remind the resident to breathe deeply and cough often. This helps prevent mucous secretions from building up in the lungs.
- Keep tissues handy. Use gloves when handling tissues with secretions. Dispose of tissues in proper containers.
- Provide comfort by fluffing pillows, giving back rubs, etc.
- Monitor the resident's vital signs and report any changes.
- Monitor their symptoms and report even a small change to the charge nurse.
- Wash your hands before and after contact with the resident.

Chronic Obstructive Pulmonary Disease (COPD).

Chronic obstructive pulmonary disease results from many years of problems with the bronchial passageways and lungs. Bronchitis, emphysema, and asthma are types of COPD. These diseases cause a chronic inflammation that narrows the bronchioles and alveoli. This narrowing results in a loss of lung elasticity.

Signs and Symptoms of Chronic Obstructive Pulmonary Disease
- difficulty breathing
- wheezing
- coughing
- increased sputum production
- cyanosis
- shortness of breath
- activity intolerance

Nurse Assistant's Role in Observation and Intervention
- Maintain adequate respiration.
- Monitor the resident for secondary conditions such as infection.
- Reduce the resident's anxiety.

Goals of Care
- Keep the resident breathing comfortably.

Interventions or Skills for Care
- Encourage a resident, if able, to take four or five deep breaths in and out several times during the day. Deep breathing helps fill the lungs with air, and helps the chest wall stay flexible.
- Encourage the resident to rest between meals, bathing, exercise, and social activities.
- Encourage the resident to breathe slowly and deeply while walking, and to rest often for a minute during longer walks.
- When the resident is seated, ask them to lean forward and cross their arms in front to make breathing easier.
- Watch for any change in a resident's ability to perform the activities of daily living. Report even a small change to the charge nurse.
- Monitor the resident's vital signs. Even a small change in temperature, pulse, respiration, or blood pressure may indicate a complication in a resident with COPD.

Respiration – exchange of oxygen and carbon dioxide in the lungs

Some residents may need oxygen occasionally or continuously. To care for residents on oxygen, you should:

- Check the resident's nasal passages. Oxygen therapy can be very irritating to tissues in the nose. Report redness, bleeding, or discomfort to the charge nurse.
- Do not change the oxygen flow-rate setting. Only the nurse may do this. Too much oxygen can depress the respiratory centers of the brain and be life-threatening.
- Elevate the head of the bed to help the resident breathe more easily.
- Never allow smoking or flames near oxygen. Make sure "No Smoking, Oxygen in Use" signs are posted.
- Check the tubing and connection to prevent twists (Fig. 11-14).

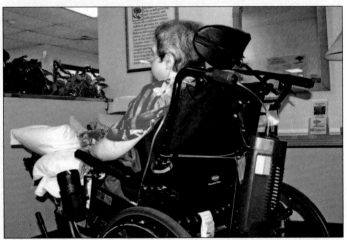

Fig. 11-14 — Always check the oxygen tubing for any twisting and make sure the connections are intact.

CIRCULATORY SYSTEM

Structures

The heart and blood vessels working together make up the circulatory system. The heart is a muscular organ with four chambers (Fig. 11-15). It is located behind the ribs and between the two lungs; the largest part lies in the left side of the chest.

The heart pumps blood through the blood vessels to every part of the body. Every time you count a resident's pulse, you are counting how fast the heart pumps blood through the body. (Counting a pulse is described in Chapter 13, Gathering Data.) Three types of blood vessels carry blood to and from the heart and organs throughout the body:

- Arteries carry oxygenated blood from the lungs and heart to the organs.
- Capillaries, which are tiny blood vessels, connect arteries and veins and exchange oxygen for carbon dioxide inside the organs.
- Veins carry deoxygenated blood from the organs back to the heart and lungs.

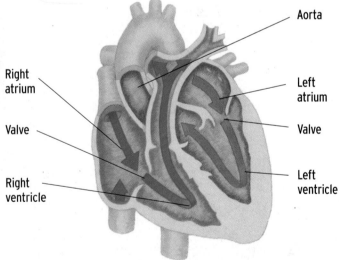

Fig. 11-15 — The heart and its components.

Functions

The circulatory system carries oxygen from the lungs and other vital nourishment to all the cells of the body. It also carries waste products to some body organs so the body can get rid of them.

The circulatory system works as follows: First, the body returns deoxygenated blood (the oxygen has been used by the organs) to the right atrium of the heart. The blood passes through an opening (valve) into the right ventricle. The right ventricle pumps it through blood vessels to the lungs, where the blood is oxygenated. Then the blood returns to the left atrium. The blood passes through a valve into the left ventricle, which pumps it out of the heart into the largest blood vessel, the aorta.

The aorta branches off to the upper and lower parts of the body and connects with smaller blood vessels that carry oxygenated blood to every organ and cell in the body.

Aging Changes

Table 11-4 lists the changes that occur in the circulatory system as a person ages.

TABLE 11-4
CHANGES IN THE CIRCULATORY SYSTEM WITH AGING

CHANGE	RESULT
The heart muscle wall thickens, becomes stiffer, and may increase in size.	The heart has to work harder to pump the same amount of blood. The heart can become overworked during strenuous activity, forcing an older person to take more frequent rest periods.
The blood vessels become more rigid and stiff.	The heart has to work harder to pump blood through rigid vessels; blood pressure is higher.
Sensors that regulate blood pressure with position changes are less sensitive.	Dizziness occurs when changing position.
The heart rate decreases.	May cause no symptoms. If the heart rate becomes too low, dizziness may result.

Abnormal Signs and Symptoms

- swollen extremities due to edema
- shortness of breath, especially on exertion
- feet may turn pale color
- weight gain or loss
- complaints of chest pain or indigestion
- increased or decreased blood pressure
- cold, damp skin
- fast, slow, or irregular pulse
- fatigue

Observations To Report

- Are the resident's feet or ankles puffy or swollen, or is the sacrum swollen in a bedridden resident?
- Has the resident suddenly gained weight?
- Is the resident suddenly unable to do things they could do before (walk to the dining room, climb stairs)?
- Is the resident's heart rate regular? Is their blood pressure normal? Does the resident complain of dizziness?

Edema – swelling because of fluid gain, most commonly observed in the legs and ankles

Sacrum – bottom part of the spine

Common Chronic Illnesses, Diseases, and Problems of the Circulatory System

Congestive Heart Failure (CHF).   Congestive heart failure occurs when the heart muscle weakens. The heart moves blood through the body less effectively. CHF is common in people who have had high blood pressure and coronary artery disease for years.

Signs and Symptoms of Congestive Heart Failure
- shortness of breath
- swelling of the legs and ankles due to edema (fluid weight gain) (Fig. 11-16)

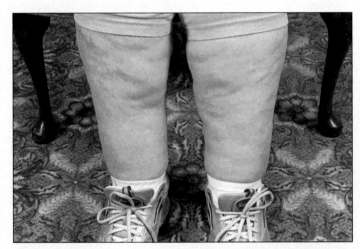

Fig. 11-16 – One sign of congestive heart failure is edema, especially in the legs and ankles.

- cyanosis
- noisy respiration
- complaints of tiring easily

Nurse Assistant's Role in Observation and Intervention
- Identify any changes in a resident that suggest the condition is worsening, such as an inability to perform the activities of daily living.
- Monitor vital signs as directed by the charge nurse.
- Monitor the resident's weight (Fig. 11-17).
- Follow the resident's dietary restrictions if any have been ordered.

Goals of Care
- Help maintain the resident's level of independence.
- Help maintain the resident's level of cardiac function.
- Help maintain the resident's weight.

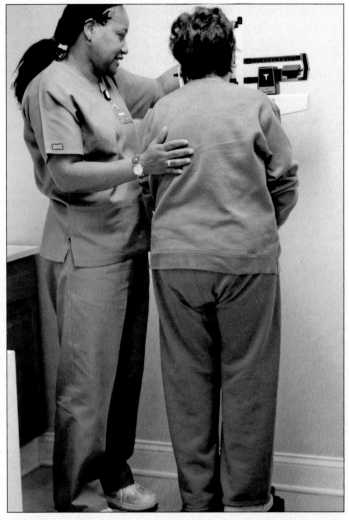

Fig. 11-17 – Maintaining the resident's weight is one goal of care.

Interventions or Skills for Care
- Give the resident opportunities to perform their own personal care.
- Encourage the resident to rest frequently.
- Encourage the resident to take deep breaths.
- Weigh the resident as ordered, and report any increase or decrease in weight to the charge nurse.
- Maintain accurate intake and output records.

To assist a resident with edema in the lower legs: Have the resident sit with their legs elevated on a footstool or lie in bed with legs stretched out for one to two hours, three times a day. Legs should be elevated higher than the buttocks, and pressure should be off the resident's heels.

- Encourage the resident to exercise and walk regularly.
- Make sure the resident's shoes are not too tight.

If the doctor has ordered support stockings, follow these guidelines (Procedure 11-2):
- Use the correct size of support stockings. The stockings should be snug enough to give support but not too tight or too loose. If a person has gained or lost much weight, check for correct stocking size. Check with the charge nurse if you are unsure.
- Be sure the stockings are clean and dry.
- Put the support stockings on the resident in the morning before they move their legs off the bed. This will help prevent fluid from pooling in the feet.
- Make sure residents know not to roll the stockings down. That could greatly reduce the circulation in their legs.
- Tell the resident to call you if they become uncomfortable.
- Check the toes every hour to ensure they are warm and a normal color. Check the stockings to make sure there are no wrinkles.
- Remove elastic stockings at least twice a day for 30 minutes or according to the care plan. Check with the charge nurse on how long the elastic stocking should be off. This lets you observe the skin and allows the legs to rest (Fig. 11-18).

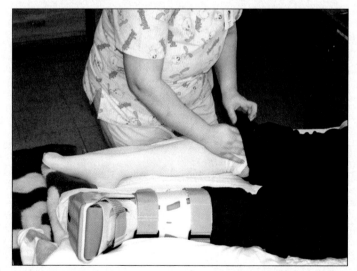

Fig. 11-18 – Check with the charge nurse and care plan about elastic stocking use.

PROCEDURE 11-2. APPLYING ELASTIC STOCKINGS

▶ **REMEMBER: BE AWARE**

Items Needed
- correct size and length elastic stockings
- baby powder (unless the person has a respiratory problem)
- basin with warm water
- soap
- washcloth
- towel

1. Assist the person to lie on their back.

2. Expose only the person's legs.

3. Observe the person's legs for swelling, moles, cuts, bruising, or other changes in skin color or appearance.

4. Clean and dry the person's legs and feet before applying elastic stockings.

5. Apply a very small amount of baby powder to the person's legs and feet unless the per son has any respiratory difficulty. The powder makes it easier to apply the stockings, which fit tightly and can be difficult to apply.

6. Apply one elastic stocking at a time. Begin by rolling the stocking with your hands so that only the toe section is exposed. Put the stocking on the person's leg, positioning the hole over the top of the toes. Make sure the heel is properly placed. Then roll the stocking up the leg as far as it will go.

7. Do the same on the other leg. The stockings should fit firmly and have no wrinkles.

8. Check for good circulation and movement by observing the person's toes for color and ability to move freely.

▶ **REMEMBER: UNDERSTAND**

Peripheral Vascular Disease (PVD). Peripheral vascular disease causes a diminished blood flow to the arms and legs. Tissues in the extremities then do not receive enough nourishment. This condition is more common in the feet.

Signs and Symptoms of Peripheral Vascular Disease
- a pale color in the feet and sometimes hands
- complaints of feet and sometimes hands being cold
- tingling sensation ("pins and needles")
- loss of feeling

Nurse Assistant's Role in Observation and Intervention
* Identify changes in a resident's skin.
* Monitor the environment to prevent injury.

Goals of Care
* Promote circulation.
* Prevent injury.
* Maintain skin integrity.

Interventions or Skills for Care
* Inspect the resident's feet.
* Feel the temperature of the resident's skin. If circulation is decreased, the skin feels cool.
* Observe the color of the skin. When circulation is decreased, skin looks bluish or pale in a light-skinned person or dusky gray in a dark-skinned person.
* Observe the color of the nail beds. Poor circulation can cause a bluish tinge to the nail beds.
* Feel for pulses in the lower extremities: the popliteal pulse behind the knee, the posterior tibial pulse at the ankle, and the pedal pulse on the upper part of the foot (Fig. 11-19). Report to the charge nurse whether or not you can feel these pulses.
* Watch for and report reddened areas, cracked skin between the toes, or skin breakdown.
* Encourage the resident to change position every one to two hours while awake. If a resident reads or watches television sitting or lying down, encourage them to get up and walk around for a few minutes every hour or so.
* Encourage the resident to take daily walks and participate in exercise programs at the facility.
* Report any changes you observe in any wounds.
* Explain to the resident why they should or should not do the following, to ensure normal circulation.

The resident should avoid the following:
— crossing legs at the knees
— dangling the feet a long time
— wearing restricting clothing such as tight garter straps or panty girdles
— smoking cigarettes or cigars
— spending time in cold environments, which narrow blood vessels
— sitting too close to a heat source

The resident should do the following:
— Keep legs elevated.

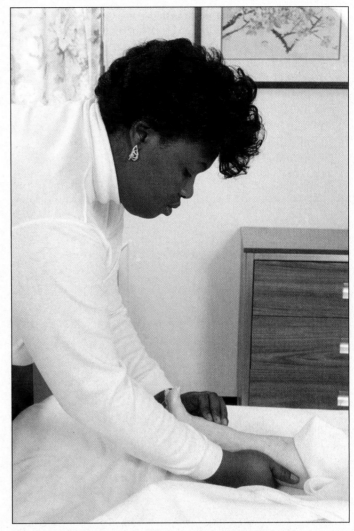

Fig. 11-19 — Feeling for the pedal pulse is a good indicator of a resident's circulation to the lower legs.

The nurse assistant should do the following:
— Encourage the resident to wiggle their toes and make circles with the feet to promote circulation.
— Keep the resident's skin clean, dry, and lubricated (moisturized).
— Provide a safe environment to prevent injury.
  — Keep a clear path for the resident when walking.
  — Keep the resident's room uncluttered.
  — Check bath water temperature for the resident.
  — Make sure shoes fit properly.

Coronary Artery Disease (CAD). Coronary artery disease results from decreased blood flow through the coronary arteries, which nourish the heart. The exact cause of coronary artery disease is not known. Several factors can contribute to its development:

- high blood pressure
- diabetes
- obesity
- family history
- smoking
- diet high in fat
- lack of exercise
- stress
- cholesterol

Signs and Symptoms of Coronary Artery Disease

- complaints of chest pain
- change in pulse rate or rhythm (palpitations)
- elevated blood pressure
- elevated cholesterol level
- feeling light-headed
- shortness of breath

Nurse Assistant's Role in Observation and Intervention

- Monitor and watch for changes in the resident's vital signs.
- Follow all treatment programs that are prescribed.

Goals of Care

- Maintain the person's independence.

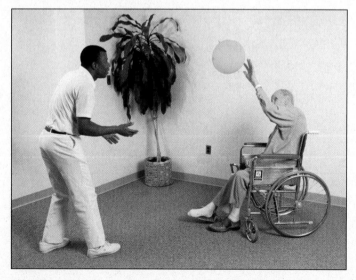

Fig. 11-20 — Exercise can improve a resident's circulation.

Interventions or Skills for Care

- Encourage the resident to exercise (Fig. 11-20).
- Encourage a low-fat diet.
- Limit stress: Talk to the resident about anything that is upsetting to them, and work with other staff to reduce the resident's stress.
- If pain occurs:
  - Have the resident immediately stop all activity.
  - Have the resident sit or lie down. When the resident is lying down, elevate the head of the bed.
  - Call the charge nurse. Follow the charge nurse's instructions.
  - Monitor the resident's vital signs.
  - Help with the delivery of oxygen.
  - Reassure the resident.
  - Communicate to other staff what factors seem to cause pain (precipitating factors).

Cerebral Vascular Accident (CVA) — Stroke.
Cerebral vascular accident, or stroke, can be caused by many things, including narrowing of a blood vessel because of plaque buildup, a blood vessel rupture, or a traveling blood clot that blocks the blood flow.

Signs and Symptoms of Cerebral Vascular Accident (CVA)

- The signs and symptoms of CVA depend on the location in the brain affected, the extent of the interruption in blood supply, and the resulting tissue damage. The most common results are:
  - weakness or paralysis on one side of body
  - difficulty in swallowing or talking
  - difficulty in communicating
  - change in mental status

It is important to quickly tell the nurse if a resident has any of these symptoms. Very prompt medical intervention can prevent or limit the effects of a stroke.

Nurse Assistant's Role in Observation and Intervention

- Support the resident's rehabilitation.

Cerebral vascular accident (CVA)– condition that occurs when blood flowing to the brain is interrupted (also called stroke)

Coronary artery disease (CAD) – condition that results from reduced flow through the coronary arteries, which nourish the heart

Goals of Care
- Prevent complications of paralysis, like **muscle atrophy** (wasting) and contractures.
- Improve the resident's level of functioning and promote independence.

Interventions or Skills for Care
To help a resident with paralysis:
- Recognize that paralysis changes a person's life drastically. Residents with paralysis may feel very angry and cheated.
- Help the resident with ROM exercises three or four times a day to prevent contractures and maintain muscle strength. The physical therapist sets the therapeutic plan. Check the care plan or ask the charge nurse for specific guidelines for the ROM exercises.
- Position and turn the resident at least every 2 hours. Support affected limbs with pillows.
- Make sure a footboard is used at the end of the bed and that the resident's affected foot or feet are against it to prevent foot drop.
- Keep things the resident uses where the resident can see and reach them.
- Check with the charge nurse about how to support the work of the physical therapist and occupational therapist to help the resident re-learn skills such as eating, moving, and dressing.

For difficulty swallowing:
- Always place the resident in an upright sitting position.
- Encourage or give small bites of food.
- Encourage or give small sips of fluid to moisten food.
- Give verbal cues when the resident is eating.
- Be prepared to perform the **Heimlich maneuver** if the resident chokes (see Chapter 20, Emergency Care).
- Offer small sips of fluid often throughout the day to ensure adequate fluid intake.

Notify the charge nurse of:
- the resident's intake for each meal and snack
- worsening of the resident's ability to swallow
- signs and symptoms of illness, such as fever or rapid pulse rate

For difficulty communicating and for residents who do not understand:
- Check the care plan.
- Talk to the resident in a calm, reassuring manner.
- Recognize that a resident may understand written messages but not spoken ones.
- Point to objects and use gestures as much as possible to reinforce what you are saying.
- Be patient and gently touch the resident often if they are comfortable with that.
- Speak slowly, using simple sentences.

To help residents who understand speech but cannot put their thoughts into words:
- Talk to them in a normal way. Explain everything you do with or to them.
- Remember that they can understand you and are not confused.
- Give them time to try to speak to you. They may be able to speak some words.
- See if they can write messages. Sometimes residents can still write when they cannot speak.

Heimlich maneuver – technique used to free a foreign object from the airway when a resident is choking

DIGESTIVE SYSTEM

Structures

The main structures of the **digestive system** are (Fig. 11-21):

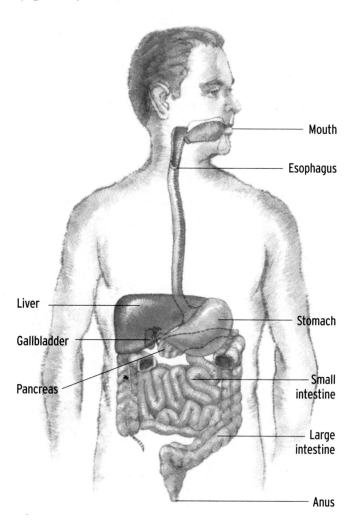

Fig. 11-21 – The digestive system and its components.

Labels on figure:
Mouth
Esophagus
Liver
Gallbladder
Pancreas
Stomach
Small intestine
Large intestine
Anus

- The mouth takes in food and fluid. Food is chewed and mixed with saliva, beginning the digestive process.
- The esophagus is a tube that passes swallowed food and fluid from the mouth to the stomach.
- The stomach is a sac-like organ that mixes food and fluid with digestive juices, preparing it for absorption.
- The small intestine is a long tube-like structure where most of the absorption of nutrients takes place.
- The liver produces bile, which helps digest fatty foods.
- The gallbladder stores bile.
- The pancreas produces digestive juices, which help break down foods for nutrients to be absorbed, and insulin, which regulates the body's blood sugar level.
- The large intestine is a long tube-like structure that moves the remaining food and waste through the body to the rectum and out of the body through the anus.
- The large intestine absorbs fluids the body needs.
- The anus is the opening from which food wastes, in the form of feces, come out in a bowel movement.

Function

The function of the digestive system is to provide the body with a supply of nutrients and fluid and to remove food waste products.

Aging Changes

Many changes occur normally in the digestive system of older persons (Table 11-5).

TABLE 11-5
CHANGES IN THE DIGESTIVE SYSTEM WITH AGING

CHANGE	RESULT
Food passes through the digestive system more slowly.	Constipation, decreased frequency of bowel movements Decreased ability to tolerate food or large meals
The amount and effectiveness of digestive juices are decreased.	Decrease in specific nutrients being absorbed

Abnormal Signs and Symptoms

- loss of appetite, food left on tray
- decreased frequency of bowel movements as reported in the resident's record or communicated by the resident
- increased bowel movements, especially with unformed, loose, or watery feces
- change in color of feces: bright red (blood), black, green
- change in texture of feces: watery, sticky, rock-like, slimy, loose
- foul odor of feces
- complaints of feeling bloated
- excessive straining during bowel movements
- nausea, vomiting, or pain
- swollen abdomen or one that feels firm or tender to the touch
- loss of bowel control (incontinence)
- weight loss

Observations To Report

- Do I know the resident's normal eating habits?
- Do I know the resident's normal bowel pattern?
- Is the resident getting enough exercise, fluid, and fiber?
- Is the resident gaining or losing weight?
- Does the resident enjoy meals?

Common Chronic Illnesses, Diseases, and Problems of the Digestive System

Constipation.   Constipation is a slowing of the bowel that results in difficulty eliminating feces. It is common among residents but occurs more often in residents who do not get enough exercise or enough fluid or fiber in their diet.

Signs and Symptoms of Constipation
- decreased number of bowel movements from the resident's usual pattern
- swollen or enlarged abdomen
- complaints of feeling bloated
- complaints of gas
- loss of appetite
- passing hard stool

Nurse Assistant's Role in Observation and Intervention
- Identify change in bowel movement pattern.
- Help the resident maintain their regular pattern of bowel movements.
- Recognize complications such as fecal impaction.

Goals of Care
- Help the resident return to a normal pattern of bowel movements.
- Prevent future problems.

Interventions or Skills for Care
- Encourage the resident to drink plenty of fluids (unless they are on fluid restrictions).
- Encourage the resident to eat fruits, vegetables, breads, and cereals, especially those high in fiber, like bran.
- Encourage exercise, especially walking.
- Follow any prescribed orders for enemas or suppositories.

Constipation – condition in which bowel movement is delayed and feces are difficult to expel from the rectum

Enema – procedure that introduces fluid into the rectum to stimulate a bowel movement

Fecal impaction – condition that may occur when constipation is not treated; hard feces are packed in the rectum

The enema may be a prepared commercial product (already mixed and ready to administer) or may have to be mixed. Different mixtures are used in enemas:

- tap water enema
- oil retention enema
- cleansing enema
- medicated enema (the nurse adds the medication and supervises the enema)

With all types of enemas, the goal and procedure are the same. First ask the charge nurse what equipment to use, how much water and at what temperature, and how to mix the solution. Procedure 11-3 describes how to give an enema.

Fecal impaction may occur if a resident's constipation is not treated. Then it is necessary to manually remove the feces. This is unpleasant for residents and may lead to a serious problem, a bowel obstruction. Fecal impaction is a serious problem, but it is preventable. You must monitor, record, and report any problems concerning a resident's bowel movements to the charge nurse. One sign of fecal impaction is that a resident may have small amounts of loose, watery stool that pass by the blockage. This loose, watery stool is sometimes mistaken for diarrhea. In addition, a resident with fecal impaction may have constipation symptoms.

PROCEDURE 11-3. GIVING AN ENEMA

 REMEMBER: BE AWARE

Items Needed
- three pairs of gloves
- plastic trash bags
- disposable enema filled with prescribed solution
- lubricant
- two disposable protective pads
- bedpan
- toilet paper

1. Put on gloves.

2. Place disposable protective pad under the resident's buttocks. Place a second protective pad at the end of the bed to place under and over bedpan when resident is finished.

3. Position the resident on their left side, helping them turn if necessary. Make sure their hips are near the edge of the bed on the side where you're working.

4. Hold the rectal tube over the bedpan. Open the clamp on the tubing and let the solution run through into the bedpan until it flows smoothly, so that no air is left in the tubing to cause discomfort for the resident. Close the clamp.

5. Turn back the bath blanket so that the resident's hips are exposed but the rest of the body is covered. Hold the lubricated rectal tube about 5 inches from the tip. Gently put it into the rectum to the red line on the tube.

6. Raise the container about 15 inches above the resident's hips. Never hold the container any higher.

7. Open the clamp and let the solution run in slowly. If the resident complains of cramps, tell them to breathe deeply through their mouth, as you clamp the tubing for a minute or so. You may also lower the irrigating bag.

8. When all the solution has run in, close the clamp.

9. Remove the rectal tube. Place the tubing in a plastic trash bag.

10. Turn the resident on their back and slip the bedpan under them. Ask the resident to try to hold the solution as long as possible. Raise the head of the bed. Ensure that the call button and toilet paper are within reach.

11. Give the resident privacy, but do not leave them for a long period of time. Check on the resident after 5 minutes.

12. When the resident feels they are done, put on gloves, and assist with wiping if necessary. Remove the bedpan and place it on a protective pad. Remove your gloves, and help the resident into a comfortable position. Put on gloves and remove the covered bedpan.

▶ **REMEMBER: UNDERSTAND**

Diarrhea. Diarrhea is caused by a number of factors: a particular food that did not agree with the person, food allergies, or the flu. These forms of diarrhea are noninfectious. Infectious diarrhea, on the other hand, can be a major problem in a facility. This form of diarrhea can spread rapidly to other residents and cause other complications.

Signs and Symptoms of Diarrhea
* frequent watery stool
* complaints of cramping
* increased gas

Nurse Assistant's Role in Observation and Intervention
* Help the resident maintain a regular pattern of bowel movements.
* Identify a change in the resident's pattern of bowel movements.

Goals of Care
* Prevent the complications of dehydration and skin breakdown.
* Prevent the spread of infectious diarrhea.

Interventions or Skills for Care
* Offer the resident clear liquids to prevent dehydration.
* Keep the resident's skin clean and dry. Apply protective cream to reddened areas to protect the skin.
* Keep the charge nurse informed about the number, color, and consistency of the resident's stools.
* Practice all infection control procedures as instructed by the charge nurse.
* Collect specimens as directed.

Bowel Incontinence. The term "bowel incontinence" means the person cannot control or is unaware of their bowel movements. Residents with dementia may not recognize the need to have a bowel movement. Some residents with a stroke or spinal cord injury may not be able to feel the urge for a bowel movement.

Signs and Symptoms of Bowel Incontinence
* involuntarily expelled feces
* inability to feel the urge to have a bowel movement
* no awareness of the passage of stool

Nurse Assistant's Role in Observation and Intervention
* Help the resident achieve and maintain a regular pattern of bowel movements.

Goals of Care
* Identify the resident's pattern of bowel movements.
* Return the resident to a regular pattern of bowel movement.
* Keep the resident clean and dry.

Interventions or Skills for Care
* To assist a resident with a bowel training program:
* Record on the bowel training flow sheet every bowel movement the resident has (Fig. 11-22). Record when the resident usually has a bowel movement, such as morning or evening, and how often they have a bowel movement, such as once a day or every other day.

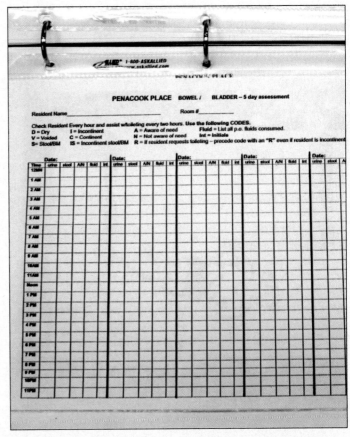

Fig. 11-22 — It is important to record a resident's bowel movements.

- Position the resident on the toilet at the time they usually have a bowel movement. Give them plenty of time to finish. Use a bedpan if no other options are appropriate.
- Provide plenty of fluids: at least eight 8-ounce glasses of liquid every day.
- Encourage the person to eat high-fiber foods such as bran cereals and bread, fruit, and vegetables.
- Encourage regular exercise, if possible, such as walking.
- Use a laxative or enema as part of the training program as the doctor orders and the nurse directs.
- Talk daily with the charge nurse about the results of the bowel training program.
- Skin care is important for incontinent residents. Monitor the resident's buttocks for reddened areas and apply a protective cream. Use disposable incontinence briefs if necessary.

Some residents may need to wear disposable incontinence briefs. Follow these guidelines:
- Never refer to an incontinence brief as a diaper.
- Check the resident often for incontinence. The resident should not wear a soiled brief.
- Give perineal care after changing an incontinence brief.
- Maintain the resident's dignity and privacy. Incontinence briefs can be embarrassing for the resident.

Incontinence briefs are usually available in small, medium, and large sizes. Make sure you use the right size for the resident. Many different products are available. Your facility's administration chooses the product used there. Talk to the charge nurse if the product does not fit a resident well. Procedure 11-4 describes how to apply a disposable brief.

PROCEDURE 11-4. APPLYING A DISPOSABLE INCONTINENCE BRIEF

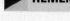 **REMEMBER: BE AWARE**

Items Needed
- disposable incontinence pads
- disposable briefs
- plastic trash bag
- underpants (if resident requests their own underpants over the brief)
- three pairs of gloves
- two washcloths
- one towel
- soap or perineal wash

1. Place an incontinence pad on the bed to protect clean linen.

2. Help the resident onto their back.

3. Put on gloves.

4. Help remove garments below the waist.

5. Discard the soiled incontinence brief in the plastic trash bag.

6. Remove and dispose of your soiled gloves.

7. Put on new gloves.

8. With the resident on their side, give perineal care, including cleaning the rectal area.

9. Remove and dispose of your soiled gloves.

10. Put on new gloves.

11. Fan-fold one-half of the briefs under the resident's buttocks.

12. Help the resident move onto their back. Unfold the side that was fan-folded, and open the adhesive tabs on both sides. Place the brief upward between the resident's legs, and join the tab from the back of the brief to the tab in the front of the brief.

13. Put on the resident's underpants and clothing.

REMEMBER: UNDERSTAND

URINARY SYSTEM

Structures

The urinary system is one of the most important systems in the body. It helps the body maintain fluid balance (the amount of water in the body) and eliminate liquid wastes. The urinary system has these major structures (Fig. 11-23):
• The right and left kidneys maintain the body's fluid balance by filtering out waste products and producing urine.
• The right and left ureters are tubes that carry urine from the kidneys to the bladder.
• The bladder is a sac-like muscle that stores urine until it is eliminated. The urethra is the tube that carries the urine from the bladder outside the body.

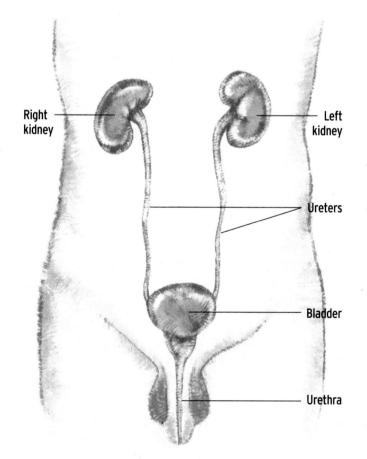

Right kidney
Left kidney
Ureters
Bladder
Urethra

Fig. 11-23 – The urinary system and its components.

Functions

The urinary system eliminates waste materials from the blood and reabsorbs the proper amount of water and salt for the body.

Aging Changes

Significant changes in the kidneys and bladder gradually occur with normal, healthy aging (Table 11-6).

TABLE 11-6
CHANGES IN THE URINARY SYSTEM WITH AGING

CHANGE	RESULT
Decreased size of kidneys	Slowing of kidneys' ability to filter the blood Less efficiency in concentrating urine
Decreased bladder capacity	More frequent urination
Decreased bladder muscle tone	Decreased ability to empty bladder: residual (leftover) urine present after urination
Decrease in hormones that regulate fluid volume	Increased risk of dehydration

Abnormal Signs and Symptoms

• very dark yellow urine (Fig. 11-24, next page)
• very small amounts of urine
• bloody or orange urine
• cloudy urine
• complaints of burning or stinging during urination
• sense of urinary urgency
• very strong odor of urine
• frequent urination in small amounts (called urinary frequency)
• loss of urine control (incontinence)

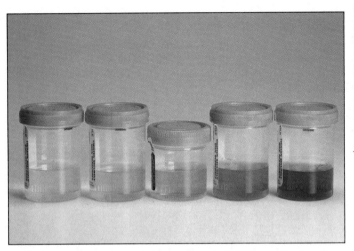

Fig. 11-24 – Urine can range in color. Very dark yellow or cloudy urine can indicate something may be wrong.

Observations To Report

- Is the resident getting adequate fluids?
- Are intake and output about equal?
- Does the resident still feel like urinating just after urinating?
- Does the female resident wipe the urethral area correctly from front (near the pubic bone) to back (toward anus) (Fig. 11-25)?
- Do I always respond fast enough to the resident's call light to meet their elimination needs?
- Does the resident have good hygiene?

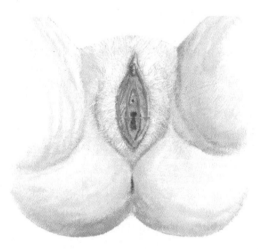

Fig. 11-25 – When assisting with perineal care on a female resident always wash from front to back (from the pubic bone down toward the anus).

Common Chronic Illnesses, Diseases, and Problems of the Urinary System

Urinary Tract Infections.   An infection in the urinary system is called a urinary tract infection. The bladder is most commonly affected. Urinary tract infections occur more often in women, incontinent residents, and residents with poor fluid intake.

Signs and Symptoms of Urinary Tract Infections
- urinary frequency
- complaints of burning or stinging during urination
- urine that is dark yellow or cloudy or has a foul odor
- blood in urine

Nurse Assistant's Role in Observation and Intervention
- Identify residents at risk for a urinary tract infection.
- Report any changes in a resident's urinary pattern to the charge nurse.

Goals of Care
- Prevent urinary tract infection.
- Help decrease the discomfort the resident feels.

Interventions or Skills for Care
- Encourage residents to drink enough fluids every day, especially water and fruit juices.
- Encourage residents to urinate at least every 3 to 4 hours when awake.
- Encourage proper perineal hygiene (such as females wiping from front to back after urination) and daily washing of the perineal area.

Urinary Incontinence.   The term "urinary incontinence" means a person cannot control when and where they urinate. Urinary incontinence can be treated or improved in most cases. The key to successful treatment is a good assessment of the resident. This assessment is done by the physician, a urinary specialist, or a nurse. You help with the assessment by observing and recording the frequency and timing of incontinence, the resident's reaction, and related environmental factors, such as when incontinence occurs in the activity room because the bathroom is too far away. The goals of the assessment are to:
- Determine the resident's usual pattern.
- Identify and treat causes.
- Determine the plan needed for the resident.

Causes of Urinary Incontinence
Causes within the urinary system:
- The bladder contracts when it should not, causing an abrupt gush of urine.
- The bladder does not contract when it should, causing the bladder to fill, and urine spills over.
- A blockage of the urethral opening causes the bladder to fill and urine to spill over.
- Weakness of the urethral opening causes stress incontinence, a leakage of urine that happens when the person coughs, sneezes, or laughs hard.

Causes outside the urinary system:
- medications
- urinary tract infection
- lack of access to a bathroom
- fecal impaction
- delirium
- immobility
- depression
- diabetes mellitus
- congestive heart failure
- vaginitis
- neurologic lesions

Signs and Symptoms of Urinary Incontinence
The resident is repeatedly found to be wet from urine. The resident is not aware they are urinating until they feel the wetness. In some cases a resident, such as a resident with Alzheimer's, may not feel the wetness at all.

Nurse Assistant's Role in Observation and Intervention
- Identify residents at risk for incontinence.
- Support the assessment process.
- Closely monitor the resident's urinary pattern.
- Report any abnormal signs or symptoms.

Goals of Care
- Help the resident regain as much control over urinary function as possible by treating the cause and using a bladder training program or prompting program, depending on the resident's needs.
- Maintain the resident's dignity by helping calmly and promptly with incontinence episodes.

Interventions or Skills for Care
Bladder Training Program. The goal of this program is to lengthen the intervals between times the resident voids (urinates). This program is successful with most residents with normal cognitive skills. Begin by keeping a record of the resident's voiding pattern, including:
- time between urination
- amount voided each time (Fig. 11-26)
- fluid intake

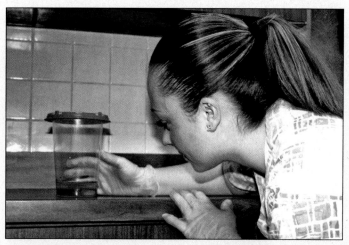

Fig. 11-26 — When recording a resident's intake and output include the amount voided each time.

You and the charge nurse set a schedule for expected voiding times based on the resident's voiding pattern. At the chosen interval, you help the resident to the toilet. This interval is used for two days and the results documented. If after two days the resident has not been incontinent, the interval is increased by 30 minutes. This cycle continues until the resident's voiding interval is 4 hours. Between times, encourage the resident to resist the urge to urinate.

It takes time, often several weeks, for an incontinent resident to regain control of their bladder. The resident needs continuous encouragement from staff. All staff must be attentive and consistent with the training schedule. Residents may also participate in a pelvic muscle exercise program. If so, remind the resident to perform the exercises.

Prompted Training Program. This bladder training program is used for residents with cognitive impairments. The goal is to prompt the resident to void at intervals short enough to prevent leakage.

1. The charge nurse establishes the start date.
2. Every two hours ask the resident if they are wet or dry. Then check for wetness and give feedback to the resident.
3. Ask if the resident wants to go to the toilet.
4. If they do, record the amount voided.
5. If they don't, try to encourage the resident. If the resident still says no, come back in an hour. Repeat the check for wetness and the request to toilet.
6. Increase the time between prompts if the resident's incontinence improves.

General Guidelines for Resident Care During Bladder Training

- Give routine personal care any time a resident is incontinent to prevent skin rashes and breakdown.
- Some incontinent residents will not be successful with bladder training. Give these residents frequent perineal care, use incontinence pads and briefs or panty liners, and provide emotional support.

Applying a Disposable Incontinence Brief or Panty Liner

When using disposable incontinence briefs, follow the steps described in Procedure 11-4 (page 192). If the resident chooses to use a panty liner, use the same procedure but instead place the liner over their buttocks. Then have the resident move onto their back, and bring the front of the liner up between their legs. Put on their underpants and garments below the waist.

Urinary Catheter Care. The physician may order an indwelling urinary catheter for a resident for medical reasons. The nurse inserts the catheter using sterile technique to prevent infection. The catheter passes through the urethra into the bladder. A small balloon inflated with sterile water keeps the catheter in place. Urine passes from the bladder through the catheter tube and into a closed collection bag hung from the bed or chair (Fig. 11-27).

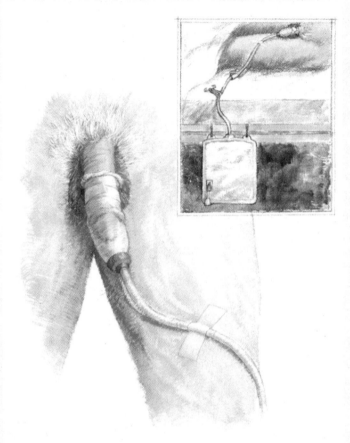

Fig. 11-27 – A urinary catheter tube is placed in the resident's bladder so that urine can drain from the bladder through the tubing into the catheter collection bag. The tube has a balloon that is inflated to keep the tubing in the bladder.

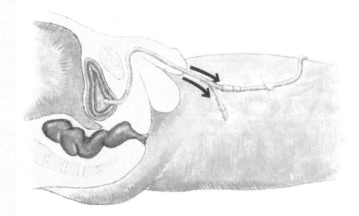

Fig. 11-28 – Clean the tubing at the urethral opening first then downward away from the opening.

Your responsibility for a resident who has a catheter is to give routine perineal care and position the external catheter tubing and drainage bag. Follow these guidelines for perineal care:

1. Put on gloves before giving perineal care.
2. Always keep the external catheter tube as clean as possible.
3. Clean the tubing with antiseptic solution and cotton balls or gauze pads. Clean the tube first at the urethral opening, and then cleanse downward and away from the opening (Fig. 11-28, previous page). Do not pull on the catheter tube while cleaning it, to prevent discomfort for the resident.
4. Use only one cotton ball or gauze pad for each downward stroke. Discard it, and use a new one to clean the next area.

5. Do the rest of perineal care as usual, cleansing with soap and water from front to back.

When you help a resident with a urinary catheter change position, follow these guidelines:

- The external part of the catheter tube can be secured with a strap to the resident's upper thigh to prevent pulling on the catheter when they move.
- The urinary catheter tube, connecting tube, and drainage bag should not be separated except by a nurse using a sterile technique to change the tubing or collect a specimen. The drainage system is kept closed to help prevent infection.
- Check the tubing for kinks and leaks.

Note: *You should empty a resident's urinary drainage bag every eight hours or more often when the bag is full (Procedure 11-5). Always record the amount of urine you drain from the bag. Most residents with a urinary drainage bag have their fluid intake and output recorded.*

PROCEDURE 11-5.   EMPTYING A CATHETER DRAINAGE BAG

▶ **REMEMBER: BE AWARE**

Items Needed
- paper towels
- gloves
- container (measuring container)
- I & O record

1. Put on gloves.

2. Place the paper towel on the floor underneath the drainage bag.

3. Place the measuring container on the paper towel.

4. The drainage bag has a closed clamp that allows the urine to flow from the bag. Open the clamp and drain all the urine into the container, making sure not to touch the clamp to the sides of the container.

5. Close the clamp and secure it to the drainage bag immediately after it is completely drained.

6. Note the amount of urine and discard the urine in the resident's toilet.

7. Remove and discard your gloves, and wash your hands.

8. Record the amount of urine on the intake and output record.

▶ **REMEMBER: UNDERSTAND**

• The urinary drainage bag is secured to the bed or chair below the resident's bladder, so that the urine flows from the bladder into the bag by gravity. Never let the drainage bag touch the floor, which is considered an "unclean" area. Never lift the drainage bag above the resident because urine could flow back into the bladder, increasing the risk of infection.

NERVOUS SYSTEM

Structures

The nervous system has three major parts (Fig. 11-29):

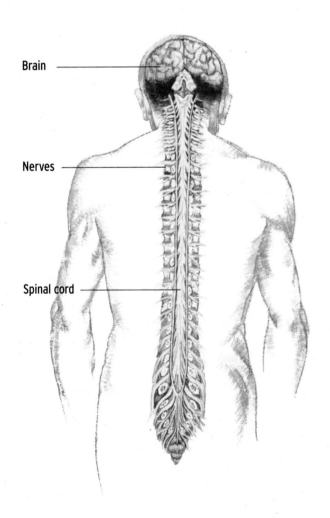

Brain

Nerves

Spinal cord

• The brain is located within the protective skull. Messages are received and interpreted in the brain, which is the body's communication center. Information is processed and stored. Thinking, reasoning, and judgment are brain functions.
• The spinal cord contains nerves that control movement. It extends down the back, protected within the spine (vertebral column).
• The nerves are fibers that extend from the spinal column to all parts of the body. The nerves carry messages in both directions between the body and brain. Information received from the outside world is taken to and processed in the brain, and messages from the brain travel back to the body to control functions.

Function

The nervous system is like a communication center. It helps you make sense of the world. The nervous system works with the sensory and endocrine systems to direct all other body systems.

Aging Changes

Table 11-7 lists the changes that occur in the nervous system as a person ages.

TABLE 11-7 CHANGES IN THE NERVOUS SYSTEM WITH AGING	
CHANGE	**RESULT**
Slowing of nerve impulses	Longer time for residents to learn new information Slower response time to situations, which may result in injury
Decreased blood flow to certain areas of the brain	Decrease in short-term memory

Fig. 11-29 – The nervous system and its components.

Abnormal Signs and Symptoms

- loss of interest in learning, confusion, feeling isolated, memory loss
- impatience
- complaints of not remembering where things are
- complaints of not reacting as quickly as in the past
- paralysis
- reduced sensation
- involuntary motions
- tremors
- unsteady walking
- speech problems

Observations To Report

- Do I reinforce the resident's recently learned behavior?
- Do I take every opportunity to go over new information with the resident?
- Can the resident move without help?
- Does the resident have any tremors or weakness?
- Is the resident steady on their feet?

Common Chronic Illnesses, Diseases, and Problems of the Nervous System

Multiple Sclerosis. Multiple sclerosis is a disease that affects nerve fibers in the central nervous system. It is a progressive, disabling disease that often starts in young adulthood.

Signs and Symptoms of Multiple Sclerosis
The symptoms depend on which nerve fibers are affected. In general they include:
- visual problems
- weakness that progresses to paralysis
- fatigue
- speech pattern changes
- loss of bowel and bladder control

Nurse Assistant's Role in Observation and Intervention
- Provide care the resident needs because of the progression of the disease.

Goals of Care
- Help the resident to maintain their independence as long as possible.
- Prevent complications.

Interventions or Skills for Care
- Help with ROM exercises of the resident's arms or legs that are affected by the disease (Fig. 11-30).

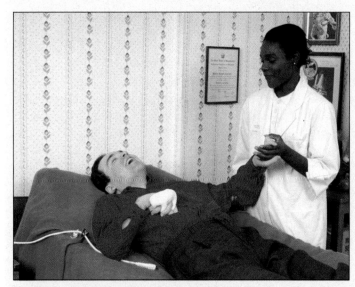

Fig. 11-30 – Range of motion exercises will help with circulation and mobility in residents with multiple sclerosis.

- Use proper positioning methods.
- Maintain the resident's skin integrity.
- Monitor proper nutrition.
- Provide adequate fluids.
- Identify the resident's bowel and bladder patterns, and ensure compliance with the resident's toileting routine.
- Support and listen to the resident's concerns about changes occurring in their body.
- Attend to the resident's requests regarding personal hygiene or with regard to social interactions with family and friends.

Parkinson's Disease. Parkinson's disease is a neurological disease that affects a person's motor skills (movement of muscles). The exact cause of Parkinson's disease is not known, although Parkinson's-like symptoms can occur as a side effect of some drugs and strokes. The disease usually begins when the person is in their 60s.

Signs and Symptoms of Parkinson's Disease
- Musculoskeletal changes:
  - muscle weakness and stiffness
  - muscle tremors
  - slumped, bent-over posture
  - shuffling walk, poor balance (falls)
  - mask-like expression

- Gastrointestinal changes:
  - constipation
  - difficulty chewing and swallowing

- Personality changes:
  - mood changes
  - confusion

Nurse Assistant's Role in Observation and Intervention
- Identify changes in a resident's status.

Goals of Care
- Help the resident maintain their mobility.
- Maintain adequate nutrition and fluids.
- Maintain a safe environment to prevent falls.
- Help the resident maintain their independence.

Interventions or Skills for Care
- Keep the resident's room free of clutter.
- Encourage the resident to use assistive walking devices as ordered.
- Encourage frequent rest periods.
- Offer small, frequent meals high in fiber.
- Encourage adequate fluid intake.
- Keep tasks simple.
- Support residents by listening to their concerns about their loss of abilities.

ENDOCRINE SYSTEM

Structures

The endocrine system includes many different glands (Fig. 11-31). Glands are organs that make and release hormones, which are substances needed by different organs. The following are the major structures in the endocrine system:

- The pituitary gland, located in the brain, secretes hormones and regulates other glands such as the ovaries and testes. It is often called the "master gland."
- The adrenal glands, located on top of the kidneys, secrete hormones that regulate metabolism. They also help regulate sodium, water, and potassium levels in the body. Adrenal glands release hormones that increase blood sugar, control blood vessel constriction, and help us to react in emergency situations.
- Cells called the islets of Langerhans, located in the pancreas, secrete insulin, which controls the breakdown of carbohydrates (sugars) in the body.
- The thyroid and parathyroid glands, located in the neck, secrete hormones that help regulate metabolism, the process of producing energy.
- The female ovaries, located in the pelvic area, secrete hormones that control sexual function and are involved in pregnancy.
- The male testes or testicles, located in a sac behind the penis, secrete a hormone controlling sexual function and sperm production.

Functions

The endocrine system makes hormones that help the body work properly. Their vital functions include the regulation of body energy, the breakdown of sugar for energy, and the ability to have children.

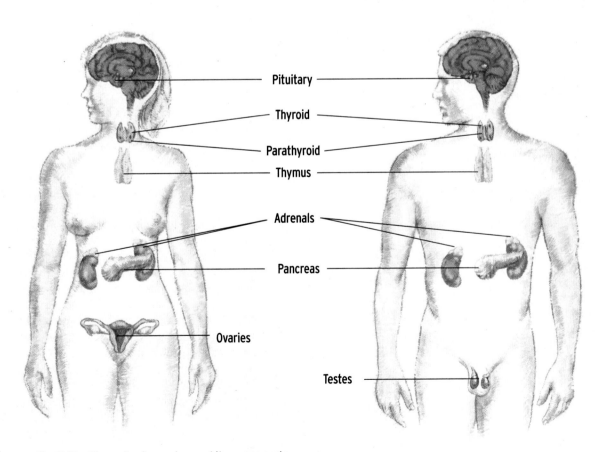

Pituitary
Thyroid
Parathyroid
Thymus
Adrenals
Pancreas
Ovaries
Testes

Fig. 11-31 – The endocrine system and its components.

Aging Changes

Table 11-8 lists the changes that occur in the endocrine system as a person ages.

TABLE 11-8
CHANGES IN THE ENDOCRINE SYSTEM WITH AGING

CHANGE	RESULT
Glands have a slower rate of releasing hormones.	This change affects the resident's blood studies but should not affect the overall health of the resident.
Decreased insulin production	The body takes longer to process sugar; resident may have less energy.
Dramatically decreased amount of hormones produced by the ovaries	Menstruation stops, along with the ability to have children; this is known as menopause.
Male hormone production decreases but does not stop.	May have decreased sexual response.

Abnormal Signs and Symptoms

- excessive thirst (drinking large amounts of fluids)
- dramatic increase in urine output
- increased food intake
- complaints of feeling tired or cold

Observations To Report

- Have the resident's requests for water dramatically increased?
- Does the resident go to the bathroom more often than normal?
- Is the resident eating lots of food?
- Is the resident lethargic?

Common Chronic Illnesses, Diseases, and Problems of the Endocrine System

Diabetes. The most common disease of the endocrine system is diabetes. According to the American Diabetes Association, in the U.S. there are 20.8 million children and adults with diabetes. In diabetes, either the pancreas does not produce enough insulin or the body does not use insulin effectively. Insulin controls the body's use and distribution of carbohydrates. When an insulin problem occurs, the person's blood sugar level becomes too high or too low.

There are four types of diabetes:
- **Type 1** is an autoimmune disease. For unknown reasons, the immune system destroys insulin-producing cells in the pancreas. Then the pancreas cannot produce enough insulin needed to live. A person with type 1 diabetes must have insulin injections.
- **Type 2** is the most common type of diabetes. In type 2 diabetes the pancreas produces insulin, but for unknown reasons the body does not use it effectively.
- **Gestational diabetes** develops only during pregnancy.
- **Pre-diabetes** occurs when a person's blood sugar is higher than normal but not high enough to be diagnosed with type 2 diabetes.

Type 1 diabetes usually occurs in youth. The person needs regular insulin injections. Type 2 diabetes usually occurs later in life. Type 2 can usually be controlled with diet, exercise, and oral medication.

People with diabetes are at risk of developing complications. Complications are generally caused by damage to nerves and/or blood vessels. The person's blood vessels narrow, causing reduced blood flow. Poor blood circulation to the legs can cause reduced sensation, changed skin color, and leg cramps. A decrease in blood flow to the eyes can cause pain and vision problems such as vision loss. Nerve damage can occur in any part of the body. A nerve problem in the legs can cause symptoms such as numbness, tingling, or a shooting or stabbing pain. Nerve damage to internal organs can affect many body functions, such as digestion or elimination.

Diabetes also slows down the body's ability to fight off infection. High blood sugar levels may lead to bacterial overgrowth or infection. Common infection sites for diabetics include the feet, kidneys, bladder, and skin. It is important to observe for and report any changes in diabetic residents. With early detection, it may be possible to slow or reduce complications.

To prevent or slow the progression of diabetic complications, the health care team helps control the resident's blood sugar level, blood pressure, and cholesterol levels.

Signs and Symptoms of Diabetes
- change in behavior, such as irritability
- excessive thirst
- excessive urination
- blurring vision
- excessive hunger
- itching of the skin
- itching of the vagina and vulva
- tingling and numbness of hands and feet
- slow healing of a sore
- fatigue
- weight loss

Nurse Assistant's Role in Observation and Intervention
- Identify any changes in the resident's behavior.
- Closely monitor the resident's nutrition. Residents with diabetes typically are on special diets.
- Monitor and encourage the resident's daily exercise program.
- Identify and report any physical changes in the resident immediately.
- Provide a safe environment to prevent injury.

Goals of Care
- Prevent complications by observing and reporting changes in the resident.
- Help maintain a proper diet.
- Encourage exercise.

Interventions or Skills for Care
- Promptly provide meals and snacks specially prepared for residents with diabetes. All residents with diabetes must eat on time and must eat the correct amount of the foods prepared for them. Carefully observe a diabetic resident's food intake. Record and report it if the resident does not eat all of their meals and snacks or if they eat foods not on their diet.
- When helping a resident with diabetes with personal care, inspect their skin daily and report any changes immediately (Fig. 11-32). Wash, rinse, dry, and inspect the resident's skin thoroughly, especially their feet. Observe the skin for any reddened areas or skin breakdown. Report any skin changes to the charge nurse. Tell the nurse if the resident's fingernails or toenails need to be cut. A nurse or physician must cut

a diabetic resident's toenails because of the high risk of injury.

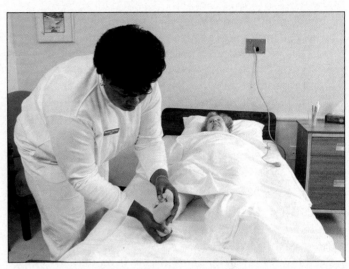

Fig. 11-32 – Be especially mindful of a diabetic resident's skin. Report any changes immediately to the charge nurse.

- Observe the resident for any skin discolorations or sores that are not healing. This may indicate decreased circulation to the area. Report any complaints of numbness or tingling in the hands or feet immediately to the charge nurse.
- Some residents must have their blood sugar (glucose) levels checked daily with a blood glucose device or monitor. Many different glucose monitoring devices are available. Become familiar with the device used in your facility. With all devices follow these general guidelines:
  – Wash your hands and put on gloves.
  – Explain the procedure, because finger sticks hurt.
  – Be sure you have all needed supplies before beginning.
  – Read the manufacturer's directions for using the blood glucose device.
  – Dispose of supplies in the appropriate containers, following facility policy.
- Although urine testing is no longer recommended for controlling blood sugar, it still gives the health care team valuable information about the person. Urine tests may show the presence of harmful ketones or protein in the urine. Ketones are byproducts when the body burns fat instead of glucose for fuel. Ketones present in the urine can signal a serious diabetic

problem. Therefore, you may test a diabetic resident's urine for ketones. The physician may also order a diabetic resident's urine to be tested for protein. Protein in the urine is an early sign of kidney disease. Record and report the results.

- Pay close attention to a diabetic resident's behavior. Note and report any changes. Changes may be important because they may indicate a problem in blood sugar level.
- Monitor the resident's physical activity. All residents with diabetes need physical exercise, but each resident's program must be designed for their individual needs.

SENSORY SYSTEM

The organs of the **sensory system** are the eyes, ears, nose, tongue, and skin. The sensory system gives us information from the outside world. The senses receive and send information to the brain. Aging influences the function of the senses. Sight and hearing are most commonly affected by aging.

THE EYE

Structures

The eye is a round ball with several major structures (Fig. 11-33):

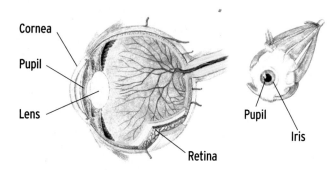

Fig. 11-33 – The eye and its components.

- The sclera is the "white" of the eye.
- The iris is the "color" of the eye. It helps regulate the amount of light that enters the eye by controlling the size of the pupil.
- The pupil is the opening through which light passes to get to the retina.
- The cornea protects the iris.

- The iris and lens direct and focus light on the retina.
- The retina is the back of the eye, where light images become nerve impulses to the brain. The brain interprets and processes the impulses into pictures.

Function

Sight gives us knowledge about our surroundings. This is important so that we can care for ourselves.

Aging Changes

The changes in the eye caused by aging are described in Table 11-9.

TABLE 11-9
CHANGES IN THE EYE DUE TO AGING

CHANGE	RESULT
The cornea flattens.	Resident has decreased ability to focus at normal reading distances.
The lens becomes more yellow.	Greens and blues are difficult to see, and reds and oranges easier to see.
The lens becomes more rigid or less elastic.	Resident can see objects clearly only at a greater distance.
The pupil becomes smaller.	Because less light reaches the inner eye, it is more difficult to see in poorly lit conditions.
The retina becomes less efficient.	Resident's spatial discrimination decreases.
The iris becomes more rigid.	Eyes do not adjust well to changes in amount of light.

Abnormal Signs and Symptoms
- discharge from the eyes
- excessive watering of the eyes
- inability to find things, bumping into things
- complaints of not being able to see well, inability to focus clearly, or burning sensations

- complaints of eye pain
- complaints of double vision

Observations To Report

- Does the resident have enough light?
- Is the resident wearing eyeglasses? Are they clean and the correct prescription?
- Do I leave things where the resident can find them?
- Do I address the resident directly?
- Is the resident concerned about loss of sight?
- Is the resident having trouble distinguishing color?

Common Illnesses, Diseases, and Conditions of the Eye

Cataracts.   Cataracts can occur in one or both eyes.

Signs and Symptoms of Cataracts
- increase in nearsightedness
- complaints of double vision
- problems with glare
- inability to distinguish color
- complaints of blurry vision (Fig. 11-34)

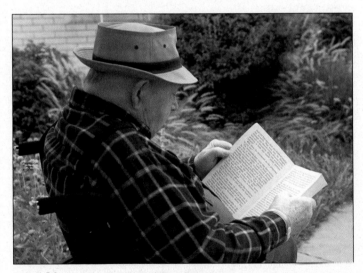

Fig. 11-34 – Cataracts cause vision changes.

Nurse Assistant's Role in Observation and Intervention
- Identify the resident's capabilities.
- Ensure a safe environment.

Goals of Care
- Improve the resident's ability to do the activities of daily living.
- Protect the resident from injury.

Interventions or Skills for Care
- Be sure the resident's things are kept in the same place and always returned there.
- Help the resident with their personal belongings. Open lids, put toothpaste on their toothbrush, help them pick out color-coordinated clothing, etc.
- Describe where foods are on the resident's plate, using "clock face directions" (Fig. 11-35). For example, "The potatoes are at 3 o'clock, the vegetables are at 11 o'clock, and the meat is at 6 o'clock."

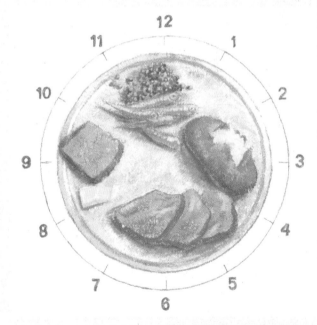

Fig. 11-35 – For residents with visual difficulty, you can describe the location of food on their plates using the face of a clock.

- Make sure the resident wears their glasses. Clean and store them properly.
- Read to the resident if necessary.
- Keep the room well lit and uncluttered.

Cataract – cloudy film that develops in the lens of the eye and reduces sight

- Let the resident know when you enter the room, and identify yourself.
- Stand where the resident can see you.
- Encourage the resident to touch and feel things.
- Support the resident emotionally if they need surgery.

Blindness.   Blindness is the inability to see. Some residents who are considered "legally blind" still have some sight.

Signs and Symptoms of Blindness
- difficulty with the activities of daily living
- difficulty moving from place to place

Nurse Assistant's Role in Observation and Intervention
- Identify the resident's capabilities.
- Ensure a safe environment.

Goals of Care
- Improve the resident's abilities to perform the activities of daily living.
- Protect the resident from injury.
- Help the resident to remain active and not become socially isolated.

Interventions or Skills for Care
- Be sure the resident's things are kept in the same place and always returned there.
- Help the resident with managing their personal belongings. Open lids, put toothpaste on their toothbrush, help them pick out color-coordinated clothing, etc.
- Describe the location of foods on their plate, using clock face directions.
- Make sure the resident wears their glasses. Clean and store them properly.
- Read to the resident if necessary.
- Keep the room well lit and uncluttered.
- Let the resident know when you enter the room, and identify yourself.
- Encourage the resident to touch and feel things.
- Help the resident walk: Have them hold your elbow or use an assistive device as you guide them along (Fig. 11-36).
- Position their furniture in a simple arrangement.
- Orient the resident to their surroundings.

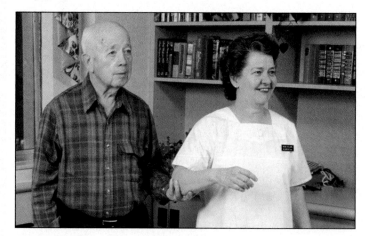

Fig. 11-36 — When helping a blind resident walk, have them hold your elbow or use an assistive device as you guide them along.

THE EAR

Structures

The ear has three areas (Fig. 11-37):
- the inner ear
- the middle ear
- the outer ear

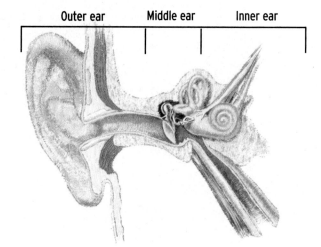

Fig. 11-37 — The ear and it components.

These areas have different structures involved in hearing. Sound enters the outer ear and is transmitted through the middle ear to the inner ear. Nerve impulses resulting from sounds go from the inner ear to the brain for interpretation. Other structures inside the ear help the body maintain its balance. If these structures are not working properly, a resident may feel dizzy.

Functions

The ear lets us hear. Hearing, like vision, helps us be aware of the world around us. Sounds provide clues to dangers as well as communication and pleasure. The inner ear also helps us maintain our balance.

Aging Changes

Table 11-10 lists the changes that occur in the ear as a person ages.

TABLE 11-10
CHANGES IN THE EAR WITH AGING

CHANGE	RESULT
Hearing structures in the ear become stiff.	Loss of hearing of high-frequency sounds
Structures in inner ear related to balance begin to degenerate.	Harder to maintain balance
Production of soft ear wax decreases.	Buildup of hard, dry wax in the ears, which can cause hearing loss

Abnormal Signs and Symptoms

• isolation or anger
• discharge from the ear
• continual tugging or scratching of the ear
• resident yells when talking
• resident turns television or radio up very loud
• complaints of ringing in ears
• complaints of feeling dizzy or unsteady

Observations To Report

• Do I speak directly to the resident?
• Do I lower the tone of my voice?
• Do I speak clearly?
• Does the nurse check the resident's ear regularly for wax?
• Does the resident use a hearing aid (Fig. 11-38)?

Is it clean and operating properly? Does the resident know how to use it? Is the battery working?
• Does the resident avoid group activities?
• Is the resident withdrawn or seem fearful?

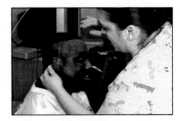

Fig. 11-38 — Encourage residents with a hearing loss to wear their hearing aids.

Common Chronic Illnesses, Diseases, and Problems of the Ear

Hearing Loss

Signs and Symptoms of Hearing Loss
• The resident may not respond to a person's voice.
• The resident may not interact with other residents.
• The resident may not participate in activities.
• When listening, the resident may turn their head or cup their hand over their ear.
• The resident may look like they do not understand you.

Nurse Assistant's Role in Observation and Intervention
• Report any changes you notice about how a resident who is hard of hearing communicates.
Goals of Care
• Maintain and improve the resident's communication with others, including caregivers.
Interventions or Skills for Care
• Stand in front of the resident at eye level when speaking to them.
• Speak slowly and clearly because the person may be reading your lips.
• Speak in your normal voice, not a louder or a high-pitched voice.
• Reduce background noise.
• For a resident who cannot hear you or read your lips, use writing to communicate.
• Point to objects you are talking about.
• If the resident uses a hearing aid, make sure they are wearing it and check the battery each day before they put it in. Be familiar with the type of hearing aid the resident uses. Hearing aids should be labeled with the resident's name. Always keep the hearing aid in a safe place when it is not being worn.

THE OTHER SENSES

Aging Changes

Table 11-11 lists changes that occur in the other senses as a person ages.

TABLE 11-11 CHANGES IN THE OTHER SENSES WITH AGING	
CHANGE	**RESULT**
Smell The ability to identify or detect odors decreases with age, more commonly in men than in women.	Resident may not be able to detect odors that signal a danger, like chemicals or smoke from a fire.
Taste The ability to taste salty and sweet tastes may decrease because of changes in the tongue.	Resident may request more seasoned foods.
Touch Decreased sensitivity of touch receptors Decreased response to painful stimuli	Resident may not be able to tell how hot an object is, leading to a burn.

Abnormal Signs and Symptoms

- inability to taste or smell food, or complaints that the food is bland
- burns on skin

Observations To Report

- Does the resident like the type of food served?
- Is water temperature adjusted correctly for the resident's personal care?
- Does the resident check water temperature with the inner part of their wrist?

MALE REPRODUCTIVE SYSTEM

Structures

The main structures of the male reproductive system are (Fig. 11-39):

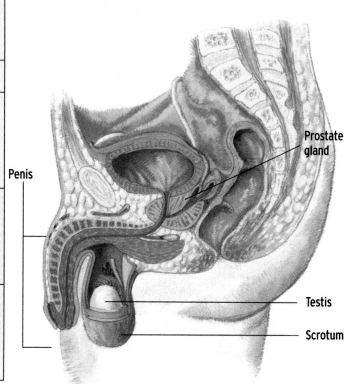

Fig. 11-39 – The male reproductive system and its components.

- The penis is used for sexual intercourse and urination.
- The testes are two oval-shaped glands, sometimes called the sex glands or gonads. They produce sperm cells and the male sex hormone testosterone. Sperm cells leave the body in semen.
- The scrotum is the sac that holds the testes outside the body.
- The prostate gland secretes one of the fluids that make up semen.
- Semen is produced by the seminal vesicle.

Functions

The reproductive system provides sexual pleasure and allows humans to reproduce.

Aging Changes

Table 11-12 describes the changes that occur in the reproductive system as a male ages.

TABLE 11-12
CHANGES IN THE REPRODUCTIVE SYSTEM WITH AGING

CHANGE	RESULT
Male hormone production decreases but does not stop.	Possibly decreased sexual response
Prostate gland enlarges.	Mild urinary retention
Testicular tissue mass decreases.	Decreased rate of sperm cell production

Abnormal Signs and Symptoms

- foul-smelling discharge from penis
- bleeding
- open sores
- difficulty with sexual intercourse
- difficulty starting to urinate

Observations To Report

- Do I consider the resident's need for physical intimacy?
- Do I consider the resident's need for privacy?

Common Chronic Illnesses, Diseases, and Problems of the Male Reproductive System

Prostate Cancer. Prostate cancer is the second leading cause of death among men. It is also the most common form of cancer in men. The key is early detection and treatment. Treatment options include surgery, radiation, chemotherapy, hormone therapy, and radioactive seed implants. Today prostate cancer can be treated and cured if detected in its early stages.

Signs and Symptoms of Prostate Cancer
- The resident has problems with urination, such as urinating at night.
- In the physical examination, the prostate gland feels enlarged and has an abnormal shape.
- The resident senses that the bladder is not completely emptied after urinating.

Nurse Assistant's Role in Observation and Intervention
- Identify any changes in the male resident's urinary pattern.
- Report any changes.

Goals of Care
- Help restore the resident to optimal health.
- Support the resident emotionally during treatment.

Interventions or Skills for Care
- Help the resident to the bathroom, especially at night.
- Record the resident's urine pattern and note changes.
- Be available to talk to the resident about his fears during treatment.

FEMALE REPRODUCTIVE SYSTEM

Structures

The main structures of the female reproductive system are (Fig. 11-40):

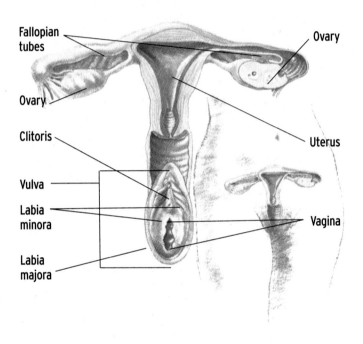

Fallopian tubes

Ovary

Ovary

Clitoris

Vulva

Labia minora

Labia majora

Uterus

Vagina

Fig. 11-40 – The female reproductive system and its components.

- The ovaries are two almond-shaped glands located in the pelvis. The ovaries hold the eggs and produce the hormones estrogen and progesterone.
- The fallopian tubes are two tubes that carry the eggs from the ovaries to the uterus.
- The uterus is the muscular organ that holds the fetus during pregnancy and sheds its lining during menstruation.
- The vagina is the muscular canal leading from the uterus used for sexual intercourse, childbirth, and the passage of menstrual flow.
- The vulva is the external female sex organ. It is made up of the labia major and minor, which are the skin flaps located on both sides of the vagina, and the clitoris, which gives sexual pleasure to females.

Functions

The reproductive system provides sexual pleasure and allows humans to reproduce.

Aging Changes

Table 11-13 describes the changes that occur in the reproductive system as a female ages.

TABLE 11-13 CHANGES IN THE FEMALE REPRODUCTIVE SYSTEM WITH AGING	
CHANGE	**RESULT**
Dramatic decrease in the amount of hormones produced by the ovaries	Monthly menstrual cycles stop, along with the ability to have children.
Decreased vaginal lubrication	Dryness in vaginal walls

Abnormal Signs and Symptoms

- foul-smelling discharge from vagina
- vaginal itching
- bleeding
- difficulty with sexual intercourse
- open sores
- mood changes

Observations To Report

- Do I consider the resident's need for physical intimacy?
- Do I consider the resident's need for privacy?

Common Chronic Illnesses, Diseases, and Problems of the Female Reproductive System

Vaginal Infections.   Bacterial vaginosis (sometimes called vaginal bacteriosis; caused by too many bacteria) and vaginal yeast infections (caused by too much yeast) are the most common types of vaginal infections. They are caused by too many bacteria or yeast growing in the vagina.

Signs and Symptoms of Vaginal Infections
* vaginal discharge
* vaginal odor
* vaginal itching
* red irritated skin around vaginal opening and labia
* pain when urinating because of urine touching irritated skin

Nurse Assistant's Role in Observation and Intervention
* Identify any changes such as odor, redness, or irritation.
* Report any signs and symptoms to the charge nurse.

Goals of Care
* Assist with treatment.
* Help relieve the resident's signs and symptoms.

Interventions or Skills for Care
* Give perineal care often to decrease odor.
* Help the nurse administer medication in the vagina.
* Pour warm water over the vaginal area while resident is on the bedpan or toilet. This sooths the irritated, swollen perineal area.

Note: *Many diseases like genital herpes, gonorrhea, chlamydia, HIV, or AIDS can affect both men and women. These diseases are acquired through sexual activity with an infected partner. These diseases are called sexually transmitted diseases (STDs).*

Common Chronic Illnesses, Diseases, and Problems of the Reproductive System

One of the most devastating problems related to the reproductive systems is HIV/AIDS. Although the HIV virus is also transmitted in other ways, the most common way is sexually.

AIDS.   Acquired immunodeficiency syndrome, AIDS, is a condition caused by the human immunodeficiency virus, HIV. HIV lives in blood, vaginal fluid, breast milk, and semen. HIV can be transmitted by sharing needles or syringes or through unprotected oral, vaginal, or anal sex. An infected mother may also transmit the virus to her baby before or during birth, or after birth through her breast milk. The infection can also be transmitted through blood transfusions, but this is now very rare today because since 1985 all donated blood is screened for HIV. HIV cannot be eliminated from the body, and there is no cure for AIDS. But many drugs are available today that allow infected people to stay healthier longer.

Signs and Symptoms of of HIV
A person can be infected with HIV for many years without feeling or looking sick. The only way to make a definite diagnosis of an HIV infection is to use a blood test. Usually the virus slowly damages the person's immune system, leading eventually to AIDS. Common signs and symptoms of HIV/AIDS are as follows:
* night sweats
* skin rashes
* swollen glands
* fever
* weight loss
* diarrhea
* fatigue

Nurse Assistant's Role in Observation and Intervention
You may care for residents who have HIV and or AIDS. But you cannot always know if a resident is HIV-positive, which means they are infected with the virus and can transmit it to others. Therefore you must use standard precautions and bloodborne pathogen precautions for every resident, as you learned in Chapter 10.

Goals of Care
* Help relieve the resident's signs and symptoms.
* Help the resident feel as comfortable as possible.
* Provide emotional support.

Interventions or Skills for Care
* Follow standard precautions at all times.
* Teach the resident to follow standard precautions.
* Elevate the head of the bed for a resident with pneumonia.
* Treat all skin conditions as directed by the care plan.
* Always treat the resident with respect and dignity
* Report any changes to the charge nurse.

IN THIS CHAPTER YOU LEARNED:
- The general characteristics of aging
- The meaning of the terms "acute," "chronic," "observation," "signs," and "symptoms"
- Why no one should be labeled by a disease or condition
- The importance of early detection of cancer
- The structures and functions of the 10 body systems
- How the body systems change with aging
- What information should be reported to the charge nurse
- How to complete a resident's chart with a description of an illness, disease, or problem; signs and symptoms; your role in observation and intervention; the goals of care; and interventions or skills for care

SUMMARY
One of your most important responsibilities is to understand, recognize, and report changes that occur in residents you care for. Therefore you need to know abnormal signs and symptoms in the different body systems and to understand acute and chronic illness. Often chronic illness also has an acute phase.

Each of the 10 body systems has important structures that carry out needed functions in the body. Changes occur in the body's structures with aging, leading to possible changes in function. Abnormal signs and symptoms you observe in a resident may be related to a common problem, illness, or disease in a body system. For these residents you have a special role using interventions and skills to help the resident meet the goals of care.

PULLING IT ALL TOGETHER
One of the most exciting parts of becoming a nurse assistant is learning new information. You will often think and talk about things that you learn in this course and especially in this chapter. Over time your family, friends, and neighbors will rely on you as a source of medical and health information.

As a nurse assistant you will not be expected to recall every detail of this medical information after this course. You will be expected, however, to get to know your residents and recognize changes in them. You must carefully observe the residents in your care and report any changes to the charge nurse. Only in this way can residents receive the care they need and deserve.

Think about this resident. Mrs. Swansee is a wonderful 89-year-old woman who was admitted to your facility three years ago. From her first day there she has shown an incredible spirit. She is alert and very bright. The staff and residents always enjoy her company. Mrs. Swansee has diabetes. She is completely blind in one eye and has poor sight in the other.

This particular morning you go into Mrs. Swansee's room and find her still in bed. She seems lethargic. She usually gets her ADLs done before breakfast and participates in the day's planned activities. When you ask her if something is wrong, she tells you she just feels tired. You help her up into a sitting position and help her get ready for breakfast. When you help her get up to go to the bathroom, you notice her legs are swollen and she seems short of breath.

You immediately call the charge nurse. The charge nurse asks you to weigh her. You report that her weight is three pounds more than yesterday. You help her back into bed to rest, and take her vital signs. Her temperature is 98.6 F, pulse 96 and weak, respiration 32, and blood pressure 180/98. You are concerned about the swelling in her legs; her shortness of breath; her weight gain; and the increases in her pulse, respiration, and blood pressure.

The charge nurse immediately calls the physician. The physician orders an increase in her fluid reduction medication, a chest X-ray, a 1000 cc fluid restriction for the next 24 hours, vital signs taken every two hours, and monitoring and recording intake and output. The charge nurse discusses this with you and tells you the physician will be here soon to do a physical examination.

The physician concludes that Mrs. Swansee is in congestive heart failure. Fortunately, because you identified these changes so quickly, she gets treatment right away. She is already beginning to respond favorably to it. Because of your observations and quick action, she will not have to go to the hospital. During the report at the change of shift, the charge nurse tells other staff about Mrs. Swansee's condition. The charge nurse also praises your work and thanks you for coming to her right away with these important changes.

CHECK WHAT YOU'VE LEARNED

1. **An acute illness usually:**
   A. Causes obvious swelling.
   B. Does not cause a fever.
   C. Lasts seven to 10 days.
   D. Develops very gradually over time.

2. **Which of these changes to the skin is a normal sign of aging?**
   A. Frequent bruising.
   B. Bleeding.
   C. Changes in the color and size of moles.
   D. Dryness and decreased elasticity.

3. **As a nurse assistant, you typically learn about a resident's symptoms by:**
   A. Interviewing the resident's roommate.
   B. Talking to the resident.
   C. Observing the resident while they sleep.
   D. Taking the resident's vital signs.

4. **Which of the following is a cancer warning sign?**
   A. Nagging cough or hoarseness.
   B. Headache.
   C. Gradual weight gain.
   D. Irritability in the early morning.

5. **The early detection of cancer is important because:**
   A. Hair loss is greater later on.
   B. The resident needs time to adjust to having cancer.
   C. Insurance does not pay for treatment of advanced cancer.
   D. The cancer may spread to other parts of the body and be more difficult to treat.

6. **Mrs. Whitman has pneumonia. She has a fever, difficulty breathing, and aches and pains in her chest. This kind of infection reaction is called a:**
   A. Silent response.
   B. Whole body response.
   C. Localized response.
   D. Absent response.

7. **The function of the endocrine system is to:**
   A. Eliminate waste materials from the body.
   B. Produce hormones that help the body work properly.
   C. Prevent germs in the environment from entering the body.
   D. Carry vital nourishment to all the cells of the body.

8. **Which of the following occurs because of nervous system changes as we age?**
   A. Slowing of respirations.
   B. Slowing of heartbeat.
   C. Decreased insulin production.
   D. Decreased short-term memory.

9. **Mrs. Shapiro has peripheral vascular disease. You should encourage her to:**
   A. Wear tight clothing.
   B. Change position frequently and not cross her legs at the knee.
   C. Sit as close as she can to a source of heat.
   D. Avoid elevating her legs.

10. **Mr. Altoid had a stroke and now has difficulty swallowing. What should you do when you help him eat?**
    A. Do not give any fluids until after the meal.
    B. Feed him in bed with the bed as close to flat as possible.
    C. Encourage or give small bites of food.
    D. Clap him frequently on the back as he chews.

(Answers to "Check What You've Learned" are in the Instructor's Manual.)

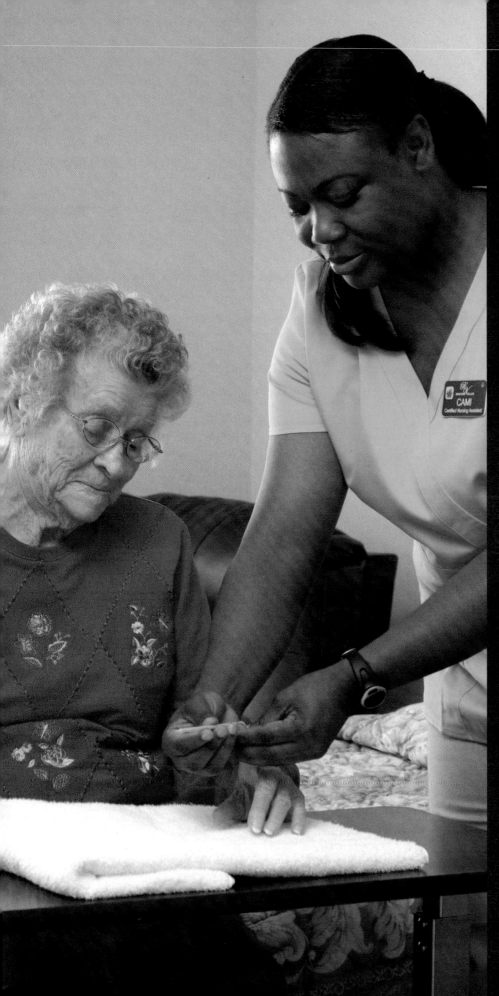

Section
4

How To Give Quality Care

Chapter 12

THEMES OF CARE

By this point you may be wondering how you are going to meet all the needs of the residents you will care for. The tasks of caring for even one person can seem overwhelming. How can you handle caring for many at the same time? As you have learned, the key to success is balancing the art of caring with the science and skills of nursing. To give quality care while promoting residents' quality of life, you have to incorporate themes of care into all your activities.

A theme is something repeated over and over. It's like a song you cannot get out of your head. The words may change between verses, but the melody, the musical theme, stays the same and keeps repeating. The tasks you perform every day are like the words of the song. The specifics may change throughout the day, or they may be different for every resident because of their preferences, but the themes of care should always stay the same. In every interaction with a resident, these themes must be part of what you do. Weave them into every daily task. Themes of care help you balance the art of caregiving with the skills you use in your job.

This chapter focuses on how to provide the very best care. The eight themes of care described here are a map for how to give the best care. You will learn how to use all of these themes when performing any skill as a nurse assistant. Remember to incorporate two vital things into all the themes of care: "Be Aware" and "Understand." As you read through this chapter you will see the meaning of each theme. The phrase "Be Aware" will remind you of the proper preparation steps to include in each task. The word "Understand" will remind you of the steps to take when ending each procedure with your residents.

OBJECTIVES
- Define the themes of care
- List general questions you should consider when beginning a skill
- List the commonly used preparation and completion steps
- List several CMS requirements for services that long term facilities must provide residents

"You constantly amaze me. You are so efficient and care for each of us as though we were your only focus."

Do you know the saying "It's not what you do, but how you do it"? Think of a simple task, like opening and closing a door. The fact of opening and closing is always the same, but how it is done can send different messages. The door can be pushed open so hard that it bangs against the wall. It can be opened so quietly that no one hears you come in. The door can be gently closed or slammed shut. How you do something even as simple as this can show your anger, frustration, or distraction—or it can show that you are considerate and caring. You must be aware as you review each theme and take note of how it is completed. The themes of care are about how you should do things. Incorporating them into all your activities helps you provide quality care in a timely, efficient manner.

THEMES OF CARE

There are eight themes of care. You should incorporate all eight into your caregiving every day with every resident. These themes of care involve both the art of caregiving and the science of nursing.

Caregiving themes include:
- communication
- autonomy
- respect
- maximizing capabilities

Nursing themes include:
- safety
- infection control
- observation

Time management, the eighth theme, is a general theme of care for performing all tasks in an efficient manner.

Be Aware of Communication

In Chapter 7 you learned how people send and receive messages. You communicate with residents throughout the day. If you did not communicate with a resident, or if you failed to notice the resident's nonverbal messages, how would you know if they were unhappy or in pain? How would a resident know that when you start taking off their clothes you are about to help them to bathe? Residents have the right to know what is happening to and around them. Communication is also important for developing a trusting relationship with residents and other staff (Fig.12-1).

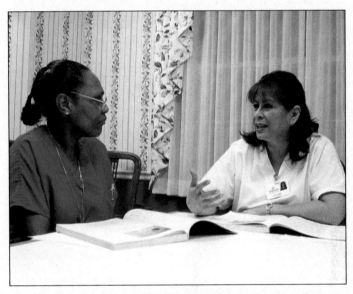

Fig. 12-1 – Communication is the foundation for creating a trusting relationship.

Autonomy – making decisions for oneself

Infection control – methods used to prevent the transmission of infection

Maximizing capabilities – working with a resident's own capabilities to their fullest

Observation – recognizing and paying attention to details

Respect – to consider worthy of high regard

Safety – being free from harm or risk and secure from threats or danger

Theme – something practiced continually

Time management – ability to organize activities and perform them efficiently

Be Aware of Autonomy

Autonomy means making decisions for oneself. This includes how to live one's life. Being autonomous means being independent. You must help each resident be as independent as possible (Fig. 12-2). Encourage them to take responsibility for their care by making their own choices. Then support residents in the choices they make, even when it means you have to change how you do a task. Residents are entitled to make their own decisions about how care will be given by themselves or by you. If you become too protective or do everything for a resident instead of letting them do it, you undermine their autonomy and take their independence away.

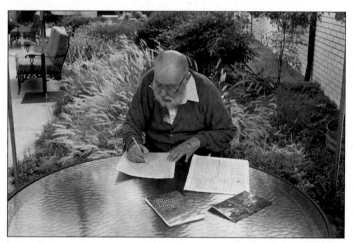

Fig. 12-2 – Residents should be encouraged to be as independent as possible.

Be Aware of Respect

Everyone deserves to be treated with dignity and respect. Simple courtesies show that you are respectful. This includes knocking on the resident's door before entering, saying please, and asking permission. Ask yourself, "If I were this resident, how would I like to be treated?" Treating each resident with respect must be part of everything you do (Fig. 12-3). Remember that all residents are human beings with their own feelings, thoughts, and beliefs. You must respect and never violate their basic human rights.

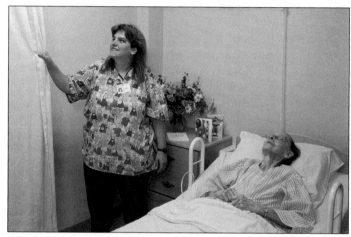

Fig. 12-3 – Maintaining the resident's privacy shows the resident you respect them.

Be Aware of Maximizing Capabilities

Maximizing capabilities means that you work with the resident's capabilities and support them to their fullest. You emphasize what the resident can still do—not what they cannot do. When you incorporate this theme into your care, you become a coach. You work with the resident to help them be the best they can be (Fig. 12-4). Check the care plan for information about what a resident can do.

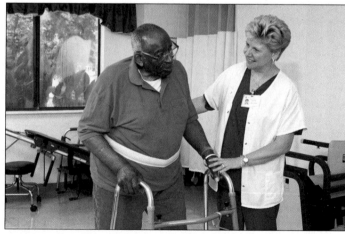

Fig. 12-4 – Always work with residents to help them achieve their goals.

Be Aware of Safety

Safety means being free from harm or risk and secure from threats or danger. The facility's environment is designed to be a safe place where the entire staff can focus on giving care in a home-like setting. But if care becomes a quick and careless routine, injuries and accidents are likely. Both residents' safety and your own depend on acting thoughtfully and carefully at all times (Fig.12-5).

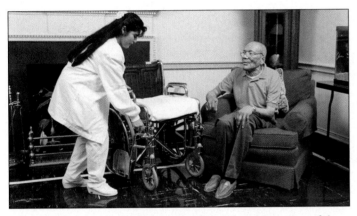

Fig. 12-5 – Locking the wheels on the wheelchair helps ensure safety.

Be Aware of Infection Control

The infection control procedures in Chapter 9 help prevent the transmission of harmful microorganisms. The transmission of microorganisms can be kept to a minimum if everyone follows these principles (Fig. 12-6). Incorporate this theme in all your caregiving actions. This helps protect both the resident and you.

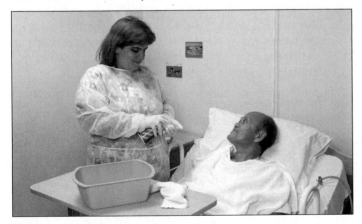

Fig. 12-6 – Using proper infection control procedures minimizes the spread of infection.

Be Aware of Observation

You have already learned that observation means to watch and pay attention to details. You must pay close attention for any changes in a resident. Report any changes immediately. Remember, since you spend the most time with residents, you will see changes before anyone else on the caregiving team does (Fig. 12-7).

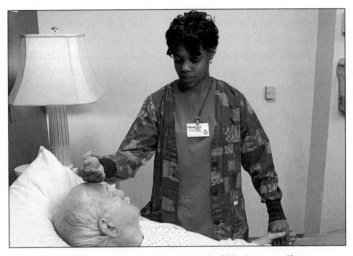

Fig. 12-7 – Paying attention to the resident will help you notice any changes that may need to be reported.

Be Aware of Time Management

Time management is the skill of organizing your activities and performing them efficiently. Take control and prioritize your tasks by deciding what is most important. This helps you become more efficient (Fig. 12-8). All eight of these themes are important. Work to incorporate them all into your everyday caregiving.

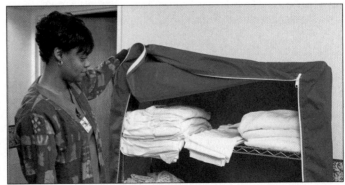

Fig. 12-8 – Gathering supplies you need to do the resident's care before you begin helps you to be organized.

HOW TO USE THEMES IN YOUR WORK

You can incorporate the themes of care into your daily work if you think of each task as having four parts:

1. You consider the resident's capabilities and get their permission.
2. You prepare to do the task.
3. You do the task or carry out the procedure.
4. You complete the task.

Remember to think about the themes of care as you do the steps of each task. *How* you perform these steps is as important as finishing the task. Ask yourself these six questions every time you begin:

- What do I need to know or consider about the resident?
- Did I get permission to do the task?
- How should I do this task?
- What do I need to do before I get started?
- What supplies or equipment do I need to get to complete the task?
- How can I incorporate the themes of care in this task?

Consider the following example. Helping a resident to take a shower is a common task for nurse assistants. If you consider the questions above, your preparation for the shower will include the following steps:

1. Check the care plan to ensure that all special instructions regarding the resident are considered before you prepare the shower.

2. Knock on the resident's door, and wait for their permission before entering. (Knocking shows your respect for the person's privacy).

3. Introduce yourself and identify the resident. Introducing yourself is respectful. Identifying the resident ensures you are helping the correct person, which is a safety issue.

4. Check with the resident to be sure they want to take a shower. Explain what you would like to do and ask if this is a convenient time.

5. Gather all supplies needed for the shower, such as a washcloth, towels, and bath blanket. Having things ready before you start is good time management.

6. As needed, prepare the resident's own supplies, such as soap, deodorant, clean clothes (if the resident will be dressing in the shower room), and lotions. This step is good time management and promotes autonomy.

7. Ask the resident how much help they need and what their preferences are. When you ask the resident about what they can do, you are maximizing their capabilities. You may have to determine this for the resident if they cannot communicate to you. These steps involve several themes of care: communicating, showing respect, promoting autonomy, and maximizing the resident's capabilities.

8. Check the shower room. Be sure it is available and clean. Hang an "Occupied" sign outside the shower.

9. Wash your hands before any patient contact. Always observe good infection control practices to prevent the spread of infections.

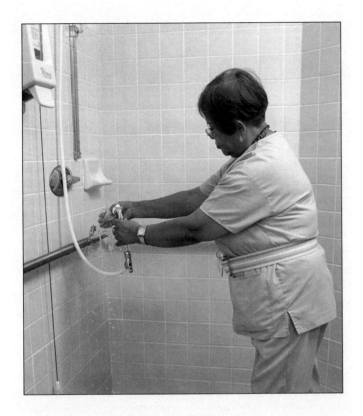

Because you prepared in advance, you can complete the shower without having to stop to get other supplies. This saves time. Nurse assistants who plan each task also enjoy their work much more. Residents are happier, and the whole experience is more enjoyable for both of you. This is a good example of how to balance the skills and art of caregiving.

Let's look at a different example in which the themes of care are *not* used. Suppose you are supposed to give Mrs. Jones a shower. Without thinking, you follow these steps:

1. You walk into Mrs. Jones' room.

2. You say hello to her.

3. You tell her what is going to happen.

4. You help her out of bed and to the shower.

10. Help the resident to the shower. Be sure they are completely covered during the transfer. This ensures the resident's safety and shows respect by protecting their privacy.

11. Help the resident get ready. Encourage them to do as much as they can do. This encourages them to be as independent and autonomous as possible. This also involves the theme of observation. Observing a resident's capabilities helps you encourage them to maintain or improve on that level.

12. Turn on the water and check the water temperature.

13. Ask the resident if the water temperature feels OK to them. This safety measure ensures the resident is not burned.

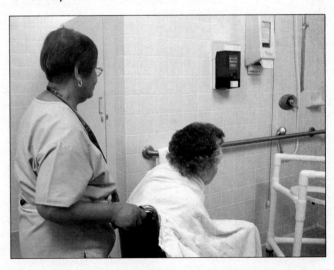

5. You open the shower room door and find that another resident's used towels and supplies are still there. You leave Mrs. Jones waiting while you clean up the mess.

6. You tell Mrs. Jones you forgot her supplies and leave to get them. You leave Mrs. Jones sitting on a chair in the shower room. While you are gone, Mrs. Jones needs to go to the bathroom. She gets up, slips on a wet spot on the floor, and falls. You come back and find her on the cold, wet floor.

(text continued on page 224)

TABLE 12-1 COMMON PREPARATION STEPS

►	**REMEMBER: BE AWARE**		
	STEP	**RATIONALE**	**THEMES**
B	Before giving care, check the plan.	The care plan gives you information about the resident, including details about their capabilities or if any additional equipment is needed before entering the room.	Maximizing Capabilities
E	Enter by knocking and introduce yourself.	Knocking respects the privacy rights of the resident. An introduction lets them know who is entering their room.	Communication, Autonomy, Respect
A	Assemble all equipment, and secure assistance if needed.	This saves you time, helps you plan the task, and prevents possible injuries to you and to the resident.	Autonomy, Safety, Time Management
W	Wash your hands, and put on additonal protective equipment as needed.	Handwashing prevents the transmission of infections. Additonal protection devices protect the resident and the staff from cross contamination and infections.	Infection control
A	Ask about the resident's preferences and needs.	Give an explanation of what you are about to do and seek the resident's input so they are more comfortable and involved with their care. Make sure that safety needs are met throughout the care by locking the wheelchair, adjusting the height of the bed, and using all equipment properly.	Communication, Safety, Autonomy, Maximizing Capabilities, and Respect
R	Respect the resident's privacy at all times.	Provide privacy by closing the door, pulling the curtain, and keeping the resident covered during care.	Respect
E	Explain the procedure, and answer any questions.	Explaining the procedure gains the resident's cooperation and creates a more relaxed atmosphere. It helps the resident feel more involved and in charge of their care needs. Courtesy and politeness are important in your relationship with your resident.	Communication, Autonomy, and Respect

TABLE 12-2   COMMON COMPLETION STEPS

REMEMBER: UNDERSTAND

	STEP	RATIONALE	THEMES
U	Understand the resident's concerns as you complete the procedure.	Courtesy and communication are important in your relationship with the resident.	Autonomy, Communication, and Respect
N	Note the resident's reactions.	By observing the resident's reactions, you are better able to determine any unusual changes that you might need to report. When you notice changes you can more effectively meet the resident's needs.	Observation, Autonomy
D	Determine the resident's preferred position for comfort.	Making the resident comfortable is a part of your responsibilities.	Autonomy, Respect
E	Examine the environment for safety concerns.	The bed should be in the lowest position. The wheelchair should be locked. It is your responsibility to make sure that you minimize any safety concerns.	Safety
R	Remove your gloves and dirty items and dispose of them properly.	Changing gloves and disposing of dirty items helps to prevent the spread of infections. All facilities have separate containers for items like linens and contaminated disposables. Proper disposal prevents transmission to both residents and staff.	Infection control
S	Secure the call light and any other needed items within reach of the resident.	Residents must be able to reach you throughout your shift.	Safety
T	Talk to the resident and let them know that you will be leaving soon.	Keeping the resident informed helps them to stay involved. Courtesy and good communication are necessary in all aspects of care.	Communication, Autonomy, and Respect
A	Always wash your hands upon completion of care.	Handwashing and use of needed protective equipment help prevent the spread of infection.	Infection control
N	Never leave without asking the resident if they need anything else.	Giving residents choices and control of their care helps them to remain independent.	Communication, Autonomy, and Respect
D	Document the procedure and report any findings to the staff in charge.	Detailed records help staff identify the resident's normal patterns. Documentation helps the charge nurse identify potential problems with a resident. Remember that often you are the first person to notice when something may be wrong with a resident.	Communication, Observation

(text continued from page 221)

If you had been thinking of the themes of care and planned the shower carefully and mindfully, you would have prevented this unpleasant and dangerous situation.

COMMON PREPARATION AND COMPLETION STEPS

Much of your job involves preparation. Preparing in advance for all tasks reduces your workload. It helps you get the job done efficiently. All nurse assistant skills—whether bathing a resident, making a bed, or moving a resident from bed to chair—involve preparation. Often you will use the same preparation steps every time you do the task. However, because different residents have different needs and preferences, and because the environment changes, small variations in preparation are often necessary.

The examples above show how important it is to be aware during the preparation steps. Being mindful and incorporating the eight themes of care are important in all steps of the task as well, not just preparation. Most of the chapters in the rest of this book describe the specific steps for doing tasks.

How you complete tasks is similar for most of the tasks that you will do daily. The completion steps let residents know that you are done and that you understand and are caring for their needs. The steps also ensure that residents are safe and comfortable and gives them an opportunity to ask questions (Fig. 12-9).

Tables 12-1 and 12-2 on the preceding pages list the common steps to take to Be Aware and prepare for each task properly, and to Understand the resident's needs when ending each activity. The themes of care are incorporated in all these areas.

The exact steps of care may differ somewhat from task to task and even from moment to moment. Remember that tasks are not exact routines done the same for all residents at all times. Quality care involves adjusting tasks to meet the individual's needs. You must be flexible and adapt your caregiving to each resident's preferences. Different equipment and settings may also require adjusting the preparation steps.

Become familiar with these preparation and completion steps. Use them daily with all tasks you perform. You can change the order of some steps because of a resident's needs, but always prepare for and finish the skill. These steps help you incorporate all eight themes of care:

- communication
- autonomy
- respect
- maximizing residents' capabilities
- safety
- infection control
- observation
- time management

If you incorporate the themes of care in everything you do, you will be successful as a nurse assistant.

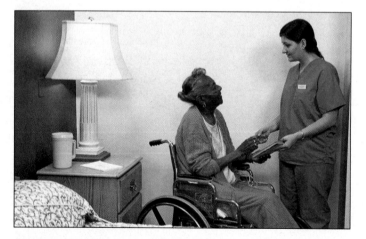

Fig. 12-9 – Completion steps include making the resident safe and comfortable.

THE FORMAT OF SKILL PROCEDURES

In the following chapters you will learn many skills. The steps in these skills are numbered to help you learn what to do first, second, third, etc. At the beginning of each skill is a reminder that looks like this:

> ▶ **REMEMBER: BE AWARE**

This is to help you use the BE AWARE acronym as shown on page 222 and summarized in Fig. 12-10.

Systematically go through each of the important preparation steps before beginning the procedure. The skill is then described, step by step. Learn the steps of procedures in the order given, but remember that you may need to be flexible in some steps based on a resident's preferences.

At the end of each procedure you will see a reminder that looks like this:

> ▶ **REMEMBER: UNDERSTAND**

This is to help you use the UNDERSTAND acronym as described on page 223 and summarized in Fig 12-11.

Follow these completion steps for each procedure so that you can provide you residents with everything they need before you leave.

When you remember these two important themes of care, you will be able to give the best quality care possible.

▶ **REMEMBER: BE AWARE**

B Before giving care, check the plan.
E Enter by knocking and introduce yourself.

A Assemble all equipment and ask for help if needed.
W Wash your hands before giving any resident care.
A Ask resident for any personal preferences during the procedure.
R Respect resident's privacy by closing the door and pulling the curtain.
E Explain the procedure as you go and answer any resident's questions.

Fig. 12-10 – The BE AWARE acronym will help you remember the common preparation steps.

▶ **REMEMBER: UNDERSTAND**

U Understand the resident's concerns as you complete the procedure.
N Note the resident's reactions.
D Determine the resident's preferred position for comfort.
E Examine the environment for safety concerns.
R Remove your gloves and dirty items and dispose of them properly.
S Secure the call light and any other needed items within reach of the resident.
T Talk to the resident and let them know that you will be leaving soon.
A Always wash your hands upon completion of care.
N Never leave without asking the resident if they need anything else.
D Document the procedure and report any findings to the staff in charge.

Fig. 12-11 – The UNDERSTAND acronym will help you remember the common completion steps.

CMS REQUIREMENTS FOR QUALITY OF CARE

The Centers for Medicare and Medicaid Services (CMS) requires facilities to provide all residents with the necessary care and services to attain or maintain their highest practicable physical, mental, and psychosocial well-being. The resident's condition must not diminish unless clinical conditions show this to be unavoidable. The resident's care must follow their plan of care. Following are CMS requirements for care:

- **Activities of daily living** must be maintained, such as bathing, dressing, grooming, eating, communicating, and moving. A resident who cannot manage their own personal care must receive these services.
- **Pressure ulcers** must not be allowed to develop. If they do, the resident must receive treatment to promote healing, prevent infection, and prevent new sores from developing.
- **Urinary incontinence** must be treated. Services must be given the resident to prevent urinary infection and to restore as much bladder function as possible. A resident should not be catheterized unless a clinical condition makes a catheter necessary.
- **Range of motion** must not diminish in a resident unless a clinical condition makes it unavoidable. If a resident has limited range of motion, treatment and services must be given to increase their range of motion or prevent any further decrease.
- **Accidents** must be prevented. Supervision must be adequate, and assistance devices available and used. The resident's environment must be free of hazards.
- **Nutrition** parameters, including body weight and protein levels, must be maintained. If a nutritional problem occurs, the resident requires a therapeutic diet.
- **Hydration** must be maintained. The resident must have sufficient fluid intake to maintain proper hydration and health.
- A **nasogastric feeding tube** should not be used in a resident who can eat enough alone or with assistance. A resident being fed by gastrostomy or a nasogastric tube must receive treatment and services to prevent aspiration pneumonia, diarrhea, vomiting, dehydration, metabolic abnormalities, and nasopharyngeal ulcers, and to restore, if possible, normal eating skills.
- **Special needs** must be met. The resident must receive proper treatment and care involving injections, parenteral and enteral fluids, tracheostomy care, tracheal suctioning, respiratory care, foot care, and prostheses.
- **Unnecessary drugs** must not be given. The facility must ensure a medication error-free environment.
- **Influenza and pneumococcal immunizations** policies and procedures must be followed. The resident must receive information regarding the benefits and side effects of influenza and pneumococcal immunizations. Every resident must be offered an annual flu shot from October through the end of March, and a pneumococcal vaccine every five years, unless it is medically contraindicated. Residents have a right to refuse all immunizations. The facility must keep documentation of education materials given the resident that outline the benefits and side effects of all immunizations. The facility must also maintain documentation of who received and who did not receive immunizations and why.
- **Mental and psychosocial services** must be offered the resident to attain or maintain their functioning.
- **Vision and hearing** screening and services must be scheduled regularly.

As a nurse assistant, you are not responsible for ensuring that your facility offers all these services. You will be responsible for helping the resident attain or maintain their highest practicable physical, mental, and psychosocial well-being.

IN THIS CHAPTER YOU LEARNED:
- The themes of care
- General questions you should consider when beginning a skill
- Commonly used preparation and completion steps, including the BE AWARE and UNDERSTAND acronyms
- The CMS expectations for residents' quality care

SUMMARY
This chapter discusses how you can meet all your residents' needs. You learned that the key to your successful nursing care involves balancing the art of caregiving with the technical skills you perform to help residents. The way to achieve this balance is to incorporate the eight themes of care in your practice. The common steps for beginning and ending any task also incorporate the eight themes of care.

PULLING IT ALL TOGETHER
Remember the saying "It's not what you do but how you do it"? You may also know the saying "Anything worth doing is worth doing right." These sayings sum up the message of this chapter. If you are going to care for residents, then do it properly. Do it with compassion, respect, and understanding. The eight themes of care should become your guide for delivering care. The themes will guide you as you perform all skills, from beginning to end. They will help you always give quality care.

Imagine you are a resident with a chronic disease. Every day is a challenge just to function. Perhaps the only thing you can count on is the staff giving you tender loving care. This means everything to you because every day truly is a challenge.

1. **Effective communication includes paying attention to a resident's:**
   A. Vital signs.
   B. Nonverbal messages.
   C. Sleeping hours.
   D. Holiday card list.

2. **Which theme of care encourages residents to make choices and be independent?**
   A. Safety.
   B. Autonomy.
   C. Observation.
   D. Self-actualization.

3. **When you maintain the resident's privacy during all aspects of personal care, which theme of care are you paying attention to?**
   A. Safety.
   B. Respect.
   C. Communication.
   D. Infection control.

4. **Time management involves:**
   A. Organizing activities and performing them efficiently.
   B. Noticing changes in a resident early on.
   C. Supporting residents in the choices they make about how they will spend their time.
   D. Emphasizing tasks that residents can still do for themselves.

5. **What does maximizing capabilities mean?**
   A. You help the resident exercise hard every day.
   B. You trust the resident to stay in the tub room alone.
   C. You coach the resident to do all they can for themselves.
   D. You always seek approval from the charge nurse before giving care.

6. **When should infection control practices be followed?**
   A. Whenever you feel you may be catching a cold or flu.
   B. In all caregiving actions.
   C. With residents known to be sick.
   D. When the charge nurse requests it.

7. **Whenever you prepare to do a task, you should ask yourself a number of questions, including which of the following?**
   A. Is this task in my job description?
   B. Should I call the resident's family to check whether they want me to do this task?
   C. Will the charge nurse respect me more for doing this task?
   D. Did I get the resident's permission to do the task?

8. **Common preparation steps include:**
   A. Washing your hands.
   B. Writing into the resident's medical record what you are about to do.
   C. Disposing of dirty items from a previous task.
   D. Putting all supplies away.

9. **Common completion steps include:**
   A. Rewarding the resident with a cookie or candy for cooperating with you.
   B. Checking the resident's wristband.
   C. Raising the resident's bed to its highest level.
   D. Making the resident comfortable.

10. **Which of these statements about the theme of observation is true?**
    A. Since you spend the most time with residents, you will see changes first.
    B. You observe only for things the charge nurse directs you to observe at the beginning of your shift.
    C. You should pay attention to large, dramatic changes in a resident, not details.
    D. The medical record tells you exactly what to look for in the resident.

(Answers to "Check What You've Learned" are in the Instructor's Manual.)

Chapter 13

GATHERING INFORMATION

In Chapter 8 you learned about your important role in gathering information that may be used in the Resident Assessment Instrument (RAI). Remember that the RAI is a data collection tool with five parts, one of which is called the Minimum Data Set (MDS). You will hear nursing staff refer to the MDS as the tool for collecting information about residents. It is important to accurately report or record your observations about your resident's physical, social, psychological, and recreational or relaxation activities for the accuracy of the MDS. All facility staff collect information about the resident. Much of it comes from the physical examination, including the resident's vital signs, height, and weight. Data collection begins when the resident is admitted to the long term care facility. Data collection is a continuous process in which you will play a critical role (Fig 13-1).

In this chapter you will learn how to assist with a physical examination, how to take vital signs, and how to measure the resident's height and weight. These important skills help determine a resident's health status and help all members of the health care team to provide resident care.

OBJECTIVES
- Explain the purpose of an accurate history
- Describe what information the health care team obtains about a resident's past medical history
- Define two interviewing techniques the health care team uses during the physical examination
- Describe two methods used by the health care team for collecting history data
- Describe questions asked by the health care team during the review of body systems
- Explain your role in the physical examination
- Explain techniques used by the physician to examine the resident
- Demonstrate how to take an oral temperature
- Demonstrate how to take a rectal temperature
- Demonstrate how to take an axillary temperature
- Demonstrate how to take a radial pulse
- Demonstrate how to take an apical pulse
- Demonstrate how to take count respirations
- Demonstrate how to take a blood pressure
- Demonstrate how to measure height and weight

MEDICAL TERMS
- **Auscultation** – a technique of listening through a stethoscope to sounds produced by organs (such as heart, lungs, or bowels) to evaluate a body area
- **Axillary** – armpit
- **Blood pressure** – pressure of blood in the arteries
- **Glaucoma** – disease of eye that can cause gradual loss of vision
- **History** – A record of a person's medical background, including lifestyle and social information
- **Macular degeneration** – eye condition that causes loss of central vision
- **Oral** – by mouth
- **Palpation** – an examination technique of touching the resident's body on the surface and more deeply in an organized manner
- **Percussion** – tapping on a body area and listening to the sound produced, used to determine if tissue is air-filled, solid, or fluid-filled
- **Physical examination** – an organized approach to learn about a resident's health status and needs by looking, listening, feeling, and smelling.
- **Pulse** – measure of heart rate
- **Rectal** – by rectum
- **Temperature** – a degree of heat that naturally occurs in the body
- **Temporal scan** – measurement of temperature of the forehead
- **Tympanic temperature** – measurement of temperature of the eardrum
- **Vital signs** – necessary for life: temperature, pulse, respiration, and blood pressure

"You constantly amaze me. You are so efficient and care for each of us as though we were your only focus."

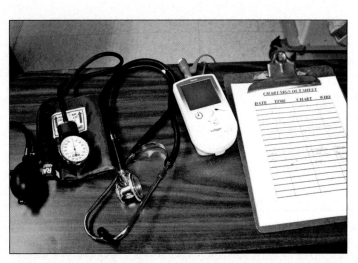

Fig. 13-1 – A blood pressure cuff, stethoscope, thermometer, and a resident's chart sign-out sheet.

Think about when you last had a physical exam. Maybe you were entering a new school or job, or you may have been ill. Now, think about how you felt during the exam. Was your privacy protected? Were you draped properly? Did the physician knock before entering the exam room? Was everything explained to you? Remember that your resident will have the exact same concerns when questioned by the physician about their medical history and during the physical exam.

PHYSICAL EXAMINATION AND HISTORY

To clearly understand a resident's total physical, psychological, and social needs, a physical examination must be performed. The examination is performed using an organized approach. As a nurse assistant your role is to assist the physician during the physical examination. Along with the physical examination, the resident's vital signs are taken, and height and weight are measured—these provide you with quick information about the person's health. Later in this chapter you will learn these skills.

A physical examination is always performed by a physician or designated health care provider when a resident is admitted to a facility. An examination is also done when a

---

📖

Medical History – A record of a person's medical background, including lifestyle and social information

Physical examination – an organized approach to learn about a resident's health status and needs by looking, listening, feeling, and smelling.

resident becomes ill. The nurse may perform a brief physical exam when required for the MDS or as required by state regulation. Your role is to assist the resident and the physician before and during the examination. You may be responsible to gather some information, equipment, and laboratory specimens ordered by the physician. During the exam, the health care team use communication, documentation, and reporting skills while collecting subjective and objective information. At the beginning of the resident's first physical examination, a history is often taken.

PURPOSE OF THE HISTORY

The purpose of obtaining an accurate history is to learn as much about the resident as possible. An accurate history is the basic foundation for collecting data and understanding the resident's needs or problems. Residents who can provide information have an opportunity to tell the physician about themselves, how they think, and how they feel. The physician gains insight into the person's habits, lifestyle, and beliefs. If possible, ask the physician if you can listen in while the history is taken. This is a good way for you to get to know the resident as well.

Sometimes the health care team cannot get the information directly from the resident due to health problems. Instead, information in the resident's record and information from family members and friends is used. In such cases, the physician will explain to the person providing information why accurate data is needed for giving the resident the best possible care.

Many residents now have, and may carry with them, a Personal Health Record (PHR). This record may be in written or electronic form. An electronic PHR may be stored at an Internet site or on a card or "drive" that can be read by a computer. Before taking a resident's history, a health care professional should always ask them or their health care representative if a PHR exists. If a PHR does exist already, the health care professional should first review the PHR and then ask questions to clarify or update that information.

OBTAINING THE HISTORY

The first step is to obtain or update the resident's health history. Be sure to provide for privacy in a quiet, distraction-free area. Introduce yourself in a courteous manner, addressing the resident by their last name. Explain the process for obtaining an accurate history or updating information, and ask the resident for permission to assist in their physical examination. Next, assist the resident to a comfortable sitting position while the physician taking the

history talks to them. You can explain that the first questions will be about their past medical history, including information about their family, psychological, and social history. Explain that these questions are asked to get a better understanding of who the resident is and how best to care for them. During this process make sure your facial expressions, body language, and tone are pleasant and nonjudgmental (Fig 13-2).

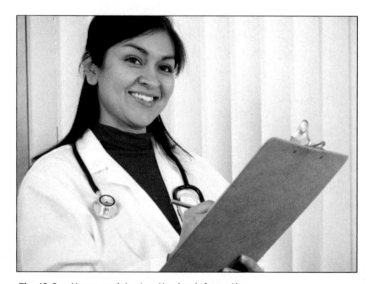

Fig. 13-2 – Nurse assistant gathering information.

The resident needs to feel that you are a good listener so that they feel free to express important facts and feelings. Interviewing techniques the physician uses when obtaining a history include:
- Explaining the questions being asked to put the resident at ease and obtain the best possible answers
- Rewording any confusing questions so that the resident understands what the physician is asking
- Repeating the resident's information to verify that it is accurate
- Never expressing their own opinion
- Being sure to quote any remarks from the resident that will help others better understand the resident
- Allowing the resident to speak freely
- Using direct questions based on the resident's complaints

COLLECTING THE HISTORY DATA

The history includes personal and social information. The resident will be asked questions about their:

- Personal life (age, birth place, education, marital status, living arrangement, sexual preferences and activity)
- Lifestyle (nutrition, sleep patterns, exercise routine, drug/alcohol/tobacco use)
- Economic status (income source, health and life insurance)

The physician then continues with the physical examination, beginning with a review of body systems.

This systematic approach provides both subjective and objective information about the residents' health. Often the physician can obtain better details about the resident's past and present health issues when the resident focuses on one area at a time. In Chapter 11 you learned specific information about each body system.

REVIEW OF BODY SYSTEMS

A systematic approach is used to obtain information about the resident's past and present symptoms in different body systems (Fig 13-3). The physician learns clues to

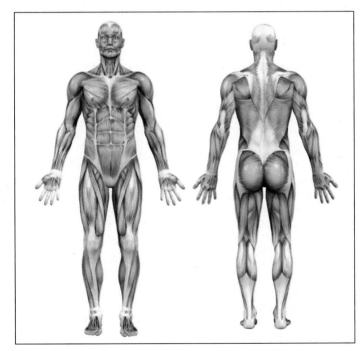

Fig. 13-3 – Human body showing systems approach to the physical exam.

diagnose problems involving multiple systems or clues that a disease has progressed to involve more than one system. The physician also asks about surgery and present or past

treatments as each system is reviewed. The review may begin by asking the resident direct questions like "Have you ever had any changes or problems relating to your skin?" Then the physician asks more specific questions about:
- any rash
- any change in color (pigmentation)
- any skin cancers
- hair or nail problems
- sweating problems
- changes in skin dryness or oiliness
- easy bruising
- lack of healing

The review proceeds through each body area and system, one at a time, as follows. Have you ever had any changes or problems with your head or nervous system? Then more specific questions about:
- headaches
- dizziness
- fainting
- feelings of depression
- memory
- coordination or balance
- **trauma**
- weakness
- hand tremors or grasp problems

Have you ever had any changes or problems with your eyes? Then more specific questions about:
- vision changes or problems
- eye pain
- itching
- burning
- infection
- **glaucoma**
- **macular degeneration**

Have you ever had any changes or problems with your ears? Then more specific questions about:
- hearing and whether or not hearing aids are prescribed and/or used
- history of infection

Glaucoma – disease of eye that can cause gradual loss of vision
Macular degeneration – eye condition that causes loss of central vision
Trauma – a physical injury such as hitting head in a fall

Have you ever had any changes or problems with your nose? Then more specific questions about:
- smelling problems
- sinus pain
- postnasal drip

Have you ever had any changes or problems with your teeth? Then more specific questions about:
- sensitivity
- pain
- bleeding gums
- regular dental care
- changes in or abnormal mouth odor

Have you ever had any changes or problems with your mouth? Then more specific questions about:
- sores
- swelling
- changes in taste of food or inability to taste food
- dry mouth

Have you ever had any changes or problems with your throat? Then more specific questions about:
- pain
- hoarseness
- ability to swallow

Have you ever had any changes or problems with your neck? Then more specific questions about:
- pain
- stiffness
- swelling

Have you ever had any changes or problems with your joints or bones? Then more specific questions about:
- stiffness in joints
- pain
- mobility problems, such as climbing stairs, reaching up or down, or walking on flat surfaces, and whether an assistive device such as a cane or walker is used

Have you ever had any changes or problems with your thyroid or pancreas? Then more specific questions about
- enlarged thyroid
- diabetes

Have you ever had any changes or problems with your breathing? Then more specific questions about:

- shortness of breath
- wheezing
- cough
- pain while breathing

Have you ever had any changes or problems with your heart, blood, or blood vessels? Then more specific questions about:
- chest pain or pain in arms, jaw, or shoulders
- fluid retention, such as swollen ankles, knees, fingers, or face
- pain in legs that may come and go

Have you ever had any changes or problems with swelling in your neck or groin? Then more specific questions about:
- tenderness or enlargement in these areas

Have you ever had any changes or problems with your stomach or digestion? Then more specific questions about:
- changes in eating habits
- weight changes
- bowel changes, such as diarrhea or constipation, "rumbling" sensation after eating, changes in color of stool, blood in stool, or pain during a bowel movement
- pain or gas after eating
- problems with eating fatty foods

Have you ever had any changes or problems with your urine or urination? Then more specific questions about:
- pain when urinating
- frequency of urinating (or "leaking" urine without warning, urinating when under stress or cold, or urinating at night)

Have you ever had any changes or problems with your sexual reproduction organs? Then more specific questions about:
- sexual dysfunction or changes in sexual enjoyment
- method of contraception if still needed (female) or at all times (male)
- (female) date or approximate date of menopause
- (female) breast problems and date of last mammogram

Diabetes — a common disease involving a problem in the body's production or use of insulin

- (male) prostate problems and date of last exam or laboratory test
- known diseases or problems

Have you ever had any changes or problems with your mood or mental health? Then more specific questions about:
- sadness or change in ability to "get up and go"
- repetitive thoughts or actions that you cannot easily control
- thoughts about hurting yourself
- outlook toward the future

After the history and review of systems, the resident is examined. The physical examination helps the physician:
- evaluate the resident's current physical and mental status.
- make a diagnosis.

Physical examinations can be performed in the physician's office or in a clinic setting. Some facilities have a designated area for physical examinations. If a resident is not feeling well, or if the facility has no designated area, the physical examination will be done at the resident's bedside.

NURSE ASSISTANT'S ROLE IN THE PHYSICAL EXAMINATION

Your role in the physical examination is to always care for the resident's safety, comfort, and privacy. You are also responsible to:
- apply the principles of standard precautions you learned in Chapter 10
- prepare the equipment the physician will use during the physical examination before the resident arrives
- cover the examination table with clean disposable paper
- provide privacy and comfort for the resident
- measure the resident's height and weight and record these on the correct form
- take the resident's vital signs and record these on the correct form
- assist the resident with undressing, putting on the gown for the examination, and dressing afterwards
- assist the resident onto the examination table, and provide pillows for comfort and a warm blanket if the resident feels cold before and after the examination
- assist the physician with positioning the resident safely during the physical examination
- drape the resident during the examination
- collect, label, and deposit specimens in the area designated by the facility for transport to the lab (Fig. 13-4)

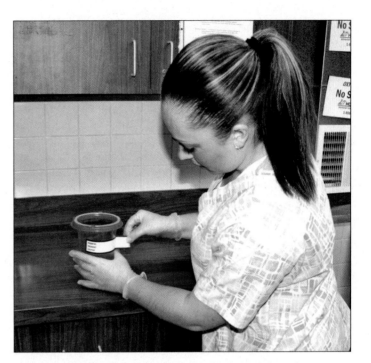

Fig. 13-4 – Nurse assistant labeling specimen immediately after collection.

- provide equipment needed during the examination
- reassure the resident
- assist the resident as needed after the examination

TECHNIQUES USED IN PHYSICAL EXAMINATION

The physician uses several techniques to assess the resident's physical health during the physical examination. Inspection, or looking at the resident's body, gives valuable visual information about the resident's health status. Palpation helps the physician determine what structures (such as bones and internal organs) actually feel like and locate any tenderness or pain. Percussion helps to determine if an area or organ is air-filled, solid, or fluid-filled. Auscultation can reveal abnormalities in function.

Auscultation – a technique of listening through a stethoscope to sounds produced by organs (such as heart, lungs, or bowels) to evaluate a body area
Palpation – an examination technique of touching the resident's body on the surface and more deeply in an organized manner
Percussion – tapping on a body area and listening to the sound produced, used to determine if tissue is air-filled, solid, or fluid-filled

The sense of smell is also used during the physical exam. Abnormal smells can help determine whether a resident has an infection, liver problems, or other abnormal conditions.

After the physical examination, you have a very important role—to listen to and acknowledge any fears of the resident and to explain what the next steps will be. The resident may be very anxious about the findings and any tests that are ordered. If you know, tell the resident when to expect answers about their condition. You can help both the resident and the physician make the process as comfortable as possible.

TAKING AND RECORDING VITAL SIGNS

As the nurse assistant helping with the physical examination or admitting the resident to the facility, you are responsible for taking and recording the resident's vital signs. **Vital signs** is a term used for the following:
- Temperature
- Pulse rate
- Respiration rate
- Blood pressure

In some facilities pain is considered the fifth vital sign. Pain is discussed in detail in Chapter 21.

Vital signs are always taken when the resident is admitted as part of the initial admission physical examination, then as ordered by the physician. The physician may order vital signs taken every four hours, every shift, once a day, or even once a month. Vital signs are always taken if a resident has any physical, mental, social, or other change that might signal an illness. Facilities often have a **protocol** for how often you take vital signs. Vital signs are recorded each time in the resident's chart or on a special form so that the health care team can evaluate the significance of any changes or abnormalities (Fig. 13–5). In some facilities vital signs are documented electronically.

The term "vital signs" shows their importance—they are crucial measurements of life functions. Take vital signs correctly and record them accurately. Nurses and physicians rely heavily on accurate records to decide whether and how to treat a resident's condition. Medications are often ordered based on the records of vital signs. If a resident's vital signs change, cannot be taken, or seem abnormal to you, tell the charge nurse immediately.

If you are ever unsure about the vital signs you take, get help from your supervisor.

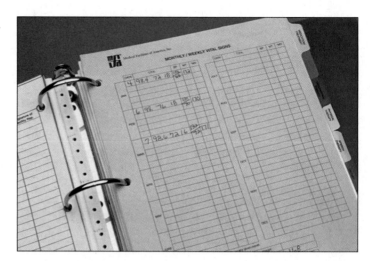

Fig. 13-5 – Vital signs are recorded on a flow chart and placed in the resident's medical record.

TEMPERATURE

Temperature is a measurement of body heat, and even when normal may vary for each person. A person's temperature normally changes during a 24-hour day. The lowest reading is usually in the morning before the person wakes. The highest is in the late afternoon and evening.

A higher than normal temperature is commonly called a fever. Fever may indicate an infection or an allergic reaction to a medication. An older resident's temperature does not change as much as a younger person's, even in these situations. A resident with a fever often also has other signs and symptoms.

There are five ways to measure body temperature with a thermometer:
- **Oral** (temperature taken in the mouth)
- **Rectal** (temperature is taken in the rectum)
- **Axillary** (temperature is taken under the armpit)
- **Tympanic** (temperature is taken in the ear with a probe)
- **Temporal scan** (temperature is taken on the forehead with a probe)

Protocol – a facility's official way of doing something, usually put in writing

Temperature – a degree of heat that naturally occurs in the body

Vital signs – necessary for life: temperature, pulse, respiration, and blood pressure

Normal temperature ranges are different at these different body sites. The thermometer is also kept in place for different lengths of time. The normal range for an oral temperature in an adult is 97.6 F to 99.6 F (the F means Fahrenheit scale). The average is 98.6 F. The normal range for an axillary temperature in an adult is 96.6 to 98.6 F. The average is 97.6 F. The normal range for a rectal temperature is 98.6 to 100.6 F. The average is 99.6 F.

Note: *Because glass thermometers are easily broken and the mercury inside would make a hazardous waste problem, many facilities do not use glass thermometers; if they do, they use non-mercury glass thermometers. If your facility does use glass thermometers, be sure you know the facility's clean-up* **policy**. *Clean-up guidelines are required by OSHA.*

There are many different types of thermometers (Fig. 13-6):

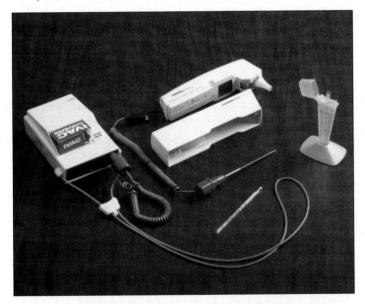

Fig. 13-6 — A resident's temperature can be measured using one of several types of thermometers.

- Oral glass thermometers. This thermometer has a blue top and long narrow or small rounded tip.
- Rectal glass thermometers. This thermometer has a red top and a more rounded tip to prevent injury to rectal tissue. Use a lubricated cover to prevent discomfort and possible injury to the rectum. Use a non-lubricated cover for axillary and oral temperatures.

- Electronic and digital thermometers. These may be used to take oral, rectal, and axillary temperatures. Following proper infection control practices, all have disposable probe covers or are disposed after each use. Normally, use a blue tip for an oral or axillary temperature, and a red tip for a rectal temperature. The temperature is displayed on the front of the device. Many digital thermometers have a battery and an automatic shut-off mechanism that turns off in 60 seconds. Other electronic thermometers are recharged on a charging base.
- Tympanic (ear) probe. This thermometer measures body temperature when the probe is placed in the ear. It measures the heat from blood vessels in the eardrum.
- Disposable thermometer. The disposable thermometer has a chemical dot that changes color when heated. The chemical change takes place within 45-60 seconds.
- Temperature-sensitive tape. The tape can be placed on the abdomen or forehead. The tape changes color in about 15 seconds in response to body heat.
- Temporal scan. The probe is placed in the middle of the forehead flush against the skin. While the scan button is pressed, the probe is slid across the forehead toward the hairline. The scan shuts off in 30 seconds and shows the temperature result.

Electronic or digital thermometers are now the most common method of taking a temperature because they decrease the spread of infection and are quick and easy to use. After you insert the thermometer, wait for the beep that means the thermometer is ready. Then read the digital display of the temperature. Because the battery inside this thermometer must be recharged, remember to return it to the base unit for charging.

Before using a glass thermometer, you must know how to clean it, how to shake it down, and how to read it. You must take special precautions if the thermometer breaks. These skills and precautions are part of the knowledge required to take a temperature.

How To Clean a Glass Thermometer.   To clean the thermometer before using it:
1. If the thermometer is stored in a disinfectant, hold the stem end under cold running water to rinse off the disinfectant. Use cold water because hot water can break the thermometer.

📖
Policy – a high-level plan for meeting goals, acceptable procedure

2. Wipe the water off the thermometer with a tissue. Wipe from the stem toward the bulb end.

To clean the thermometer after use:
1. Wipe the thermometer with a piece of gauze soaked with a cleansing or disinfectant solution (such as alcohol), or use a pre-moistened disinfectant (alcohol) pad.
2. Wipe the thermometer from the stem end to the bulb end. The bulb end is considered dirty because it is the part that was in contact with the person; the stem end is considered cleaner. Twist the thermometer as you wipe it off to ensure full cleaning. Be sure to rinse it thoroughly.
3. Replace the thermometer in the dirty or used container in the utility room, or follow your facility's protocol.

How To Shake Down the Thermometer.   You must shake down a thermometer to get an accurate reading. Hold the thermometer by the stem. With a quick wrist motion shake the thermometer as if shaking something off the bulb. Be careful not to hit the thermometer on anything. Shake the thermometer down to 95 F or lower.

How To Read a Thermometer.   The thermometer is marked with lines that indicate degrees. Between large lines showing single degrees F are five small lines, each indicating 0.2 F. To read the thermometer, follow these steps:
1. Hold the thermometer at eye level to clearly see the lines (Fig. 13-7).
2. Slowly turn the thermometer until you can see the place where the liquid inside the glass (silver or red) stops.
3. Read the temperature and write it down.

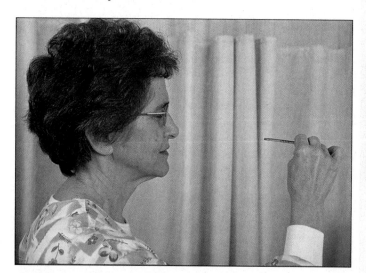

Fig. 13-7 – To read a glass thermometer hold it at eye level.

PROCEDURE 13-1.
TAKING AN ORAL TEMPERATURE

▶ **REMEMBER: BE AWARE**

Items Needed
- glass or electronic thermometer with cover
- watch with a second hand
- paper and pencil

Note: *Check with the person to make sure they have not just eaten or drunk something hot or cold or smoked a cigarette in the last 10 minutes. These activities change the temperature of the mouth and give you a false reading. If they did, wait 5-10 minutes.*

1. Shake the thermometer down to 95 F or to the lowest number, and then put on the plastic cover.

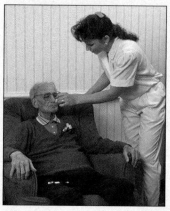

2. Insert the bulb end of the thermometer under the resident's tongue, and ask them to close their lips around it.

   The resident may want to hold onto the end of the thermometer to keep it in place. The resident should not walk with the thermometer in their mouth.

3. Wait at least three minutes. As you wait, you can take the person's pulse and respiratory rates. Remove the thermometer and the plastic cover. Read the temperature.

Note: *If there is an excessive amount of mucus on the thermometer when you remove it, use a barrier such as gloves to remove the cover.*

4. If you use an electronic thermometer, wait until it beeps.

5. Record the result.

▶ **REMEMBER: UNDERSTAND**

Oral Temperature.   An oral temperature is the most common method. An oral temperature should not be taken when:

- A resident is receiving oxygen with a mask or has trouble breathing.
- A resident is confused or combative.
- A resident has a mouth disorder or gum disease or has had recent mouth surgery.
- A resident is paralyzed on one side of the mouth (such as after a stroke) and cannot hold the thermometer in place.

Ask the nurse if you have any questions. Follow the steps outlined in Procedure 13-1, previous page.

Review Tables 12-1 and 12-2 in Chapter 12, Common Preparation and Completion Steps, before you learn each of the skills in this chapter. These tables are also found at the very end of this book.

Rectal Temperature.   The rectal temperature is considered to be the most accurate temperature because it registers the body's "core" temperature. A rectal temperature is taken when:

- A resident is confused or very restless and may bite the thermometer if placed in the mouth.
- A resident can breathe only through their mouth.
- The physician orders a rectal temperature.

PROCEDURE 13-2. TAKING A RECTAL TEMPERATURE

▶ **REMEMBER: BE AWARE**

Items Needed
- glass thermometer and cover
- watch with a second hand
- paper and pencil

1. Be sure to wear gloves.

2. Shake down the thermometer to 95 F or lower.

3. Position the resident on either side. Help the resident bend up the upper leg as far as possible.

4. Put a plastic cover over the thermometer and lubricate it. Separate the person's buttocks with one hand while with the other you insert the bulb 1 inch into the rectum.

5. Hold the thermometer in place 1 to 3 minutes, remove it, and wipe any excess lubricant from the rectum with a piece of tissue paper. Remove the cover, and read the thermometer.

6. Record the result.

Note: *Always cover a resident while taking a rectal temperature. Never leave them during this time because they may roll off their side and be injured by the thermometer. Talk with the person while waiting for the temperature reading to take their mind off the procedure.*

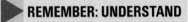

▶ **REMEMBER: UNDERSTAND**

PROCEDURE 13-3. TAKING AN AXILLARY TEMPERATURE

▶ **REMEMBER: BE AWARE**

Items Needed
- glass thermometer and cover
- watch with a second hand
- paper and pencil

1. Shake down the thermometer to 95 F or lower.

2. Loosen the resident's clothing to be able to reach the armpit. Dry the armpit.

3. Place the thermometer in the resident's armpit. Have them place the arm along their side.

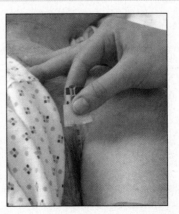

4. Wait 10 minutes. Remove the thermometer and read the temperature.

5. Record the result.

▶ **REMEMBER: UNDERSTAND**

There are situations when taking rectal temperature is not advised or where you must use extreme caution and care:
- A resident has diarrhea.
- A resident has had recent rectal surgery.
- A resident has hemorrhoids.

In these situations, check with the nurse to make sure the temperature should be taken rectally. Be sure to use a rectal thermometer. It usually has a red stem and a short, rounded bulb. Some facilities use disposable thermometer covers. Procedure 13-2 (previous page) outlines the steps.

Axillary Temperature. The axillary temperature is the least reliable method. Use it only when the other two methods cannot be used, for example with a confused resident who will not allow you to take a temperature by other methods. To take an axillary temperature, use an oral thermometer in the armpit. Procedure 13-3 (previous page) outlines the steps.

Pulse Rate. The pulse rate is the number of times the heart beats in a minute. You can feel the pulse in several body areas. Figure 13-8 shows common pulse sites.

Usually you take the pulse at the wrist. This is called the radial pulse. It is quick and easy to take and usually gives an accurate reading.

You feel the pulse as a throbbing in an artery over a bone each time the heart pumps blood through the body. The normal rate in an adult at rest is 60-90 beats per minute. The pulse normally has a regular rhythm, beating at regular intervals with pauses between.

The pulse might be fast because of:
- exercise
- anxiety or anger
- a heart condition
- some medications

The pulse rate might be slow because of things such as:
- condition of the heart
- some medications
- a pacemaker
- a calm resting state

Things to note when taking a pulse:
- The person should be calm or feel relaxed.
- Pay attention to any irregularities in the pulse rhythm, or pattern of beats. Note how strong the pulse is. If you can easily feel the pulse with your fingertips, it is strong. If the pulse feels very faint under your fingers, it is weak. Report any irregularities to the charge nurse. The best way to learn pulse strength is to practice on a lot of people.

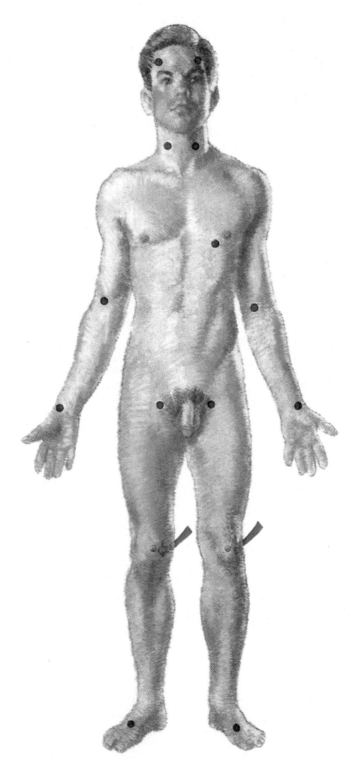

Fig. 13-8 – There are a number of places on the body where you can feel a resident's pulse.

PROCEDURE 13-4.
TAKING A RADIAL PULSE

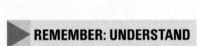

REMEMBER: BE AWARE

Items Needed
- watch with a second hand
- paper and pencil

1. Place your second and third fingers gently over the radial artery (on the thumb side of the wrist) and note the rhythm of the pulse.

2. Look at your watch, and when the second hand is on the 12, start counting the pulse for 1 minute. Count each beat you feel. Check for abnormalities in the rhythm.

3. Record the result.

REMEMBER: UNDERSTAND

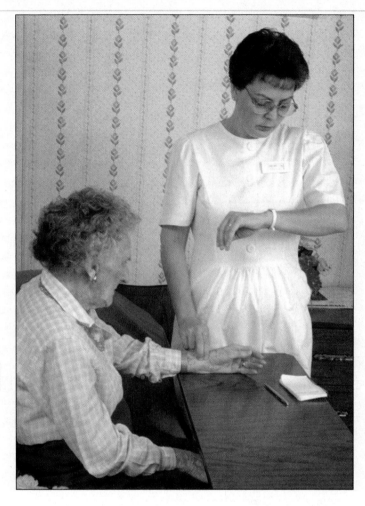

- Count the pulse rate, which is how many beats per minute you feel.
- Do not use your thumb to take a pulse because your thumb has a pulse that could be confused with a resident's pulse.

Procedure 13-4 (above) outlines the steps for taking a radial pulse.

RESPIRATORY RATE

Counting respirations is another part of taking a resident's vital signs. Respiration is the process of inhaling air into the lungs and exhaling air out of the lungs.

Count the respiratory rate by watching a resident breathe in and out. One respiration is equal to one inspiration (breathing in) and one expiration (breathing out). A person's normal respiratory rate changes with physical and emotional activity and with sleep. The normal respiratory rate for an adult at rest is 12-20 breaths per minute. When counting a resident's respiratory rate observe if the resident is taking in deep slow breaths, or shallow rapid breaths. Are the breaths in a regular pattern, or are some deep and slow and some shallow and rapid? Record your findings and report any irregularities to the charge nurse. Procedure 13-5 (next page) outlines the steps for counting the respiratory rate.

BLOOD PRESSURE

Blood pressure, abbreviated BP, is the last vital sign. Changes in blood pressure may signal a change in a resident's health condition or disease process. A blood pressure that is too high all the time or sometimes can lead to a stroke, heart attack, or other problems. A blood pressure that is too low can lead to conditions such as fainting (especially on standing), fatigue, or weakness. It may also indicate the need to evaluate or change the resident's medications.

PROCEDURE 13-5. TAKING A RESPIRATORY RATE

 REMEMBER: BE AWARE

Items Needed
- watch with a second hand
- paper and pencil

1. Count the respiratory rate immediately after counting the pulse rate.

2. Keep your fingers on the resident's radial pulse but without pressure. (Do this so the resident will breathe normally. Often residents hold their breath or breathe deeper if they know you are counting.) Watch the chest go up with inspiration and down with expiration.

3. Count the respiratory rate for 1 minute.

4. Record the result.

 REMEMBER: UNDERSTAND

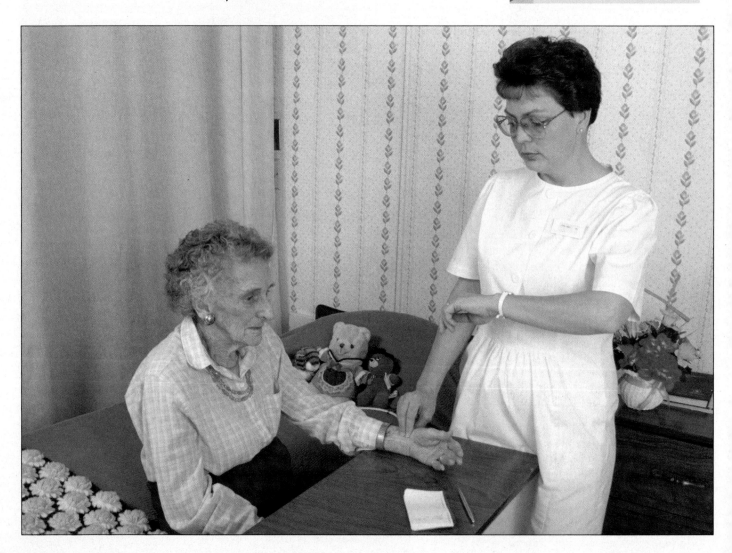

Blood pressure is the pressure of blood in the arteries. The pressure is affected by the force of the heart's contraction, the rigidity of the arterial blood vessels, and the amount of circulating blood. Two numbers are recorded for a blood pressure, such as 170/80. The top (first) number is called the systolic pressure, which is the pressure in the artery when the heart is pumping. The bottom (second) number is called the diastolic pressure, which is the pressure when the heart is at rest between beats.

Blood pressure differs from person to person and in the same person from time to time. Many factors can affect a person's blood pressure, such as:

- stress
- medications
- weight and diet
- family history
- exercise
- smoking
- physical position
- arm in which blood pressure is taken

Some factors can be controlled and some cannot. A resident's BP might be higher on admission because of anxiety. A resident's BP and other vital signs are generally taken often during the first week to determine what is a normal baseline for this person.

The normal blood pressure range for adults is <120mm Hg systolic and <80mm Hg diastolic. In someone over age 50, a systolic blood pressure above 140mm Hg is a much more important cardiovascular disease risk than a high diastolic blood pressure.

The systolic BP in older adults tends to be higher than in younger individuals because the arteries become narrower and more rigid with age. An older adult may have a high BP range of:

Systolic: 140–160 (top number)
Diastolic: 90 (bottom number)

Table 13-1 shows the classification and the management of blood pressure for adults.

If the person's blood pressure is always high, this is called hypertension. Low blood pressure is called hypotension. Blood pressure should be measured when a resident is sitting or lying down. You can take the blood pressure in either arm. Blood pressure should not be taken in an arm with an intravenous (IV) tube present or in an arm that is injured or has recently undergone surgery.

ACCURATE REPORTING AND RECORDING OF VITAL SIGNS

Vital signs are always taken if a resident has any change that might signal illness. Vital signs are recorded in a resident's chart on a special form each time they are taken so that the nurse and the physician can evaluate any changes or abnormalities. Always take vital signs carefully and record them accurately. Vital signs are usually recorded with abbreviations: T for temperature, P for pulse, R for respiration, and BP for blood pressure. For example:

T 98.6, P 86 R 20 and BP 120/80

Baseline – beginning observations used for later comparisons
Blood pressure – pressure of blood in the arteries

TABLE 13-1
BLOOD PRESSURE CLASSIFICATION AND MANAGEMENT

BP CLASSIFICATION	SYSTOLIC BP MMHG	DIASTOLIC BP MMHG	LIFESTYLE MODIFICATION	MEDICATION NEEDED
Normal	<120	And <80	Encourage	No
Prehypertension	120-139	Or 80-89	Yes	No
Stage 1 Hypertension	140-159	Or 90-99	Yes	May need one medication
Stage 2 Hypertension	>=160	Or >=100	Yes	Two or more medications needed

PROCEDURE 13-6. TAKING A BLOOD PRESSURE

▶ **REMEMBER: BE AWARE**

Items Needed
- BP cuff of correct size
- sphygmomanometer
- stethoscope
- paper and pencil

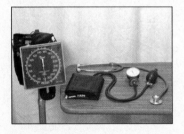

Note: *To take a blood pressure you use a stethoscope, a blood pressure cuff, and a sphygmomanometer. You will learn the equipment used in your facility.*

1. Have the resident place their arm on the bed, bedside table, or arm of the chair, with their palm up and elbow at the same level as the heart. (If the arm is higher than the heart, the blood pressure can register too high. If the arm is lower than the heart, the blood pressure can register too low.)

2. Expose the resident's arm by rolling the sleeve up to the shoulder, taking care that the sleeve is not too tight on the arm, which might increase the blood pressure. Wrap the blood pressure cuff evenly around the upper arm 1 inch above the elbow. Make sure the arm is not lying on the tubing and the tub-

ing is not kinked. The tube that is attached to the bulb should be on the side closest to the resident's body. The tube to the sphygmomanometer gauge should be on the other side of the arm, away from the body. Be sure to use the correct size cuff for the resident. The wrong size cuff can give you an incorrect reading. The cuff should fit over the center of the resident's upper arm. It should not extend to the elbow or to under the resident's armpit.

3. Close the valve in the air pump by turning it clockwise. The valve is the little metal knob on the bulb.

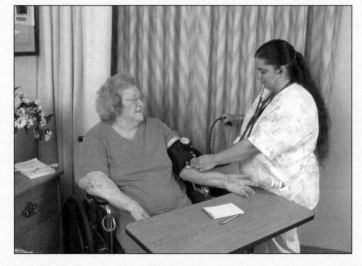

4. Place the stethoscope earpieces in your ears.

5. Locate the pulsation in the brachial artery by placing your second and third fingers over the area. When you find the pulse, place the diaphragm of the stethoscope firmly over the area and hold it in place with your left hand. Use your right hand if you are left-handed.

6. With your right hand, pump air into the cuff by squeezing the bulb until the gauge measures 180–200.

Note: *If you hear the pulse immediately after stopping pumping, begin again and pump the cuff so the gauge reads higher than 200 mm Hg (Hg=symbol for mercury). One way to avoid pumping the cuff too high is to feel the pulse at the brachial artery and pump the cuff slowly until you no longer feel the pulse, making sure to remember where you last felt the pulse and to add 30 mm Hg when beginning to take the blood pressure.*

7. Slowly open the valve on the bulb and watch the cuff pressure decrease on the gauge.

8. Listen for the first thumping sound and note the pressure reading; remember this number. This is the systolic pressure.

9. Continue to listen for a distinct change in sound (muffled sounding) or the last sound and note the pressure reading. This is the diastolic pressure.

10. Record the results.

▶ **REMEMBER: UNDERSTAND**

If ever you are unsure about taking vital signs or the results you obtain, get help from your supervisor. Always report any irregularities you note in the vital signs.

HEIGHT AND WEIGHT

A resident's height is measured on the admission physical examination and then once a year. A resident's weight is measured on admission and usually once a week for four weeks following admission to establish a baseline, and then at least once a month or more often if ordered by the physician or if the resident's weight has been unstable. These measurements help the nursing staff, dietitian, and others on the health care team know if a resident's weight is normal for their height, sex, and age. They are then weighed regularly to see if they are gaining or losing weight. Weight measurements are sometimes also used to calculate drug dosages or to monitor the success of diet, drug, or dialysis therapy.

Weight is one of the most important indicators of nutritional status. Evaluation of a resident's weight status involves comparing their current weight with their usual weight. Weight loss changes for some residents may be desirable, such as for residents who have been retaining fluid. A resident's weight loss is compared to their usual body weight.

Weight

A resident's weight can be interpreted in several ways. Weight is often calculated as either a percentage of (ideal) weight or a percentage of (usual) weight. Both are important. The percentage of ideal weight gives a benchmark comparison for evaluating the resident's weight. For example, if a man is 30% above his ideal range, he is considered obese. Obesity is determined only by comparing a person's weight with the normal, or ideal, weight range. The dietitian or dietary manager calculates ideal weight.

A person's percentage of usual weight is also important. If a female resident's previous normal weight was 120 pounds but she weighs 100 pounds on admission to the facility, she has lost 17% of her usual weight and can be considered at risk for poor nutritional status. But if she has not weighed over 100 pounds for the last 10 years, this weight may be accepted as normal for her, and then her weight would simply be monitored closely.

Measuring a resident's weight is an important part of the physical exam on admission. The physician orders a resident's weight depending on their needs or physical condition. The physician may order a weight to be measured

every day or every shift if:
- The resident has a recent weight loss or gain.
- The resident is on medication that increases or decreases body weight.
- The resident is not eating well.

In long term care residents are routinely weighed every month unless otherwise ordered by the physician.

Accuracy is important because weight is an indication of a resident's health. Underweight residents are less resistant to infection, are more sensitive to cold, and may be weaker overall. Tell the nurse immediately about a resident's weight loss. A weight change is considered severe in these conditions:
- loss of 5 pounds in one month
- loss of 7.5% of body weight or more in three months (for a 120 lb person, this would be a 9 lb loss)
- loss of 10% of body weight or more in six months (for a 120 lb person, this would be a 12 lb loss)

Because accuracy is so important, a weight change of 2-5 pounds or more should be rechecked and confirmed before you record and report it.

Weight can be measured in several ways, depending on a resident's mobility. If they can stand, use a standard bathroom scale or upright scale (Fig. 13-9, next page). Scales for wheelchairs are also available. For residents confined to bed, lift scales are used (Fig. 13-10, next page).

You will learn to use all types of scales in your facility. Follow these guidelines:
- The scale must be checked periodically for accuracy. Follow the manufacturer's procedure for checking the scale's balance. There may be a lever or knob you can adjust.
- Always weigh a resident on the same scale. There may be slight differences between scales.
- Try to weigh a resident at the same time of day and wearing the same amount of clothing.
- If a resident's weight changes more than 2-5 pounds from the previous month, weigh them again and report the weight change to the nurse.

Dialysis – a medical procedure given to some patients with kidney disease

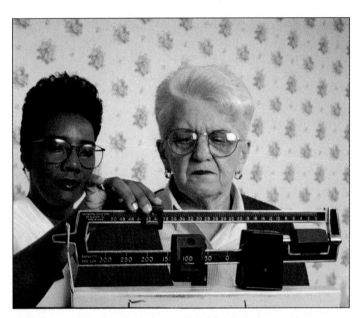

Fig. 13-9 – An upright scale can be used when the resident can stand up and maintain their balance.

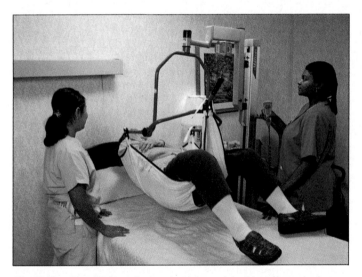

Fig. 13-10 – A resident on bed rest can be weighed by using a scale similar to a mechanical lift.

The dietitian may also calculate and use the resident's **body mass index (BMI)** to evaluate their nutritional status. A standard formula is used to determine whether a resident is at a desirable weight, severely underweight, overweight, or obese based on their sex, height, and current weight.

Height

Weight cannot be properly evaluated without a height measurement. Height is difficult to measure for residents who cannot stand erect or who have a disease such as arthritis or osteoporosis.

An alert, oriented resident can be asked to report their height, but height must still be measured because it may decrease with age. The resident's previous height gives you an idea whether your measurement is accurate. For example, if Mr. Smith states his height as 5 feet 8 inches and your measurement is 5 feet 7 inches, your measurement is probably correct. If, however, your measurement shows him to be 5 feet 11 inches, you should measure again.

The method used to measure a resident's height, like their weight, depends on their mobility. Ambulatory residents should be measured standing, preferably without shoes. Take the measurement with the resident standing against the wall or standing on an ambulatory scale with a vertical measuring device (Fig. 13-11, next page). If a resident is confined to bed, check with the nurse to make sure you can measure their height as they lie face up and flat on the mattress. Residents with breathing difficulties may not be able to lie flat in bed. Using a tape measure, measure from the crown of their head to the bottom of their heel, recording the measurement in feet and inches. The dietitian will then add 1.5 inches to this measurement as an estimate of the resident's standing height.

Residents with contractures or other disabilities that make it difficult to measure height may need to be measured by special means such as a knee-height caliper or by arm span. Alternative ways to measure height may be used by the dietitian. The dietitian or the charge nurse will tell you what they need you to do.

Residents with amputated lower limbs (one side or both sides, at any leg level) need careful measurements of their height on admission, or after any surgical amputation after admission. A full or partial loss of limb or height affects their BMI and caloric requirements.

Height and weight measurements made at the time of admission are used as baseline data. Later measurements of the resident are compared to these. If this baseline data is wrong, this can affect the person's data collection and plan of care. Procedure 13-7 describes the steps for measuring height and weight using an upright scale.

Body Mass Index (BMI) – a measurement of a person's body fat

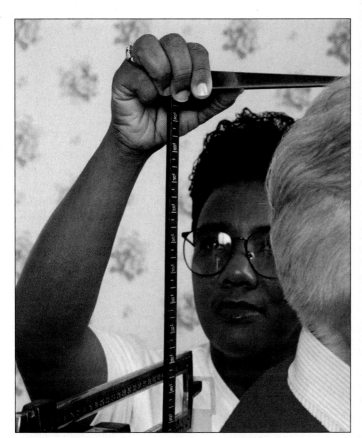

Fig. 13-11 – Measuring a resident's height allows the staff to better evaluate the resident's weight.

PROCEDURE 13-7. MEASURING HEIGHT AND WEIGHT USING AN UPRIGHT SCALE

 REMEMBER: BE AWARE

Items Needed
- scale with a height measure
- paper towel

1. Determine if the resident can walk to the scale or whether you need to bring a portable scale to their room.
2. Before they step on the scale, adjust the height measurement bar so it is higher than the resident's height.
3. Ask the resident what their height is as a check for accuracy.
4. Clear the scale and make sure it is balanced. It should register 0 when the weights are moved all the way over to the left.
5. Place a paper towel on the scale platform. Ask the resident to remove their shoes. Help them stand on the scale. Make sure they are not holding anything.
6. Have the resident stand up straight, with their arms by their side and their eyes looking forward. Slowly lower the height measurement bar to the top of their head. Record their height in feet and inches.
7. Measure the resident's weight by moving the weights to the right until the balance needle is centered.

Note: *If the weight is 5 pounds or more different from the previous measurement, weigh the resident again before reporting it to the charge nurse. If the resident is wearing a cast or brace when they are weighed, also report this to the nurse.*

8. Help the resident off the scale.
9. Record the resident's height and weight on the worksheet and report the findings to the charge nurse. Example of charting: Height: 5 feet 6 inches, Weight: 135 lbs

Note: *Your facility may have special scales for weighing residents while they are in a wheelchair or confined to bed. Follow your facility's policy and the manufacturer's instructions for using different scales.*

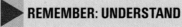 **REMEMBER: UNDERSTAND**

IN THIS CHAPTER YOU LEARNED:
- Your role in a resident's history and physical exam and why it is important
- Why a physical examination is important
- How and why it is important to measure and record vital signs
- How and why it is important to measure and record a resident's height and weight

SUMMARY
Gathering accurate information about a resident is one of the best ways to get to know them. It also allows the entire team to give the best possible care. As the person who spends the most time with the resident, you play a vital role in assuring that the resident receives necessary care and support. Taking and recording accurate information can make a big difference in the resident's life.

PULLING IT ALL TOGETHER
Just imagine what could happen if a resident is admitted to the facility and inaccurate information is recorded or valuable information is not documented. Most likely, the resident will not receive the proper care. In addition, reimbursement for services is based on information documented in the MDS, and part of this information comes from the history and physical examination.

Imagine that the resident or a family member gave you information and you forgot to document it or to tell other team members about it. This could result in the resident not receiving medication or an infection getting worse.

Accurate documentation and communication to other team members is critical for success when caring for residents.

CHECK WHAT YOU'VE LEARNED

1. **You should check a resident's vital signs:**
   A. Only on the first day of each month.
   B. Whenever a change occurs that might signal an illness.
   C. Everyday at the beginning of your shift.
   D. Only when the charge nurse tells you to.

1. **A higher than normal temperature may mean the resident has:**
   A. An infection.
   B. Cancer.
   C. Diabetes.
   D. Alzheimer's disease.

3. **For how long do you count the resident's pulse to obtain an accurate rate?**
   A. 10 seconds.
   B. 30 seconds.
   C. 60 seconds.
   D. 120 seconds.

4. **When you take a resident's respiratory rate, you should:**
   A. Announce that now you will start counting their breaths.
   B. Put your hand on their chest to feel their breathing while you count.
   C. Keep your fingers on their wrist as if you are still taking their pulse.
   D. Count breaths for 10 seconds and multiply by 6 for the rate per minute.

5. **How much weight loss by a resident is considered serious?**
   A. A loss of 1 pound in 1 month.
   B. A loss of 5 pounds in 1 month.
   C. A loss of 1% of body weight in 3 months.
   D. A loss of 2% of body weight in 3 months.

6. **When collecting information about a person during the physical exam, what questions will the health professional ask?**
   A. About a fight the person had with her brother when she was young.
   B. Personal life questions (age, birth, education).
   C. What television shows the person enjoys.
   D. How the person feels about stem cell research.

7. **When the health professional reviews the integumentary system during the physical exam, what specific questions will be asked?**
   A. Questions relating to dizziness.
   B. Questions relating to skin rashes.
   C. Questions relating to breathing.
   D. Questions relating to blood pressure.

8. **When the health professional reviews the digestive system during the physical exam, what specific questions will be asked?**
   A. Questions relating to chest pain.
   B. Questions relating to pain or gas after eating.
   C. Questions relating to enlarged lymph nodes in the neck.
   D. Questions relating to tremors.

9. **What is your role during the physical examination?**
   A. To examine the heart.
   B. To obtain a pap smear.
   C. To care for the person's safety, comfort, and privacy.
   D. To perform a rectal exam.

10. **Which is your responsibility during the physical examination?**
    A. To take, report, and record vital signs.
    B. To obtain a urine sample if the health professional orders one.
    C. To assist the person with undressing and dressing if needed.
    D. All of the above.

(Answers to "Check What You've Learned" are in the Instructor's Manual.)

Chapter 14

THE IMPORTANCE OF CREATING A HOME

What you do when a resident enters your facility sometimes makes the difference between life and death. Some residents feel great stress when they enter a long term care facility. This can cause a decline in their health, an inability to care for themselves, disorientation, and confusion. These symptoms can become worse if they are not recognized and addressed. This problem is very common but may be overlooked. You should watch for signs of this problem so you can help the resident adjust to their new home. If the resident does not adjust well, their health can get worse within a few weeks after entering the facility, but what you and other staff do can make a dramatic difference. As the person who spends the most time with the resident, you can make a big difference in helping residents adjust to their new home.

This chapter will help you to learn how to create a home for residents in a long term care facility. You will learn about admitting residents to the facility and your role in transferring or discharging a resident. You will learn why it is important to respect residents' privacy. You will also learn skills such as how to make a resident's bed and make their room more comfortable and how to teach residents to use the call system.

OBJECTIVES
- Describe your role in admitting a resident
- List three ways to make a resident's room home-like
- Describe your role in caring for a resident's belongings
- Explain ways to ensure the resident's privacy
- Demonstrate how to make an unoccupied and an occupied bed
- Demonstrate the use of the call system
- Describe your role in transferring and discharging a resident

MEDICAL TERMS
- **Relocation stress syndrome** – reaction of an unprepared resident entering a long term care facility

PROCEDURE 14-1
Making an Unoccupied Bed

PROCEDURE 14-2
Making an Occupied Bed

"I was so scared the day I came, but your smile and kindness made all the difference."

People move to new homes for many different reasons—they marry, have children, or start or change jobs. Residents move to a facility for many reasons, too. Some move to the facility because a family member or their physician feels they should not live alone due to a change in their health. Others move because they are too frail to carry out the activities of daily living without support. They may not be able to cook, clean, and manage their day-to-day activities independently. They may be moving to the facility because they lost their spouse or other family member or friend, or because of their health. You should understand why the person is moving to the facility. You need to know how the person feels about the move and how they are adjusting to the change.

People often have difficulty adjusting to the changes that happen when they enter a facility. Think about those changes. Most residents formerly lived alone or with family members, and now in the facility they must live among many strangers. Perhaps for the first time in their lives, they may share a room with someone who is not their spouse or another family member. They have to follow new rules, like eating meals at certain times or telling staff where they are going. They may not like other rules like not playing music or the television too loud or too late, not dressing too casually outside their rooms, or not smoking or drinking.

Have you ever moved to a different house or apartment? What did you unpack first? How did you make your new space feel like your home? How long did it take before you felt it was truly your home? At first you probably felt uncomfortable. You might have wondered, "Where will I put all my things? Will I make new friends around here? Will I ever become comfortable here?" Most people can adapt to changes if they feel they have some control over their surroundings. If you can make decisions about how you live and have your familiar things around you, you feel more secure and in control. This helps you feel better about your life.

ADMISSION OF RESIDENTS

Residents are usually admitted to a long term care facility when their physical or mental condition makes it too difficult to stay at home. Usually the family decides that 24-hour nursing care is needed. This is often very stressful for both the resident and the family.

Sometimes a resident comes directly from their own home or a family member's. Sometimes a resident comes from a hospital or another facility. Each resident who is being admitted has their own needs and concerns. From the minute the admission process begins, keep in mind the loss the person feels and their need to adjust to their surroundings.

Being admitted to a long term care facility is a very emotional experience and often causes anxiety. Some residents experience **relocation stress syndrome** when they enter a long term care facility (Fig. 14-1). Relocation stress syndrome can happen whenever a person moves from one place to another. A resident's health can **deteriorate** within a few weeks after entering a long term care facility because of a poor **adjustment** to the facility, but what you and other staff do can make a dramatic difference. You can make this experience much less difficult and trying for the resident. Remember that a resident is often upset about moving. A friendly, home-like, caring, and welcoming atmosphere may help them feel more comfortable (Fig. 14-2, next page). The resident may feel fearful about the unknown. They may have many questions like these:

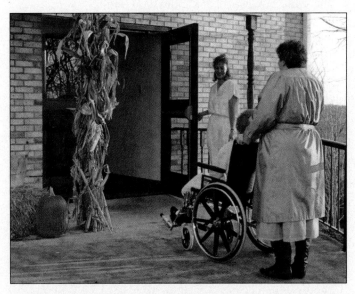

Fig. 14-1 – When it is determined that 24-hour care is required for a loved one, it may cause stress for both the new resident and the family.

📖
Adjustment – a correction or modification for actual conditions
Deteriorate – to grow worse
Relocation stress syndrome – reaction of an unprepared resident entering a long term care facility

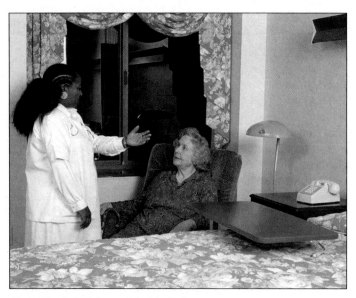

Fig. 14-2 — Orient the resident to their room.

- Will staff know who I am and what I need?
- How will I know what I can do here?
- Will my family and friends visit me here?
- Can I keep doing the things I've always enjoyed doing?
- Can I get up in the morning and go to bed when I want?
- Can I bathe when I want?
- Can I eat what I want and when I want?

The Interdisciplinary Approach for Admission

Facilities have forms to fill out and procedures for admitting residents. Admission is a complex effort. The whole staff team is involved. When you begin work in a long term care facility, you will learn its specific procedures for admitting residents. The following personnel may all be involved in the admission of a resident:

- **Admission Coordinator.** This person's main responsibility is to help residents through the admission process. This person may be a social worker, nurse, or someone else trained in admission policies. They often work with discharge planners at hospitals.
- **Social Worker.** This person may work as the admissions coordinator. The social worker also helps fill out the admission paperwork and take a social history of the resident. They may also help the family with financial issues.
- **Housekeeping Department.** They help clean and set up the new room. They might also help residents move in.
- **Dietary Department.** They interview residents or family members to find out the resident's food preferences.

- **Maintenance Department.** They may help move residents into the facility and put in a phone for residents who want one.
- **Front Office.** These employees assist with financial concerns and payment schedules. They might also give the family information about how to apply for Medicaid.
- **Nurses.** The charge nurse makes sure all equipment and medications are ready for a resident on admission. They assess each resident carefully and document all findings. The charge nurse starts the resident assessment process. The nurse answers the resident's and family members' questions and helps them feel as comfortable as possible. The nurse also obtains or confirms orders with the resident's physician.

All team members work closely together to make the admission a successful experience.

What Can You Do To Prepare for the New Resident?

Because you will spend the most time with the resident, you have an important role in helping the resident feel welcome upon arrival. Before the resident arrives you may do the following:

- Check that the bed is made, a pillow is on the bed, and a blanket is available in the room.
- Check that a chair and working reading light are present and that the light is working.
- Check that the call light is in place and working properly.
- Check that the bed's electric or manual cranks are working.
- Check that personal care supplies such as washcloth, towel, soap, and soap dish are in place. If you already know the person cannot get to the bathroom, have a clean bed pan, and a urinal for a male resident, in the bedside table.
- Check that a water glass and water pitcher are ready to fill after the resident has been admitted.
- Be sure the resident's name is on the door.

A room that is properly prepared helps the resident and family feel welcome. It shows that you are ready, organized, and capable of giving good care (Fig. 14-3, next page).

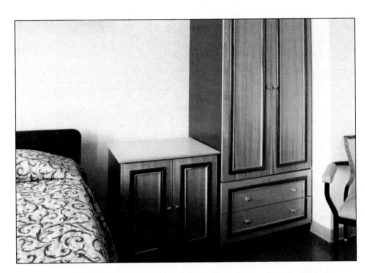

Fig. 14-3 – Having the room prepared for the new resident will help them feel welcome to the facility.

Greeting Residents

Greeting a resident warmly when they first come to the facility helps make admission more pleasant. Introduce yourself in a way that inspires confidence in the family and resident and creates a sense of well-being. Remember how you like to be treated.

To help a resident feel comfortable, you should:
- Greet them by name, for example, Miss or Mrs. Smith. Some residents may prefer to be called by their first names. Ask what name they want you to use. This lets them know you care about who they are as an individual.
- Appear poised and assured, but warm. Remember, you are part of the facility's first impression on residents and family members.
- Introduce yourself by name. Let the resident know you are a nurse assistant and will be helping them get settled. Assure them you are there to help if they have questions.
- Introduce the new resident to their roommate if they share a room. This helps both residents feel more comfortable.
- Greet any family members or friends who come with the resident.

This is a good time to get to know them. Remember, this is probably a difficult time for the resident and the family. Although the admission process is routine to you, it is not routine for them. Tell them that the nurse on duty can also answer their questions related to their care.

After a resident has unpacked and you finish filling out forms, such as a personal item inventory list and the resident's basic assessment, show them around the facility (Fig. 14-4) and explain equipment. This should include:
- bathroom facilities
- nurses' call light
- television or radio
- dining area
- visitors' or residents' lounge
- location of the nurses' station
- location of the telephone

If a resident cannot leave the room or bed, show them everything in the room. Describe other areas in the facility that they can visit at another time.

It often takes awhile, sometimes as long as six months, for new residents to feel comfortable in their new home. Remember that it can be very frightening to move from a familiar home to a new place where there are many strangers. Plan to spend extra time with and pay special attention to a resident during this time.

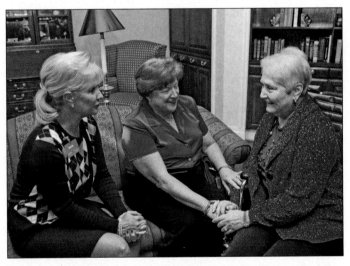

Fig. 14-4 – Every resident and their family should be shown around the facility when they are admitted so that they will be comfortable with their new surroundings.

CREATING A HOME IN A LONG TERM CARE FACILITY

When someone enters a long term care facility, they may feel many losses. They lose their home and many cherished belongings. You need to help create and maintain a home for residents in the facility. To meet this challenge, you must first learn how a resident wants the room arranged so that it feels like their own place. A resident may want pictures of grandchildren on the walls, for example, or a special bedspread on the bed. They may want personal things in a special place. Meeting a resident's wants is your highest priority. Make sure each resident feels like the facility is their home.

You can promote a home-like feeling by encouraging residents and their families to bring in their own things. These may include small furniture if there is room, wall hangings and decorative items, pictures and mementos of loved ones, plants, and personal grooming items. Familiar things help create a positive environment and the secure feeling of home. Follow these guidelines for residents' personal things:

- Treat a resident's belongings as if you are a visitor to their home.
- Comment positively on pictures and furniture.
- Encourage residents to use their own things.
- Help safeguard the resident's personal things.
- Talk with every resident to see how they want the room cared for. Together set a schedule that meets their needs as well as the facility's policy.
- Some residents choose not to bring in personal items. Treat the furniture in their room as if it were their own, and encourage them to treat it like their own.

RESPONSIBILITIES IN CARING FOR RESIDENTS' PERSONAL BELONGINGS

Although space is limited in most long term care facilities, residents have the right to bring with them and use personal items as space permits. Residents often bring both necessary things such as clothes, hearing aids, etc. and personal things that have special meanings for them.

If belongings are damaged, lost, or stolen in the facility, this can cause great distress for a resident and family and a feeling of loss. The resident may feel vulnerable and think staff don't care for them. Residents and family must be able to count on staff to respect and protect special belongings. Always think: "How would I feel if that happened to me?"

A list (inventory) of all their belongings is part of a resident's chart (Fig. 14-5). Personal items brought into a resident's room after admission must also be recorded on this list, and removed items noted on the record.

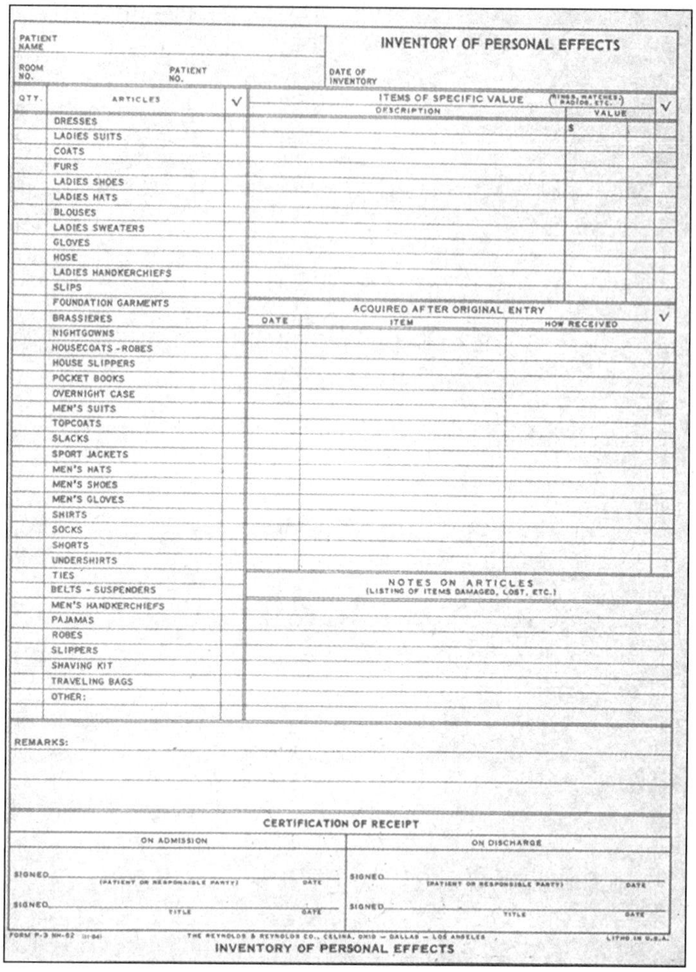
PATIENT NAME
ROOM NO. PATIENT NO.
INVENTORY OF PERSONAL EFFECTS
DATE OF INVENTORY

QTY.	ARTICLES	✓
	DRESSES	
	LADIES SUITS	
	COATS	
	FURS	
	LADIES SHOES	
	LADIES HATS	
	BLOUSES	
	LADIES SWEATERS	
	GLOVES	
	HOSE	
	LADIES HANDKERCHIEFS	
	SLIPS	
	FOUNDATION GARMENTS	
	BRASSIERES	
	NIGHTGOWNS	
	HOUSECOATS - ROBES	
	HOUSE SLIPPERS	
	POCKET BOOKS	
	OVERNIGHT CASE	
	MEN'S SUITS	
	TOPCOATS	
	SLACKS	
	SPORT JACKETS	
	MEN'S HATS	
	MEN'S SHOES	
	MEN'S GLOVES	
	SHIRTS	
	SOCKS	
	SHORTS	
	UNDERSHIRTS	
	TIES	
	BELTS - SUSPENDERS	
	MEN'S HANDKERCHIEFS	
	PAJAMAS	
	ROBES	
	SLIPPERS	
	SHAVING KIT	
	TRAVELING BAGS	
	OTHER:	

ITEMS OF SPECIFIC VALUE (RINGS, WATCHES, RADIOS, ETC.)

DESCRIPTION	VALUE	✓
	$	

ACQUIRED AFTER ORIGINAL ENTRY

DATE	ITEM	HOW RECEIVED	✓

NOTES ON ARTICLES (LISTING OF ITEMS DAMAGED, LOST, ETC.)

REMARKS:

CERTIFICATION OF RECEIPT

ON ADMISSION	ON DISCHARGE
SIGNED (PATIENT OR RESPONSIBLE PARTY) DATE	SIGNED (PATIENT OR RESPONSIBLE PARTY) DATE
SIGNED TITLE DATE	SIGNED TITLE DATE

FORM P-3 NH-62 (11-64) THE REYNOLDS & REYNOLDS CO., CELINA, OHIO — DALLAS — LOS ANGELES LITHO IN U.S.A.
INVENTORY OF PERSONAL EFFECTS

Fig. 14-5 – At the time of admission, an inventory form is completed to track the resident's personal items.

Keeping track of personal belongings is a responsibility of the whole team. For example, if a resident's eyeglasses are missing, inform housekeeping, laundry, and dietary staff. The glasses may be in the laundry in a shirt pocket or mixed in with dirty dishes on a dining tray.

Care of a Resident's Clothes

A resident's clothing is important for the resident's self-esteem. Follow these guidelines to care for the resident's clothes:

• Ensure all clothing is labeled with the resident's name where it can be easily found but not on public display, such as on the inside, on a tag (Fig. 14-6).

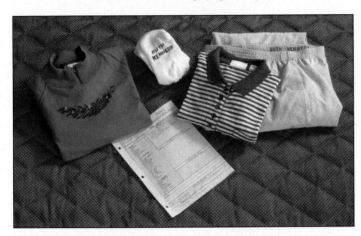

Fig. 14-6 – The resident's clothes should be labeled.

• Watch for new clothing family members and friends bring to a resident, and make sure every item is labeled.
• Be especially careful on special occasions, such as holidays and birthdays. Imagine how a resident and family would feel if a beautiful gift blouse worn only once was sent to the laundry or misplaced and never seen again.
• Try to keep a resident's clothing from becoming soiled and stained. If a resident tends to spill food, use a large napkin or other protector to prevent stains from meals or snacks.
• If an item of clothing becomes soiled, wash it in a sink as soon as possible to prevent staining. You may also ask the laundry department to treat the area, depending on your facility's protocol.
• Put laundry in the appropriate bag or container when soiled, following your facility's protocol.

Care of a Resident's Other Belongings

Belongings like hearing aids, eyeglasses, and **dentures** are necessary for the well-being of residents. Follow these guidelines:

• These items should be labeled or marked with the resident's name. (Kits are available for marking dentures.)
• Keep these items in appropriate containers when not in use. Encourage residents to do the same.
• Record the serial number of a hearing aid in the resident's record for future reference.
• Routinely check pockets when collecting clothes for the laundry. Prevent valuables such as a watch, hearing aid, or wallet from going through the laundry.
• Watch that dentures, eyeglasses, or hearing aids are not left on bedding or food trays.

Follow these guidelines for other personal belongings:
• Have the attitude that a resident's things are important and valuable. Treat them like your own.
• Be careful when cleaning or tidying the room not to damage special belongings. Open the closet and drawers only with the resident's **permission**.
• If possible, valuable items such as cash, jewelry, heirlooms, etc. should not be kept in the facility. The family should take them home. However, if such items are in the room, check with the charge nurse and follow the facility's protocol. Be sure they are on the inventory list.
• Follow your facility's policy for food left in the resident's room. Family members often bring food the resident likes. Tell them what type of container the food must be in to prevent spoiling and infection. Offer to help with storing food if needed.
• If a belonging is lost or broken, report it to the charge nurse immediately.

It can be a challenge to keep track of residents' personal belongings. Use your common sense and mindful care to lower the chance of loss or damage.

📖
Dentures – false teeth
Permission – the act of giving formal consent

RESPECTING RESIDENTS' PRIVACY

Even though many people go in and out of residents' rooms, you and all staff must respect their privacy. Remember the facility is their home. Residents have private lives—they are not just part of your routine. As you get to know residents, be careful not to let this familiarity become routine. Always be mindful. Consider this example:

> You have been caring for Mrs. Jones for a month. You know her usual morning routine: she brushes her teeth, eats breakfast in her room, and then showers and dresses for the day. Once she is up and about, she likes her room straightened and her bed made before her daughter's daily visit. You know that everyday by 10 a.m. Mrs. Jones is out of her room.
>
> Today at 10:30 a.m. you walk into Mrs. Jones' room without knocking or speaking, pull the curtain open, and find Mrs. Jones in a private conversation with a clergy member. Everyone is embarrassed, and you have violated Mrs. Jones' right to privacy. You did three things wrong:
>
> 1. You assumed Mrs. Jones' routine would never change.
> 2. You did not knock on the door and wait for her permission to enter.
> 3. You did not announce yourself.
>
> Remember that residents are people, not machines—never take their actions for granted. If you had knocked on Mrs. Jones' door, called out your name, and said you were there to make the bed, Mrs. Jones would have been able to tell you that now was not a good time. She could ask you to come back later. In this way you respect Mrs. Jones' home and her right to privacy.

To show respect for residents' privacy, always follow these principles:
- Knock on the door (Fig. 14-7).
- Ask permission to enter. If the resident cannot respond, enter the room and introduce yourself.
- Ask how residents want their rooms.
- Never move items without a resident's permission.
- Encourage residents to help care for and arrange their room.
- Maintain residents' privacy with respect and clear communication in everything you do.

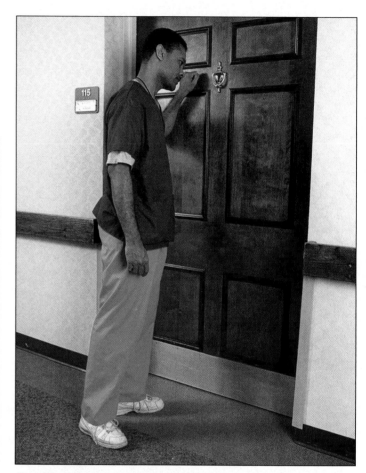

Fig. 14-7 – Always knock on the resident's door and wait for permission to enter.

BED MAKING

As a nurse assistant, you are responsible for caring for all items in a resident's room, especially the bed. Always remember to ask the resident's permission before caring for any item in their room. Some facilities have hand-crank beds, and others have electric ones. Crank beds take some effort to raise or lower the entire bed, or just the head or foot. Residents may ask for your help with crank beds. The cranks are at the bottom of the bed and are pulled out for use. Be careful always to return the crank after use so that no one bumps into it or trips over it. Electric beds have either foot pedals or controls on the side of the bed. Electric beds are easier for residents to use.

Making a neat, wrinkle-free bed is important for the resident's comfort and dignity. It also helps prevent skin irritation and breakdown. Most residents can get out of bed while you make it. This is called making an *unoccupied* bed. But some residents cannot get out of bed, and then you need to make an **occupied bed**. Follow these guidelines when making any bed:

- Always ask the resident's permission first.
- Make sure there are no wrinkles.
- Wear gloves if the linen is soiled.
- Raise the bed to a good working height.
- Make one side of the bed at a time to reduce the steps you have to take.
- Follow the facility's policy for putting soiled linen in proper laundry bags.
- Never put linens on the floor.
- Keep soiled linens away from your uniform.
- When making an occupied bed, always roll a resident toward you, which is safer than rolling the resident away from you.
- Follow the facility's policy about when to change linens. Often the routine is a complete change of linens once or twice a week or when soiled.

Procedure 14-1 (pages 258-259) outlines the steps for making an unoccupied bed. Procedure 14-2 (pages 260-261) outlines the steps for making an occupied bed.

FINISHING TOUCHES

The bed is only one part of a resident's environment. You also take care of the bedside table, over-bed table, other furniture, and the resident's belongings. Also think about finishing touches you can add to make a resident's room feel warm, friendly, and more comfortable. These include:

- Eliminate clutter, like disposable cups, tissues, old newspapers, and magazines. Ask the resident before you throw anything away.
- Adjust lighting as the resident likes it, such as drawing window shades in the evening and raising them in the morning.
- Adjust the room temperature and ventilation the way the resident likes it if possible.
- Help keep noise down.
- Help care for residents' plants and flowers if needed.
- Dust pictures and other mementos.
- Display cards.

These simple things can really make a difference in how residents feel about their home in the facility.

📖
Occupied bed – the resident is in the bed
Unoccupied bed – the bed is empty

CALL SYSTEM

You cannot be with every resident all the time. To make sure residents get help when they need it, facilities have call systems for all residents. The call system has these parts:

- A call button on a cord plugs into an outlet over or near each resident's bed. A resident pushes the button when they need help. The cord has a clip that can be attached to the pillow or sheet to keep the button from falling on the floor out of reach.
- A light outside the resident's door comes on when they push the call button (Fig. 14-8).

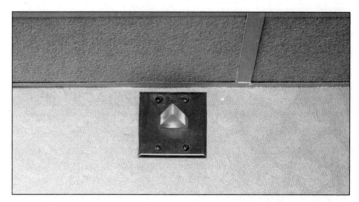

Fig. 14-8 – A light goes on outside the resident's room when they press the call button.

- On the call board at the nurses' station, the resident's room number lights up when a resident pushes the button (Fig. 14-9). (The board may also buzz or ring.)

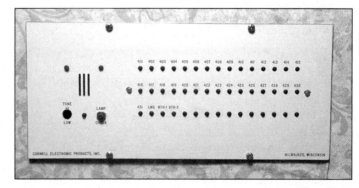

Fig. 14-9 – In some facilities the resident's room number lights up at the nurses' station.

(text continued on page 262)

PROCEDURE 14-1. MAKING AN UNOCCUPIED BED

▶ **REMEMBER: BE AWARE**

Items Needed

- two flat sheets or one fitted and one flat sheet
- draw sheet (if used)
  (an extra sheet that lies on top of the bottom sheet used to position residents)
- blanket and spread, if needed
- pillowcases

1. Look for any belongings in the bed. Residents may fall asleep with personal belongings under their pillow or elsewhere in the bed.

2. Lower the head of the bed and raise the whole bed to a comfortable position, usually about hip level.

3. Remove the spread and any blankets, and fold them on the chair.

4. Remove soiled linen, including the pillowcase. Loosen sheets from under the mattress and carefully roll them into a ball, keeping the soiled side inside the ball and away from your body. (This keeps the cleaner side close to you. Rolling linens prevents the spread of organisms from dirty linens.) Put the sheets in the laundry bag.

5. Check the mattress for any soiling or wetness. Wash and dry it with paper towels if necessary. Change the mattress pad if it is soiled or scheduled for change.

6. *If you are using a fitted sheet (shaped to the mattress by elastic edging), follow these steps:*
   Starting at the top corner of the mattress, wrap the edge of the mattress with the corner of the sheet, then go to the bottom of the bed on the same side and wrap that edge. Do not shake the linen while unfolding it. (Shaking the linen raises dust and organisms.) Go to the opposite corner at the top of the bed and wrap that edge, and then wrap the last edge over the last corner. The sheet should fit the mattress snugly.

7. *If you are using a draw sheet, follow these steps:* place it in the center of the bed so it covers the middle part of the bed. Tuck in the draw sheet on both sides. A draw sheet is often used for residents needing help with moving and positioning, or to keep bottom sheets clean and dry.

8. *If you are using a flat sheet follow these steps:*

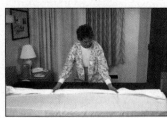

   a. Unfold the bottom sheet lengthwise down the bed's center. Do not shake the linen while unfolding it. (Shaking linen raises dust and organisms.)

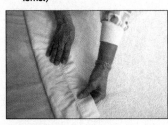

   b. Put the hem seams toward the mattress. This keeps rough edges from touching the person.

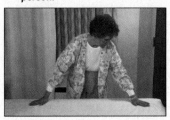

   c. Slide the sheet so that the hem is even with the foot of the mattress. Keep the fold in the exact center of the bed from head to foot. (You want the extra length of sheet at the top to tuck it under the mattress).

   d. Open the sheet from the fold so that the sheet covers the entire mattress and hangs evenly on both sides. Tuck the top hem in tightly under the mattress at the head of the bed by lifting the head of the mattress and sliding the sheet under the mattress. Make a mitered corner (also called a hospital corner):
   i. Face the side of the bed.

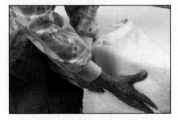

   ii. With one hand, pick up the top of the sheet hanging down the side of the bed, and lay it on top of the bed so that it looks like a triangle.
   iii. Tuck the remaining sheet under the mattress.

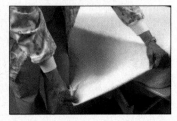

   iv. Drop the section of sheet from on top of the bed over the side of the bed, and tuck it in.

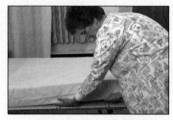

e. Tuck the remaining sheet under the mattress neatly, starting from the mitered corner down to the foot of the mattress.

f. If a draw sheet is used, open it up and place it in the center of the bed so it covers the middle part of the bed. Tuck in the draw sheet on the side where you are working. A draw sheet is often used for residents needing help with moving and positioning, or sometimes to keep bottom sheets clean and dry. You may also put any needed disposable incontinence pads over the draw sheet. Products used for incontinence are discussed in Chapter 18.

Continue with the top sheet:

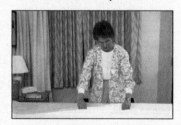

9. Place the top sheet on the bed. The wide hem should be even with the head of the mattress, with the seam on the outside. When you fold the hem over, the smooth side will be next to the resident's skin, preventing irritation from any rough edges. The excess sheet will be over the foot of the bed.

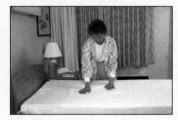

10. Open the sheet from the fold so that the sheet covers the entire mattress and hangs evenly on both sides.

11. Place the spread on top of the sheet in the same manner. Make sure the sheet does not hang below the spread on the sides.

12. Tuck in the sheet and spread at the foot, making a mitered corner on the bottom end (Step 8d above).

13. Smooth the sheet and spread from the bottom to the top of the bed, and fold down the top hem of the sheet over the spread.

14.a. Move to the other side of the bed and finish in the same way, starting with the bottom sheet, the draw sheet if used, and finishing with the top sheet and spread.

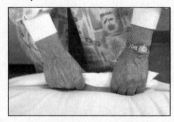

b. Pull the bottom sheet tight before each tuck to remove wrinkles. (Tuck in the draw sheet tightly if used.)

15. Place a clean pillow case on the pillow:

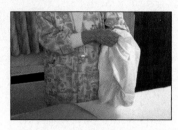

a. Hold the center of the closed end of the pillow case with your hand and turn it inside out over your hand;

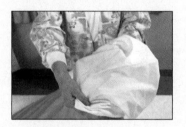

b. then grab the pillow with your hand inside the pillowcase and slide the case over the pillow. Make sure the corners of the pillow fit into the corners of the case.

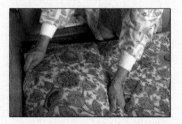

c. Place the pillow(s) at the head of the bed, and fold the spread over them.

16. Put the blanket at the foot of the bed or in the closet if a resident prefers.

17. Return the bed to low position.

▶ **REMEMBER: UNDERSTAND**

PROCEDURE 14-2. MAKING AN OCCUPIED BED

 REMEMBER: BE AWARE

Items Needed
- two full sheets or one fitted and one flat sheet
- draw sheet (if needed)
- blanket and spread, if needed
- pillowcases

1. Lower the head of the bed, and remove the pillow from under the resident's head. (Do this only if the resident is comfortable in a completely flat position.)

2. Remove the spread and any blankets, and place them folded on the chair.

3. Loosen the top and bottom sheets from under the mattress.

Note: *Side rails may be used for support in moving. If there is any risk that the resident could be injured by hitting the side rail, do not use it. Have another nurse assistant on the opposite side to support the resident if there is any risk of injury; make sure this person is ready to help before you begin.*

4. Help the resident roll over on their side toward you. Raise the side rail and ask them to hold onto it for support. Go to the other side of the bed. Be sure the resident stays covered throughout the procedure.

5. Check for any belongings in the bed.

6. Roll lengthwise (top to bottom) the bottom soiled sheet from the side of the mattress to the center of the bed close to the resident's body. (If the linen is wet or very damp, place a barrier like a plastic-covered padding over the sheet.) Change the mattress pad if it is soiled or scheduled for changing.

7. *If you are using a fitted sheet (shaped to the mattress by elastic edging), follow these steps:*
Starting at the top corner of the mattress, wrap the edge of the mattress with the corner of the sheet; then go to the bottom of the bed on the same side and wrap the edge. Be sure half the mattress is covered and the sheet is tucked close to the resident.

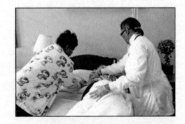

8. *If you are using a draw sheet follow these steps:* Place it in the center of the bed so it covers the middle part of the bed and is tucked close to the resident. Tuck in the draw sheet on the side you are working. A draw sheet is often used for residents needing help with moving and positioning, or sometimes to keep bottom sheets clean and dry. You may also put any needed disposable incontinence pads over the draw sheet.

9. *If you are using a flat sheet follow these steps:*
a. Unfold the bottom sheet lengthwise, centered on the bed. Do not shake the linen while unfolding. (Shaking the linen raises dust and organisms.) Be sure the hem seams face the mattress. (This prevents any rough edges from touching the resident.)

b. Slide the sheet so that the hem is even with the foot of the mattress. Be sure to keep the fold in the exact center of the bed from head to foot. (You want the extra length of sheet at the top so that you can tuck it under the mattress.)

c. Open the sheet and fan-fold it lengthwise so that one half of the sheet is next to the rolled dirty sheet.

d. Tuck the top hem in tightly under the mattress at the head of the bed by lifting the mattress edge and sliding the sheet under it. Make a mitered corner:

  i. Face the side of the bed.

  ii. With one hand, pick up the top of the sheet hanging down the side of the bed, and lay it on top of the bed so it looks like a triangle.

  iii. Tuck the remaining sheet under the mattress.

  iv. Drop the section of sheet that is lying on top of the bed over the side of the bed, and tuck it in.

e. Tuck the remaining sheet under the mattress neatly, starting with the mitered corner down to the foot of the mattress.

f. *If you are using a draw sheet,* place it in the center of the bed so it covers the middle part of the bed. Fan-fold the excess and tuck it in with the sheet. Tuck in the draw sheet. A draw sheet is often used for residents needing help with moving and positioning, or sometimes to keep bottom sheets clean and dry.

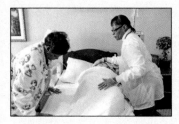
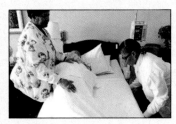
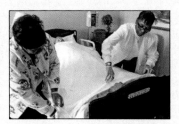
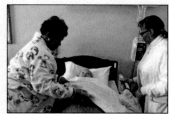

Continue with the next steps:

10. Flatten the rolled or fan-folded sheets and help the resident roll over the linen toward you, using the procedure for turning them (see Chapter 15, Learning to Position and Move Correctly). Don't forget first to tell the resident that the roll of linen is behind them.

Note: Side rails may be used for support in moving. If there is any risk that the resident could be injured by the use of the rail, do not use it. Put up the side rail and ask the resident to hold onto it for support.

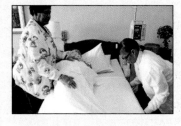

11. Go to the opposite side of the bed, lower the side rail, and remove the dirty bottom sheet.

Note: Never leave the resident unattended to take away dirty laundry. Put the dirty sheets in the laundry bag (if it is in the room) or at the bottom of the bed between the mattress and footboard.

12. Pull the clean linen toward you until it is completely unfolded, and tuck the sheets in tightly the same way as you did on the other side. Tuck in the draw sheet if used.

13. Help the resident roll back to the center of the bed.

14. Place the top sheet on the bed over the sheet covering the resident. Open the sheet from the fold so that the sheet hangs evenly on each side of the bed. The wide hem should be at the top with the seam on the outside. When you fold the hem over, the smooth side will be next to the resident's skin, preventing any rough edges from touching them. The excess sheet is over the foot of the bed.

15. Ask the resident to hold onto the clean sheet, then carefully remove the dirty top sheet by placing your hand under the clean top sheet and rolling the dirty sheet down toward the foot of the bed. Remove it and put it with the other dirty linen.

16. Place the spread on top of the sheet in the same way you did the top sheet. Make sure the sheet does not hang below the spread on the sides.

17. Tuck in the sheet and spread at the foot of the bed, and make a mitered corner at the bottom ends:
    a. Face the side of the bed.
    b. With one hand, pick up the top sheet hanging down the side of the bed, and lay it on top of the bed so it looks like a triangle.
    c. Tuck the remaining sheet under the mattress.
    d. Drop the sheet lying on top of the bed over the side of the bed, and tuck it in.

18. Smooth the sheet and spread from the bottom to the top of the bed, and fold down the top hem of the sheet over the top of the spread. Be sure the top linens are not so tight that they are pressing on the resident's feet. To be sure, make a toe pleat. This is done by pulling the top linen up to form a pleat.

19. Remove the dirty pillowcase, and put a clean case on the pillow. Hold the center of the closed end of the pillow case with your hand, turn it inside out over your hand, and then grab the pillow with the hand inside the pillow case and slide the case over the pillow. Make sure the corners of the pillow fit into the corners of the case. Put the pillow under the resident's head.

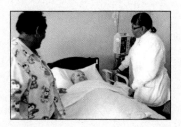

▶ **REMEMBER: UNDERSTAND**

(text continued from page 257)

Some facilities also have an intercom system from the station to residents' rooms.

Help residents learn how use the call system:
- Explain the purpose of the call system.
- Show how to use the call button. Then have a resident show that they can use the call button (Fig. 14-10).

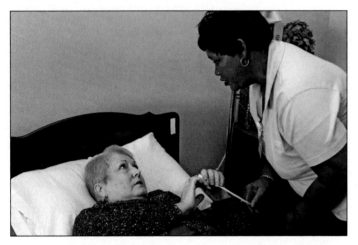

Fig. 14-10 – Make sure the resident knows how to use the call light button.

- Watch for call lights and answer quickly when you see one, even for residents you are not caring for that day. Turn off the call light when you enter the room so that another staff person does not also come to help.
- Make sure each resident's call button is always plugged in, working properly, and within reach when they are in bed or sitting near the bed.
- If a resident's call light is not working, report it to the charge nurse immediately. A bell can be used until the light is repaired.
- If a resident does not understand the call system or cannot pull the cord or push the button, work with the charge nurse to find another way for them to call for help.

Note: *Additional call buttons are located in residents' bathrooms and shower areas. Teach residents how to use these safety systems too.*

TRANSFER OF A RESIDENT

Residents may be **transferred** to a different unit or wing in a facility for different reasons. The resident, family, and physician decide this in consultation with other team members. Residents are often transferred because of a change in their needs or level of care. For example, a resident was admitted for rehabilitation after having a stroke. This resident was first admitted to a skilled area in the facility where licensed professionals such as physical therapists, speech therapists, and occupational therapists worked closely with them along with nursing staff to help them regain as many abilities as possible. After the resident regains skills, they have less need for such intense work. Then the resident is transferred to another wing or unit that meets their needs just as well.

Even though a person who is being transferred is already a resident in the facility, the transition can still be difficult. It can still cause anxiety, concerns, and questions. You can help minimize these effects on the resident with good communication and a caring attitude.

Interdisciplinary Approach for Transferring a Resident

Transferring a resident can be an involved procedure. Nursing has a role along with other departments in the facility. Everyone works together to transfer a resident:
- **Social Worker.** The social worker gets permission from a resident and family before a transfer or a room move can take place. The social worker also communicates with other departments and staff, such as the dietary department, front office, medical records, etc.
- **Housekeeping Department.** Housekeeping cleans the new room to prepare it for the resident. Sometimes housekeeping, along with nursing staff, helps pack the resident's belongings and moves them to the new room. Sometimes nurse assistants help, too.
- **Nurses.** The charge nurse helps staff in the new unit or wing get to know the resident. The nurse writes a note in the nursing record about the resident's mental and physical condition at the time. The nurse helps transfer the resident and takes all treatments and medications to the new wing or unit.

Transfer – process that occurs when a resident moves from one area to another

When you are transferring a resident to another unit, wing, or room, keep these things in mind:

- As with a discharge, a resident may have feelings of loss.
- A resident may be upset and concerned about the move. The resident may be comfortable with and attached to the former staff, other residents, and even the environment. The resident may not want to leave their roommate.
- A resident may be concerned that they will not like the new unit or wing as much as the former one.
- It can be very confusing to switch environments.

Transfer procedures are usually routine for staff, but we must remember they are very stressful for residents.

How You Can Prepare for the Transfer of a Resident

Just as nurses in the two units communicate about the resident being transferred, nurse assistants of the two units must communicate too. Share information about a resident's likes and dislikes. Pass on ideas and techniques that have proven helpful in caring for them. Try to think of any information that would make the transition to the new unit easier. Before the transfer, be sure the right person in the facility has the resident's and family's permission. Be sure that the new room is ready the same as for a new admission. Do all this before a resident is transferred. It often helps to call ahead and ask staff on the new unit to come meet the resident before the transfer.

Transferring Residents

The transfer should be handled professionally and warmly. If you are doing the transfer, reassure the resident. Help them get over any fears or concerns. If you are receiving the resident on the new unit, greet them warmly and genuinely. Use the name the resident wants used and introduce yourself. Introduce them to their new roommate and help both residents feel more comfortable (Fig. 14-11). Treat the resident like a new admission. Help them unpack and orient them to the new room:

- bathroom facilities
- nurses' call light
- television and radio
- dining areas and mealtimes
- visitors' or residents' lounge
- location of the nurses' station
- location of the telephone

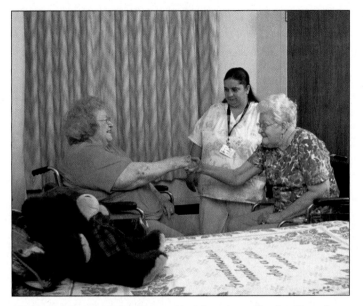

Fig. 14-11 – Be sure to handle a resident transfer professionally and warmly. Introduce the resident to the staff and their new roommate.

Orient a resident to these areas even if they cannot leave the room or bed, because they may be able to in the future. Make sure their personal belongings and medical records are transferred.

DISCHARGE OF A RESIDENT

Discharge is the process that occurs when a resident leaves the facility. Residents may feel many different emotions. Often the discharge is a joyful occasion, such as when a resident has improved enough to go home or to a less restrictive facility. But sometimes discharge is not a happy occasion. In all cases, do your best to help residents and family feel good about their decision by what you say and how you respond to them. The most common reasons for discharge are:

- Because a resident's condition has changed, a different setting is required.
- A resident has improved enough to go to a less restrictive setting.
- A resident or family dislikes the facility and desires a move.
- A resident is moving to a facility closer to the family and more convenient for them to visit.

Many team members are involved in discharge planning. For some residents, discharge planning begins the day of admission to the facility. This commonly happens for residents admitted for rehabilitation and subacute care.

Interdisciplinary Approach for Discharging a Resident

A resident's discharge involves other departments in the facility:

Social Worker The social worker arranges a discharge planning meeting to help decide what is best for the resident. For a resident going home, the social worker helps set up community services to meet their needs. If a resident is moving to another facility, the social worker networks with it for a smooth discharge and transition. The social worker tells other staff when the discharge will take place.

Housekeeping Department Housekeeping may help pack up the resident's belongings. They also help clean and prepare the room after the discharge.

Nurses The nurse works closely with the physician, resident, family, and social worker to ensure the discharge is correct. The nurse obtains the necessary discharge order from the physician. The nurse communicates with the resident and family regarding care instructions. If a resident is going to another facility, the nurse works closely with nursing staff there to ensure continuity of care. The nurse writes a discharge note, coordinates the discharge care plan, and sends the resident's medications and records.

Helping Residents Adjust During the Discharge

If a resident is going home to a less restrictive setting, be encouraging and let them know you are happy about it. If for any reason you have negative feelings about the discharge, don't let these feelings show or affect your attitude or your help. Be professional and warm. You may be the last impression a resident and family have of the facility.

Moving to a different place is a change for a resident, even when it's a positive move, and change can be frightening. A resident may be anxious and may demand more attention than usual. They may also feel sad because of leaving other residents and staff, or may feel angry about the change. To help a resident accept this change, you can:
- Accept that a resident may have feelings such as sadness, anger, or fear. Don't try to convince them that these feelings are not OK or will go away.

- Keep a positive attitude. Even if a resident is leaving because they do not like the facility, you can say, "Another facility may be better able to meet your needs."
- Encourage the person to say goodbye to residents and staff.
- Ask the social worker to tell the resident about the place where they are going, if it is unfamiliar to them. Include:
  − the name of the place
  − how big it is
  − where it is
  − what services are available
  − what it looks like

Day of Discharge

When it is time for a resident to leave, you should:
- Have a wheelchair available if needed.
- Ask the resident for permission to pack their personal belongings, unless they wish to do it themselves. Have a cart ready to transport belongings.
- Check the personal items inventory list, and account for each item.
- Check that the resident is appropriately dressed and groomed.
- Go with the person to the exit (Fig. 14-12).

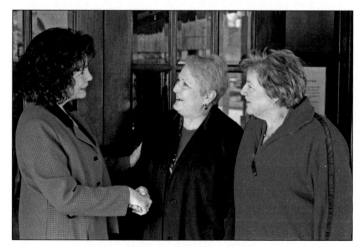

Fig. 14-12 − When the resident is discharged, the staff work together to make sure that the transition is a positive one.

- Say goodbye, and wish them well.

After a resident leaves, the room is prepared for the next resident. Usually housekeeping cleans and disinfects the room, but you may help with preparation of the room.

Take all the linen off the bed and place it in the laundry bag. Remove unnecessary articles, including disposable personal care items. Throw away any trash. Take any utensils kept at the bedside table, such as the wash basin and bedpan, to the service room.

Housekeeping removes the mattress, cleans the bedsprings, washes the bed frame and all furniture (Fig. 14-13),

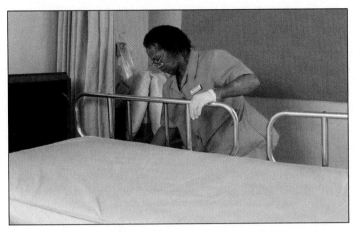

Fig. 14-13 – After a resident is discharged, housekeeping prepares the room for the next resident.

and replaces the mattress. After the room has been cleaned, you should make the bed with clean linen. Arrange the bedside table. Put everything in it for the next resident. You are now ready for the next resident to be admitted.

Note that this same cleaning is done regularly while a resident is in the facility. The charge nurse will show you how to move the resident out of the room so that it can be cleaned. As always, take care that a resident's belongings are not lost or broken. Treat them as if they were yours. Never throw away anything belonging to a resident without asking first.

IN THIS CHAPTER YOU LEARNED HOW TO:
- Help admit a resident
- Make a resident's room home-like in three ways
- Care for a resident's belongings
- Ensure the resident's privacy
- Make an unoccupied and an occupied bed
- Teach residents how to use the call system
- Help in the transferring and discharge of a resident

SUMMARY
Helping a resident adjust to a long term care facility is one of the most important things you can do as a nurse assistant. All staff must try to prevent relocation stress syndrome. Know what your facility does to help the resident adjust to their new home. Pay attention to the resident. Ask family members if they see changes in the resident's behavior, and report all changes to the charge nurse.

Knowing your role in the admission, transfer, and discharge of residents is also important. Knowing how the whole staff team works together will help you understand this complex process.

Creating a home-like environment helps the resident feel safe and comfortable. Always remember how important your home is to you so you can help the resident feel like their room space is their home.

PULLING IT ALL TOGETHER
This chapter involves learning your role when a resident is admitted to your facility and how to maintain a home-like environment for the resident.

Think about this:

You arrive to work and your assignment is to take care of six residents who have been in the facility between six weeks and one year. You also have two new residents being admitted today. One of the new residents is expected at 9 a.m. and the other at 2 p.m. Mrs. Smith, who is arriving at 9 a.m., will be the roommate of Mrs. Jones, a recently admitted resident. Mrs. Jones has been crying every day since she arrived at the facility. You have concerns about putting the new resident in the room with her. You decide to talk with the charge nurse about this. You suggest to the charge nurse that Mrs. Smith room with another resident who has lived in the facility for a year. The charge nurse asks you why you feel this will help. You explain that you think Mrs. Jones misses her home and husband. You think she needs to adjust before she gets a new roommate. You think the new resident will have a better transition if she lives with a resident who is comfortable with the environment.

The charge nurse is pleased with your suggestion and makes this change. She also calls Mrs. Jones' family to discuss her unhappiness and addresses the issue with the whole staff team. Together everyone works to help Mrs. Jones deal with the loss of her husband and her relocation stress. As the person who spends the most time with the resident, your valuable information and care make the difference in a resident's life.

CHECK WHAT YOU'VE LEARNED

1. **Mrs. Paulsen is being admitted to the unit today. You want her to feel okay about being here. How can you help her adjust?**
   A. Introduce her to staff and other residents.
   B. Insist on unpacking and putting away her belongings for her.
   C. Leave her by herself so she can get used to being alone in the facility.
   D. Suggest that the family not visit her right away.

2. **What could cause a new resident to develop relocation stress syndrome?**
   A. Making too many new friends.
   B. Enjoying new activities at the facility.
   C. Eating different foods.
   D. Not adjusting to a changed environment.

3. **What can you do to protect yourself from contamination from soiled linen when making an unoccupied or occupied bed?**
   A. Place a barrier between you and your uniform.
   B. Hold linen so it does not touch your uniform.
   C. Put the linen on the floor and let a co-worker pick it up.
   D. Hold the linen close to you so you do not strain your back.

4. **What is one of the most important tasks you should do before leaving a resident's room?**
   A. Take the resident's vital signs.
   B. Hand the call light to the resident or make sure it is within reach.
   C. Make sure there is a no smoking sign outside the resident's door.
   D. Explain the meal schedule to the resident.

5. **When caring for a resident's room, what is important for you to do?**
   A. Ask permission.
   B. Throw the old newspapers away.
   C. Rearrange the resident's family pictures.
   D. Remove the beautiful spread a family member made and place it in the closet where it will not get soiled.

6. **What is the best thing to do when making an occupied bed?**
   A. Make the bed alone.
   B. Put an extra draw sheet at the end of the bed.
   C. Ask for another nurse assistant to help you turn the resident over on their side to make one side at a time.
   D. Ask for another nurse assistant to help you transfer the resident out of bed so you can make the bed.

7. **Why is it important to make a neat, wrinkle-free bed?**
   A. Wrinkles give germs places to grow.
   B. It is more difficult to launder sheets that are wrinkled.
   C. Wrinkled sheets can cause skin irritation and breakdown.
   D. Old-fashioned charge nurses think neat beds look best.

8. **How should you prevent spreading dust and microorganisms as you make a bed?**
   A. Shake out the soiled sheets before disposing of them.
   B. Pile the soiled sheets on the floor by the bed for Housekeeping to pick up later.
   C. Store the soiled sheets in the clean utility room.
   D. Roll the soiled sheets into a ball with the soiled side inside, and put them in the laundry bag.

9. **What can you do to be sure the resident is comfortable and the bed linens do not restrict their feet?**
   A. Do not tuck the top linen in.
   B. Make a toe pleat.
   C. Make a mitered corner.
   D. Remove the top linen.

10. **Mrs. Dyson has just been admitted as a new resident. When explaining the facility's call system to her, you should say:**
    A. She should use the call light only in an emergency.
    B. She should use the call light frequently to make sure it's always working.
    C. At night the button will be clipped to the sheet or pillow so that it does not fall out of reach.
    D. She should not expect staff to keep coming to her room if she uses it too often.

(Answers to "Check What You've Learned" are in the Instructor's Manual.)

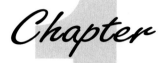

Chapter 15

LEARNING TO POSITION AND MOVE CORRECTLY

Helping a resident move and be comfortably positioned is one of the most important things you do as a nurse assistant. Remember that CMS Guidelines say that all long term care facilities must ensure that a resident's abilities for the activities of daily living do not diminish unless their health deteriorates. A primary activity of daily living is moving about freely. As a nurse assistant, you work with the charge nurse and physical therapist to meet resident's mobility needs (Fig. 15-1). Learning to move and position residents correctly makes sure both you and residents are comfortable and safe. According the U. S. Bureau of Labor Statistics, the leading cause of injury in long term care is incorrect body mechanics when moving and lifting. This causes overexertion of the back. These injuries often happen because of poor planning when moving or positioning a resident.

In this chapter you will learn why moving and positioning are so important. You will learn how to determine a resident's mobility in different situations and how to help them move safely and efficiently. You will also learn how to help residents into various body positions for their comfort and safety when they cannot change positions by themselves through the day.

OBJECTIVES

- State the importance of moving and positioning residents correctly
- List at least five questions to consider when preparing to move or position a resident
- Demonstrate how to move a resident:
  - up in bed
  - to the side of the bed
  - onto the resident's side or back for personal care
  - into a sitting position
  - from bed to chair, wheel chair, commode, or toilet
- Demonstrate how to help a resident move from bed to chair and back with the help of a coworker (with or without a mechanical lift), and how to move a resident up in a chair

- Demonstrate how to help a resident into the supine, Fowler's side-lying, and sitting positions
- Explain what to do if a resident falls

MEDICAL TERMS

- **Fowler's position** – lying on the back with the head of the bed raised 30 to 90 degrees, most commonly about 45 degrees
- **Postural hypotension** – Reduced blood flow (blood pressure) upon sitting or standing, causing dizziness
- **Supine** – lying on the back

"Some days I'm so stiff. But even then, your firm yet gentle guidance always helps me move more easily."

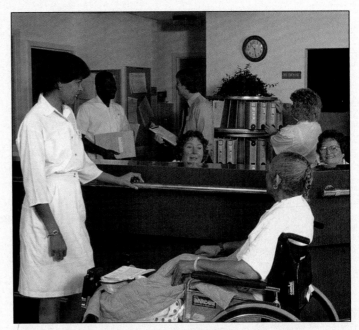

Fig. 15-1 – You will work with many staff members to determine a resident's mobility needs.

Did you ever fall asleep in one position, such as on your back with your arms at your sides and your legs straight, and wake up in a totally different position, such as on your stomach with your arms across the bed? Did you wonder how you got there?

Our bodies normally move often to stay comfortable. Sometimes we move on purpose, such as when we change positions to feel more comfortable sitting on a park bench. Sometimes we move without thinking about it, such as when we change position to keep the blood flowing freely to all parts and to prevent stiffness (Fig. 15-2, next page). Movement of our limbs and our whole body is very important. Although residents have different physical needs and abilities, moving is important for all residents. Each resident's need for support in moving can be different, but your goal is always to help them optimize their mobility. Some residents have difficulty helping with their own care because they have limited ability to move. Then you need to find ways for them to participate in their care and be as independent as possible.

📖

Independent – not subject to control by others, not dependent
Limb – arm or leg
Mobility – capable of moving or being moved

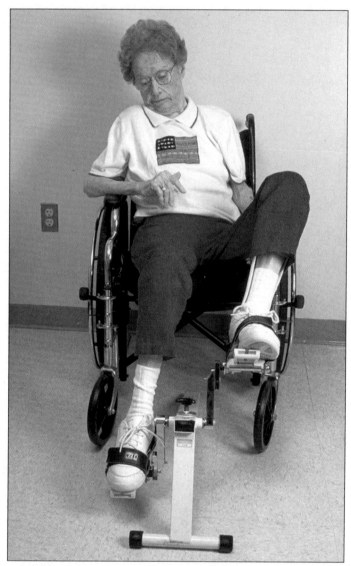

Fig. 15-2 – Movement keeps the blood flowing and prevents joints from becoming stiff.

decreased appetite or become constipated (digestive system). They may feel short of breath or dizzy when moving (circulatory and respiratory systems). Their skin may become red in places (integumentary system). Their movement may slow down (nervous system). Movement is essential for keeping all body systems functioning well.

Positioning is how you help residents sit, lie down, or change position when they cannot move independently. Even residents who can move by themselves may need help with positioning. They may have trouble getting comfortable or have skin problems from not changing positions often enough. The best positions for a resident depend on their (Fig. 15-3):

- body type
- medical needs
- equipment needs
- skin condition
- comfort

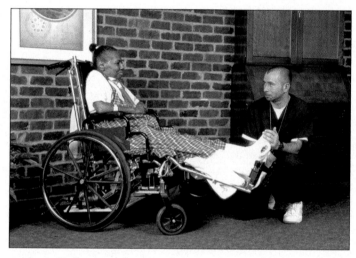

Fig. 15-3 – Even if a resident can move by themselves, you may have to help them with positioning.

HOW MOVEMENT AFFECTS BODY SYSTEMS

The human body is designed for continual movement. Each body system is constantly changing. When a person stops moving or has restricted movement, the body adapts and slows down to accommodate for this. Because body systems are interconnected, even a small change in movement can affect all body systems. Because aging also slows down many body functions, long term care residents are affected even more by movement restrictions.

Someone who has been in bed for even a short time may feel stiff or weak (muscular system). They may have a

📖

Adapt – change to fit new conditions
Positioning – an act of placing or arranging

WHY MOVING AND POSITIONING ARE IMPORTANT

Certain body areas are more likely to be damaged by pressure. This can cause a pressure ulcer. Usually pressure ulcers can be prevented by proper moving and position changes. Other benefits of moving and positioning include:

- helps reduce swelling in an arm or leg
- prevents stiffness in a limb
- helps keep tubes or equipment lines from being pulled
- helps residents be as comfortable as possible
- helps prevent pain and discomfort resulting from stiffness, pressure, and poor circulation

Moving and positioning our bodies is also emotionally important. Without freedom of mobility, a resident has trouble meeting basic needs. Often a resident's self-esteem depends on at least some independence in mobility.

As with all other care, you must observe residents and work with the charge nurse and physical therapist to choose the best way to move or reposition them. For example, when positioning a resident, consider these factors:

- spinal deformities (such as rounded back, forward head, leaning to one side)
- areas of skin redness
- bandaged areas, casts, or splints
- arms, legs, hands, or feet in a stiff position or swollen
- intravenous tubes or other medical lines
- oxygen being given
- recent surgery

PREPARING TO MOVE OR POSITION A RESIDENT

Before you help move or position a resident, observe the resident's abilities and ask the charge nurse and your coworkers about their needs. Be sure you know what the physician and charge nurse expect. Ask yourself these key questions about yourself, the resident, and the environment:

1. **Think about your own capabilities and limitations:**
   - Can you do what's needed?
   - Do you need help?
   - Do you understand the physician's orders and the charge nurse's expectations?

2. **Think about the resident:**
   - How much help does this resident need to move?
   - How large or heavy is this resident?

- Does this resident have any special needs or behaviors to consider before you start the move?
- Does this resident have any physical condition that affects moving, such as fragile skin or bones?
- How much weight is the resident allowed to place on the limb?
- How much limb motion is allowed?
- Does this resident use an assistive device such as walker, cane, or brace?
- Can this resident understand what you are asking them to do?
- Can this resident see and hear you? Do they need glasses or a hearing aid to see or hear better?
- What equipment do you need to most easily move this resident?
- Where are this resident's shoes and socks?
- What tubes or equipment is connected to this resident, such as an IV tube or oxygen line?
- Does this resident have any dressings or open wounds?
- Can this resident tolerate all positions?

3. **Think about the environment:**
   - Could the lighting, noise level, or distractions such as family members, or ongoing nursing care of another resident affect moving and positioning?
   - Are any obstacles, such as medical equipment, appliances, extra linens, personal possessions, or furniture in the way?
   - Is the bed at the proper height?
   - Is everything needed close at hand?
   - Can you move around any tubes or equipment near the resident?
   - What chair or seating device does the resident use?

Know the answers to these questions before you move or position a resident.

Review Tables 12-1 and 12-2 in Chapter 12, Common Preparation and Completion Steps, before you learn each of the skills in this chapter. These tables are also the last pages of this book.

Fragile – easily broken or destroyed, delicate

Considering Ergonomic Principles

Remember in Chapter 10, Personal Protection and Injury Prevention, you learned that you should use equipment to support you when moving or positioning a resident. This equipment helps reduce the risk of injury to both you and your resident. Review Table 10-1 before you learn each of the skills in this chapter. The description will help you know what equipment to use with which skill.

When To Get Help

Before you move or position a resident, decide whether you need help. If you are not sure, then always get help. You may need help for many reasons. Always be safe and get help if:
- you are not sure how a resident will respond to your help
- you do not know the resident well
- you are uncomfortable lifting the resident by yourself

COMMUNICATING WITH RESIDENTS

Communicating with residents and your coworkers is important. Serious injury can occur if someone does not understand how the move is to be done. Giving clear directions is important. Everyone must know what to do and when to start to do it. Be sure to talk clearly with a resident about their role. Ask them to do things "on the count of three," such as to push off the bed to help you raise them to a standing position. For example, ask them to grasp the side rail while you are turning them toward you, or to lift their head up as you start to move them. Remember that the resident should be an active participant in the move. Never do for residents what they can do for themselves.

Note: *You can use the side rail of the bed during moving and positioning as long as it benefits the resident. But side rails that restrict a resident's mobility are considered restraints and cannot be used without a physician's order except temporarily in moving and positioning.*

MOVING

Any move will be successful if you first think about the resident and situation. Remember the questions listed earlier when preparing to move a resident. Apply what you learned in Chapter 10 about using good body mechanics and the right equipment to prevent injury to residents and yourself. Box 15-1 highlights the principles of body mechanics. Follow these principles when lifting and moving the resident. Consider each situation individually, and adapt your approach to meet each resident's needs. Work closely with the charge nurse and the physical therapist to meet each resident's own needs.

BOX 15-1.
PRINCIPLES OF BODY MECHANICS

- Get help if needed.
- Keep one foot slightly in front of the other.
- Always maintain a broad base of support by keeping your feet 10-12 inches apart.
- Always bend your knees and keep your back neutral.
- Use counting as a communication tool for other helpers and the resident. The nurse assistant with the heaviest part of the resident's body does the counting.
- Hold the resident close to your body when transferring.
- When transferring, turn your whole body as a unit. Do not lift and twist.

Note: *Never move a resident by pulling on their arm or the skin under their arm. There are many arteries, nerves, and veins under the armpit. Pulling can damage blood vessels or nerves. Many older residents also have osteoporosis or fragile joints or bones that can be easily dislocated or broken.*

If a resident is **supine** and needs help moving up, down, or to the side of the bed for personal care or repositioning, use the positioning procedures described here. Remember to first position the bed for the move. For example, put the bed in a flat position to move the resident up in bed, and raise the head of the bed when helping a resident out of bed.

(text continued on p. 277)

Supine – lying on the back

PROCEDURE 15-1.
MOVING UP IN BED WHEN A RESIDENT CAN HELP

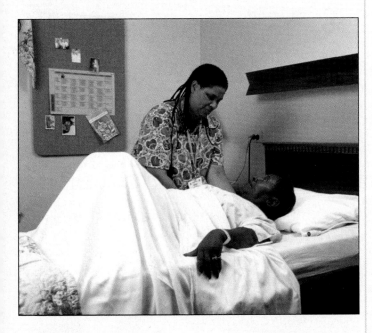

1. Put the head of the bed flat if the resident can tolerate it. Move the pillows against the headboard.

    Note: *Placing a pillow against the headboard will prevent the resident from injuring their head when moving up in bed.*

2. Help the resident bend their knees up and place their feet flat on the bed. Place one arm under the resident's upper back behind the shoulders and the other under their upper thighs.

3. On the count of 3, have the resident push down with their feet and lift up their buttocks (bridging) while you help move them toward the head of the bed.

    Note: *You may also try having the resident help by using the side rails. Remember to put the side rails down when done.*

PROCEDURE 15-2.
MOVING UP IN BED WHEN A RESIDENT IS UNABLE TO HELP (TWO NURSE ASSISTANTS)

1. Call another staff person to assist you.

2. Put the head of the bed flat if the resident can tolerate it. Remove the pillow and place it against the headboard.

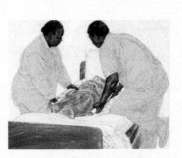

3. Help the resident to cross their hands over their chest.

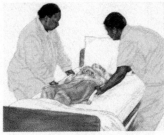

4. Roll the draw sheet up from the side toward the resident until you and your helper both have a tight grip on it with both hands. Keep your palms up if that gives you more strength for moving.

    Note: *You can put one knee on the bed to get as close to the resident as possible.*

5. Count aloud to 3, and you and your helper lift the resident up to the head of the bed, using good body mechanics. You can do this in stages until the resident is in position.

    Note: *If the resident is able, ask them to lift their head off the bed during the move.*

6. Unroll the draw sheet and tuck it in.

PROCEDURE 15-3.   MOVING TO THE SIDE OF THE BED WHEN A RESIDENT CAN HELP

▶ **REMEMBER: BE AWARE**

1. Stand on the side to which you plan to move the resident.

2. Help the resident bend their knees up and place their feet on the bed.

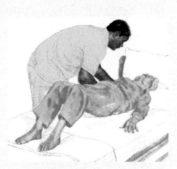

3. Help the resident to bridge (lift up their buttocks), and move their buttocks to the side of the bed.

4. Help the resident move their legs over, and then their head and upper body, by sliding your arms under them and gliding them toward you if they need help.

5. You can do this in stages to reach the desired position.

▶ **REMEMBER: UNDERSTAND**

PROCEDURE 15-4.   MOVING TO THE SIDE OF THE BED WHEN A RESIDENT IS UNABLE TO HELP
(Do this only if you are sure you will not damage a resident's skin.)

▶ **REMEMBER: BE AWARE**

1. Stand on the side to which you plan to move the resident.

2. Ask the resident to fold their arms across their chest or do this for them if needed.

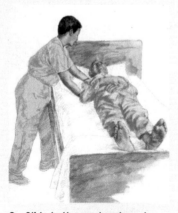
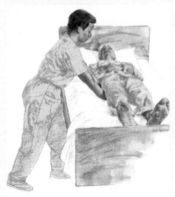
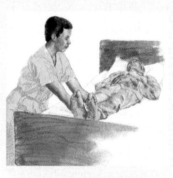

3. Slide both your hands under the resident's head, neck, and shoulders and glide them toward you on your arms.

4. Slide your arms under the residents' hips and glide them toward you.

5. Slide your arms under their legs and glide them toward you.

Note: *Keep the resident in proper body alignment.*

▶ **REMEMBER: UNDERSTAND**

PROCEDURE 15-5. MOVING A RESIDENT TO THE SIDE OF THE BED USING A DRAW SHEET

> **REMEMBER: BE AWARE**

1. Call another staff person to help you.

2. Help the resident place their arms across their chest.

3. Both you and your helper roll up the draw sheet from the sides toward the resident until you both have a good tight grip with both hands. (If the linen is soiled, use a barrier to prevent contaminating your uniform.)

Note: *The staff person who is moving the resident away may want to put one knee on the edge of the bed to prevent injury caused by reaching too far. This person also leads the count because they have the heaviest part of the move.*

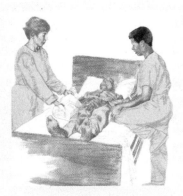

4. Count aloud to 3, and on 3 you both lift the resident to the side of the bed. You can do this in stages until the desired position is reached.

5. Unroll the draw sheet and tuck it in.

> **REMEMBER: UNDERSTAND**

PROCEDURE 15-6. TURNING A RESIDENT FROM SUPINE TO SIDE-LYING FOR PERSONAL CARE

> **REMEMBER: BE AWARE**

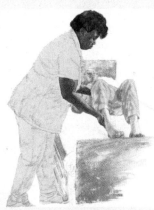

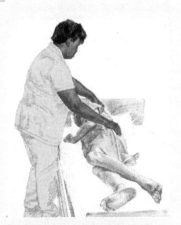

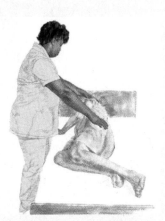

Note: *Some residents may be more comfortable guiding the turn by holding onto the side rails.*

1. Help the resident bend their knees up one at a time and place their feet flat on the bed.

2. Place one hand on the resident's shoulder farther away from you and the other hand on the hip farther from you.

3. On the count of 3, help the resident roll toward you. Continue personal care.

> **REMEMBER: UNDERSTAND**

PROCEDURE 15-7.   MOVING THE RESIDENT FROM SUPINE POSITION TO SITTING

▶ **REMEMBER: BE AWARE**

IN THIS PROCEDURE, THE RESIDENT BEGINS ON THEIR BACK.

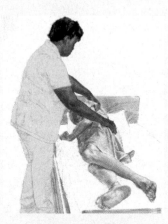

1. Help the resident roll onto their side facing you, or elevate the head of the bed.

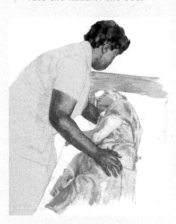

2. Reach under the resident's head and put your hand under their shoulder (using your arm closer to the head of the bed). The resident's head should be supported by and resting on your forearm.

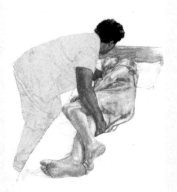

3. With your other hand, reach over and behind the resident's knee farther from you.

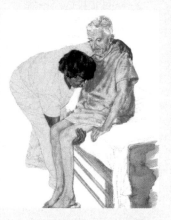

4. Using your legs and arms to do the lifting, bring the resident's head and trunk up as you swing their legs down to the sitting position. Hold the resident's legs, letting their knees rest in the crook of your elbow.

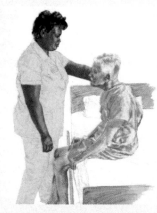

Note: *Your arm behind the resident's head and body must stay in contact with the resident once they are sitting up to prevent them from falling backward. Remember to stay directly in front of the resident so you can block them with your body if needed for safety.*

Note: *If you need a second staff person to help you assist the resident to sit up, both of you stand on the same side. One of you lifts the resident's head and body, while the other lifts their legs.*

5. Help the resident get comfortable in the sitting position.

ANOTHER OPTION IS TO:

1. Help the resident roll onto their side facing you, or elevate the head of the bed.

2. Slide their feet over the edge of the bed.

3. Reach under the resident's head and put your hand under their shoulder (using your arm closer to the head of the bed). The resident's head should be supported by and resting on your forearm.

4. Place your other hand on the resident's hip. As you help the resident sit up, place gentle but firm pressure on their hip (using leverage) and help raise the resident's head to a sitting position.

Note: *Your arm behind the resident's head and body must stay in contact with the resident once they are sitting up to prevent them from falling backward. Remember to stay directly in front of the resident so you can block them with your body if needed for safety.*

▶ **REMEMBER: UNDERSTAND**

PROCEDURE 15-8.   MOVING THE RESIDENT FROM SITTING TO SUPINE POSITION

> **REMEMBER: BE AWARE**

Note: *Before moving a resident from sitting to the supine position, be sure they are centered in the bed with the backs of their knees against the mattress. Help them push down on the floor with their feet and down on the bed with their hands to move their body back onto the bed in a sitting position.*

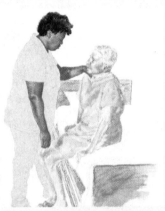

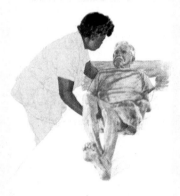

Note: *You might want to elevate the head of the bed before helping the resident into the supine position. Once they are in bed, you can lower the head of the bed.*

1. Place one hand behind the resident's shoulder, and let their head and neck rest on your forearm. Place your other hand under their knees, and let their legs rest in the crook of your elbow. Position your arms as if you were carrying someone in front of you.

2. Use your legs to lift and breathe out as you help the resident lift their legs up onto the bed. Gently lower their trunk and head onto the bed.

> **REMEMBER: UNDERSTAND**

(text continued from p. 272)

POSITIONING

When residents cannot change positions by themselves, you need to do this for them. Make a positioning schedule that ensures the resident is comfortable and has good blood flow to all body parts. Usually you change their position every two hours. As you read about different positions, think about a 24-hour period and how you would reposition a resident every two hours. Some positions are better for some residents. Some could cause problems for some residents. For example, a resident who is short of breath may have problems breathing when supine (on their back with the head of the bed flat). Discuss all positions with the charge nurse to make sure they are allowed for the resident. As always, pay attention to your body mechanics when moving residents. Always use available positioning devices to help avoid injuries to either you or the resident. Remove any wrinkles from the resident's clothing before positioning them because wrinkles can cause pressure ulcers.

Fowler's Position

Some residents have breathing problems caused by obesity, pulmonary disease, heart disease, or other causes. For these residents, the physician or charge nurse may order the Fowler's position. In the Fowler's position, the person lies on their back, and the head of the bed is raised 30 to 90 degrees. The most common angle is about 45 degrees. Other terms for Fowler's position include semi-Fowler's and high-Fowler's. When you elevate the head of the bed, this raises the resident's head, neck, and body (Fig. 15-4, page 279). You can place the resident in Fowler's position by elevating the head of the bed or by placing pillows under their back, head, and neck. If possible, keep the resident's head and neck only slightly higher than their chest.

Also use this position when you want to feed a resident or help them with personal care procedures. It is also used when the resident wants to sit in bed to read, watch television, or visit with relatives.

Side-Lying Position

The side-lying position may be used when a resident must be turned at least every two hours. Which side you position a resident on depends on the resident's comfort, their ability to hold the position, and any areas of skin breakdown.

Procedures 15-1 to 15-10 describe the steps for helping residents move from one position to another. (Procedures 15-1 to 15-8, pp. 273-277; 15-9, p. 280; 15-10, 281)

Using a Guard Belt (Also Called a Gait Belt)

A guard belt placed around the resident's waist helps you move them safely and prevents injury. The belt prevents residents from straining or injuring their arms or legs. Residents feel more secure moving when a guard belt is used. Be sure you explain the use of the guard belt to the resident before you put it on.

Note: *Do not use a guard belt with residents who have a broken rib, abdominal wound, an abdominal tube such as a G-tube, or an abdominal opening such as a colostomy.*

Putting a Guard Belt on a Resident

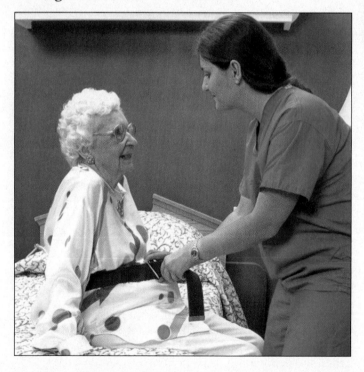

1. Hold the belt with the label on the outside (most manufacturers label the outside).

MOVING A RESIDENT FROM ONE PLACE TO ANOTHER (TRANSFER)

When transferring a resident, safety is a key factor. You must make sure that both you and the resident do the transfer safely. Many facilities require using a guard belt

Transfer – moving a resident from one surface to another, such as from bed to chair, chair to toilet, bed to commode, and so on.

2. Place the belt around the resident's waist over their clothes while they are either lying or sitting.

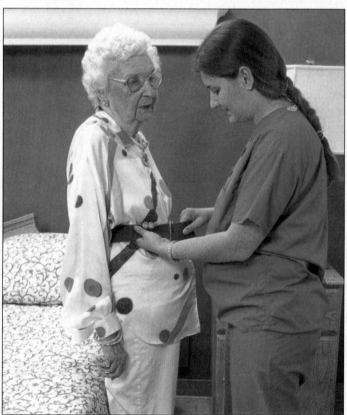

3. With the belt around the resident's waist, put the end through the buckle (or attach the Velcro or connect the plastic latch), and tighten the belt firmly. Do not make it so tight that you cannot get your fingers under it to hold it when transferring the resident. Be sure to tighten it again after they stand.

4. Now you are ready to continue with any of the transferring procedures.

(also called a safety, gait, or transfer belt) and other equipment made for transferring a resident.

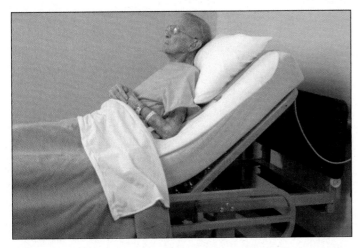

Fig. 15-4 – Fowler's position is often used for residents who are short of breath.

Considerations for Transfers

Before transferring a resident, get ready:
- A resident's wheelchair should be locked and set sideways to the bed with the arm of the chair next to the bed. The chair should be on the resident's stronger side. For example, if the resident had a stroke that weakened their left side, put the chair on their right side. If they had a hip fracture on the right side, put the chair next to their left side.
- A resident's walker or cane should be next to or in front of them.
- A resident's brace or other special equipment should be correctly in place.
- The bed usually should be at its lowest position, or raised if needed for a tall resident.
- When transferring a resident out of bed, be sure to let them dangle their legs for a few minutes while sitting on the edge of the bed before standing. This helps prevent dizziness due to a sudden change in posture. If the resident complains of dizziness, help them to lie down and call the charge nurse. Do not leave a resident unattended unless they are secure.

When starting to transfer a resident from bed to chair, watch for any problems that may occur. Here are some things that could happen:
- You lose your grip on the resident.
- The resident's legs cannot support them.
- The resident gets dizzy. Sometimes a position change causes dizziness because blood pools in the extremities, and for a moment less reaches the brain. If you wait a few minutes, the dizziness should go away. This is called postural hypotension.

These problems may also occur:
- If you are helping a resident stand, and you feel you do not have a good grip or enough leg support, help them sit down again and change your position for more support.
- If a resident's legs start to collapse or extend past your legs, put your legs in front of theirs and help them sit again. You may need to get help.
- If a resident becomes weak and unsteady, or starts to pass out, help them sit. Then lower them to the supine position if needed, and call the charge nurse. (See the later section on stopping a resident's fall.)

If any of these problems occurs, use a different technique or get help.

There are several types of transfers:
- stand pivot transfer
- transfer with an assistive device
- sliding board and seated transfers (less common)
- mechanical lift transfers
- dependent lift using two or more staff

The stand pivot transfer and assisted transfer with an assistive device are the methods most commonly used. Moving someone out of bed and into a chair or wheelchair uses the same method as transferring them onto a bedside commode. A chair is used in these procedures.

Note: *Before you can transfer a resident from bed to a chair, the resident first needs to sit up on the side of the bed. The resident first rolls onto their side and then sits up. Procedures 15–11 to 15–13 (pages 282, 285, 286) describe the steps for transferring residents in different situation (text* *continued on p. 283)*

Postural hypotension – Reduced blood flow (blood pressure) upon sitting or standing, causing dizziness

PROCEDURE 15-9.   POSITIONING A RESIDENT ON THEIR BACK

Residents generally lie on their back when sleeping or resting in bed. Usually their arms and legs are out straight.

 REMEMBER: BE AWARE

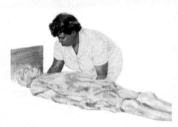

1. First move the resident's trunk and lower body so that their spine is in a neutral position. Do the positioning from the top of the body to the bottom.

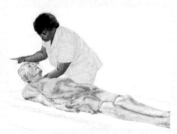

2. Position the resident's head and neck. Place a pillow under the resident's head and neck extending to the top of their shoulders. Do not elevate their head too high. Keep it as close to even with the chest as possible or as is comfortable.

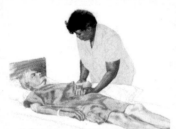

3. Position the resident's arms. The backs of the shoulders and elbows are common places for pressure ulcers in residents who cannot change positions by themselves. Vary their arm positions to prevent this. Keep their arms straight and resting on the mattress away from their sides, or bend their arms slightly at the elbow with a pillow between the inner arm and their side so that their arm rests on the pillow and their hand on top of the abdomen. Always support the arms in two places when moving them, and move them gently.

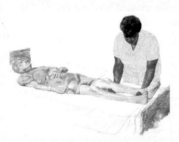

4. Position the resident's legs. The sides of the hips, the buttocks, the sacrum and coccyx (the tip of the spine at the buttocks, or "tailbone"), and the backs of the heels are common places for pressure ulcers. Position the resident's legs straight and slightly apart. Always support the legs in two places when moving them, and move them gently. For those residents who tend to keep their legs tightly together or crossed, you may place a pillow between the resident's legs.

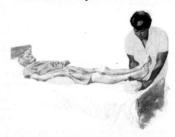

Note: *If a resident has ulcers on the sides of the hips, place a towel roll along the hip between the hip and the mattress on the affected side. If a resident has redness or ulcers under their heels, support their legs with a pillow lengthwise to raise their heels from the bed, or put a towel roll under their legs just above the heels.*

Note: *Support casts, splints, or swollen arms or legs by placing them on a pillow lengthwise to support the hand or foot higher than the rest of their arm or leg.*

 REMEMBER: UNDERSTAND

PROCEDURE 15-10.   POSITIONING A RESIDENT ON THEIR SIDE (SIDE-LYING POSITION)

1. Stand on the side to which the resident will be turning.

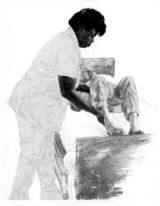

2. Help the resident to bend their knees up.

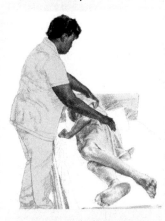

3. Place one hand on the resident's shoulder farther from you and the other on the hip farther from you. On the count of 3, help the resident roll toward you. Position the resident comfortably with proper body alignment.

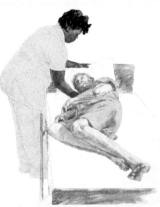

4. Position the resident's head and neck. Place the pillow under their head so that their top ear is almost level with their top shoulder.

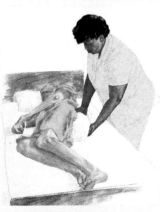

5. Fold a pillow lengthwise and place it behind the resident's back. Gently push the top edge of the pillow under their side and hip.

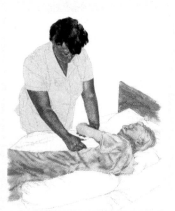

6. Position the resident's arms. Gently pull the bottom arm out from under the resident's body if it is not already in front of the body. Place a pillow diagonally under the top arm between the arm and the resident's side. Bend the top arm or the elbow and shoulder to rest the arm on the pillow.

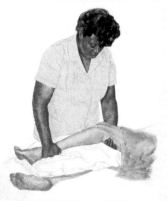

7. Position the resident's legs. Bend the top hip up and rotate it slightly forward. Place a pillow lengthwise between the resident's knees to separate their legs down to their ankles.

Note: *Depending on the resident's condition, you can modify any of these positions to prevent pressure ulcers and make the resident comfortable.*

PROCEDURE 15-11.   THE STAND PIVOT TRANSFER

1. Stand in front of the resident. Make sure the wheels of the wheelchair are locked.

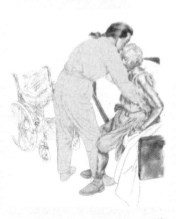

2. Place one of your legs between the resident's legs and the other close to the target you are moving toward, such as a chair. (This gives you better control over the speed and the direction of the movement.)

3. Hold onto the guard belt at the resident's back, slightly to either side. If you are not using a guard belt, put your arms around the resident's waist.

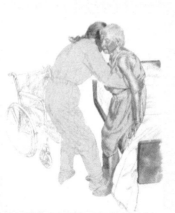

4. Ask or help the resident to push down on the bed with their hands, lean forward, and stand up. If they are not able to do this, you can have them hold your waist during the transfer. Do not let the resident hold you around your neck, which could injure you.

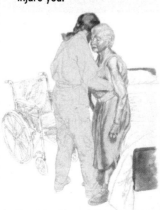

5. On the count of 3 help the resident stand by leaning your body back and up, thereby bringing the resident's body forward. Ask them to lean forward and stand up.

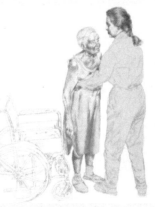

6. Once the resident is standing, keep your back neutral and body facing forward, and pivot (turn on your feet or take small steps) to turn them until the backs of their knees are against the chair.

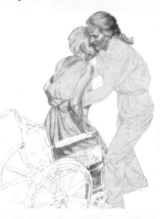

7. Ask the resident to reach back for the arm of the chair with one or both hands if possible.

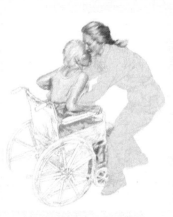

8. Help the resident bend their knees and sit.

9. Once the resident is sitting, ask or help them to push back in the chair by pushing down with their feet on the floor and their arms on the armrests.

(text continued from p. 279)

Two-Person Assistive Device Transfer

If the resident cannot help with a transfer, a second staff person may be needed to help you. Decide first how this person can best help you. You may have the second person on the other side of the resident holding onto the guard belt and walker. Or this person may just hold the chair in place during the transfer and be there in case the resident gets dizzy or some other problem occurs (Fig. 15-5).

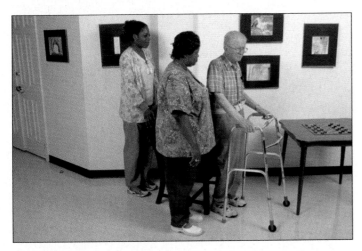

Fig. 15-5 — If the resident is unsteady, be sure you have another nurse assistant available to help.

Mechanical Lift Transfer

If a resident cannot help with any of the transfers described above, they need to be lifted from the bed to the chair, and back to the bed. You can do this with two or more staff or a mechanical lift.

There are various types of mechanical lifts. Some require more work than others. The type of lift you use depends on the devices the facility has and the resident's ability. Used properly, all lifts keep residents safe during a transfer and reduce the stress on your own body when you move a dependent resident.

Most lifts have a base and frame on wheels that can be locked and unlocked, a sling in different sizes that you place under the resident, and an arm that attaches the sling to the lift. You control the lift with a crank, button, or lever pump control. At least two people are needed to transfer a resident with a mechanical lift. You need to know how the mechanical lift in your facility works. Always

follow the manufacturer's instructions. Never use any piece of equipment you are not familiar with. Procedure 15-14 (p. 287-288) describes the steps for moving a resident with a mechanical lift. Procedure 15-15 (p. 288) describes the steps for moving a resident up in a chair after transferring them to it, and Procedure 15-16 (p. 289) describes the steps for returning a resident to bed using a mechanical lift.

Positioning a Resident in a Chair

Anytime you position a resident in a chair, follow these guidelines:

• Observe the resident's sitting posture throughout the day (Fig. 15-6). You can prevent skin problems and pressure ulcers by padding any areas the resident leans on with sheets or pillows. These may include the elbows, calves, heels, one side of their body, the backs of their thighs, or buttocks. If a resident in a wheelchair has skin problems, such as redness or pressure ulcers on the buttocks, ask the physical therapist to assess this resident for a wheelchair cushion if one is not already being used.

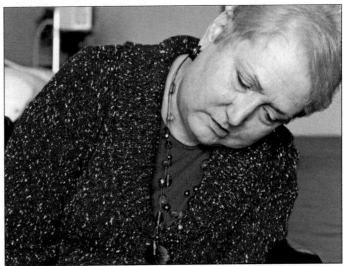

Fig. 15-6 — Report to the charge nurse if the resident has any problems with posture when sitting in their chair.

• A resident's legs and feet must always be supported. In a wheelchair, put their feet on the footrests. Position the calf pads of the leg rests down behind their calves. Their knees should be at the same height as their hips. Ask the maintenance department, charge nurse, or physical therapist to adjust the leg rests to the proper height if needed.

Consider these things when positioning a resident in a chair:

- If a resident is in a regular chair and their feet do not reach the floor, put a stool or pillow under their feet to support them. Dangling feet are uncomfortable and can cause leg swelling.
- Support the resident's arms and back with the chair's armrests and chair back. If a resident has a leg cast or a swollen leg, it should be elevated. Elevate the leg rest of the wheelchair or recline the resident in a recliner chair, or prop their leg up on a stool or chair.
- If a resident has a swollen hand, place a pillow on their lap and the armrest under their forearm and hand to support the hand higher than the elbow.
- If a resident has had a hip fracture and tends to bring their knees together or cross their legs, put one or two pillows between their knees. If this does not work, discuss the situation with the charge nurse or physical therapist. This resident may need a special pillow to hold their knees apart.
- If a resident with a rounded back is sitting in a recliner, support their head with pillows so their ears are directly above their shoulders. Sitting with the head and neck extended is very uncomfortable and may dangerously obstruct the blood supply to the brain.

STOPPING A FALL

If you are transferring or walking a resident and they start to fall, what do you do? This can be a frightening experience for both of you. Always be prepared for a possible fall. If the resident starts to fall, use these steps to help them:

1. First, pull up on the guard belt and ask the resident to try to stand up (Fig. 15-7).
2. If you cannot stop a resident from continuing to fall, move behind them, hold onto the guard belt with both hands or gently hold them around the chest, and support them against your knee. Use good body mechanics. Call for help.

If you cannot hold a falling resident up until help arrives:

1. Gently lower the resident to the floor as best you can and as slowly as possible to prevent injury to both of you.
2. Once the person is in a safe, stable position such as sitting or lying on the floor, call again for help. Do not leave the resident, because they are likely to be frightened and feel helpless. Always ask if they are OK and reassure them that help is on the way.

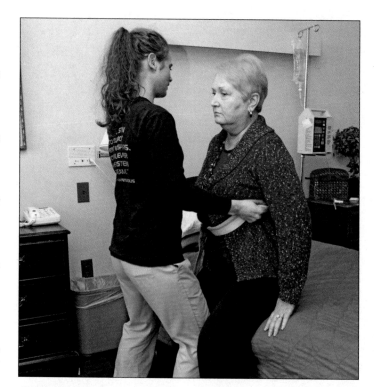

Fig. 15-7 – Hold the resident by the gait belt to prevent falls.

3. If you must leave a resident to get help, first ask if they are OK and help them lie down with their head supported. Explain you are going to get help and will be right back. Try to keep an eye on them as you seek help. In a busy area, be sure the person is not in anyone's path, or ask someone else to get help so you can stay with the resident.

If a Resident Falls and Seems Injured

If a resident seems to be hurt, or if you are unsure if they are OK, do not move them. Leave the resident on the floor until a nurse or physician examines them. Call for help. Do not leave the person alone unless absolutely necessary, such as if you feel their condition is serious and no one is answering your call for help.

When help arrives and it is OK to move the resident, help them back to a sitting position on the floor. If the person can walk fairly well, you and another staff person can help them stand with one of you on each side pulling up on both sides of the guard belt.

If a resident needs to be moved onto a stretcher or back into a chair, use a mechanical lift or other devices the facility has for this purpose. *(text continued on p. 290)*

PROCEDURE 15-12. ASSISTED TRANSFER WITH AN ASSISTIVE DEVICE (ONE PERSON)

REMEMBER: BE AWARE

1. Once the resident is sitting on the side of the bed without difficulty, place the assistive device in their hand (cane) or in front of them (walker).

2. Stand to the side of the resident on the side opposite the device.

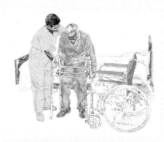
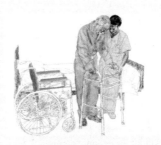
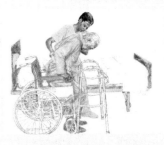

4. For residents using a walker, after they are standing, help them put both hands on the walker.

5. Help the resident move toward the chair. Guide them with statements like these: "Turn, turn, take a step toward me, now back up."

7. When the resident is in front of the chair, ask them to reach back and put one hand on the armrest.

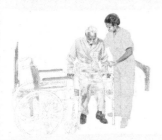

3. Ask or help the resident to push down on the bed with their hands and stand on the count of 3. You can help them by pulling up and forward on the back of the guard belt with one hand while pushing down on the walker or cane to keep it stable while the resident stands. Encourage a resident using a walker to stand before grabbing onto the assistive device.

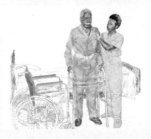

Note: *Have the resident stand for a few minutes before trying to move, especially if they are dizzy.*

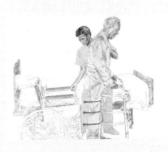

6. Help the resident back up to the chair. Ask if they can feel the chair against the back of their legs. Explain that they should not sit until they feel this.

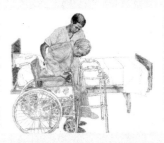

8. Help the resident reach back with the other hand for the arm of the chair and slowly sit down.

REMEMBER: UNDERSTAND

PROCEDURE 15-13.   TRANSFERRING A RESIDENT FROM A CHAIR TO A BED, COMMODE, OR TOILET

Whether you are helping a resident move from a chair back to bed or to the toilet or commode, use the stand pivot transfer or assistive device transfer if they can help with the transfer. (If a resident cannot help, use the mechanical lift, as described later, or have a co-worker help with the transfer.) Follow these steps.

1. Position the chair with the resident's stronger side closer to the bed, commode, or toilet.

2. If the resident is in a wheelchair, ask them to move their feet off the footrests. Raise up the footrests.

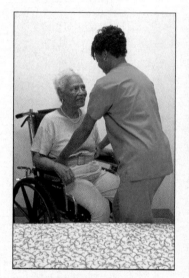

3. Ask the resident to slide forward to the edge of the chair. This is often difficult, and the resident may need help.

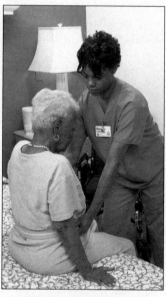

4. Use either the stand pivot or assistive device transfer procedure in reverse to move the resident from the chair and into bed.

PROCEDURE 15-14.   MOVING A RESIDENT WITH A MECHANICAL LIFT

▶ **REMEMBER: BE AWARE**

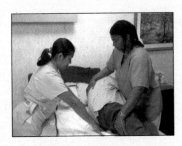

1. Adjust the head of the bed as flat as possible if the resident can tolerate it. To put the sling under the resident, first turn the resident toward you. Help the resident move toward you while your helper on the other side of the bed pushes the fan-folded sling under the resident as far as possible. Then help the resident back and toward the other side and pull the sling under them.

Note: *The sling should be placed from under the resident's shoulders to the back of the knees. Have the same amount of sling material on both sides of the resident so that the resident is centered.*

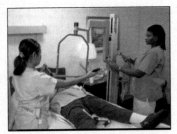

2. Place the lift frame facing the bed with its legs under the bed. Lock the wheels on the base.

3. Elevate the head of the bed so the resident is partially sitting up.

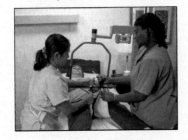

4. Attach the sling to the lift following the manufacturer's directions.

5. Ask the resident to cross their arms over their chest before operating the lift.

Note: *If a resident cannot keep their hands in their lap or across their chest, try having them hold onto an object on their lap.*

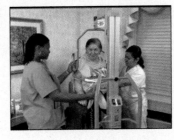

6. Follow the manufacturer's directions to raise the resident up to a sitting position with the lift. While you operate the lift, your helper should help you guide the resident.

Note: *Repeatedly ask the resident if they are OK. Reassure the resident because this can be a frightening experience, especially the first time.*

7. Once the resident is sitting, keep raising the lift until they are 6 to 12 inches over the bed and chair height.

8. Unlock the swivel, if the lift has one, or use the steering handle to move the resident directly over the chair. You may need to guide the resident's legs.

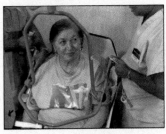

9. Tell the resident that you are now going to lower them slowly into the chair. Your helper guides the resident into the chair by moving the sling. Press the release button to slowly lower them down.

PROCEDURE 15-14.   MOVING A RESIDENT WITH A MECHANICAL LIFT (*CONTINUED*)

10. Once the resident is securely in the chair, unhook the sling and remove the lift frame.

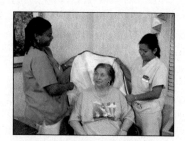

▶ **REMEMBER: UNDERSTAND**

11. Position the resident in the chair, leaving the sling under them (unless the sling is removable) until it is time to return to bed. Pull the metal bars of the sling out so that the resident does not lean against or sit on them.

PROCEDURE 15-15.   MOVING A RESIDENT UP IN A CHAIR

▶ **REMEMBER: BE AWARE**

Note: *These steps are for moving a resident up in the chair after a transfer procedure to the chair. You need a helper for this procedure.*

1. Place the guard belt on the resident.

2. Standing on both sides of the resident, you each grasp the guard belt with one hand and and put the other hand under the resident's knees. Ask the resident to cross their arms in front of their chest.

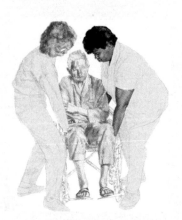

3. On the count of three, breathe out and lift the resident back in the chair. Be sure to use good body mechanics.

▶ **REMEMBER: UNDERSTAND**

PROCEDURE 15-16.   RETURNING A RESIDENT TO BED USING A MECHANICAL LIFT

The process for returning a resident to bed reverses the steps for transferring a resident from the bed.

1. Position the lift facing the chair.

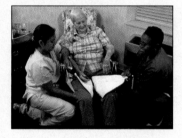

2. Attach the sling to the lift following the manufacturer's directions.

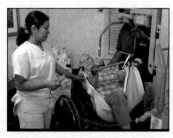

3. Crank (or raise) the resident up with the lift. Your helper guides the resident by holding the sling.

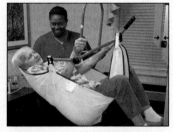

4. Swing the frame of the lift over the bed and slowly lower the resident down onto the bed.

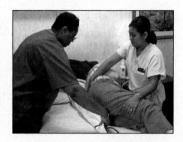

5. Unless the resident will spend only a short time in bed, roll them from side to side to remove the sling. (The sling could cause skin irritation if left under the resident.)

6. Position the resident as preferred.

(text continued from p. 284)

Follow these steps to lift the resident if a mechanical lift or other device is not available:

1. Get as many staff to help as needed.
2. Prepare for the lift by first moving the resident into a sitting position on the floor with their knees bent up and feet flat on the floor. Ask the resident to fold their arms across their chest.

4. The team leader asks if everyone has a good grip and is ready. Then the leader says, "On the count of 3, lift." Then, "Ready, 1, 2, 3, and lift." You may find it easier to do the lift in two steps, saying, "1, 2, 3, and lift to stand," and then "1, 2, 3, and lift into the chair" or onto the stretcher.

Note: *Anytime a resident falls, report the situation to the charge nurse.*

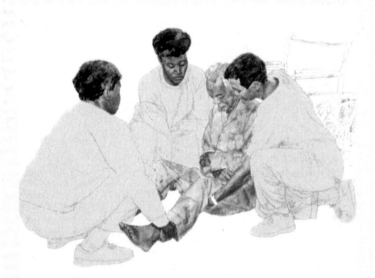

3. Before lifting the resident, one person kneels on each side of the resident and holds onto the guard belt with one hand and puts their other hand under the resident's leg. A third person puts their hands under both the resident's legs while kneeling in front of the resident or facing the resident. A fourth person may hold the chair or stretcher.

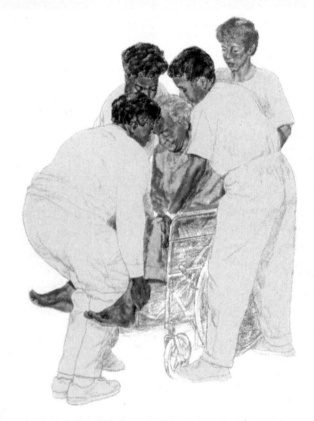

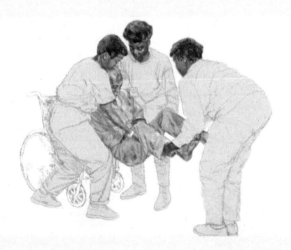

IN THIS CHAPTER YOU LEARNED:

- The importance of moving and positioning residents
- Questions to consider when preparing to move or position a resident
- How to move a resident:
  - up in bed
  - to the side of the bed
  - onto the resident's side or back for personal care
  - into a sitting position
  - from bed to chair, wheelchair, commode, or toilet
- How to to help move a resident from bed to chair and back with a coworker's help (with or without a mechanical lift), and how to move a resident up in a chair
- How to help a resident into the following positions:
  - supine
  - Fowler's
  - side-lying
  - sitting
- What to do if a resident falls

SUMMARY

The information in this chapter is very important for you to learn well. Remember that a leading cause of injury on the job is overexertion when lifting. But if you learn to use good body mechanics and the proper equipment as described in Chapter 10, Personal Protection and Injury Prevention, and learn the skills in this chapter, you can prevent injury to both yourself and residents.

The human body is designed for frequent movement. Movement is essential for all body systems to function well. It is your job to make sure residents move in a safe, comfortable manner. Remember the things you need to consider before beginning to move or position a resident. Determine each resident's individual needs before you decide how to continue. Once you have considered the situation, follow the steps of the procedure carefully. Each procedure is designed to move or position residents in a careful, safe fashion.

PULLING IT ALL TOGETHER

One of the residents you are caring for on the day shift is Mrs. Casey. She is an 85-year-old woman who has had several strokes. She now has limited ability to move and position herself independently. Moving and positioning to prevent skin breakdowns and other problems caused by immobility are among the most important tasks in her care plan. She is one of eight residents you are caring for. What should your plan be for moving and positioning her?

Think about this:

7:15 a.m. Check in with her to say good morning. Tell her it will soon be breakfast time and you now want to change her position to get ready for breakfast. You move her from the right side-lying position onto her back with her head elevated.

8:30 a.m. Breakfast arrives, and you help Mrs. Casey with her meal.

9 a.m. Mrs. Casey says she would like to rest before getting ready for the day. You position her on her left side.

10 a.m. You schedule another nurse assistant and the mechanical lift for 10:30.

10:30 a.m. You transfer Mrs. Casey from the bed to the wheelchair with the help of another nurse assistant using the mechanical lift.

11 a.m. Mrs. Casey attends recreational activities.

12 p.m. You walk Mrs. Casey to the bathroom using a guard belt, walker, and another nurse assistant. She returns to her wheelchair.

12:30 p.m. Mrs. Casey has lunch in the dining room.

1:30 p.m. Mrs. Casey returns to her room for a short nap. You transfer her to the bed with help from another nurse assistant. You position her on her right side.

3 p.m. You tell the next shift that Mrs. Casey's position needs to be changed by 3:30. You let them know that she did well today using the guard belt, walker, and support from a second nurse assistant.

1. **Any time you are about to move a resident you should first:**
   A. Check the resident's medical record.
   B. Call the family to ask about their preferences.
   C. Think about your own capabilities and limitations.
   D. Ask their roommate to leave the room.

2. **When should you get help to move a resident?**
   A. Always.
   B. Only if the resident weighs considerably more than you do.
   C. If you are unsure how a resident will respond.
   D. At the beginning of your shift before you've stretched your muscles.

3. **Good body mechanics when moving a resident in bed should include:**
   A. Keeping your feet 10-12 inches apart.
   B. Keeping your knees straight.
   C. Bending your back.
   D. Holding the resident as far from your body as you can when transferring them.

4. **Which statement is true when you move a resident up in bed who is unable to help?**
   A. Put the head of the bed at about 30 degrees.
   B. Put the pillow under the resident's knees during the move.
   C. Ask another staff person to help you.
   D. Slide the resident along the sheet as quickly as possible.

5. **What should you consider before transferring a resident from the bed to a wheelchair?**
   A. Check to see if the wheelchair is locked.
   B. Position the guard belt around the resident's shoulders.
   C. Put the wheelchair on the resident's weaker side.
   D. Ask a co-worker to help only if you are unsuccessful in your first attempt.

6. **If a resident starts to feel dizzy as you help them stand up from their bed to get to their walker, you should:**
   A. Move them quickly before they have a chance to fall.
   B. Help them to lie down and call for the charge nurse.
   C. Keep them standing until the dizziness passes.
   D. Have them sit on the edge of the bed while you go to talk to the charge nurse.

7. **Why is it good practice to use a guard belt when transferring a resident?**
   A. You never need other helpers.
   B. It supports the resident's body during the transfer.
   C. It keeps the resident's clothing in place.
   D. It makes the transfer go twice as fast.

8. **Which of the following statements is true about the use of a mechanical lift?**
   A. Put the sling under the resident from under the shoulders to the back of the knees.
   B. Raise the head of the bed before positioning the sling under the resident.
   C. Another staff member is needed to assist the resident out of bed so that they can sit down in the sling.
   D. Place the sling over the resident like a blanket and have them roll over onto it.

9. **Which of the following is the correct description of Fowler's position?**
   A. Head and feet elevated about 45 degrees.
   B. Head elevated about 45 degrees.
   C. Head and shoulders elevated about 45 degrees.
   D. Head, neck, and trunk elevated about 45 degrees.

10. **What is important when positioning a resident in a chair?**
    A. Leave their legs free to dangle and swing.
    B. Their arms are supported with the armrest, their back supported by the chair back, and their legs positioned comfortably.
    C. If a resident has a leg cast or a swollen leg, strap it down to the footrest of the wheelchair.
    D. Use a lap restraint so that the resident cannot get up.

(Answers to "Check What You've Learned" are in the Instructor's Manual.)

Chapter 16

PERSONAL CARE

Many people enter a long term care facility when their health declines and they are less able to care for themselves. Often family members say things like, "My mother's hair was always curled and so neat. She would never let herself go like this." The individual's lack of personal care often triggers a concern by family members and friends that the resident needs the support of a long term care facility. Personal care includes bathing, oral hygiene, shaving, nail and hair care, and dressing. How you help residents do these tasks shows the family the quality of services the facility is providing their loved one. These are things people notice about the care that is given in a facility.

Successful personal care means much more than just learning how to help residents with these skills. You must really learn and feel what it means to the resident to have someone else do or help with their personal care. You must understand what is important to the resident—such as shaving twice a day or being up and dressed by 8 a.m. every day.

Because personal care makes up so much of your work with residents, you must be mindful when helping with personal care. This is a great time to really be with the residents, to observe them, to talk with them, and have fun with them.

In this chapter you will learn how the word "personal" relates to the care you give. You will also learn how to make routine activities mindful. You will learn how to give personal care while respecting residents' autonomy and individuality.

OBJECTIVES
- Define personal care
- Give examples of ways to make routine activities mindful and to consider the resident's preferences in personal care
- State why observation is important during personal care
- Demonstrate how to help with the following skills:
  — complete bed bath
  — perineal care
  — back rub
  — tub bath
  — shower
  — whirlpool bath
  — shampoo and conditioning
  — brushing and flossing
  — caring for dentures
  — mouth care for a comatose resident
  — shaving
  — trimming facial hair
  — hair care
  — care of fingernails
  — care of toenails
  — assisting with dressing and undressing

MEDICAL TERMS
- **Antiseptic** – a substance that reduces the growth or action of microorganisms
- **Anus** – the posterior opening from the large intestine (rectum)
- **Aspirate** – to breathe in or draw in by suction
- **Comatose** – someone in a coma, unconscious
- **Foreskin** – a fold of skin that covers the tip of the penis in an uncircumcised male
- **Labia** – the outer and inner fatty folds around the vulva
- **Perineal** – area of body between the anus and the external genitals
- **Podiatrist** – physician specializing in the care and treatment of the feet
- **Scrotum** – the external pouch in males that contains the testes
- **Urethra** – the canal in males and females that carries urine from the bladder; in males, it also serves as the duct for sperm

"I really do feel better when I look my best, and your help makes all the difference."

Think about the word **personal**. What does it really mean to you? Some people think personal means private, something you do for yourself, something no one else should see, know about, or touch. When you help residents with personal care, keep in mind that residents think and feel as you do about personal things and their body. Remember that some residents have to let you help them with things they always did on their own, in private, with no help. Think about how that must feel.

Everyone has the right to be treated with respect and dignity. If a resident wants to wear a red dress, help her put on that dress. If a resident wants to comb and style their hair a certain way, help them do so. Your responsibility is to give individualized care to improve the quality of life for each resident.

Think about these ideas:
- Most people care how they look.
- When you like the way you look outside, you feel better inside.
- Everyone has their own style and preferences.
- What you like may be very different from what others like.
- How people style their hair is very personal.
- Being free from odor is important to most people.
- Clean teeth and a nice smile are inviting to look at and feel good.

Remember these ideas when you help residents with personal care. Personal care involves cleanliness and appearance and includes bathing, mouth care, grooming, and dressing. How much help you give a resident depends on their needs. You help residents create who they are on the outside based on how they view themselves on the inside.

Personal – private, or referring to a person's body

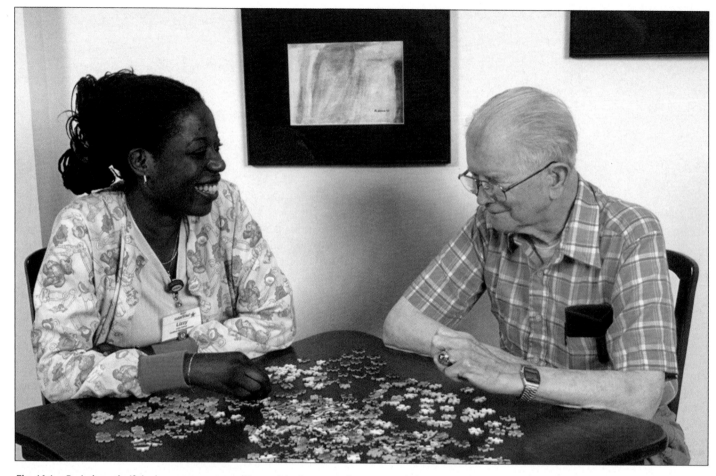

Fig. 16-1 – By being mindful whenever you are with a resident, you can learn a great deal about them.

MAKING ROUTINE ACTIVITIES MINDFUL

Long term care facilities often call daily care activities "routine care." This means you give the care every day. Even so, do not let your care become "routine" or the same for all residents. Instead, help with routine care based on each resident's individual needs. Look back to the section on providing care in Chapter 2. As you read this chapter, think about mindfulness and learning each resident's own needs. Apply these principles in all the types of care described in this chapter.

When you help with care every day, think of what you can do for residents to keep it from seeming routine or boring. For example, ask residents what they would like to do first: "Would you like to read today for an hour before taking a shower?" or "Would you like to have a foot soak before (or after) physical therapy today?" Just by asking simple questions and encouraging residents to participate

and make choices, you are more mindful in your everyday care (Fig. 16-1). Plan your day according to each resident's preferences, not your own.

Daily Routines Based on Personal Preferences

Before you help with personal care, you need to know each resident's likes and dislikes. Learn this information first to help meet each resident's needs. One resident may like their hair styled very differently from another. One resident may enjoy bright, dressy clothes, and another may prefer casual clothes in pastels.

Think about how you like to dress, bathe, brush your teeth, and style your hair. Now think about someone else, like your best friend, your spouse, or a relative. Does this person do things exactly the same as you? The exact same hair style and the exact same clothing? Everyone has their own preferences. They are unique and individual. Residents too have their own ideas about dressing, cleanliness, and grooming. Always base the personal care you give on the resident's personal preferences. If a resident cannot express their preferences, ask their family and friends about their personal preferences (Fig. 16-2). For example, ask Mrs. Jones' daughter how her mother likes to wear her hair.

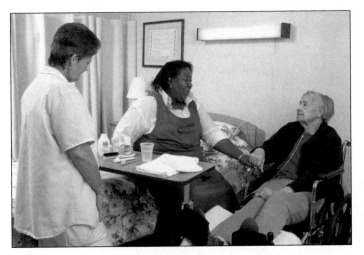

Fig. 16-2 – If your residents are unable to tell you what they like or dislike, ask family members about their preferences.

Determination of Assistance Needs and Observation During Personal Care

As you learn how to help with personal care, you are learning about oral hygiene, bathing, and grooming. But your job involves much more than just this. You need to determine the resident's capabilities before each task and observe them while you are giving care. This means looking at the situation to see how to do the task best. For example, you need to know if a resident needs help with bathing or only needs you to help them out of the tub. If a resident does need help, you need to determine how much help and exactly what to do.

By determining the resident's needs for assistance, you become better prepared and organized. Residents also will find the experience more pleasant and will appreciate your attention. Here are two examples:

You are about to help a resident with a tub bath. The person cannot stand without help. You determine how much assistance is needed ahead of time and arrange for another nurse assistant to help you assist this resident into and out of the tub.

You are about to help a resident with a complete bed bath. The resident's legs are paralyzed. You determine how much assistance is needed and realize you need another nurse assistant to help you turn the resident for back care and perineal care.

Observation is also important when helping with personal care. You observe residents for any physical and psychological changes (Fig. 16-3). Think of your observation as a head-to-toe look at a resident. You may do a quick check of each body system to see, hear, smell, and feel for any changes. Of all staff in the facility, you have the best opportunity to observe residents. Record and report any changes you observe.

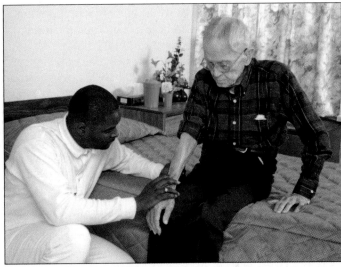

Fig. 16-3 – During personal care you have an opportunity to observe your residents for physical and psychological changes.

For example:
- During a bed bath you notice a reddened area the size of a quarter on a resident's left hip.
- You notice a resident is quieter than usual.
- When helping a resident shave, you notice a rash on his neck.
- While shampooing a resident's hair, you see a dry, flaky scalp.
- When helping a resident brush and floss their teeth, you notice their gums are bleeding more than usual.

Perineal – area of body between the anus and the external genitals

Your follow-up actions with your observations are very important. First, write down your observations so you do not forget to report and record them. You must tell the charge nurse about any change in a resident so that treatment can be given if needed. You must also report any resident complaints. Remember to state what information is subjective and what is objective. Never think that any change you observe is insignificant. All changes are important.

Observation is your responsibility during personal care. Residents depend on you to see changes so that they get the best possible care.

USE OF GLOVES IN PERSONAL CARE

As you learned in Chapter 9, Prevention and Control of Infection, always wear gloves when helping with personal care that involves a resident's body secretions or excretions. This includes perineal care and oral hygiene. Also wear gloves when bathing a resident who has skin sores, a rash, or a wound. Wear gloves if you have an open sore, rash, or skin sore on your hands. You do not have to wear gloves for care that does not expose you to a resident's body secretions or excretions, such as giving a back rub. Be sensitive to how residents may feel when you put on gloves. Tell them that gloves must be worn for certain personal care skills for all residents, regardless of who they are.

PERSONAL CARE ROUTINES

The next sections describe many personal care skills. You will do these on a regular schedule, based on your facility's practices and routines and the residents' preferences. On some days you may do them all, but on other days only a few. You may help residents with some types of personal care at different times of the day or to prepare for different activities. For example, staff sometimes call the care given residents before breakfast "a.m. care." This may include helping residents with washing their face and hands, toileting, and oral hygiene. This care helps prepare them for the day. You give "p.m. care" to help prepare them for bedtime. Helping residents with washing their face and hands, oral hygiene, back rubs, undressing, and toileting are common p.m. care skills. Always keep a resident's preferences in mind to help you decide what care to give, how to give it, and when to give it.

Note: *A resident's preference may sometimes conflict with your facility's practices. If you have any concerns about how or when to help with personal care, talk with your charge nurse.*

During all personal care activities, encourage the resident to participate as much as possible. Explain each step to the resident. This is a good time to provide range-of-motion activities (see Chapter 27, Restorative Activities), inspect the resident's skin, and engage in conversation with the resident.

BATHING

Bathing helps keep skin healthy and prevents skin problems. The three main purposes of bathing are:
* to remove dirt, perspiration, and microorganisms that build up on the skin
* to increase circulation to the skin
* to help the resident feel better and more comfortable

If a resident can leave the bed, help them with a bath or shower. Facilities have schedules for residents who need help with bathing, based on their hygiene needs and comfort. Bathing too often may cause skin dryness, which can cause skin breakdown. Give partial baths between complete baths as needed.

Remember, bathing is a very personal activity, and a resident may feel very uncomfortable being helped. Help them be more comfortable by giving them privacy during bathing and encouraging them to make their own choices about how to bathe.

Some residents who cannot get into and out of bed need bed baths. Procedure 16-1 describes the steps for a complete bed bath. Procedure 16-2 describes the steps for a tub bath, and Procedure 16-3 for a shower.

Using a Resident's Personal Products

A resident or family member may want you to use certain bath or personal hygiene products for personal care. Honor their requests and become familiar with their products. These may include bathing oils, special fragrance soaps, deodorants, powders, lotions for dry skin, perfumes, and aftershave lotions (Fig. 16-4). Most products come with directions for use. Check the directions and talk with the resident about how they like to use them.

(text continued on page 304)

Perspiration – a saline fluid secreted by sweat glands

PROCEDURE 16-1. COMPLETE BED BATH

▶ REMEMBER: BE AWARE

Items Needed
- two washcloths
- towel
- bedpan
- basin half filled with water
- soap
- gloves
- plastic trash bag or waste basket
- lotion
- plastic-covered pad or protective covering
- bath blanket
- clothing

Note: Before beginning the bath, remove the resident's blanket and bedspread and put them on a clean surface. Put a bath blanket over the top sheet and then pull down the top sheet to the foot of the bed, leaving the bath blanket covering the resident. Expose only the part of the resident's body you are washing. This gives the person privacy and prevents them from becoming cold. Remove their clothing also under the bath blanket. The best position for the resident is flat in bed, if they can tolerate it. Fill the water basin halfway with water that is warm to your touch. Test the water with your bare hand—not with gloves on. The water temperature should be 98.6 F to

103 F. You can use a thermometer if one is available, or test the water temperature with the inside of your wrist, and then have the resident feel the water to be sure it is comfortable. Wash, rinse, dry, and inspect each body part. Be gentle.

Start by making a bath mitt.

Making a Bath Mitt
Make a bath mitt with the washcloth. The mitt provides a soft surface for the person's skin and is easier to use than an unfolded washcloth. The edges of an unfolded washcloth may get cold and make the resident uncomfortable.

1. After wringing out the wet washcloth, put your hand in the center of the washcloth.

2. Fold the side of the washcloth over from your little finger, and hold the fold with your thumb.
3. Fold the remaining cloth over and hold it firmly with your thumb.
4. Fold the top edge of the cloth down and tuck it into your palm. Hold it with your thumb.

5. The mitt is now ready to use. Rinse the cloth and refold the mitt as needed during the bath.

Giving a Complete Bed Bath

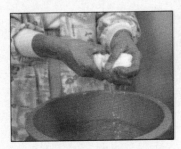

1. Begin with the resident's eyes, using only water—no soap.

Start with the eye that is farther from you. With one corner

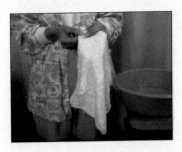

of the washcloth, wash from the inner corner of the eye outward toward the ear. Clean away any crusting that may be

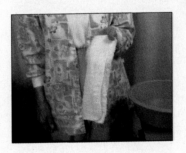

stuck to the lower part of the eye. Use another corner of the washcloth to wash the near

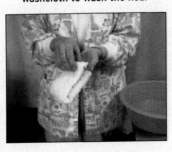

eye. Be sure to move the

📖
Tolerate – to put up with, to endure

washcloth from the inner corner of the eye outward.

2. Wash the resident's face. Some residents prefer not to use soap on their face. If so, use water only. Rinse, dry, and inspect the area.

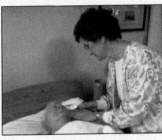

Note: To wash with soap, wet the washcloth and apply a small amount of soap on it. Be sure to rinse the soap off. When you dry the resident's skin, pat it dry, being careful not to rub too hard.

3. Wash the resident's ears and neck. Rinse, dry, and inspect the area.

Note: When washing the resident's ears, wash behind the ear as well as inside. Wring out the wash cloth so that excess water does not enter the ear canal.

4. Wash the arms, underarm areas, and hands. Expose only the areas to be washed. Use a bath blanket to cover the resident. Use soap sparingly.

(Remember: soap dries the skin.) Wash the side away from you first, then the side near you, so that you are moving from a clean area to a dirty area, unless you feel you have to stretch too far and might injure yourself. (If so, wash one side of the resident's body, then move to the other side and wash it.)

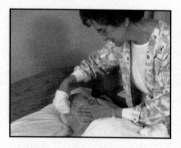

Rinse, dry, and inspect the area.

5. Fold the bath blanket down and cover the resident's chest with a towel. Wash the chest and abdomen down as far as the pubic area. Rinse, dry, and inspect the area. Pay particular attention to the skin under

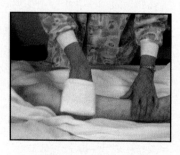

a female resident's breasts and or any skin folds on the chest and abdomen. These are common areas for skin irritation and breakdowns. Note any redness, odor, or skin

breakdown.
Cover the chest with the bath blanket.

6. Expose one leg and foot. Cover the exposed leg with a towel. Wash the legs and feet. Don't forget to wash between the toes. Rinse, dry, and inspect the area. Check between the toes for any redness, irritation, or cracking of

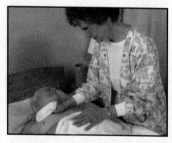

the skin. Note any swelling of the feet and legs.

Note: *Change the water at this time or at any time during the bath if the water gets too cold, soapy, or dirty. (Using the same water after foot washing could potentially spread a foot fungus.) Cover up the resident before leaving to change the water.*

7. Help the resident to turn to one side (see procedures for moving residents in Chapter 15). Keep the resident covered with a bath blanket.

8. Expose the resident's back and buttocks. Wash the resident's back and buttocks. Rinse, dry, and inspect the area.

9. Give the resident a back rub. Rub a small amount of lotion into your palms. Starting at the resident's lower back, gently move your hands up

toward the shoulders, then downward to the lower back. Give the back rub for at least three minutes. Back rubs are comforting and relaxing and stimulate circulation, helping prevent skin breakdown.

Note: *You may also give a back rub on request or as part of p.m. care.*

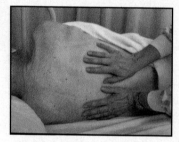

10. Help the resident move back onto their back.

11. Give **perineal** care (wash the genital and anal area of the body), as described below.

Note: *After the back rub and before perineal care, put a plastic-covered pad under the resident to absorb water used to wash the perineal area, and put on a new pair of gloves. You can also use a bedpan for this. The bedpan allows a good view of the perineal area because it raises the resident's pelvis and lets you use more water for washing and rinsing. Since it might be uncomfortable for a resident, ask first. Sometimes you can use a fracture pan or a folded towel under the buttocks to raise the pelvis. Remember these guidelines:*

- *Always change the water before perineal care.*
- *Always change the washcloth and towel.*
- *Always wear gloves when giving perineal care.*

Note: *Perineal care is described here as part of a complete bed bath. If you do it separately, perform preparation and completion steps before and after the perineal care.*

12. Help the resident get dressed.

Perineal Care for Female Residents

1. Help the resident onto the bedpan or pad.

2. Put on gloves.

3. **Drape** the resident by folding back the bath blanket to expose only her legs and per-

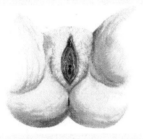

ineal area. Ask the resident to bend her knees.

4. Have the resident check the water temperature to ensure that it is not too warm.

5. Apply soap to a wet wash-cloth.

6. Wash the **pubic** area with a downward stroke from the front to the back on each side of the **labia**. Make sure to use a clean area of the washcloth with each stroke.

7. Wash downward in the middle over the **urethra** and vaginal opening. Always wash down-ward toward the **anus** with a clean area of the cloth to pre-vent the spread of infection.

8. Using a second clean wash-cloth, rinse the soap from the pubic area using the same technique. Wipe front to back using a clean area of the cloth

with each stroke.

9. Dry the pubic area with a towel, and inspect the area for any redness, swelling, odor, drainage, or areas of irritation.

10. After washing the pubic area, turn the resident onto their side and then wash and rinse the anal area moving with upward strokes toward the back. Make sure to use a clean area of the cloth for each stroke.

11. Dry with a clean towel.

12. Reposition the resident for comfort.

Perineal Care for Male Residents

1. Put on gloves.

2. Drape the resident to expose only his legs and perineal area by folding back the bath blanket.

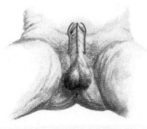

3. Wash the penis from the ure-thral opening or tip of the penis toward the base of the penis, and then wash the **scrotum**. Take care to wash, rinse, and dry between any

skin folds. Pull back the fore-skin on **uncircumcised** males and clean under it. Return the foreskin. Check for any redness, swelling, or areas of irritation.

4. Help the resident turn onto his side. Wash, rinse, and dry the anal area, moving upward toward the back.

▶ **REMEMBER: UNDERSTAND**

📖

Anus – the posterior opening from the large intestine

Drape – to cover

Foreskin – a fold of skin that covers the tip of the penis in an uncircumcised male

Labia – the outer and inner fatty folds bounding the vulva

Perineal – area of body between the anus and the external genitals

Pubic – the region of pubic hair, genital area

Scrotum – the external pouch in males that contains the testes

Stimulate – to arouse a function

Uncircumcised – not circumcised, the foreskin remaining at the tip of the penis

Urethra – the canal in males and females that carries urine from the bladder; in males also serves as the duct for sperm

PROCEDURE 16-2. TUB BATH

Items Needed
- gloves
- two washcloths
- three towels
- clothes for resident
- soap, lotion, shampoo, etc.
- bath mat

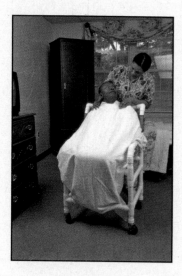

1. Assist the resident to the tub room with all supplies.

Note: *Some facilities may use chairs on wheels that may be taken to the resident's room. If you use this chair to bring the resident to the tub room, make sure that they are properly dressed and draped to protect their privacy and use the safety straps if needed and available.*

2. Help the resident sit on the chair. Fill the tub halfway with warm water.

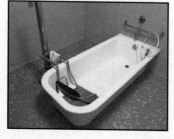

3. Remember, always turn the hot water off first.

Note: *The tub water should be in the range of 98.6 F to 103 F. Use a thermometer if available, or test the water temperature with the inside of your wrist, and then have the resident feel it with their hand or foot. The resident's physician may order special medication to be added to the bath water, such as bran, oatmeal, starch, sodium bicarbonate, Epsom salts, pine products, sulfa, potassium permanganate, or salt. Always check with the charge nurse about the proper use of any of these substances.*

4. Help the resident remove their clothing.

5. Check that the bath mat is in place. Help the resident into the tub.

6. Help with bathing as needed. (Put gloves on if you will be assisting with perineal care.)

Note: *Never leave the resident alone while bathing in a tub. Always encourage residents to use safety rails. Be sure to check the water temperature during the tub bath to be sure it has not cooled down. Add hot water as needed.*

7. Place a clean towel on the seat of the chair.

8. Help the resident out of the tub. Encourage them to use safety rails. Cover them with a bath blanket.

9. Help the resident with drying, applying personal hygiene products, and dressing.

Note: *You may give them a back rub before dressing, if the resident desires.*

10. Help the resident back to their room. Bring any of their personal hygiene products back to their room.

PROCEDURE 16-3.   SHOWER

▶ **REMEMBER: BE AWARE**

Items Needed:
- gloves
- two washcloths
- three towels
  (four if shampooing)
- clothes for resident to wear
- soap, lotion, shampoo, etc.
- shower cap if needed
- shower chair
- shower mat
- bath blanket

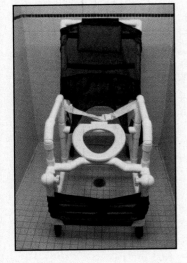

1. Help the resident to the shower room with all necessary supplies.

2. Help the resident sit on the chair, using safety straps if needed and available.

3. Turn on the shower with warm water. Test the water on the inside of your wrist and have the resident feel it with their hand or foot. Adjust the temperature as needed.

4. Help the resident remove their clothing.

5. Help the resident into the shower. Encourage them to use the safety rails.

Note: *Most facilities have shower chairs that lock in place. If the resident needs to shower sitting down, be sure the shower chair is locked before they sit down.*

6. Help the resident with showering as needed. (Wear gloves if you help with perineal care.) Encourage the resident to participate in bathing as much as possible. Give help and verbal cueing as needed. Wash from head to toe. Rinse the washcloth as needed.

Note: *Bathing is a good time to observe the resident's skin for any skin conditions, to conduct range-of-motion exercises, and to engage in conversation with the resident. These acts add restorative care into the resident's daily routine.*

Note: *If the resident is not shampooing, use a shower cap to prevent their hair from getting wet.*

7. Place a dry towel on the chair outside the shower.

8. Help the resident out of the shower and onto the covered chair. Cover the resident with a bath blanket.

9. Turn off the shower. Turn the hot water off first to prevent a burn.

10. Help the resident dry off, use personal hygiene products, and get dressed.

Note: *You may give a back rub at this point if desired.*

11. Help the resident back to their room. Bring their personal hygiene products back to the room and put them away.

▶ **REMEMBER: UNDERSTAND**

(text continued from page 298)

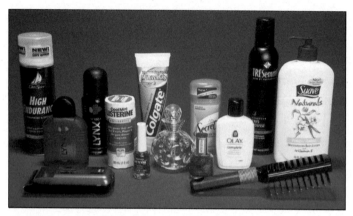

Fig. 16-4 – Always ask the resident what products they want to use for bathing and grooming.

Waterless Products

Products are available for bathing a resident without water. You may use premoistened cloths to clean the resident's body without having to rinse or dry the skin. These are packaged individually with enough cloths to wash the resident's entire body. These products save time. Waterless products are also available for hair care.

Whirlpool Bath

A whirlpool bath is a special **therapeutic** bath that comforts and bathes a resident. The physician may order the bath as part of the resident's treatment plan. For example, a resident may have a wound that needs daily cleaning or poor circulation that needs stimulation. Whirlpool baths move the water to help meet these goals. Some whirlpools have a mechanical lift to move residents into and out of the tub. Follow the facility's guidelines for using the whirlpool, including cleaning guidelines and infection control measures before and after using the whirlpool. You will learn these guidelines on the job. Procedure 16-4 describes the steps for helping a resident with a whirlpool bath.

Partial Bath

A partial bath is used to wash only certain body parts. On days a resident is not having a complete bed bath, tub bath, shower, or whirlpool bath, you may give a partial bath. When giving a partial bath, help a resident wash their face, hands, and underarms, and then provide perineal care.

Shampooing and Conditioning

Shampooing can be done in the bed, shower, tub, or sink. Shampooing once a week is usually enough to keep a resident's hair and scalp clean. Some residents prefer to shampoo more often.

Many facilities have a beauty parlor and a hairdresser who shampoos and styles hair. Some have a barber shop or bring in an outside barber to give haircuts to men. Often you are the one who shampoos a resident's hair, especially those who cannot go to the beauty or barber shop. Procedure 16-5 describes the steps for helping residents with shampooing and conditioning.

ORAL HYGIENE

Mouth care helps prevent gum disease and tooth loss. Mouth care also improves a resident's sense of well-being, appearance, appetite, and ability to chew food properly. Mouth and gum problems can be contributing factors to many different diseases.

Brushing and Flossing

Help a resident brush at least twice a day and floss their teeth at least once a day. Always encourage the resident to do their own brushing and flossing if they can. During mouth care inspect the gums for any paleness, discoloration, bleeding sores, or irritation. Inspect the teeth for decay or looseness. Flossing stimulates the gums and removes particles of food from between the teeth that brushing cannot remove. Procedure 16-6 describes the steps for helping residents with brushing an flossing.

Note: *Because of changes like loose teeth or inflamed or receded gum lines, not all residents can have their teeth flossed. Check with the charge nurse before you floss a resident's teeth.*

(text continues on page 308)

Therapeutic – referring to a treatment

PROCEDURE 16-4. WHIRLPOOL BATH

▶ **REMEMBER: BE AWARE**

Items Needed
- gloves
- three towels
- two washcloths
- personal hygiene products
- clothes for the resident to wear
- bath blanket

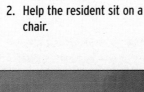

1. Help the resident to the whirlpool room with all supplies.

2. Help the resident sit on a chair.

3. Turn on the water in the whirlpool following the facility's procedure. The water temperature should be 98.6 F to 103 F. Test the water temperature on the inside of your wrist, and have the resident feel it with their hand or foot. Adjust the temperature as needed.

4. Help the resident remove their clothing.

5. Help the resident into the whirlpool bath. Encourage use of safety rails.

Note: *Follow the manufacturer's and facility's guidelines. If you use a mechanical lift, be sure you know how to use it properly.*

6. Help the resident bathe. Encourage the resident to participate in bathing as much as possible. Give help and verbal cuing as needed. Wash from head to toe. Rinse the wash cloth as needed. Wear gloves if you help with perineal care. Never leave the resident unattended.

Note: *If the resident has a wound dressing, ask the nurse to remove it before the bath and apply a clean one afterward. If the physician has ordered an antiseptic solution in the whirlpool bath, the nurse will add the solution or give you specific instructions.*

7. Place a dry towel on the chair.

8. Help the resident out of the whirlpool bath and onto the covered chair. Encourage them to use the safety rails. Cover them with a bath blanket.

9. Help the resident dry off, apply personal hygiene products, and get dressed.

Note: *You may give them a back rub at this point if desired.*

10. Help the resident back to their room.

▶ **REMEMBER: UNDERSTAND**

Antiseptic – a substance that reduces the growth or action of microorganisms

PROCEDURE 16-5. SHAMPOOING AND CONDITIONING

▶ **REMEMBER: BE AWARE**

Items Needed
- comb or brush
- one or two towels
- shampoo
- conditioner (if used)
- face cloth

1. Help the resident into a chair.

2. Comb or brush out any tangles before shampooing.

3. Turn on the water to a warm temperature, no more than 103 F. Test the water temperature on the inside of your wrist, and have the resident feel it with their hand.

4. Help the resident take off their clothes for showering or tub bathing. Wash the resident's hair as the resident prefers (some residents want it done first, and some last). If a resident is shampooing at the sink, put the back of the chair against the front of the sink. Pad the rim of the sink with a towel. Position the resident for the method you are using: upright in a shower chair, flat in bed with pillows placed under their shoulders, or tilted in shampoo chair. Protect their clothes with a towel draped over the shoulders. If you are shampooing in bed, you need a shampoo trough, basin, or pail, and a waterproof bed protector.

5. Wet the hair entirely. Place a face cloth over the resident's eyes to prevent shampoo from getting into the resident's eyes.

6. Pour a small amount of shampoo into your palm and apply it to the resident's wet hair. Massage the shampoo gently throughout hair and scalp.

7. Rinse the hair well with warm water.

8. Apply conditioner, if used.

9. Rinse the hair well with warm water.

10. Help the resident out of the shower or tub into the chair. Cover them with a bath blanket. Wrap a towel around their hair. Help them dry off and get dressed. If the resident is in bed, help them wipe their face with the towel used to protect their eyes. Remove the trough or basin from beneath the resident's head. Remove the waterproof sheet from under their head and shoulders. Change the linen as necessary. Position the resident with the head of the bed up.

11. Dry their hair thoroughly and quickly to prevent chilling. Use a hair dryer on a low setting if available.

12. Style the resident's hair as they like it. Check for any flaking, reddened areas, or other scalp problems.

Note: *Some residents use special shampoos or conditioners, often with medicine the doctor orders for a specific condition. Ask the nurse for instructions and read the labels carefully before using them.*

13. Help the resident back to their room.

▶ **REMEMBER: UNDERSTAND**

PROCEDURE 16-6.   BRUSHING AND FLOSSING

▶ REMEMBER: BE AWARE

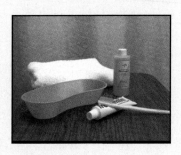

Items Needed
- towel
- soft-bristle toothbrush
- toothpaste
- paper cup half filled with cool water
- mouthwash, if desired
- dental floss
- emesis basin
- towel
- gloves
- plastic trash bags

Note: *You can help residents with brushing and flossing at the bedside table or the resident's sink, as they prefer.*

1. Apply a small amount of toothpaste to the wet toothbrush and set it aside. Mix water and mouthwash in a cup. A solution of half water, half mouthwash is best. Set this aside. Mouthwash is strong and could be harmful to sensitive gums.

2. Break off or least 18 inches of floss. Set this aside.

3. Put on gloves.

Note: *If you know that the resident's gums bleed, talk with the charge nurse about other personal protective equipment you may need, like protective eye wear and face mask.*

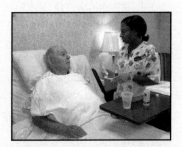

4. Put a towel over the resident's chest to protect their clothing.

5. Give the resident a small amount of mouthwash solution to swish around in their mouth to rinse it. Place the emesis basin under the resident's chin so they can spit out the solution.

6. Brush the resident's upper teeth and gums first, moving the brush from the gums to the teeth downward. Then brush the lower teeth and gums moving again from the gums to the teeth upward. Be sure to brush the back of the teeth. Inspect the teeth and gums while brushing.

7. Brush the tongue gently.

8. Help the resident rinse their mouth with a little mouthwash solution.

9. Wrap the ends of the floss around your middle fingers of each hand to get a good grip. Gently insert the floss between each tooth and the next. Move the floss to the gum line and down between the teeth. Wrap the floss around your fingertips to keep using a clean section as you move from tooth to tooth.

10. Have the resident rinse their mouth thoroughly.

11. Dry any solution around the resident's mouth or chin.

▶ REMEMBER: UNDERSTAND

(text continued from page 304)

Dentures

Dentures (false teeth) are worn by people who have lost some or all of their natural teeth. A resident may have full dentures (both upper and lower) or partial plates that replace some teeth (Fig. 16-5, next page). Partial plates are usually held in place by an attachment to remaining teeth.

Dentures and plates are expensive. Handle them carefully to prevent breaking them. Encourage residents to wear their dentures as often as possible to avoid gum shrinkage, to improve their speech, to help them chew food, and to improve their appearance. Dentures should be cleaned at least twice daily (Procedure 16-7). When dentures are removed for a time, always store them in a denture cup in cool water or a commercial denture cleansing solution if the resident prefers.

PROCEDURE 16-7.   CARING FOR DENTURES

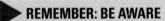 **REMEMBER: BE AWARE**

Items Needed
- denture cup (or paper cup half filled with cool water)
- swab moistened with water and mouthwash
- plastic bag for disposable items
- one or two pairs of gloves
- towel
- denture adhesive (if used)
- tissue or paper towel
- toothpaste
- emesis basin
- mouthwash

1. Put on gloves.
2. Ask the resident to remove their dentures and place them in the denture cup. If the resident cannot remove their own dentures, follow these steps.
   a. Place a towel over the resident's chest.
   b. Rinse the resident's mouth with mouthwash solution to moisten it. Ask them to swish the solution around, and put the emesis basin under their chin so the resident can spit out the solution.

   c. Remove the upper denture using a paper towel for a better grip. Loosen the denture by gently rocking it back and forth to help break the seal. Put it in the denture cup.
   d. Remove lower denture using a paper towel for better grip. Loosen it by gently rocking it back and forth. Put it in the denture cup.
3. Rinse the resident's mouth with mouthwash solution.
4. If the resident cannot rinse, use a swab moistened with water and mouthwash to clean the whole mouth, including the tongue and gums.
5. Explain that you will clean the dentures and then return them.
6. Take the denture cup with dentures, toothbrush, and toothpaste to the resident's bathroom.
7. Put toothpaste on the toothbrush.

8. Turn on cool water (hot water can damage dentures), put a small towel or face cloth on the bottom of the sink, and fill the sink halfway. (This helps prevent dentures from breaking if they slip from your hands.)

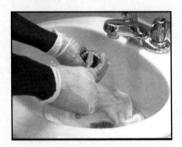

9. Hold the dentures over the sink and brush all surfaces.
10. Rinse the dentures with cool water.
11. Return the dentures to the denture cup.

12. If the resident uses denture adhesive, apply it to the dentures before putting them back in their mouth. If the resident does not want the dentures put back at this time, store them safely. Put them in a denture cup labeled with the resident's name and half filled with cool water.

Note: *Inspect the resident's mouth for bleeding, sores, a dry, coated tongue, and mouth odor. Report any changes to the nurse. If the resident has a partial plate with only a few artificial teeth, handle it the same way as a complete set of dentures. Be careful when you remove the partial plate, which has wires that support the teeth in place.*

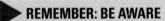 **REMEMBER: UNDERSTAND**

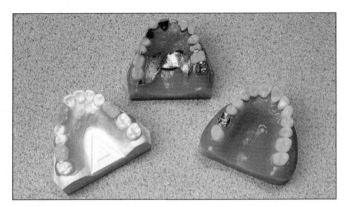

Fig. 16-5 — Some residents have partial dentures while others have full dentures.

Mouth Care for Comatose Residents

You may care for residents who are comatose. These residents are not aware of their surroundings and cannot respond. Comatose residents need mouth care every two hours (Procedure 16-8). Because they often breathe through their mouths, their mouths and lips become dry.

📖
Comatose – someone in a coma, unconscious

PROCEDURE 16-8.   MOUTH CARE FOR COMATOSE RESIDENTS

▶ **REMEMBER: BE AWARE**

Items Needed
- towels
- gloves
- toothettes
- cup with mouthwash
- protective jelly or lip balm
- plastic trash bag

1. Gently turn the resident's head toward you and elevate the head of the bed (if they can tolerate it) to prevent **aspiration**.

2. Put a towel over the resident's chest to protect their clothing.

3. Put on gloves.

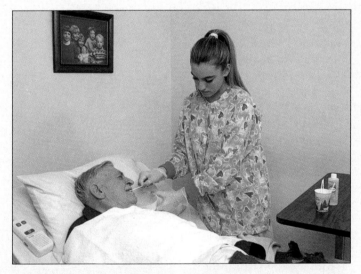

4. Gently open the resident's mouth and inspect the mouth, teeth, gums, and tongue for changes or signs of injury: bleeding sores, loose or broken teeth, dry coated tongue, or mouth odor. Using a toothette dipped in mouthwash, clean the inside of the mouth (gums, tongue, teeth, roof of the mouth, and insides of the cheeks).

Note: *Tap excess mouthwash off the toothette. Excess fluid can drip back into their throat and potentially cause aspiration.*

5. Using a corner of the towel draped over the resident's chest, dry any solution from around their mouth and chin.

6. Dispose of toothettes as you use them into the plastic trash bag.

7. Put protective jelly or lip balm on their lips to moisten them.

▶ **REMEMBER: UNDERSTAND**

📖
Aspirate – to breathe in or draw in by suction; in this case inhaling fluid or food into the lungs

GROOMING

Grooming care includes shaving (which may include the face, legs, and underarms), trimming facial hair, hair care, and care of fingernails and toenails.

Shaving

Shaving is a daily activity for many male residents. Some female residents may want their legs and underarms shaved during a shower or bath. Male residents can use an electric razor or a safety razor. Never share the same razor among different residents or recap disposable razors. Discard disposable razors in a sharp's container. Always check with the charge nurse before shaving a resident to learn if there are any special considerations. For example, some residents must use electric razors because their medication could cause too much bleeding if they were accidentally cut with a safety razor. Procedure 16-9 describes the steps for helping shave a male resident's face. Procedure 16-10 describes the steps for helping shave a resident's underarms, and Procedure 16-11 for helping shave a resident's legs.

Facial Hair

Some female residents have facial hair. This is common on the chin, on the upper lip, and under the lower lip. Never trim or shave this facial hair unless the resident requests it. Always check with the charge nurse before trimming facial hair (Procedure 16-12). Some residents or family members may request hair removal using a cream remover (depilatory). Follow the manufacturer's guidelines for storage and use of such products. A physician's order may be required.

PROCEDURE 16-9.   SHAVING A MALE RESIDENT'S FACE

▶ **REMEMBER: BE AWARE**

Items Needed
- razor
- shaving cream
- aftershave (if used)
- basin, half filled with warm water
- towel
- washcloth
- mirror
- plastic bag
- gloves

1. Observe the resident's face for any moles, rashes, or cuts. Do not shave those areas, or use extra care.

2. Place a towel over the resident's chest to protect their clothing.

3. Put on gloves.

4. Using a face cloth, wet the entire beard with warm water and apply shaving cream with your hands.

5. When the beard is well **lathered** and softened, start shaving. Shave in the direction the beard grows. Hold the skin tight and smooth by pulling the skin upward with one hand and shaving with a downward stroke with your other hand. Use short, even strokes. Be particularly careful with the neck, chin, and upper lip. Use upward strokes for the neck, downward and slightly diagonal strokes for the chin, and very short downward strokes above the lip.

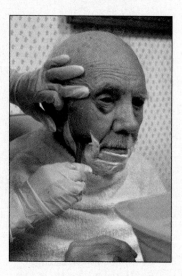

6. Rinse the razor in warm water after each stroke.

7. Wash and rinse the resident's face with the washcloth, dry his face, and apply aftershave lotion if he prefers.

8. Give the resident a mirror to look at his face.

9. Remove the towel from the resident's chest.

▶ **REMEMBER: UNDERSTAND**

📖
Lather — foam or froth when shaving cream or soap is mixed with water

PROCEDURE 16-10.   SHAVING A FEMALE RESIDENT'S UNDERARMS

▶ REMEMBER: BE AWARE

Items Needed
- razor
- soap
- basin half filled with warm water
- towel
- washcloth
- plastic bag
- gloves

1. Put the towel under the resident's shoulder on the side you are working from.

2. Raise the resident's arm up along their ear to expose the underarm.

3. Wash the area with warm water.

4. Lather some soap and apply it over the area to be shaved.

5. Carefully shave the area, moving the razor downward from the arm toward the chest.

6. Rinse the soap away thoroughly and pat the area dry.

7. Move the towel to under the opposite shoulder and repeat the steps above.

▶ REMEMBER: UNDERSTAND

PROCEDURE 16-11.   SHAVING A FEMALE RESIDENT'S LEGS

▶ REMEMBER: BE AWARE

Items Needed
- razor
- soap
- basin half filled with warm water
- towel
- washcloth
- plastic bag
- gloves

1. Place a towel under the resident's leg to be shaved.

2. Wash the part of the leg to be shaved with warm water.

3. Lather some soap or use shaving cream. Spread it over the entire area to be shaved.

4. Carefully shave the area, moving the razor upward from the ankle to the knee.

Note: *Ask the resident if she wants the area above her knee shaved.*

5. Be sure to rinse the soap thoroughly and pat the area dry.

6. Move the towel under the other leg and repeat the steps above.

▶ REMEMBER: UNDERSTAND

PROCEDURE 16-12.   TRIMMING FACIAL HAIR

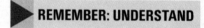

REMEMBER: BE AWARE

Items Needed
- safety scissors
- mirror

1. Using safety scissors, carefully trim the facial hair. Be careful not to trim too close to the skin.

2. Give the resident a mirror to look at her face.

REMEMBER: UNDERSTAND

Hair Care

Hair care includes regular shampooing and daily brushing, combing, and styling. Daily brushing or combing, along with good nutrition and adequate fluid intake, promotes healthy hair and scalp. Hairstyle is a personal matter. Many long term facilities have beauty shop services. Offer these services to the residents and follow the facility's procedures for notifying the beautician if a resident wishes to have their hair, cut, washed, or styled. Different cultures have different hair and scalp care preferences, and you should try to honor their requests. Ask the resident or a family member about their hair care preferences. For example, an African-American resident may want a deep protein conditioner put in her hair once a week and a moisturizer applied daily to prevent dryness and breakage. Always ask residents their preference in hairstyles. Encourage residents to brush and comb their own hair. If a resident cannot brush or comb their own hair, follow the steps in Procedure 16-13.

Care of Fingernails

Fingernail care includes daily cleaning and regular nail trimming. Although the visible part of the nail is not living tissue, the skin around and under it is, and you must protect this area from injury and infection. Trimmed, smooth nails also prevent a resident from accidentally scratching and injuring their skin. If a resident cannot clean and trim their own fingernails, follow the steps in Procedure 16-14. You can do this as part of a resident's complete bed bath or tub bath.

Care of Toenails

Toenails are usually thicker than fingernails, especially in older adults. Foot care is important because older residents are more likely to have an infection if skin breakdown occurs because their circulation in their feet may be poor. Foot care includes cleaning and trimming the toenails (Procedure 16-15). A podiatrist, nurse, or physician usually trims toenails. Follow your facility's policy. Inspect residents' feet and between the toes for skin condition. Look for **corns**, **calluses**, or other problems. Report any signs of poor circulation (pale color of the nail bed, feet very cold, swelling), reddened areas, skin breakdown, or cracking of the skin between the toes.

(text continued on p. 314)

Callus – a thickened or hard area of skin

Corn – a local hardening and thickening of the epidermis, or outer layer of skin (as on a toe)

Podiatrist – physician specializing in the care and treatment of the feet

PROCEDURE 16-13.   HAIR CARE

▶ **REMEMBER: BE AWARE**

Items Needed
- resident's own brush or comb
- mirror
- personal items for styling

1. Brush hair gently. If the resident's hair is long and tangled, remove tangles first with a comb. Start at the ends and work your way up to the scalp.

2. Gently brush and style the hair to the resident's preference. Use any personal items they may request, such as hair spray, clips, or gel.

3. Give the resident a mirror so they can see their hair.

▶ **REMEMBER: UNDERSTAND**

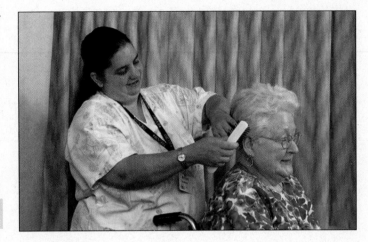

PROCEDURE 16-14.   CARE OF FINGERNAILS

▶ **REMEMBER: BE AWARE**

Items Needed
- bath basin half filled with warm water
- towel
- washcloth
- soap
- lotion
- orangewood stick
- nail clippers
- nail file (or emery board)

1. Place the basin of warm water on the over-bed table.

2. Ask the resident to soak their hands in the basin 3-5 minutes.

3. Leaving one hand in the water, wash and rinse the resident's other hand. Dry the hand and place it on a dry towel.

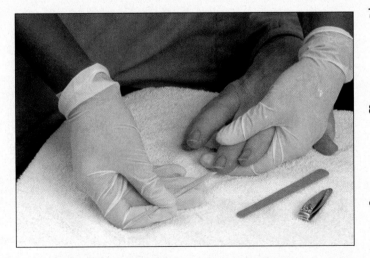

4. Clean under the nails with the orangewood stick.

5. Repeat with the other hand.

6. Inspect the resident's hands for cracks in the skin, unusual spots or discoloration, and rough areas.

7. Trim the resident's fingernails using the nail clipper. Clip nails straight across. Shape and remove any rough edges using an emery board or nail file.

8. Put lotion on the resident's hands and gently massage the hands from fingertips toward the wrists to stimulate circulation.

9. Tell the nurse about any redness, irritation, broken skin, or loose skin.

▶ **REMEMBER: UNDERSTAND**

PROCEDURE 16-15.   CARE OF TOENAILS

> **REMEMBER: BE AWARE**

Items Needed
- bath basin half full with warm water
- two towels
- soap
- washcloth
- orangewood stick
- lotion
- shoes and socks

1. To give foot care to a resident sitting in a chair, put a towel on the floor and the basin of water on the towel.

Note: *Foot care can be done while a resident is in bed, usually during a bed bath. Put a towel on the bed and the basin on the towel. Ask the resident to flex their leg and soak one foot at a time.*

2. Help the resident to remove their shoes and socks.

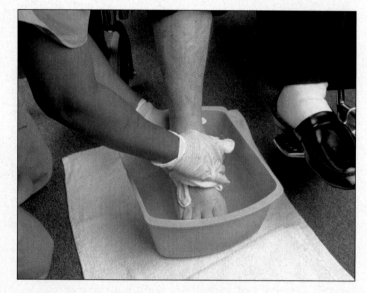

3. Place the resident's feet in the basin of warm water.

4. Soak the feet for 3-5 minutes.

5. Clean under the toenails with the orangewood stick to remove any dirt. Scrub calloused areas with a warm wash cloth.

6. Wash, rinse, dry, and inspect the feet thoroughly. Report any redness, irritation, or cracked, broken, loose, dry, or discolored skin. Report any calloused areas, corns, or loose or broken nails.

7. Apply lotion to the tops of the feet, soles of the feet, and heels. Do not apply lotion between the toes.

8. Help the resident put on clean stockings or socks and shoes.

9. Tell the charge nurse if the resident needs toenail trimming.

> **REMEMBER: UNDERSTAND**

(text continued from p. 312)

ASSISTING THE RESIDENT WITH DRESSING AND UNDRESSING

Some residents can dress and undress by themselves, while others need help. It depends on the individual. For example:
- A blind resident may need help choosing color-coordinated clothes and getting clothes from their closet.
- A resident with limited shoulder mobility may need help zipping up a dress.
- A resident who gets dizzy when bending over may need help putting on and taking off their shoes and stockings.
- A confused resident may need help putting on clothes properly. Always encourage a resident to choose the clothes they want to wear.

Procedure 16-16 describes the steps for helping a dependent resident get dressed. Procedure 16-17 describes the steps for undressing a dependent resident.

PROCEDURE 16-16.
DRESSING A DEPENDENT RESIDENT

> ### ▶ REMEMBER: BE AWARE

Items Needed
- clothes, undergarments
- stocking, socks, shoes
- accessories resident wants to wear (belt, tie, jewelry)
- plastic-covered pad (if resident is in bed)

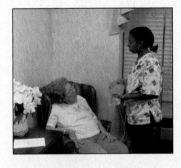

Note: *If a resident has a weak or paralyzed arm or has an IV in one arm, help them to put a shirt or dress sleeve on that arm first. With an IV, move the solution through the sleeve first and hang it on the pole. Gently guide the resident's arm through the sleeve, being careful not to dislodge the IV needle or tube. If the resident has an IV pump, call the nurse for assistance. Use this method also for a weak leg. Dress the weak side first.*

1. Remove the resident' gown or pajamas. Offer the resident a choice of clothing.

Note: *For privacy and to prevent chill, remove the top portion of the resident's gown or pajamas first. Help the resident dress on top with clean clothes, and then move to the bottom.*

2. Help the resident put on their undershirt or bra, shirt or blouse, or dress.

3. Help the resident put on underwear, stockings or socks, and pants or a skirt. Depending on the type of garment, follow these steps:

To put on a garment that opens in the back:
a. Slide the garment onto the resident's arm and shoulder on the weaker side.
b. Slide the garment onto the arm and shoulder of the stronger side.
c. Bring the sides of the garment to the back.
d. Turn the resident toward you, and bring the side of the garments to the back.
e. Turn the resident away from you, and bring the other side of the garment to the resident's back.
f. Fasten the buttons, snaps, ties, or zipper.
g. Place the resident in the supine position.

To put on a garment that opens in the front:
a. Slide the garment onto the resident's arm and shoulder on the weaker side.
b. Bring the resident to a sitting position, and bring the garment around the back. Lower the resident to the supine position.
c. Slide the garment onto the resident's arm and shoulder on the stronger side.
d. Fasten buttons, snaps, ties, or zipper.

To put on a pullover garment:
a. Place the resident in the supine position.
b. Bring the neck of the garment over the resident's head.
c. Slide the arm and shoulder of the garment onto the resident's weaker side.
d. Raise the resident to a semi-sitting position, bring the garment down over the their shoulder, and slide the arm and shoulder of the garment on the resident's stronger side.

Note: *If the resident cannot assume a sitting position, turn the resident toward you and pull the garment down on the back. Then turn the resident to the other side, and slide their stronger arm and shoulder into the garment. Pull the garment down in the back.*

e. Fasten the buttons, snaps, ties, or zipper.

To put on pants or slacks:
a. Slide the pants over the resident's feet and up their legs.
b. Ask the resident to raise their hips and buttocks off the bed.

c. Bring the pants up over their buttocks and hips.

Note: *If the resident cannot raise their buttocks and hips, turn them onto their stronger side. Then pull the pants up over their hips and buttocks on their weaker side. Turn the resident onto the other side and repeat the process.*

d. Fasten the buttons, snaps, ties, or zipper.

4. Help the resident put on socks, shoes, or non-skid slippers before they stand, so that they do not slip on the floor. When you put their shoes on in bed, put a pad on the bed to protect the bedding.

5. Help the resident stand so you can smooth out their clothing and fasten and neatly tuck in their shirt or blouse.

6. Help them put on any accessories they want to wear.

7. If a resident has a prosthesis or adaptive equipment (such as eyeglasses, dentures, hearing aid, or an artificial limb), help the resident to put the item on.

8. Collect soiled garments, and place them in a hamper for the laundry according to the facility's procedure.

Note: *Residents are usually helped out of bed after dressing for the day.*

> ### ▶ REMEMBER: UNDERSTAND

PROCEDURE 16-17. UNDRESSING A DEPENDENT RESIDENT

Items Needed
- clothing to be worn after undressing

Note: *This procedure is easier if the resident is sitting on the side of the bed.*

Note: *If a resident has a weak or paralyzed arm or an IV, remove clothing from other side first and then from the weak side or the side with the IV. If the resident has an IV, carefully guide the tubing and solution through the sleeve as the resident's arm moves.*

1. Help the resident remove upper garments (shirt, dress, blouse, and undergarments).

2. Help the resident put on the top half of their pajamas or nightgown.

3. Help the resident remove their shoes or stockings and pants or skirt.

4. If wearing pajamas, help them put on the bottoms.

5. Help the resident into bed.

PREPARING FOR AN EVENT

Just as you like to look nice when you have visitors or go out, residents also like to look good for special events (Fig. 16-6). Help a resident feel good about a coming event by helping them get ready. If visitors are coming, you may help them with grooming and personal care before the visit. Remove any clutter and bring in extra chairs if needed.

If a resident is leaving the facility on an outing, talk with the family in advance. A family member may want to help the resident prepare that day. If not, find out what time the resident needs to be ready. Find out where they are going. Do they need to wear special clothes? If the weather is rainy or cold, be sure they have the right outer wear and accessories, including hat, gloves, boots, and so on.

Preparing for a big event may be confusing for some residents. Remind them what is going to happen, especially if the resident has memory loss. This keeps them from being surprised and gives them something to look forward to. If a resident will be away overnight, prepare an overnight bag of essential things. Make a checklist to be sure you do not forget anything.

The extra attention you give a resident preparing for a visit or an outing helps both the resident and the family feel good. They will appreciate your effort.

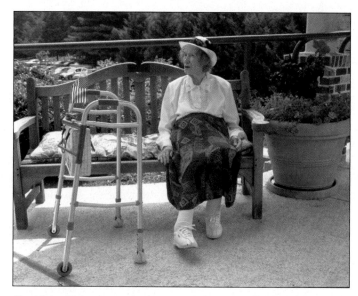

Fig. 16-6 – Make sure residents are dressed appropriately when going to an event.

IN THIS CHAPTER YOU LEARNED:

- What personal care is
- How to make routine activities mindful and to include the resident's preferences in daily routines
- Why it is important to determine a resident's needs for assistance during personal care
- Why observation is important during personal care
- How to perform the following skills:
  - complete bed bath
  - perineal care
  - back rub
  - tub bath
  - shower
  - whirlpool bath
  - shampoo and conditioning
  - brushing and flossing
  - caring for dentures
  - mouth care for a comatose resident
  - shaving
  - trimming facial hair
  - hair care
  - care of fingernails
  - care of toenails
  - assisting with dressing and undressing

SUMMARY

This chapter discusses how important it is for you to get to know the resident's likes and dislikes about personal care. Keep routine care activities from becoming mindless, automatic activities. Give personal care using your observation skills, and determine residents' needs for assistance. Encourage as much independence as possible.

Learning personal care skills is a major part of your job. Your work will often be evaluated by other staff and family members based on how you give personal care. Remember to always provide privacy when giving personal care. Treat each resident with respect and dignity. A good way to remember how important privacy, dignity, and respect are is to always think how you would want to be treated or how you would want a loved one treated.

PULLING IT ALL TOGETHER

You are assigned to care for six residents in rooms 1, 2, and 3. During report, you write down all the information about your assigned residents. The charge nurse tells you that two of your residents are scheduled for showers today, and Mrs. Jones and Mrs. Smith have hairdresser appointments at 10 a.m.

First you greet all six residents and let them know that you are the nurse assistant caring for them today. Before breakfast you help each resident with toileting, washing their hands and face, and oral hygiene. After breakfast you schedule the shower room at 8:30 a.m. and 9 a.m. for the two residents needing showers. At 8 a.m. Mrs. Billings and Mrs. Waters want to get washed and dressed. Mrs. Billings can care for herself, but she has vision problems and asks you to help her pick out matching clothes. Mrs. Waters needs help bathing. You help her get started and stay close by so she can call you when she is ready for you to wash her back and help her get dressed. At 8:30 and 9 a.m. you help Mrs. Wright and then Mrs. Evans to the shower room for their showers and then help them get dressed.

Mrs. Jones told you at breakfast she would like to rest for an hour after eating. At 9:15 a.m. you tell Mrs. Jones the time and say that she may want to get ready for the hairdresser. Mrs. Jones likes to go into the bathroom to wash and can do her own personal care. Mrs. Smith had a stroke and is paralyzed on her right side. She needs a complete bed bath and oral hygiene and needs help getting dressed. Before starting Mrs. Smith's bath you schedule another nurse assistant to help you turn Mrs. Smith on her side to wash her back, help her get dressed, and transfer her from the bed to her wheelchair. After Mrs. Smith's bath, you take her and Mrs. Jones to the hairdresser. When you come back, you have time to do nail care for Mrs. Wright, Mrs. Evans, and Mrs. Waters. When all six residents' personal care is done, you can now care for each resident's room before lunch.

As you look back at what you have done in such a short period of time, you see how you can pull it all together to meet each resident's needs. Gather information about each resident you care for, organize your time, and remember that every day will be different.

1. **When you provide personal care, it is important to:**
   A. Have all morning care done before 8 a.m.
   B. Never give care that has not been explicitly requested by the family.
   C. Keep on schedule, even if you have to rush slow residents.
   D. Encourage the resident to do all that they can for themselves.

2. **Mrs. Cortez's family is coming to visit today. How would you begin getting Mrs. Cortez ready?**
   A. Style her hair the way you think looks best.
   B. Skip her bath to give her more time to get dressed.
   C. Plan her a.m. care with her preferences in mind.
   D. Quickly pick out her clothes for her and schedule a tub bath right away.

3. **What is a benefit of observing residents carefully while providing personal care?**
   A. It frees you from having to observe residents at other times.
   B. You have the opportunity to talk with residents about family members.
   C. You may note both physical and psychological changes in residents.
   D. You can decide whether or not to give residents their medications, depending on how they feel.

4. **During Mrs. Mahler's bed bath she complains of a burning feeling in the perineal area. What should you do?**
   A. Call the family and ask them to bring an ointment.
   B. Report this to the charge nurse.
   C. Leave her alone in the bath and go find a doctor.
   D. Tell her the burning is normal and will go away soon.

5. **When should you wear gloves?**
   A. While giving a back rub.
   B. While brushing the resident's hair.
   C. When providing oral hygiene or perineal care.
   D. Whenever the resident's hands feel dry or chapped.

6. **What should the water temperature be in a tub or whirlpool?**
   A. 90 to 98.6 F.
   B. 98.6 to 103 F.
   C. 103 to 106 F.
   D. 90 to 106 F.

7. **What is a possible problem resulting from bathing too often?**
   A. The resident smells like soap.
   B. The resident becomes over-hydrated
   C. The resident often feels chilled.
   D. The resident's skin becomes dry.

8. **You are about to shave a male resident's face. Which of the following statements is true about how you should do this?**
   A. The resident's razor is missing, so it's OK to use his roommate's razor as long as the roommate agrees.
   B. Hold the skin tight and smooth by pulling the skin upward with one hand and shaving with a downward stroke with your other hand.
   C. After shaving the resident with a disposable razor, carefully replace the cap on the razor.
   D. Apply shaving cream to just a small portion of the face at a time to prevent the resident's skin from becoming too cold.

9. **Mrs. Weinberg is comatose. Her mouth care procedure includes:**
   A. Using a toothette dipped in mouthwash.
   B. Encouraging her to do all she can for herself.
   C. Using the brand of toothpaste her family prefers.
   D. Brushing her teeth with a soft-bristle toothbrush.

10. **You are providing foot care for Mr. Daly. Which of the following do you normally do?**
    A. Clip his toenails.
    B. Soak his feet in cold water.
    C. Apply powder between his toes.
    D. Clean under his toenails with an orangewood stick.

(Answers to "Check What You've Learned" are in the Instructor's Manual.)

Chapter 17

ASSISTING WITH NUTRITION

Food and nutrition are an important part of life. When people age or become ill, however, their appetite often changes. This can create a challenge for their care. The nutritional status of residents in long term care has been studied a lot in recent years. Because residents' weight is easy to track and often reveals much about their care and health, weight is considered an indication of the residents' quality of life and care in a long term care facility.

Weight loss can also occur due to acute or chronic disease. Some residents do not feel well or have chronic diseases that lead to loss of appetite. Their chronic illnesses may also affect their ability to eat by themselves or to swallow or chew. Many residents also take medications that alter their appetites. Because of memory loss caused by dementia, some residents forget to eat or question why they are being fed. These problems can also lead to weight loss and deteriorating health. The goal is to prevent weight loss by timely interventions.

Poor nutritional status has negative effects on residents. The resident and family members may be shocked by the resident's frail, thin body. Poor nutritional status also lowers their resistance to infection, can contribute to pressure ulcers and other diseases, and reduces their quality of life.

As a nurse assistant you play an important role in maintaining or improving residents' nutritional status. You can support them when they need help, offer them supplements or snacks if appropriate throughout the day, and interact with them while they are dining to make eating a more pleasant experience. You can also report any change in their appetite so that they receive appropriate medical care.

This chapter discusses how you can help improve residents' nutritional health. You have a responsibility to help make residents' dining experiences pleasant. You also need to know how to feed residents.

OBJECTIVES
- Explain the role of the food service department and how you work with that department
- List ways to provide and encourage good nutrition
- Give examples of ways to make dining a pleasant experience
- Demonstrate how to properly record residents' intake and output

MEDICAL TERMS
- **Dehydration** – a serious condition that can occur if a resident does not have adequate fluid intake
- **Dysphagia** – a condition that causes a problem chewing or swallowing food, liquid, or medication
- **Esophagus** – the muscular tube that leads from the mouth to the stomach
- **Hydration** – maintaining adequate fluid in the body
- **Supplement** – a concentrated form of nutrition given to a resident in addition to their meals
- **Therapeutic diet** – special diet that is a treatment for a disease or condition
- **Turgor** – the normal ability of the skin to change shape and return to its normal position, such as after being gently pinched up ("tented")

"Your encouragement and cheerful conversation make me look forward to my meals."

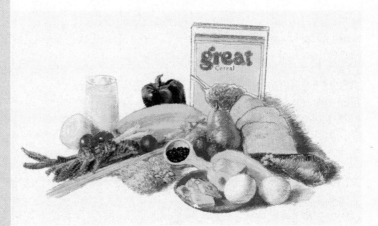

Fig. 17-1 — Eating a variety of food helps people stay healthy.

Think about what food means to you. Do you know the saying "You are what you eat"? This means that what you put in your body affects how you look and how you feel. Consider how our culture emphasizes food on television and in magazines. Most people associate food with pleasant activities such as being with friends. Food and **nutrition** help people stay healthy and happy (Fig. 17-1). We all have our own food preferences and customs. Think about why you eat what you eat. People have different reasons for their eating habits. All the following factors affect our eating:

- cognitive abilities: to recognize food and to remember how to eat
- taste: a person's own likes and dislikes for foods
- culture: how a person has been raised and their cultural practices
- state of health: people often eat less when they feel ill
- emotional state: people often enjoy food more when they are happy and relaxed but enjoy it less when sad or depressed
- ability to chew and swallow: a person's appetite or ability to eat may change after dental work, a sore throat, or a stroke
- social situation: people often eat differently when they are alone than with friends and family

As you can see, our feelings about food and our appetite are affected by many things. Everyone is affected by these factors in different ways. These factors can help you understand how residents' eating may be affected. As a nurse assistant, you have an important effect on the nutritional status of residents you care for.

THE ROLE OF THE FOOD SERVICE DEPARTMENT

The food service department in a long term care facility has many tasks. It provides residents with food that is safe, nutritional, and appealing. It must also ensure that every resident receives the correct diet ordered by the physician in a form that meets their needs. Most facilities use a cycle menu. This means the same meals are repeated, or cycled, over a time period, usually 3 to 6 weeks. Many long term care facilities allow residents to select from a menu based on their own preferences.

Different facilities make different types of diets available. Most facilities have **therapeutic diets** that offer choices based on residents' preferences. This is important because residents on therapeutic diets often do not enjoy all the foods they are allowed. If they do not enjoy their food, they may not eat enough and may lose weight, leading to negative health effects. The trend in long term care is to "liberalize" residents' diets, which means making

Nutrition – the act of nourishing or being nourished
Therapeutic diet – special diet that is a treatment for a disease or condition

them as normal as possible. As a nurse assistant, you will work closely with the food service department to meet the nutritional needs of each resident.

ASSESSING RESIDENTS' NUTRITION

Nutrition and hydration affect residents' quality of life and quality of care in many ways. Good nutrition and hydration:

- help maintain skin integrity to prevent or heal pressure ulcers
- help the body fight infections and disease
- maintain the person's overall strength and preserve functional abilities such as the abilities to walk, to eat independently, and to perform other activities of daily living
- maintain normal bowel and bladder functions
- maintain normal weight and energy stores

A person's nutritional needs increase at certain times. For example, needs change when the person has a fever, a recent fracture or surgery, or pressure ulcers. A person also needs more fluid with fever, a urinary tract infection, persistent vomiting or diarrhea, or wound drainage. Hot weather also increases residents' fluid needs because they lose fluid through perspiration.

Because adequate food and fluid intake are essential for residents' health and well-being, intake measurements are important. Later in this chapter you will learn how to measure residents' food and fluid intake and output. These measurements help determine if a resident needs nutritional intervention.

WORKING TOGETHER TO PROVIDE THE BEST FOR THE RESIDENT

Like you, residents have food preferences. These may be based on personal, religious, regional, or ethnic factors. The best way to learn what a resident likes and dislikes is to ask them or family members.

A resident's personal preferences may involve the appearance, familiarity, or taste of a food. Ask questions like these:

- What foods do you like?
- What do you dislike?
- What does a specific portion size look like to you?
- How often do you eat and when?

Some preferences result from religious traditions. For example, some Catholics do not eat meat on Fridays, and some Jews eat only kosher foods.

A resident may have regional preferences, such as grits in the South.

Ethnic preferences usually come from a resident's cultural heritage, such as an Italian, Latin American, or Asian heritage (Fig. 17-2).

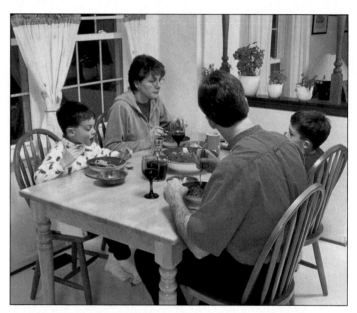

Fig. 17-2 – A resident's food choices are influenced by their cultural heritage and what they ate growing up.

All these factors play a major role in what residents want to eat, how they like their food prepared, and when they like to eat. Work with the resident, family members, and the food service to meet each resident's preferences.

Residents have a right to make choices and to express their food preferences and dislikes. The food service and nursing departments use a team approach to respond to these needs. The food service staff asks about a resident's preferences soon after admission. They will substitute foods for those the resident does not eat. If a resident refuses food, you must offer to get them something else. This is important for all residents and is critical for those who are underweight or who do not eat well. Early after admission, monitor the resident's preferences and the amounts they eat. This information helps the dietitian plan meals for the resident. An early understanding of the resident's food preferences will help prevent future problems.

Hydration — maintaining adequate fluid in the body

HELPING RESIDENTS WITH A SPECIAL DIET

Because the facility is the resident's home and the resident may be on the diet for a long time, the goal is to meet their dietary needs with as few food restrictions as possible. Residents dislike restrictions when they can no longer have their favorite foods or seasonings. For example, a resident with diabetes may tell you that at home they ate a pastry every day, and that helped them accept their other restrictions on sweets. Giving the charge nurse this information is important. It may be decided that changing this routine could cause the resident distress.

As another example, a resident with heart disease may be on a low-cholesterol diet. If they love butter on their toast, they may become upset when they can no longer eat buttered toast. Because of restrictions, the resident may eat less or become depressed. They may feel that everything they enjoy is changing. Therefore it is important to tell the charge nurse the resident's preferences so the team can balance restrictions in a therapeutic diet with those preferences.

Although many residents eat a regular diet, some require special types of diet, called a therapeutic diet. This is usually part of their therapy for a disease or condition. A therapeutic diet, such as a diabetic diet, is ordered by the resident's physician. A therapeutic diet can sometimes reduce or eliminate the need for medication. In addition, the consistency or texture of foods in any diet may be modified to meet the person's needs. Food may be chopped, ground, thickened, or pureed for residents with problems chewing. Chewing problems may come from ill-fitting or not having dentures, or a tooth or gum condition. Chewing or swallowing problems caused by a stroke or other digestive difficulties may also require a changed food consistency (Fig. 17-3).

The food service department prepares therapeutic diets along with any special considerations for residents with food allergies, food intolerances, or other special needs or preferences. The cook may also grind, chop, thicken, or puree some portions of each meal to meet the food consistency needs of some residents.

The facility usually tries to limit restrictions on a resident's diet, because the outcome is clearly negative if the resident does not eat. Discussing their diet with residents can help to find a balance. Therapeutic diets commonly ordered by the physician are:

• **Calorie-restricted diets.** These diets usually range from 1200 to 1800 calories per day and are often ordered for weight reduction.

• **No-concentrated-sweets (NCS) diet.** This is a liberal version of a diabetic diet that restricts only foods that are high in simple sugars, such as many desserts, foods prepared with sugar, and sugar packets.

• **No-added-salt diets.** These diets are usually ordered for residents with fluid retention or high blood pressure (Fig. 17-4). These residents do not receive salt on their trays and do not receive foods containing a lot of sodium, such as canned soups; salted crackers; or cured meats such as ham, bacon, or corned beef.

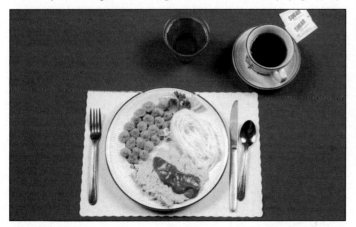

Fig. 17-3 – The consistency of food can be changed to meet the resident's needs.

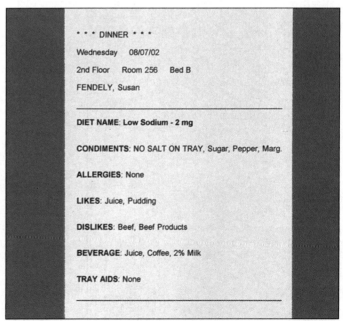

Fig. 17-4 – Some residents are on therapeutic diets.

📖
Sodium – salt

- **Fat-restricted and/or cholesterol-restricted diets.** Fat-restricted diets may be ordered for residents with diseases of the liver, gallbladder, pancreas, or cardiovascular system or for residents who have a malabsorption syndrome (difficulty absorbing nutrients) and cannot tolerate fat. Low-cholesterol diets are used to reduce blood fat levels. Foods high in fat, such as bacon, sausage, cream, gravy, margarine, whole milk, and high-fat desserts, are restricted.
- **Renal diets.** These diets are ordered for residents with kidney or liver disease and may make it possible to postpone dialysis or transplant surgery. Sometimes there are protein, sodium, phosphorus, and potassium restrictions as well. These diets can be difficult for a resident to follow if the restriction is severe. Restricted foods may include meat, eggs, dairy products, and some breads and other foods that contain small amounts of protein. A renal diet must be carefully calculated.

Serving food at the correct temperature also involves a team approach. Food must be kept at the correct temperature. Once food leaves the kitchen, you must serve it as quickly as possible: while hot foods are still hot and cold foods cold. This reduces the risk of foodborne illness as well as making the food more appetizing.

MAKING THE DINING EXPERIENCE PLEASANT

A meal is much more than just eating. Mealtimes should be pleasurable and enhance the resident's well-being (Fig.

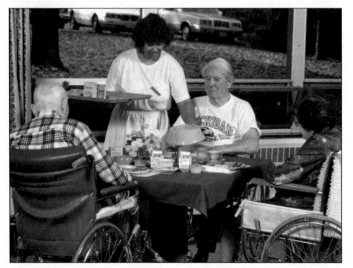

Fig. 17-5 — The environment, service, and social factors influence the dining experience for the resident.

17-5). Think about factors that affect how you feel when you dine out. Attractive surroundings, pleasant company, and courteous service all increase your enjoyment. The dining experience in a nursing facility is similar. Many factors can influence how residents feel about the experience and affect their food intake. Environmental, service, and social factors are all important.

Environmental Factors

Environmental factors involve the physical surroundings. Residents have a right to expect the dining room to be clean, uncluttered, and free of unpleasant odors. Table linens, if used, should be clean and pressed. The room temperature should be comfortable. Lighting should be soft, not glaring. The sun should not shine in anyone's eyes.

Table height is also important for residents' comfort. If a table is too high, residents must reach up. This can cause fatigue and lead to eating too little. Residents in wheelchairs should sit at tables high enough to allow wheelchairs under the table so that residents can get close to the table. Tables are arranged so that residents can come and go freely, even with walkers or wheelchairs.

Soft music, flowers, and pretty dishes also add to the pleasure of dining. Dishes should be sparkling clean and free of chips and cracks. There should be no distractions such as a loud TV or radio. Do not stack plate covers on the table or scrape dishes while residents are still eating.

Service Factors

Also consider dining service factors. Has a rude waiter ever spoiled a restaurant meal for you? Your attitude toward residents can similarly affect their dining experience.

Speak to residents in a polite, pleasant voice. Your caring, patient attitude adds to their enjoyment of the meal. Encourage residents to take their time to finish, without hurrying or rushing them. Some residents will stop eating if they think you are waiting for them to finish.

When serving the meal, refer to the food in a positive way. Your tone of voice and attitude can have a positive or negative influence on how residents view the meal.

Social Factors

Social factors also directly affect the dining experience. Encourage residents to sit with their friends. If a resident has no friends, such as when they are new to the facility, direct them to a table of residents of similar mental status. Do not seat alert and oriented residents with confused, disruptive ones. Try to create a pleasant, home-like atmosphere where residents will look forward to meals and enjoy the experience.

All these factors are also important for residents eating in their rooms. Remove any clutter from the over-bed table, prevent any unpleasant odors, and adjust the table height correctly. Remove food from the tray and position it properly on the plate. Do not carry out nursing tasks, such as taking vital signs, during meals. If possible, encourage the resident to come to the dining room.

ASSISTING RESIDENTS WITH MEALS

One of your most important duties as a nurse assistant is to help residents with meals (Fig. 17-6). Although you might think this is a simple matter of common sense, it actually requires a lot of attention. Your ability to do it well directly affects residents' nutritional status and overall health.

Preparing Residents for Meals

Residents more fully enjoy their meals when they are properly prepared for them. Before the meal, if desired, comb a resident's hair and help female residents with their makeup. If needed, help the resident with toileting before taking them to the dining room. Encourage residents to use their dentures, glasses, and hearing aids. These devices improve residents' functional abilities and help them be more independent. Also help residents with handwashing and oral care as needed. Oral care before meals may improve residents' taste sensitivity to some food flavors. If a resident is eating in bed, elevate the head of the bed to at least 30 degrees. Make each resident as comfortable as possible. Use clothing protectors or napkins to protect their clothing.

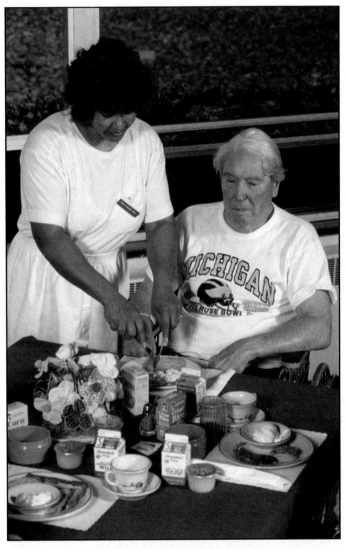

Fig. 17-6 — Always check the diet card, remove the food from the tray, and remove any covers, lids, plastic wrap, or foil. Some residents may need help cutting their food.

Tray Preparation

Before assisting with a meal, wash your hands thoroughly. This is an important part of infection control. Deliver trays as quickly as possible to help cold foods stay cold and hot foods hot. Put yourself in the resident's place. How would you feel if you were hungry and your tray was ready, but no one came to serve you for 20 to 30 minutes?

When you remove the tray from the cart, first check the diet card. This tells you which tray goes to which resident. Do you have the right tray for the person you are serving? Is the diet correct? For example, there should not be a salt packet on a tray for a resident on a low-sodium diet. Also check whether the resident has special feeding instructions.

Remove the food from the tray. Put the plate directly on the table for a more home-like feeling. Remove any covers and underliners from the plate unless the person is not ready to eat. It is better for residents to be ready for the meal before it is served, but some residents may arrive late. Serve the resident their food when they arrive.

After you remove plate covers and underliners, put them back on the tray and return them to the service cart or to another cart. Put the plate within the resident's easy reach. This is a good time to review the meal with residents who may not see well or may be unfamiliar with some foods. Describe foods enthusiastically so that the resident looks forward to eating. How you would feel if a restaurant waiter remarked "The chili looks terrible!" when serving you? Would you want to eat it?

Once the plate is within the resident's easy reach, ask the resident if they need help removing any plastic wrap, lids, or foil. Open condiments and cartons. Ask residents if they want seasoning (if permitted for them). Encourage residents to express their preferences.

Serving Residents

Slow eaters are often served first. After you have served the first resident at the table, move on to others at the same table. Serve all residents at a table before moving to the next table. Again, think of yourself in a restaurant. Have you ever been served later than everyone else at your table? It is frustrating to watch others eat and maybe even finish their meal while you are still waiting. Such a delay reduces the pleasure of eating together.

Assisting Residents With Meals

1. Prepare residents before the meal. Help them as needed with grooming, handwashing, and oral care. Residents should sit upright at a 90-degree angle, with their feet touching the floor.

2. Help residents to the dining room or make them comfortable in their rooms. If possible, transfer the resident from a wheelchair to a dining room chair.

3. Wash your hands.

4. Position napkins and clothing protectors.

5. Pass trays quickly to ensure cold foods stay cold and hot foods hot.

6. Check tray cards: Make sure the name matches the person and the diet appears correct and complete. Check for any special feeding instructions.

7. Put the plate on the table, open cartons, remove wrappings, cut meats, and season food as the resident prefers.

8. While serving the meal, describe foods positively.

9. Make sure each resident is close enough to the table to reach their food and silverware.

10. Encourage residents to feed themselves as much as possible.

11. Serve all residents at one table before moving to the next.

12. Check with residents frequently to offer assistance or substitutes for foods they are not eating.

13. Be sure each resident has enough time to finish their meal.

14. Remove the tray and make sure each resident's hands and face are clean and that they are comfortable.

Give residents any help they need, such as cutting their meat or other food. Encourage residents to be as independent as possible, but watch for residents who need help. If you cut the meat for them, cut it in small pieces to prevent choking.

After you have served residents, check with them often to offer help as needed or to encourage them to eat. Some residents respond to prompting. Give all residents enough time to finish their meal. Some residents eat much more slowly than others. If a resident does not eat well or rejects a particular food, offer to get a substitute, especially if the resident is underweight or poorly nourished. Food substitutes are available through the food service department or from food supplies on each unit in the facility.

A resident may have certain food likes and dislikes based on their personal, religious, regional, or ethnic background. Every resident has the right to expect a substitute for something they do not want to eat. By federal regulation you must offer a substitute, and the food service department must provide it. A resident should never leave the dining room hungry or be given food they cannot eat. Offering substitutes also shows your caring attitude.

Note: *Residents should not take food from the dining room to eat later. Unrefrigerated food increases the risk of foodborne illness.*

Assisting With Feeding Residents

Many residents can eat independently or with a little help from the staff. Other residents must be fed. These residents totally depend on the staff to meet their nutritional needs. An occupational therapist may assess residents who are difficult to feed or who have special problems. The therapist will train you to use special feeding techniques if needed.

Remember that the resident depends completely on you and others for their nutrition. Imagine your own family member in this situation. Before leaving the resident, ask yourself:
- Have I done all I can to encourage this resident to eat?
- Have I provided the best nutrition possible?

General Guidelines for Feeding Most Residents

1. Prepare each resident for the meal. Provide oral care, wash the resident's hands, and make the resident comfortable. Check the resident's positioning. Elevate the head of the bed to at least 75 to 90 degrees. Cover the resident with a clothing protector or a large napkin. Remember to preserve the resident's dignity at all times. Make sure to check the tray card and ask the resident to ensure accuracy of the meal being served.
2. Take foods off the tray and put them on the table in front of the resident, and describe each one. Encourage residents to help themselves eat in any way possible, such as by holding their own cup.
3. Use a spoon from which the resident can easily remove the food. Usually a teaspoon is better than a soup spoon. Fill the spoon no more than half full. Feed residents in a manner as close to normal as possible to preserve their dignity. Sit down next to the resident while feeding them. Speak softly to the resident, and maintain eye contact. Let the resident decide what to eat and in what order.
4. Be aware of food temperatures. If the food seems too hot, give it time to cool. Do not mix foods together unless the resident requests this.
5. Encourage the resident to eat more nutritious foods first. Save dessert until last if possible. Offer small bites, making sure the resident swallows each bite before offering another. Do not rush the resident. Offer liquids between bites to keep their mouth moist.
6. Have a caring attitude.
7. Encourage residents to eat all of their meal. As with all residents, offer to get a substitute if they are not eating or refuse some food.
8. When the resident is finished eating, remove the clothing protector, any remaining food, and the tray.
9. Give oral care.
10. Report to the charge nurse any changes in the resident that occur with feeding, such as nausea, stomach ache, choking, or decreased appetite.

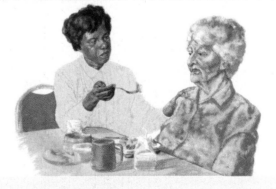

Assisting Residents with Dysphagia

Dysphagia is not a disease but a condition that affects chewing or swallowing. Dysphagia can be caused by stroke or a head injury.

Residents with dysphagia may choke or aspirate some of their food. This means that some of the food they eat falls into the lungs rather than passing through the **esophagus** into the stomach. Pneumonia or a lung infection may result, which can be fatal. A resident may be reluctant to eat if they are afraid of choking. As a result, they may not eat enough and may lose weight.

Many problems caused by dysphagia can be corrected with proper diagnosis and treatment. The therapist or nurse may give you special instructions for feeding a resident in a way that prevents problems. Positioning the resident is very important. Follow the therapist's instructions carefully to help the resident swallow without choking.

The therapist may also recommend a modified diet. A pureed diet or thickened liquids may make swallowing easier. A powdered product may be added to liquid to thicken it. Consistency depends on how much powder is added. Note that often liquids will continue to thicken for some time after the powder is added, so wait a minute or two before adding more thickener. Some residents tolerate thick liquids better than thin liquids. Thickeners can also be added to water and coffee. Many facilities offer pre-thickened liquids.

How do you recognize dysphagia? Observe residents for symptoms such as the following. Report any of these to the charge nurse:

- coughing before, during, or after swallowing food, liquid, or medications
- having to swallow three or four times after each bite
- hoarse, breathy voice or gurgling breathing
- drooling
- a feeling that something is caught in the throat
- pocketing food in the side of the mouth
- a repetitive rocking motion of the tongue from front to back
- continuous throat clearing

A resident may also be a "silent aspirator." This means that dysphagia may be present even though the resident does not have obvious symptoms. Silent aspiration may be indicated by:

- unexplained weight loss
- decreased appetite
- a lasting low-grade fever

If a resident has one or more of these symptoms, dysphagia could be a contributing factor. Discuss your observations with the charge nurse.

Important Observations While Eating

As you help residents with meals, monitor their intake as part of caring for them. If a resident avoids any major food group, ask them why. For example, they may find the meat too tough to chew. Food and fluid intake is usually documented when you observe the resident's tray in the dining room, not at the end of the day. Report it to the nurse when a resident:

- avoids any major food group, such as not eating meats or not drinking milk
- consistently eats less than 75% (or 3/4) of meals, especially if the resident is underweight or losing weight
- complains of repeatedly receiving food they do not like and will not eat
- experiences a changed status, such as needing more help with meals
- behaves differently, such as playing with food or taking food from the trays of other residents
- has any swallowing problems, including coughing or choking while eating
- has any chewing problems caused by mouth pain or dentures that do not fit well
- seems to have trouble chewing or swallowing
- complains about food or their diet
- has trembling hands that make eating difficult
- has a changed attitude, such as becoming depressed or lethargic

Identifying Residents at Risk

You play an important role in helping the interdisciplinary team identify residents at risk for nutritional problems. When admitted to your facility, the resident will be assessed for nutritional risk. Later on you may be asked about your observations of the resident's eating habits. You have an important responsibility to help prevent unintended weight loss by observing and reporting

---

Dysphagia – a condition that causes a problem chewing or swallowing food, liquid, or medication

Esophagus – the muscular tube that leads from the mouth to the stomach

changes. If you notice any change in the resident, report this information immediately. Watch for these things:

- a change in the resident's ability to eat independently, such as the resident needing help to eat or drink
- any chewing problems, such as those caused by mouth pain or dentures that do not fit
- any swallowing problems, such as coughing or choking while eating
- any weight loss
- a sudden change in the amount of food the resident eats, such as eating less than half of meals or snacks served
- complaints that food tastes funny
- sadness, crying spells, or withdrawal from others
- confusion, wandering, pacing, or leaving the dining room without eating

Reporting even very small changes in a resident's eating habits is important. The interdisciplinary team then can intervene early before a problem occurs. Following are some things you can do if the resident experiences any of these signs:

- As with any change in the resident, report your observations to the nurse.
- Do whatever you need to do to help the resident eat. Encourage, cue, or hand-feed them if necessary.
- Remember what the resident likes to eat.
- Offer substitutes when the resident does not like a food.
- Help residents who have trouble feeding themselves.
- Allow the resident time to finish eating.
- Tell the charge nurse if the resident has trouble using silverware.
- Accurately report the resident's intake of meals and snacks.
- Prepare the resident based on their previous mealtime routine.
- Position the resident correctly for feeding.
- Report a loss of appetite or if the resident seems sad.

Special Devices for Eating

Residents who have difficulty feeding themselves may benefit from using special spoons and forks, cups, and plates (Fig. 17-7). Residents need to be taught to use these devices. Usually the occupational therapist teaches the resident and staff how to use them.

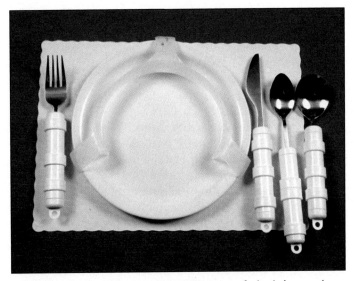

Fig. 17-7 – Special eating utensils include spoons, forks, knives, and plates.

DIETARY SUPPLEMENTS

Many residents cannot eat enough food to supply the calories and protein they need. This may result from a physical change, such as a gastrointestinal problem or cancer treatment, or an emotional change, such as depression. Often supplements are then ordered. Supplements provide concentrated nutrition. Many different kinds are available. Some provide calories and protein, and some are fortified with vitamins and minerals. Some facilities prepare their own supplements. Supplements include shakes, puddings, and frozen bars or "pudding pops."

Adding supplements to a resident's diet is often called "calorie packing" or "power packing." The goal of calorie packing is to give the resident large amounts of calories or protein in the smallest amount of food. For example, you may give a resident a milkshake made of ice cream and protein powder rather than a glass of milk. "Packed" foods include super cereal, fortified potatoes, "souper" soup, and high-protein milk. The addition of gravy, butter, sugar, or sauces helps pack ordinary foods. The food service department will guide you. Supplements may also include extra feedings, such as a small sandwich between meals.

Fortified – strengthened by adding some additional ingredient
Supplement – a concentrated form of nutrition given to a resident in addition to their meals

Examples of residents who benefit from supplements include residents:
- who accept liquids better than food
- who cannot consume large amounts of food
- with an altered sense of taste and smell
- who are very thin and underweight

Although supplements often play an important role in maintaining a resident's nutritional status, you should think of the supplement as an addition to the meal. The meal is the first priority. Except in extreme cases, supplements do not replace the meal but are given in addition to it. Encourage residents to consume as much of the meal as possible before offering the supplement.

Like food and fluid intake, supplement intake is important. If a resident often refuses a supplement, report this to the nurse so that another supplement can be offered.

RESIDENTS WITH FEEDING TUBES

Some residents cannot eat any food at all or enough food to keep them alive. The resident or responsible family member may then decide that tube feeding is appropriate. A special tube is placed either directly into the stomach or into the stomach through the nose.

The nurse will tube-feed residents, but you need to be sure that the resident is positioned with the head of the bed up at least 30 degrees, in the semi-Fowler's or Fowler's position, while the person is being fed and for at least 30 minutes afterwards (Fig. 17-8). This keeps the liquid from

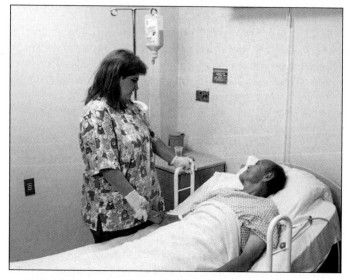

Fig. 17-8 – The head of the resident's bed must be elevated when they are being fed through a tube.

flowing back and causing them to choke on or aspirate the fluid.

Complications may occur from tube-feedings. Report any of the following:
- nausea, vomiting, or diarrhea
- swollen stomach
- constipation or cramping
- coughing, wet breathing, or a feeling that something is caught in the throat
- discomfort or dryness in the throat
- at the site where the feeding tube enters the body:
  – pain, redness, heat, or swelling
  – crusty or oozing fluid
- the resident pulls the tube out

You can do the following to help prevent these problems:
- Maintain the resident's position with the head of the bed elevated 30 degrees or more as tolerated during feedings.
- Maintain the resident's position for 30 minutes after feedings.
- Report immediately any change in the resident's bowel routine.
- Report any complaint from the resident.
- Observe the insertion site of the tube on every shift and report any redness, drainage, or other change.
- Report anything the resident may tell you about the tube. The resident may feel the tube has moved or is twisted. It is important that the nurse checks to be sure the tube is in the proper place.

DEHYDRATION

Residents must take in enough fluids to keep their bodies healthy. Diseases that cause mental or physical decline may keep a resident from feeling thirsty or expressing their thirst. If someone does not drink enough, even if they are healthy, they may experience a very serious condition called **dehydration**. Dehydration in a resident can be devastating or even cause death. Many factors can contribute to dehydration, including:
- a resident's reduced ability to recognize thirst
- the kidneys' reduced ability to retain fluid when needed
- a resident's inability to communicate the need for fluid because of their mental status
- medications such as laxatives and diuretics

Dehydration – a serious condition that can occur if a resident does not have adequate fluid intake

Dehydration can occur quickly in an elderly resident. The signs and symptoms of dehydration may include:

- not drinking at least 6 cups of fluid per day
- dry or cracked lips
- sunken eyes
- dark urine
- sudden confusion
- more sleepiness than usual
- changed ability to do tasks
- sudden weight loss
- skin on the resident's chest or forehead is easily "tented" (you can pull up skin between your thumb and forefinger to form a "tent" that does not immediately smooth out)
- decreased urine output
- excessive urine output
- dry eyes and dry mouth
- constipation
- frequent falls
- frequent urinary tract infections

If you notice any of these things in a resident, report it immediately. This is an emergency situation that requires treatment.

The following examples illustrate how quickly a person can become dehydrated:

- If a resident is thirsty but shows few signs of dehydration such as poor skin **turgor**, they may already need fluid replacement equal to 2% of their body weight. A 70 kg (154 lb) man would need 1400 cc (cubic centimeters) of fluid at this point.
- If a resident has consumed no water for three or four days, has a dry mouth, and little urine output, fluid replacement needed may be equal up to 6% of body weight, or 4200 cc.

Preventing Dehydration

Providing residents with fluids is a key part of your daily tasks. Carefully monitor all residents to ensure they are getting enough fluid even if they are not requesting it. To help ensure adequate fluid intake, you should:

- Ask the resident what they like to drink and have it on hand in the refrigerator.
- Make sure every resident has a water pitcher. Place the pitcher within easy reach of the resident.
- Make sure the water is changed at least once each shift. Make sure there is a clean cup next to the water pitcher.
- Place a clean flexible straw next to the cup of residents who may have difficulty drinking from a cup.

- Encourage the resident to drink every time you interact with them, helping as needed. Tell the charge nurse immediately about any resident who refuses your offering of fluid.

FOOD AND FLUID INTAKE

Evaluating Food Intake

Reporting the amount of food a resident eats is your responsibility. This can sometimes be a challenge because you must estimate how much they ate from what is left on their plate. Different facilities have different ways of recording the amounts of food a resident eats. During your orientation you will learn how the facility records the amounts.

Consider these examples of two different residents:

- Resident #1 has lost 10 pounds in the past two months. He is eating 100% of his meals.
- Resident #2 has also lost 10 pounds in the past two months. He is eating less than 25% of his meals.

Their food intake records tell us that these two residents may have very different problems. Because resident #1 is eating all his meals, he may be losing weight due to a disease rather than too little food intake. Although additional calories will be added to his diet, lab work or medical tests may be necessary. On the other hand, resident #2 does not seem to be getting enough calories. The approach for him is to find ways to increase his intake, such as using supplements or tube-feeding. Without accurate intake records, these residents cannot be evaluated correctly.

Intake is often recorded as the percentage the resident eats of the food given: 100%, 75%, etc. This allows the dietitian to calculate the number of calories or amount of protein consumed. Facilities use many different formats to record dietary intake. Recording intake usually involves observing the meal and judging the percentage of food the resident eats. Since it is not easy to actually measure the amount of food eaten, an estimate is often used. Take the time to evaluate each resident's intake carefully and to record the percentage eaten immediately (Fig. 17-9, next page). You might use a pocket notepad and transfer the information to the flowsheet later.

Turgor – a characteristic of skin that indicates hydration: tight skin that does not "tent" shows good hydration

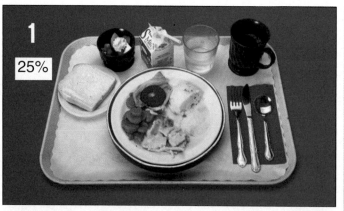
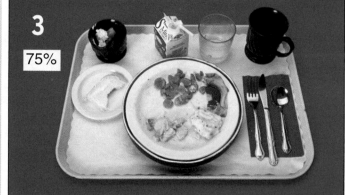
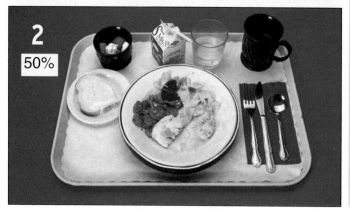
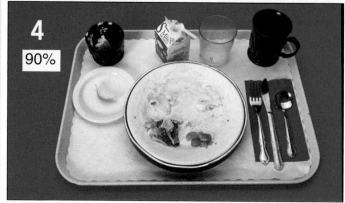

Fig. 17-9 – Reporting the amount of food a resident eats is your responsibility: 1 = 25% eaten, 2 = 50% eaten, 3 = 75% eaten, 4 = 90% eaten.

Evaluating Fluid Intake

Like food intake, adequate fluid intake is vital. Exact fluid needs depend on the person's age, size, physical condition, and level of activity, but most residents need 1500 to 2000 cc of fluid per day (Fig. 17-10). Residents with diseases such as congestive heart failure (CHF) or renal disease may be restricted to less fluid. In these residents too much fluid can result in edema. Edema is too much fluid building up in places like the legs and ankles, which become swollen.

The physician determines the resident's proper intake and gives instructions about how much fluid to allow. Unless a resident is on a fluid restriction, offer fluids often and encourage the resident to drink.

To record fluid intake, you need to know how much fluid is in common containers. Table 17-1 (next page) lists the amounts in common containers.

At times it is critical to monitor a resident's fluid intake and output (called I & O). A person's output—the amount of their urine—depends on how much fluid they take in.

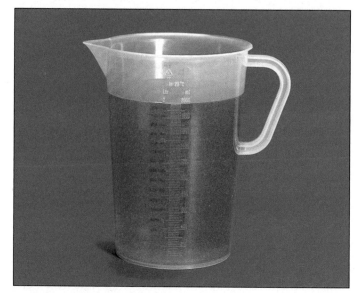

Fig. 17-10 – Residents who are not on any fluid restriction should have 1500 to 2000 cc of fluid a day.

Most people produce about 1500 cc of urine per day. Output is usually recorded on an I & O sheet after meals and immediately after serving fluids and assisting with toileting (Fig. 17-11). A resident's I & O record is often kept on their door or their bed's footboard. When recording intake and output, you should:

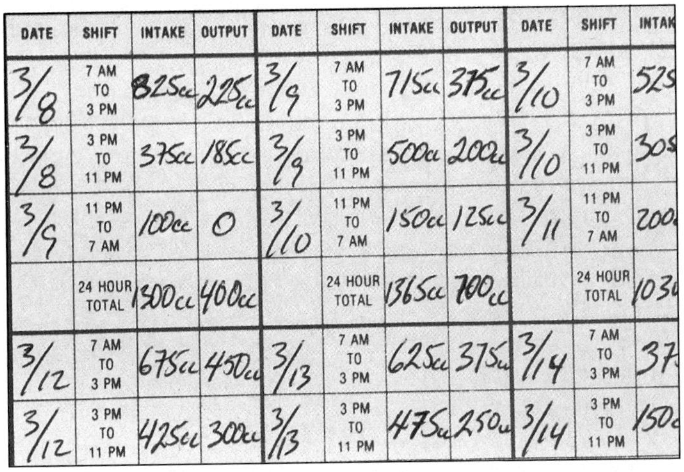

DATE	SHIFT	INTAKE	OUTPUT	DATE	SHIFT	INTAKE	OUTPUT	DATE	SHIFT	INTAKE
3/8	7 AM TO 3 PM	825cc	225cc	3/9	7 AM TO 3 PM	715cc	375cc	3/10	7 AM TO 3 PM	525
3/8	3 PM TO 11 PM	375cc	185cc	3/9	3 PM TO 11 PM	500cc	200cc	3/10	3 PM TO 11 PM	305
3/9	11 PM TO 7 AM	100cc	0	3/10	11 PM TO 7 AM	150cc	125cc	3/11	11 PM TO 7 AM	200
	24 HOUR TOTAL	1300cc	400cc		24 HOUR TOTAL	1365cc	700cc		24 HOUR TOTAL	1030
3/12	7 AM TO 3 PM	675cc	450cc	3/13	7 AM TO 3 PM	625cc	375cc	3/14	7 AM TO 3 PM	37
3/12	3 PM TO 11 PM	425cc	300cc	3/13	3 PM TO 11 PM	475cc	250cc	3/14	3 PM TO 11 PM	150c

Fig. 17-11 – A resident's fluid intake and urine output is recorded on the I & O record.

- Know how much fluid is in the glasses and cups in your facility.
- Count any liquids given throughout the day.
- Accurately record all fluid intake in the appropriate space on the I & O sheet for your shift.
- Because output may be difficult to measure, offer a bedpan or urinal. Then pour the urine into a measuring cup and measure it. Record the output in the appropriate space on the I & O sheet for your shift.

If a person is incontinent, you will have to:
- Check the resident frequently for wetness.
- Change the resident each time they are wet.
- Count the number of times they are incontinent and put an "X" on the output sheet for each time. Estimate the volume of urine as small, moderate, or large.

Note: *If a resident is incontinent with diarrhea, it is difficult to determine their urine output. Discuss this situation with the charge nurse.*

If a resident has an indwelling Foley catheter, the amount of urine is measured in the collecting bag at the end of each shift, or when the bag is full.

TABLE 17-1
CAPACITIES OF COMMON CONTAINERS

CONTAINER	CC
1 oz	30 cc
Water tumbler	240 cc
Iced tea glass	240 cc
Juice glass–4 fluid oz	120 cc
Coffee cup	180 cc
Individual coffeepot	240 cc
Individual pot of broth	240 cc
Ice cream–3 fluid oz	90 cc
Sherbet–4 fluid oz container	120 cc
Styrofoam cup, 3 in. tall–6 fluid oz	180 cc
4 oz juice cup	120 cc
6 oz can orange juice	180 cc
Soup bowl–6 fluid oz	180 cc
Cereal bowl–8 fluid oz	240 cc
Individual carton of milk	240 cc
Jell-O–1/2 cup	120 cc

HEIGHT AND WEIGHT

As you learned in Chapter 13, Gathering Data, height and weight measurements are made when a resident is admitted. This is used as baseline data, and later measurements are compared to these. If these baseline data are wrong, this can affect the person's assessment and plan of care for months or years. Measuring a resident's weight is an important part of maintaining good nutrition. A resident is weighed more frequently if there is a change in their nutritional intake or the resident has a medical issue that can cause weight fluctuations. See Chapter 13 to review how to measure height and weight.

IN THIS CHAPTER YOU LEARNED:

- The role of the food service and how you work with that department
- Ways to provide and encourage good nutrition
- How to make dining a pleasant experience
- The proper recording procedure for intake and output (I & O)

SUMMARY

This chapter discusses how you can help maintain or improve a resident's health through good nutrition. You have a responsibility to make residents' dining experiences pleasant. You can also do much to help ensure a resident does not lose weight unintentionally or become dehydrated. How you help residents eat is critical, along with how you observe changes in them. Measuring the resident's weight accurately is also important because weight may be the only indication you have of a change in a resident's nutritional status.

PULLING IT ALL TOGETHER

Watching someone waste away because they are not eating is a terrible experience. Have you ever observed someone with an unintentional weight loss? It can be very upsetting to everyone involved. Think about the value our society places on food and nutrition. We want everyone to enjoy food and to be healthy. It can be a great challenge to help residents in long term care facilities who have difficulty maintaining their health or changed nutritional status.

Think about this:

A resident with congestive heart failure is admitted to the facility. He is placed on a no-added-salt diet. You notice this resident does not eat much food when you serve him his meals. You ask him if he is eating as much food as he typically eats at home, and he says yes. You decide that his eating habits now are not unusual, and you do not report this to the charge nurse. Two weeks later you measure his weight and discover he has lost 6 pounds. This unintended weight loss is very upsetting to the resident and his family.

How could you have prevented this? Could you have asked the resident additional questions like "Does the food taste good? Do you like it? Are these foods familiar to you?" These questions would have led you to discover that this resident does not eat anything without salt and that he never shared this information with his physician.

1. **Which of the following conditions may result from poor nutrition?**
   A. Pressure ulcers.
   B. Alzheimer's disease.
   C. Lung cancer.
   D. Bladder infections.

2. **Mrs. Allard is on an NCS diet. This means she should avoid:**
   A. Salt.
   B. Sugar.
   C. Milk.
   D. Gluten.

3. **Your role in helping maintain a resident's nutrition includes:**
   A. Planning meals for the week.
   B. Helping food service staff prepare meals.
   C. Insisting that residents eat everything on their plate.
   D. Serving meals while hot foods are still hot and cold foods are cold.

4. **You should report to the charge nurse if a resident:**
   A. Says that her coffee is cold.
   B. Complains that the spinach does not taste as good as last week.
   C. Seems to have difficulty handling her utensils.
   D. Offers to share her dessert with her roommate.

5. **How can you make a resident's dining experience more enjoyable?**
   A. Turn the dining room lights on as bright as possible.
   B. Try to create a pleasant homelike atmosphere.
   C. Turn the television up loud so that everyone can hear it.
   D. Encourage residents to sit at a different table every meal.

6. **Residents with dysphagia may have trouble:**
   A. With food allergies.
   B. With constipation.
   C. Digesting their food.
   D. Swallowing their food.

7. **Mrs. Mayfield tells you she does not like the pie that is served for dessert tonight. You should:**
   A. Offer to get a substitute.
   B. Suggest that she try it anyway because it might be better than she thinks.
   C. Say you're sorry you can't do anything this time, but you'll tell the food service so it doesn't happen again.
   D. Ask others at the table if they'd like to trade another food item for Mrs. Mayfield's pie.

8. **The signs and symptoms of dehydration may include:**
   A. Blurred vision.
   B. Rosy pink skin color.
   C. Decreased urine output.
   D. Elevated blood pressure.

9. **In some cases you must monitor a resident's fluid intake accurately. To do this you must:**
   A. Never take your eyes off the resident.
   B. Ask the resident's roommate to record everything the resident drinks.
   C. Know the capacity of glasses and cups in your facility.
   D. Trust that the resident will remember at the end of the day how many cups of fluid they consumed.

10. **How long should a resident sit up after being tube fed?**
    A. 10 minutes.
    B. 30 minutes.
    C. 60 minutes.
    D. 90 minutes.

(Answers to "Check What You've Learned" are in the Instructor's Manual.)

Chapter 18

ASSISTING WITH ELIMINATION

"Elimination" refers to how the body gets rid of waste products. Urine is the liquid waste, and stool is the solid waste. Elimination is a body function we usually think about only when we have to go to the toilet or when we experience a change. It is usually a routine matter. Most people have gone to the toilet independently since being a toddler.

Everyone wants to be independent with their bodily functions. Many residents enter long term care facilities able to go to the toilet by themselves. As a nurse assistant, you should help them maintain their normal elimination pattern and independence.

Many things affect a person's ability to have normal bowel and bladder functions. A simple change in diet or fluid intake can upset a resident's normal elimination pattern. The normal changes of aging discussed in Chapter 11 can also affect elimination. As we age, food passes through our digestive tract more slowly, and digestion slows. This results in a slowed bowel pattern and decreased absorption of nutrients. Think about these normal changes of aging as you care for residents. A lack of independence or incontinence—the inability to hold urine or stool for controlled elimination—is devastating for a resident. This affects their quality of life and their care. You need to understand how to support residents with their elimination needs. Determining the resident's elimination pattern, supporting good nutrition, helping with elimination when needed, and reporting any changes are important ways you can help residents maintain a healthy elimination pattern.

In this chapter you will learn about helping residents to maintain their dignity with elimination. You will learn about equipment used for elimination and procedures to help residents with elimination. You will also learn what changes to pay attention to and what techniques to use to collect elimination specimens.

OBJECTIVES
- Describe how to determine residents' elimination patterns
- List ways to help residents maintain their dignity when you help them with elimination
- Identify equipment used to help with elimination
- Demonstrate correct ways to help a resident use a bedpan, urinal, and portable commode
- State how to identify changes in residents' elimination patterns
- Demonstrate specimen collection techniques
- Describe your role in ostomy care

MEDICAL TERMS
- **Bladder** – sac inside the body that holds urine
- **Bowel** – large and small intestines
- **Continent** – able to control elimination of urine and stool
- **Elimination** – process of ridding the body of urine and stool
- **Gastrointestinal** – related to the stomach and intestines
- **Guaiac test** – procedure for checking blood in the stool or vomit
- **Ileostomy** – surgery that leads the opening of the ileum to the stoma. The ileum is a part of the small intestine.
- **Incontinence** – inability to hold urine or stool
- **Occult** – cannot be seen
- **Ostomy** – a surgical opening from the intestine to outside the body
- **Parasite** – an organism living in or on another organism
- **Stoma** – a surgically created opening
- **Stool** – human waste, feces from the bowel
- **Urinate** – to pass urine
- **Urine** – waste liquid secreted by the kidney
- **Void** – to eliminate liquid waste from the body; commonly used to describe urination

"It's hard for me to accept that I can't control some basic bodily functions. But your professional manner helps me to keep my dignity even at times like this."

Elimination—we all do it, but usually we don't think about it much. When you feel the urge to go to the bathroom, you usually just go. But have you ever been in a situation where you couldn't find a bathroom or you felt uncomfortable about where you were? Not being able to go probably kept you from thinking about anything else until you took care of this very basic need.

Think about how you might feel if you could not get to the bathroom easily. What if someone questioned whether you really had to go again so soon? Imagine having to plead or explain that you really do have to go. How would you feel if you had to depend on someone else to help you with something so personal—something you've always done on your own in private? Think about how the residents you care for feel about this, too.

Helping with elimination and talking about it with residents may not be one of your favorite roles as a nurse assistant. But keep in mind residents' feelings. Try to make their situation as private, dignified, and independent as possible.

DETERMINING ELIMINATION PATTERNS

Every resident has their own pattern of elimination. Their pattern involves their **frequency** of elimination and usual amount of **urine** and **stool**. Some residents **urinate** more often than others. Some residents have bowel movements daily, while others have them every other or every third day. You learn a resident's normal pattern so that you can base your care on their needs. This way you will also know when a problem occurs or illness changes their pattern. A change in elimination can result from a simple change in food or fluids or from a serious condition.

To learn about a resident's elimination pattern, gather information from the resident, family members, and the resident's chart. This information is part of the resident's **bowel** and **bladder** assessment. The nurse typically gathers this information, but you may be asked to assist with this. Be sure you understand what information the nurse needs. Residents use many different words to refer to

---

Bladder – sac inside the body that holds urine
Bowel – large and small intestines
Elimination – process of ridding the body of urine and stool
Frequency – how often something happens, a habitual pattern
Stool – human waste, feces from the bowel
Urinate – to pass urine
Urine – waste liquid secreted by the kidney

urine and stool elimination. Get to know what words they are most comfortable with as you care for them. You may ask the resident or family what words they prefer to use. Although residents may use many different words, you must always be professional when you communicate with the resident and the resident's family. For example, a resident may use slang words to refer to urine or stool, but you should not use these terms when communicating with the resident.

The Resident

When you gather information about a resident's elimination, keep in mind that talking about this is uncomfortable for everyone involved. Help ease this situation by asking questions only in private. Show you really want to get to know the resident so you can help them when they need help. Work to develop a trusting relationship with them. Elimination is a private act, but a resident who trusts you feels more at ease answering your questions.

Ask these questions about the resident's bowel movements:

* How often do you have a bowel movement?
* What time of day do you normally have a bowel movement?
* Is there anything I should know that will help you keep your normal schedule?

Ask these questions about the resident's urination pattern:

* How often do you urinate?
* Do you usually urinate in large or small amounts?
* Do you have a pattern such as before breakfast, after lunch, before dinner, or at bedtime?
* Do you wake up at night needing to urinate?
* Do you ever urinate and then find you have to go again soon after?
* Do you drip urine on your way to the toilet?

The Resident's Family

If a resident cannot tell you about their elimination pattern, ask family members. Ask the same questions you would ask the resident.

The Resident's Chart

Review a resident's chart to learn their elimination patterns. This information is collected starting on the day of admission. If the resident has any problems with elimination, the care plan has information about how to care for them. The chart usually contains the following information:

Bowel Pattern Information:
* A record sheet of how often the person has a bowel movement (Fig. 18-1)

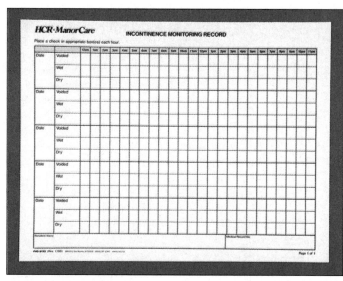

Fig. 18-1 – A resident's bowel movements are recorded on a flow chart similar to this chart for incontinence.

* The shift when a resident usually has a bowel movement
* The amount, color, and consistency of the resident's stool
* Information on **incontinence**. (Being incontinent means that for some reason they cannot control the flow of urine or stool. Your role in managing incontinence is covered in Chapter 11, The Aging Process and Disease Management.)

Urination Pattern Information:
* The resident's urination pattern
* The amount of urine

Incontinence – inability to hold urine or stool

- The color of the urine
- Any odor or pain with urination

Once you know a resident's normal bowel and urination patterns, do all you can to help the patterns stay normal. Changes in patterns can lead to problems, especially changes in bowel elimination.

TIPS FOR PROMOTING REGULAR ELIMINATION PATTERNS
- Help residents to the bathroom as soon as you are asked. If a resident cannot ask, help them to the bathroom:
  - on awakening
  - before and after meals
  - at bedtime
  - when they wake at night
  - any other time you think they may have to go based on your information
- Respond to call signals promptly.
- Make sure residents eat a balanced diet and drink plenty of fluids, especially water.
- Make sure residents get enough rest and exercise.

MAINTAINING RESIDENTS' DIGNITY WHEN HELPING THEM WITH ELIMINATION
Elimination is a very private act. Like bathing or grooming, this is something the resident has always done in private. Residents have the right to dignity, respect, and privacy even when they need your help. Help maintain their dignity when helping them with elimination, in these ways:

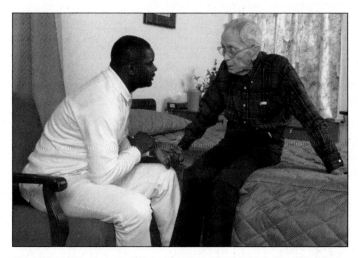

Fig. 18-2 – Always respect the resident's privacy when discussing their bowel and bladder routine.

- Ask questions about elimination only in private (Fig.18-2).
- Have a professional attitude. Never use nicknames, slang words, or unprofessional gestures to refer to elimination. As you get to know a resident, you will learn more about their sensitivities. Some residents will become more relaxed with you over time. Pay attention to their cues, and try to create a comfortable atmosphere. Sometimes humor can help reassure a resident in an awkward situation.
- Help residents in private. Close the door, pull the bedside curtains around the bed, and cover the person. Ask others to leave the room, if possible. Explain that your wearing gloves is important for infection control with all residents and protects them as well as you.
- Empty bedpans, commodes, and flush toilets immediately after elimination. Use an odor control spray if needed. Never let a resident see you with a look or gesture of disgust.

ASSISTING WITH ELIMINATION
Help a resident with elimination by using a bedpan, urinal, or portable commode (Fig. 18-3 A/B). Which one you use depends on the person's needs. For example, a male resident who is continent but cannot or does not want to walk to the bathroom at night may use a urinal. If a male resident cannot communicate his needs, try offering the

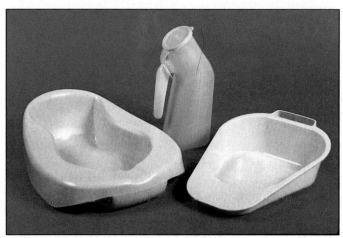

Fig. 18-3 A – Various types of bedpans and urinals.

Commode – a box-like structure with a chamber pot under an open seat; usually portable

Continent – able to control elimination of urine and stool

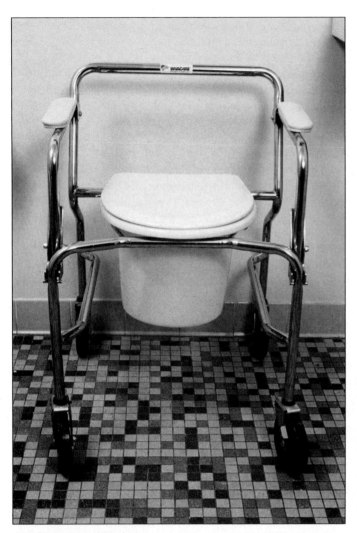

Fig. 18-3 B – A commode can be used for residents who cannot walk to the bathroom.

the most familiar. A resident who cannot get to the bathroom may use a bedpan (Procedure 18-1), urinal (Procedure 18-2), or portable commode (Procedure 18-3). With any of these, try to create an environment that feels as private and normal as going to the bathroom.

Bedpans are used by both male and female residents. A smaller **fracture pan** is often used for residents with hip or back problems. The bedside commode is a portable toilet. It is positioned beside the bed so the resident needs only to move from the bed to it. Most commodes are like a chair with a toilet seat cover and a container under the seat that catches the urine and stool.

Some residents use disposable products such as panty liners or disposable briefs if they are worried about having an accident (Fig. 18-4). Talk with the resident about what they need. Talk with the charge nurse to see if the resident may have a medical problem that can be solved. The use of disposable briefs is described in Chapter 11, The Aging Process and Disease Management.

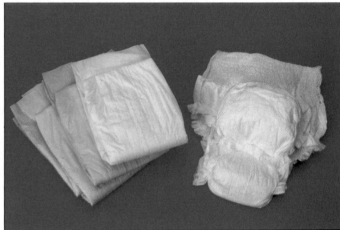

Fig. 18-4 – Disposable products can be used for residents who are incontinent.

use of a commode or the urinal. Do your best to determine a resident's needs. Offer female residents the use of a bedpan or commode. Offer male residents the use of a urinal for urinating only, and a bedpan or commode for bowel elimination or both. Follow the care plan. If the resident's elimination patterns are different from what is in the care plan, tell the nurse.

Equipment for Elimination

Some residents need help with elimination. They may need to use special equipment. They may use the toilet, bedpan, urinal, or bedside commode. Using the bathroom toilet for urination and bowel movements is easiest and

(text continued on page 344)

📖

Fracture pan – a type of bedpan that is smaller and has a lower front lip so it is easier to slide under a resident. It is usually used for residents with hip or back problems, or a broken hip or leg.

PROCEDURE 18-1. HELPING A RESIDENT USE A BEDPAN

Items Needed
- bedpan and bedpan cover
- wash basin
- two towels
- two washcloths
- soap
- toilet paper
- three pairs of gloves
- two plastic-covered pads or protective covers

1. Put on gloves.

Note: *If you contaminate your gloves in any way during the procedure, you must change to a new pair of gloves.*

2. Put a pad or cover on the surface where you will put the bedpan after it is used.

3. Fold the bedspread and blanket down to the bottom of the bed, leaving the top sheet in place to cover the resident's lower legs. Help the resident lift their nightgown or remove pajama bottoms or underpants.

4. Put a protective cover under the resident's buttocks to protect the bed linen.

5. Ask the resident to bend both knees and lift their buttocks up while you slide the bedpan underneath them. Adjust it for the resident's comfort. Sometimes using powder or cornstarch on the bedpan prevents the resident's skin from sticking to it when the bedpan is removed.

Note: *If the resident does not have the strength to lift their buttocks, ask them or help them turn onto one side (as described in Chapter 15). Hold the bedpan flush against their buttocks and have the resident turn back onto the bedpan. (You may need help from another nurse assistant.)*

6. Remove your gloves and dispose of them. Wash your hands.

7. Cover the resident with the top sheet for privacy.

8. Elevate the head of the bed slowly until the resident is in a sitting position. (Remember: You are trying to create a normal setting.) Ask the resident if they are as comfortable as they can be. Change the position of the bedpan if needed to make them comfortable.

9. Provide toilet paper and position the call light button so the resident can reach it. Tell them to call you when finished. If a resident cannot tell you they are finished, check on them every five minutes. Because a bedpan puts pressure on the skin, do not leave a resident on a bedpan longer than needed.

To help a resident from the bedpan:

10. Put on gloves.

11. Lower the head of the bed. Ask the resident to lift their buttocks up while you slide the bedpan out. If needed, help them roll onto one side while you hold the bedpan to prevent a spill. Move the bedpan to the covered surface.

12. If needed, help with wiping the perineal area. Put the used toilet tissue in the bedpan. You may need to wash the perineal area for some residents. (Remember to wash, rinse, and dry thoroughly.) Wash or wipe from front to back. Remove and dispose of the protective pad over the bed linen.

Note: *Some facilities may have premoistened disposable washcloths for perineal care or use a commercial cleanser that is put in a bottle. You squeeze this solution from the bottle over the perineal area.*

13. Remove your soiled gloves and put on clean gloves.

14. Help the resident wash their hands.

Note: *If perineal washing was necessary, change the water and use a fresh washcloth and towel for hand washing. Remove your gloves, dispose of them, wash your hands, and put on a new pair before proceeding.*

15. Help the resident get dressed.

16. Put the bedpan cover on the bedpan and dispose of the contents in the resident's toilet. Clean the bedpan and return it to the bedside table. Remove and dispose of the protective pad on which you put the bedpan.

Note: *Most facilities have a water sprayer attached to the toilet for cleaning bedpans, urinals, etc. You will learn the procedure for emptying and cleaning equipment in your facility. When you clean the equipment, be careful not to splash the contents.*

17. Remove and dispose of your gloves in the disposable trash bag, throw the trash bag away, and wash your hands.

PROCEDURE 18-2. HELPING A MALE RESIDENT USE A URINAL

Items Needed
- urinal
- three pairs of gloves
- wash basin
- soap
- towel
- toilet paper
- protective cover

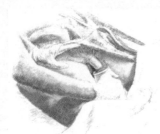

1. Put on gloves.

Note: *If you contaminate your gloves in any way during the procedure, you must change to a new pair of gloves.*

2. Put a pad or cover on the surface where you will put the urinal after use.

Note: *If the resident can stand beside the bed to use the urinal, help him to stand, and provide privacy. Put the call light button within reach so he can call you when finished; then continue with Steps 6-12.*

If a resident uses the urinal while in bed, follow these steps:

3. Fold the bedspread and blanket down to the bottom of the bed, leaving the top sheet over the resident. Help the resident lower his bottom clothing.

4. Place the urinal between the resident's legs at an angle to avoid urine spillage. Gently place the penis into the urinal.

5. Take off your gloves and put them in a plastic trashbag. Cover the resident with the top sheet and give him the call light. Tell him to call you when he is done. Check in a few minutes if he does not call you.

6. Wash your hands and put on new gloves.

7. When the resident is finished, remove the urinal and place it on the covered surface.

8. If needed, help the resident wipe off excess urine with toilet tissue. Dispose of tissue and your gloves in the plastic trash bag.

9. Wash your hands and put on new gloves.

10. Help the resident wash, rinse, and dry his hands.

11. Empty the urinal, clean it, and replace it in the bedside table.

Note: *most facilities have a water sprayer attached to the toilet for cleaning bedpans, urinals, etc. You will learn the procedure for emptying and cleaning equipment in your facility. When you clean the equipment, be careful not to splash the contents.*

12. Remove and dispose of your gloves in the disposable trash bag, throw the trash bag away, and wash your hands.

▶ **REMEMBER: UNDERSTAND**

PROCEDURE 18-3.   HELPING A RESIDENT USE A PORTABLE COMMODE

▶ **REMEMBER: BE AWARE**

Items Needed
- toilet paper
- two pairs of gloves
- washbasin
- soap
- towel

1. Put on gloves.

Note: *If you contaminate your gloves in any way during the procedure, you must change to a new pair of gloves.*

2. Help the resident out of bed to a standing position (as described in Chapter 15, Learning to Position and Move Correctly). Help pull down the resident's lower clothing. Help them sit on the commode positioned by the bed.

Note: *Position the commode so it will not move when you help the resident out of bed. Put the commode against the wall or against the bedside table to keep it from moving.*

3. Provide toilet paper and put the call light button within reach. Remove gloves.

4. If the resident needs help with wiping when finished:
   a. Put on gloves.
   b. Help with wiping, and throw the tissue into the commode or plastic trash bag.
   c. Take off your gloves and put them in the plastic trash bag.

5. Help the resident with their clothing and to get back into the bed or chair.

6. Put on new gloves.

7. Help the resident wash, rinse, and dry their hands.

8. Remove the container from the commode and empty its contents into the toilet in the bathroom.

Note: *Most facilities have a water sprayer attached to the toilet for cleaning bedpans, urinals, etc. You will learn the procedure for emptying and cleaning equipment in your facility. When you clean the equipment, be careful not to splash the contents.*

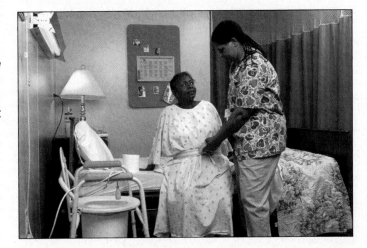

9. Clean and dry the container and put it back in the commode.

10. Remove and dispose of your gloves in the disposable trash bag, throw the trash bag away, and wash your hands.

▶ **REMEMBER: UNDERSTAND**

(text continued from page 340)

PROBLEMS WITH ELIMINATION

When you help a resident with elimination, watch for anything unusual. Listen to any problems a resident describes. Any changes or even a minor complaint could mean something serious. Box 18-1 lists problems with elimination that you should report to the charge nurse.

Some of the problems listed in Box 18-1 might be easily solved. Others require immediate medical attention. For example, a change in the color of a resident's stool from brown to black can be a sign of bleeding. This is a serious problem that you must report immediately. You need to know what is normal for residents you care for so that you can tell when things are not normal. Then you will know to report them.

BOX 18-1.
PROBLEMS WITH ELIMINATION
Report any of the following to the charge nurse.

URINATION CONCERNS
- pain or burning sensation when urinating
- foul-smelling urine
- blood in the urine
- more frequent trips to the bathroom
- voiding small amounts of urine
- cloudy urine
- lower abdominal discomfort or back pain
- A resident has not urinated during your shift.
- A resident who usually is not incontinent becomes incontinent.
- A resident who has never been incontinent has an accident.
- The urine is not a light amber color but is dark and **concentrated**.

BOWEL ELIMINATION CONCERNS
- A resident has difficulty moving their bowels.
- A resident strains more while having a bowel movement.
- blood in a resident's stool, either bright red or black
- frequent, watery stools
- foul-smelling stool
- Stool is not brown and soft but greenish, black, hard, or watery.
- A resident's abdomen is bloated or swollen and they have not had a bowel movement recently.
- swollen, bleeding tissue around the anus
- A resident has more difficulty getting to the bathroom.
- A resident is not eating.

Common chronic illnesses and problems of the urinary and **gastrointestinal** systems are described in Chapter 11, The Aging Process and Disease Management.

COLLECTING SPECIMENS

You may be asked to help the charge nurse collect a urine or stool specimen from a resident. Specimens are often collected as part a routine physical exam or if the resident's condition changes.

Specimens are typically **analyzed** in a lab or at the facility to help identify a problem. A urine or stool sample collected for this purpose is a specimen. A physician's order is needed to collect each specimen.

For the specimen to be analyzed correctly, you must follow the proper procedure. When collecting specimens:
- Explain the procedure to the resident first.
- Specimens are considered "dirty." They should not be collected or stored in "clean" areas such as nurses' stations. Specimens can be collected in the resident's bathroom and then stored according to the facility's policy.
- Wear gloves and wash your hands before and after obtaining a specimen.
- Never touch the inside of a specimen container.
- Most specimens must be as fresh as possible. Some need to be refrigerated if there will be any delay before the lab gets them.
- Specimens must be labeled correctly and promptly. Include the resident's name, room number, and the date and time you collect the specimen. This prevents any later confusion about whose specimen it is. Follow your facility's protocol for labeling.
- Put lids on specimen containers securely to prevent leakage.

After collecting and labeling a specimen, follow your facility's protocol for it to be transported to the lab. Place the specimen in a plastic bag that is labeled as a biohazard. This bag makes an additional barrier to prevent contamination if the specimen cup or container leaks.

Analyze – to study, to determine chemical parts or the presence of disease

Concentrated – less diluted, more intense in color

Gastrointestinal – related to the stomach and intestines

Urine Specimens

Urinalysis. A urinalysis, often called a UA, is a laboratory analysis of a urine specimen. You may routinely collect urinalysis specimens from some residents (Procedure 18-4). Urinalysis may reveal problems in the urinary system or some other problems. Usually the specimen should be as fresh as possible when analyzed.

When collecting a UA specimen, ask the charge nurse what container and method to use. Ask to see the procedure if you are unsure how to do it. Follow your facility's infection control policies. Sometimes you collect urine from a bedpan, urinal, or special device called a "hat" (or a "urine hat" or a "collection hat") that fits in a toilet (Fig. 18-5). Any equipment used must be as clean as possible.

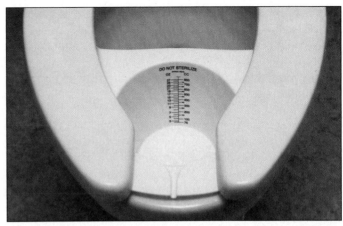

Fig. 18-5 — Urine can be collected when the resident uses the toilet by placing a collection hat in the toilet.

PROCEDURE 18-4. COLLECTING A URINALYSIS SPECIMEN

▶ **REMEMBER: BE AWARE**

Items Needed
- proper collection container
- cleaning solution if needed
- gloves
- labels
- disposable trash bag
- testing equipment

1. Have the resident void or urinate into a bedpan, urinal (if male), or clean hat in the toilet.

2. Put on gloves.

Note: *If you contaminate your gloves in any way during the procedure, you must change to a new pair of gloves.*

3. Pour about 60 cc of urine in the specimen container. Discard the urine left over by emptying it into the toilet.

4. Write the resident's name, room number, and date and time you collected the specimen on the container's label.

5. Place the specimen container in a biohazardous plastic bag and close it properly.

6. Remove and dispose of your gloves in the disposable trash bag, throw the trash bag away, and wash your hands.

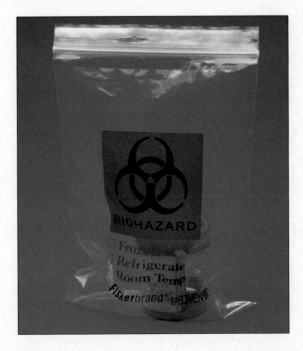

▶ **REMEMBER: UNDERSTAND**

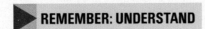

Void – to eliminate liquid waste from the body; commonly used to describe urination.

Clean-Catch Urinalysis. A clean-catch urinalysis specimen is used to check for a urinary infection. It is called a clean catch because the specimen is collected after the urethral opening is cleansed (Procedure 18-5). This cleansing prevents organisms around the urethral opening from contaminating the sample.

Collecting a 24-Hour Urine Specimen. This is a collection of all urine a resident voids in a 24-hour period. The physician may order a 24-hour urine specimen to help diagnose a problem in the urinary system (Procedure 18-6). Ask the charge nurse for directions on how to manage the specimen. A preservative may be added. The bottle may be kept cool in a refrigerator or packed in ice in a bucket in the bathroom until the 24-hour period is over (Fig. 18-6).

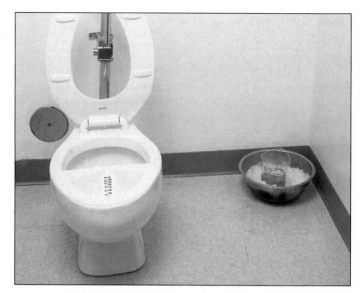

Fig. 18-6 – 24-hour urine collection–the urine container is in a bucket of ice in the resident's bathroom, next to the toilet.

PROCEDURE 18-5. COLLECTING A CLEAN-CATCH URINALYSIS SPECIMEN

▶ **REMEMBER: BE AWARE**

Items Needed
- proper collection container
- cleaning solution if needed
- gloves
- labels
- disposable trash bag

1. Put on gloves.

Note: *If you contaminate your gloves in any way during the procedure, you must change to a new pair of gloves.*

2. Clean the urethral opening.
   a. For a female resident, use one wipe to clean one side of the labia, a second wipe to clean the other side of the labia, and a third wipe to clean down the middle. Always clean in single strokes from front to back. Use each wipe only once and then dispose of it.
   b. Clean the penis following the procedure used for perineal care. For an uncircumcised male resident, pull back the foreskin of the penis to clean it.

3. Have the resident begin to urinate and then stop if they can. Do not collect this first urine.

Note: *If the resident cannot stop the flow of urine, you have to put the container under the stream before they finish to get enough urine.*

4. Hold the specimen container under the urethra, ask the resident to begin voiding again, and collect the remainder of the specimen.

5. Write the resident's name, room number, and the date and time you collected the specimen on the specimen container.

6. Place the specimen container in a plastic bag labelled for biohazards and close it.

7. Remove and dispose of your gloves in the disposable trash bag, throw the trash bag away, and wash your hands after handling each specimen.

▶ **REMEMBER: UNDERSTAND**

PROCEDURE 18-6. COLLECTING A 24-HOUR URINE SPECIMEN

> ► **REMEMBER: BE AWARE**

Items Needed
- 24-hour urine container
- container to catch urine (bedpan, urinal, or hat)
- gloves
- labels

1. Remind the resident not to throw out any urine. Place a sign in the bathroom to alert other staff or family. (Everyone involved needs to understand that if any urine is lost, the test may need to be restarted.) All urine must be collected in the same container.

2. Always put on gloves before handling specimens.

3. Discard the first voided urine of the day. At this time the collection period of 24 hours begins. (The test would be inaccurate if the first voided urine was not discarded, because it contains urine that collected in the bladder before the starting period.) During the collection period the resident should use a bedpan, commode, urinal, or collection hat on the toilet. Remind the resident to call you each time they urinate so that you can be sure all urine specimens are collected.

4. Remove and dispose of your gloves in the disposable trash bag, throw the trash bag away, and wash your hands after handling each specimen.

When the 24 hours are up:

5. Put on a new pair of gloves.

6. Write the resident's name, room number, and the date and the collection time period on the specimen container.

7. Place the specimen container in a biohazardous plastic bag and close it.

8. Remove and dispose of your gloves in the disposable trash bag, throw the trash bag away, and wash your hands after handling each specimen.

> ► **REMEMBER: UNDERSTAND**

Using Reagent Sticks (Dipsticks) for Testing Urine. Residents having a routine physical exam or experiencing a health change may have their urine tested. Tests can check for substances like blood, ketones (acetone), protein, or pH (whether the urine is acidic or alkaline). These tests are easily done. They may reveal a disease or a need for additional tests.

These tests use a paper dipstick that is dipped in the resident's urine. The dipstick then shows a change of color or other change to show the test's result. Ask the nurse what substance you are checking for. Read the instructions on the test strip bottle for how long to wait before you read the strip's result. After you dip the strip in the resident's urine, compare the result with the range of results in the chart on the bottle.

Ketone Testing. The urine of diabetic residents may be checked for ketones (acetone). This test may also be done for a resident with a change such as increased urine output. When the body burns fat, ketones may be present in the urine. You may be asked to check a resident's urine for ketones. Procedure 18-7 describes the steps for this testing.

This test is done with special test strips early in the morning before the resident eats. After dipping the strip in urine, you compare it to the color chart on the strip bottle. Some strips use + and – symbols instead of color changes to show the presence or absence of ketones.

PROCEDURE 18-7. TESTING URINE FOR KETONES

▶ **REMEMBER: BE AWARE**

Items Needed
- container to catch urine (bedpan, urinal, urine hat)
- gloves
- watch with second hand
- test strip bottle

1. Put on gloves.

Note: *If you contaminate your gloves in any way during the procedure, you must change to a new pair of gloves.*

2. Have the resident void in the bedpan, urinal, or hat on a toilet.

3. Either dip the end of the strip in the fresh urine or pass it through the urine stream.

4. Pull the edge of the strip over the rim of the container you are collecting the urine in to get rid of excess urine.

5. Wait 15 seconds (follow the bottle's directions for the time) and compare the ketone portion of the test strip with the ketone color chart on the test strip bottle. Or the strip may show a + or − symbol.

Note: *Checking for other substances in the urine, such as blood or protein, is done in a similar way. Check the directions for what time of day to do the test and how long to wait for the result.*

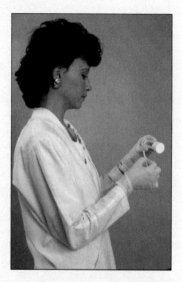

6. Remove and dispose of your gloves in the disposable trash bag, throw the trash bag away, and wash your hands after handling each specimen.

▶ **REMEMBER: UNDERSTAND**

Stool Specimens

Stool specimens help physicians diagnose gastrointestinal problems. Stool specimens also can be collected to check for **parasites** that can make a resident sick. The lab analyzes the specimen.

Bleeding in the gastrointestinal tract may be visible or invisible. **Occult** blood is not visible to the human eye. Visible blood in the stool may be bright red or may make the stool look black and sticky (called tarry stool), depending on where the bleeding is in the gastrointestinal tract.

Stool specimens are sometimes collected to test for occult blood (Fig. 18-7). You may be asked to perform this test (Procedure 18-8, next page). This is sometime called guaiacing the stool, or doing a **guaiac test** on the stool. Ask the charge nurse if you have any questions.

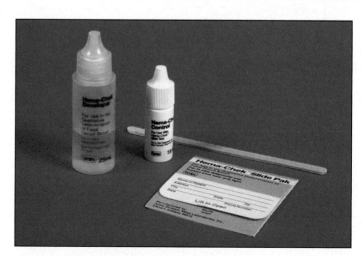

Fig. 18-7 − Equipment used to test stool for blood.

PROCEDURE 18-8. TESTING A STOOL SPECIMEN FOR OCCULT BLEEDING

Items Needed
- bedpan
- toilet paper
- specimen collection application
- gloves
- container for specimen
- testing materials

1. Put on gloves.

Note: *If you contaminate your gloves in any way during the procedure, you must change to a new pair of gloves.*

2. After the resident has a bowel movement, use an applicator to obtain a small sample of the fecal material.

3. Put a thin smear of the fecal material on the kit's test slide in the designated area. Some test slides have two sections so that you can test smears from two different areas of the stool.

4. After putting the smear on the slide, wait 3-5 minutes. (This allows the slide to better absorb the fecal matter.)

5. Put two drops of the developer solution on the back of the slide directly behind the stool sample.

6. Read the results in 60 seconds (or follow the directions in the kit). If any blue or blue-green color appears around the edge of the sample, the test is positive for occult bleeding.

Note: *Testing is often done with three consecutive stools because bleeding may occur only at times rather than continuously. Checking three stools at different times can better identify occult bleeding.*

7. Remove and dispose of your gloves in the disposable trash bag, throw the trash bag away, and wash your hands after handling each specimen.

HELPING A RESIDENT WITH AN OSTOMY

Residents may have had surgery that created an ostomy. An ostomy is a surgical opening in the abdomen to bring waste outside the body. Ostomies can be done to divert a resident's urine (ureterostomy) or stool (colostomy). The opening is called the stoma. The stoma is normally red and has a round shape. Immediately after surgery the stoma may be swollen. After surgery the stoma is measured for fitting the proper pouching system. You may care for a resident who has an ostomy. In many cases this is the resident's permanent method of elimination.

Many residents with ostomies are very sensitive and concerned about how others perceive them. They are often afraid of being avoided or treated differently. Always show a good attitude to the resident. Treat them with respect and dignity. Be careful to avoid any facial expressions or comments they may find negative.

📖
Guaiac test – procedure for checking blood in the stool or vomit
Occult – cannot be seen
Ostomy – a surgical opening from the intestine to outside the body
Parasite – an organism living in or on another organism
Stoma – a surgically created opening

Types of Ostomies

A ureterostomy is surgery that leads both ureters to the stoma in the resident's abdomen. This procedure may be done because of a disease like cancer. The resident's urine is excreted through the stoma into a bag or pouch attached to their abdomen.

A colostomy connects the colon or bowel to a stoma on the surface of the abdomen. This surgery is done for many reasons, such as colon cancer and other diseases that cause colon inflammation. Bowel elimination then occurs through this opening into an ostomy bag.

A resident with a colostomy may have one or two stomas. Some colostomies are permanent, but some are only temporary. The fecal contents eliminated may be semi–liquid or fairly well formed, depending on the site of the surgery in the intestine.

The main difference between care for a colostomy and an **ileostomy** involves stool consistency. Ileostomy fecal contents are usually much more liquid. They also contain more digestive juices, which can irritate the skin. An ileostomy is often permanent.

Ostomy Care

Follow your facility's policies and procedures when caring for someone with an ostomy. Many residents do their own care independently. They may need you only to provide supplies. How much support you give depends on the resident's level of independence. With all residents, however, pay attention to their elimination pattern for any change. Observe the stoma for changes. Because the stoma has a rich blood supply, it will bleed easily if irritated or injured. Even when injured, the resident will not feel pain or other sensations in the stoma because no nerve endings are present in the stoma. The skin around the stoma must be protected from irritating digestive enzymes. Observe the skin around the stoma for any signs of irritation. Report any problems to the charge nurse. The exact care you give depends on the resident's needs, what the charge nurse says, and the care plan.

Most residents with an ostomy use a bag device called an appliance or pouch (Fig. 18-8). Your observations related to the ostomy are very important. When helping a resident with dressing, undressing, or bathing, take time to observe the appliance and resident's skin. Ask yourself these questions:

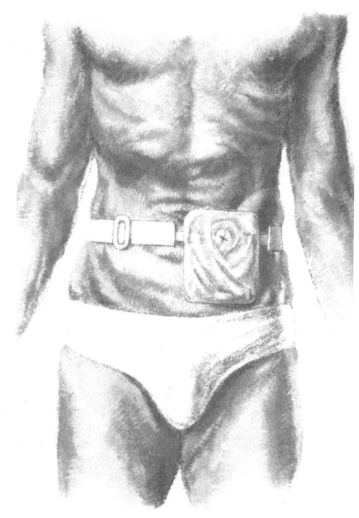

Fig. 18-8 – Most residents with an ostomy use some type of pouch.

- Is the appliance leaking?
- Is the seal around the stoma secure?
- Is the ostomy draining well?
- Are the consistency and color of the stool or urine normal?
- Are the stoma and surrounding skin intact, or is there redness, bleeding, or other skin breakdown?

Ileostomy – surgery that leads the opening of the ileum to the stoma. The ileum is a part of the small intestine.

Emptying an Ostomy Bag.   If the resident does not independently care for their ostomy, you may be asked to empty and measure the contents from their ostomy bag. When emptying an ostomy bag, follow these guidelines:

1. Always wear gloves.
2. Measure the contents of the bag at least once during a shift. To empty the bag, undo the clip on the bottom of the bag and empty the contents into a bedpan. Some bags do not have clips and must be changed after each use. Know the appliance your resident uses and how to empty it (Fig. 18-9).
3. Rinse out the bag each time you empty it. You may use a large irrigation syringe. Add a deodorizer if needed.
4. Wipe off the end of the bag.
5. Reseal the bag with the clip.

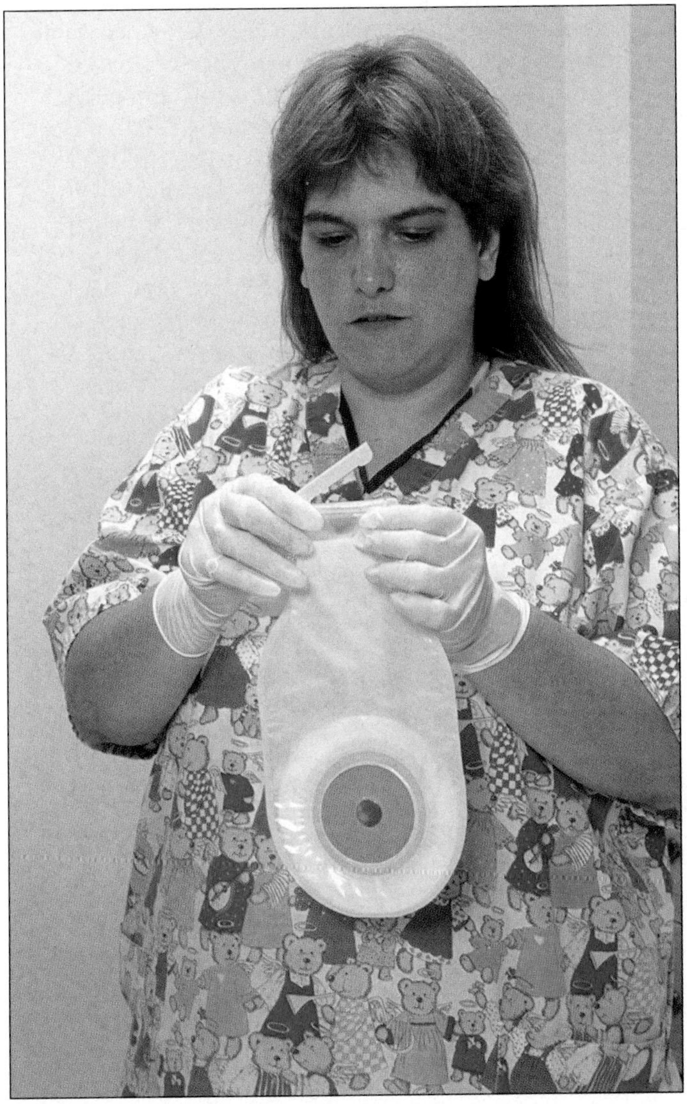

Fig. 18-9 – Be sure to read and follow the manufacturer's directions for how to empty or change an ostomy bag.

IN THIS CHAPTER YOU LEARNED HOW TO:

- Determine residents' elimination patterns
- Maintain a resident's dignity when helping with elimination
- Use equipment for elimination
- Help residents use the bedpan, urinal, and portable commode
- Identify changes in residents' elimination patterns
- Collect elimination specimens
- Help with ostomy care

SUMMARY

This chapter is about helping residents meet their elimination needs. You need to learn residents' elimination patterns and how to help them maintain their normal routines. Create an environment in which the resident is treated with dignity. Your skills for supporting residents with toileting are important. Also know what to watch for and report to the charge nurse.

You also have a role in collecting specimens to help the nurse and physician identify any problems related to elimination. Residents with ostomies may also need your support, depending on their level of independence. Treating them with respect helps them feel more comfortable with their condition.

Always remember: Everyone wants to maintain their independence with bodily functions. When many residents enter long term care facilities, they are able to do their own toileting. Work to create an environment that helps them maintain their normal elimination pattern and independence.

PULLING IT ALL TOGETHER

You are assigned to care for Mrs. Smith, an 86-year-old woman just admitted to your facility. During your interview with Mrs. Smith and her daughter you ask about elimination. You see that Mrs. Smith is uncomfortable answering your questions about her elimination patterns. Her daughter interrupts and tells you that this is a very sensitive area for her mom. Her biggest worry in coming to the facility is being able to get to the bathroom.

Mrs. Smith is recovering from a hip fracture and was admitted for rehabilitation. She is worried because she needs help to go to the bathroom. She does not want to have any accidents. You talk about her normal patterns for urinating and bowel elimination. You tell her that together you will make a plan that will help make sure she does not have accidents. You explain that all the staff caring for her will know the plan and it will meet her needs. You tell Mrs. Smith that you will talk to the physical therapist, who will tell staff the best way to help her to the bathroom. You say that maybe a commode by the bed will help when she feels she cannot make it to the bathroom. Now you see that Mrs. Smith is becoming more relaxed and open.

At the end of the interview Mrs. Smith and her daughter thank you for being so considerate and sensitive to her needs.

1. **Why is it important to be familiar with a resident's elimination pattern?**
   A. So that you never have to clean up an accident.
   B. So that you can recognize and report any changes.
   C. To keep the family informed at every visit.
   D. Because you discuss every resident's elimination at the end of your shift.

2. **What is the best way to put a resident at ease when talking about elimination patterns?**
   A. Tell elimination jokes.
   B. Have the conversation in private.
   C. Ask the resident's roommate to be present when you discuss elimination.
   D. Use the slang terms children use for elimination.

3. **Ketone testing is often used for residents with:**
   A. Diabetes.
   B. Alzheimer's disease.
   C. Constipation.
   D. An infection.

4. **Which of the following should you report to the charge nurse?**
   A. A resident urinated twice during your shift.
   B. A family member poured two glasses of water for a resident during a visit.
   C. A resident's urine is a light amber color.
   D. A resident's urine is cloudy.

5. **You are assisting Mrs. Romberti as she uses the bedpan. What is the best way to protect her dignity and privacy?**
   A. Hold her hand while she relieves herself.
   B. Reassure her by telling her how often you've changed infants' diapers while babysitting.
   C. Close the door, pull the bedside curtain, and cover her legs.
   D. Leave her alone and say you'll be back in an hour.

6. **You are a new nurse assistant at your facility. How might you learn that a certain resident has frequent incontinence?**
   A. By checking the resident's medical record.
   B. By interviewing all family members that come to visit.
   C. By checking the sheets for dampness.
   D. By checking the resident's clothing for urine stains.

7. **Mr. Noland has an ostomy and uses a disposable bag which you must empty. What is an important aspect of his care?**
   A. Noting the brand of ostomy bag he uses.
   B. Checking the condition of his skin around the stoma.
   C. Asking him frequently if his bag needs changing.
   D. Requesting family members to empty the bag.

8. **The staff is collecting a 24-hour urine specimen on Mrs. Matson using a "hat" in her toilet. You see her leaving the visitor's restroom shortly after dinner, and she admits she urinated in the toilet there but did not flush it yet. What should you do?**
   A. Tell the charge nurse the test has to be restarted.
   B. Tell Mrs. Matson that's OK.
   C. Pour about a cup of water into the specimen container to make up for it.
   D. Using a clean cup, dip some of the fluid from the toilet and add it into the specimen container.

9. **You are obtaining a clean-catch urine specimen from Mrs. Mancini. At what stage in the procedure do you clean her perineum?**
   A. Before she urinates.
   B. After she has urinated a little.
   C. After you've collected the specimen.
   D. Not until the test results come back.

10. **To collect a stool specimen, you should:**
    A. Have the resident not eat anything for 24 hours.
    B. Store the specimen wrapped in paper towels in the lunchroom refrigerator.
    C. Label the specimen container correctly and promptly.
    D. Ask the resident's roommate to hold the bedpan.

(Answers to "Check What You've Learned" are in the Instructor's Manual.)

19

MAINTAINING AND IMPROVING SKIN INTEGRITY

The condition of a resident's skin often reflects their overall health status. Maintaining intact, healthy skin is a major goal of care in all health care settings. In Chapter 11 you learned that the skin is the largest organ of the human body and is a major defense against infection. Bacteria normally live on the skin surface. Once this protective skin layer is broken, these bacteria and other disease-causing pathogens can enter the body. A skin infection or other body infection may result. One of the biggest challenges and goals of all health care providers is to prevent the formation of pressure ulcers. If you work in a long term care facility, you will be part of the team who actively works to prevent pressure ulcers.

The reasons for this major health care goal are clear: pressure ulcers are a source of much pain and suffering, as well as cost, for residents and their families. The treatment of pressure ulcers is complex and takes much nursing time. All members of the interdisciplinary team must do everything they can to help prevent pressure ulcers. This chapter is about what you can do to help care for residents' skin. It describes what you need to know and report about residents at risk for pressure ulcers. You will learn about the stages of pressure ulcers and your role in preventing them. You will also learn about other types of wounds. A wound is any break in the tissue. A pressure ulcer is one type of wound. Other wounds can occur from injury, diseases such as cancer, or surgery.

OBJECTIVES
- Describe factors that influence skin health
- Describe why maintaining skin integrity can be a problem for residents in long term care
- List at least five strategies for keeping residents' skin healthy
- Describe what can happen when a resident's skin integrity is not maintained
- Describe other common kinds of wounds
- Demonstrate how to remove a wound dressing, clean a wound, and dress a wound

MEDICAL TERMS
- **Contusion** – a type of wound made by blunt force, causing bruising and swelling but usually the skin is not broken
- **Decubitus ulcer (pressure ulcer)** – an opening or wound that appears in pressure areas of skin overlying a bony area in an immobile person
- **Incision** – a type of wound with straight edges, made by a sharp instrument or object, including surgical incisions
- **Laceration** – a type of wound made by an object causing an irregular, jagged wound
- **Puncture** – a type of wound down into the skin, made by something pointed

PROCEDURE 19-1
Removing a Wound Dressing

PROCEDURE 19-2
Cleaning a Wound

PROCEDURE 19-3
Dressing a Wound

"My skin feels so soft after you've put on my lotion. Your constant watchfulness keeps me healthy."

Have you ever noticed how some people's skin seems to radiate health? It looks soft, has just the right amount of color, and is smooth and clear. Think about a baby's skin—a perfect example of what healthy skin looks like. Healthy skin is also intact, which means it has no openings, such as cuts or wounds. Healthy skin is also free of bruises.

Healthy skin often reflects healthy lifestyle choices, such as good nutrition, drinking enough water, and getting enough sleep and exercise. Skin is healthier also when tobacco and drugs are avoided, alcohol consumption is limited, and the skin is protected from sun exposure. Think of someone you know whose skin does not look healthy. Do they smoke? Do they eat well? Do (or did) they sunbathe without using sunscreen? (Getting some sun is important for overall health, especially for the bones, but the skin must be protected from ultraviolet rays.)

Your skin often reflects your health (Fig. 19-1). Maintaining skin health and integrity as a person ages is a challenge. In your role as a nurse assistant you must understand what is needed to keep the resident's skin healthy.

THE CHALLENGE OF SKIN CARE

Remember the descriptions of long term care residents in Chapter 1. Many residents are women with a chronic illness who can no longer manage their health at home.

Usually they need help with one or more of the activities of daily living. They may need help with bathing, dressing, transferring, toileting, and eating.

If a resident needs help because they are cannot move or use the toilet independently, they are at risk for a problem with skin integrity. Being immobile or staying in the same position for even short periods of time puts a resident at risk. A resident with reduced cognitive abilities, who may be confused or forgetful, is also at a greater risk. They may not be able to tell you about symptoms they are experiencing. They may forget to change positions, or may forget to go to the bathroom. In addition, the natural aging changes you learned about in Chapter 11, The Aging Process and Disease Management, increase the risks for skin problems.

MAINTAINING SKIN INTEGRITY

As you have already learned, you must observe residents carefully and report any problems or changes you find. These include changes in skin color or temperature. You may also find a rash or other "bumps," which are signs of dermatitis. You should report immediately the slightest

📖
Dermatitis – inflammation of the skin, which may look like redness or a rash and cause itching

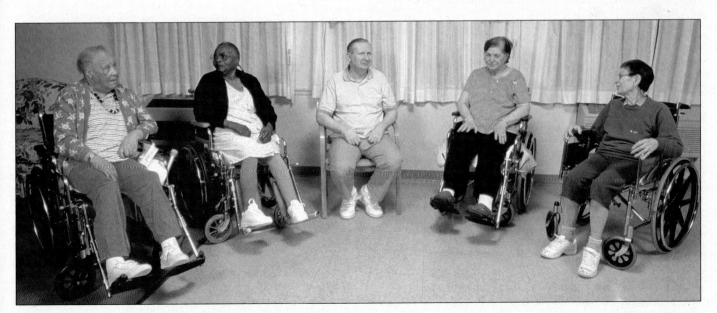

Fig. 19-1 – Skin tone and condition often vary widely among different residents.

change in a resident's skin (Fig. 19-2). Once a wound forms and there is a break in the skin, extensive treatment may be needed. Wounds can be very slow to heal.

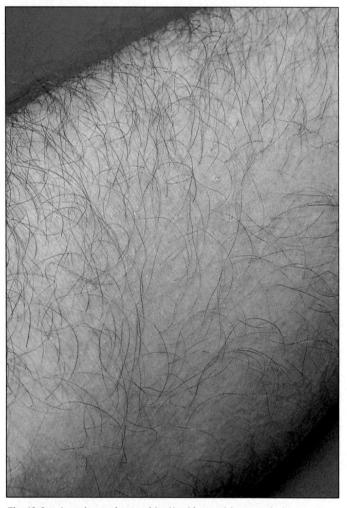

Fig. 19-2 – Any change in a resident's skin must be reported.

Your role in caring for the resident's skin includes maintaining or improving the resident's health overall as well as using strategies to prevent skin breakdown.

The keys to maintaining skin integrity are to:
- promote circulation, for example by moving the resident, encouraging mobility, and helping the resident with exercise
- keep the resident clean and help with going to the toilet, especially when incontinent, because the moisture and acidity of urine can contribute to skin breakdown
- ensure that the resident has good nutritional and fluid intake

Most facilities use an assessment tool to determine a resident's risk for a problem with skin integrity. When doing this assessment, the interdisciplinary team may ask you questions about the resident. This is usually done on admission and whenever the resident's health changes. The team may categorize residents based on the assessment information. For example, the resident may be categorized as a high or low risk for problems with skin integrity. Typically a resident is at a high risk if they cannot move about, eat, or go to the toilet by themselves. They are also at a high risk if they have cognitive loss and may forget to eat or drink or go to the toilet.

Table 19-1 outlines strategies you can use to help prevent skin problems. As you think about the actions described there, notice that almost everything you do as a nurse assistant can affect the resident's skin health. Also apply what you have learned in previous chapters.

OBSERVATION AND REPORTING

As a nurse assistant, you are in the best position to observe the resident's skin from head to toe. Be especially alert with these residents who are at greater risk:
- residents who are very thin
- residents who need help eating and drinking fluids
- residents who cannot move by themselves or are not motivated to move
- residents who are cognitively impaired or cannot communicate well

As you examine the resident's skin, especially over bony areas, check its color. If you find an area of red skin that does not return to normal color after the resident is repositioned, tell the nurse. Also check any area that is swollen, because skin that is stretched is more likely to have a problem. Report any breaks or tears in the skin to the nurse and ask for special instructions. Remember that in dark-skinned people, changes in skin color may not be apparent, but the skin may change in texture, have bumps, or be swollen.

TABLE 19-1
STRATEGIES TO PREVENT SKIN PROBLEMS

PREVENTIVE STRATEGIES	NURSE ASSISTANT'S ROLE
Mobility	Help the resident walk. Walking increases the circulation of blood to the skin, supplying nourishment the skin needs to be healthy. If a resident cannot walk, frequent changes in position are needed to relieve pressure and keep blood flowing to all areas of the body. Never slide the resident across the bed sheets. Always use available lifting devices.
Nutrition	Ensure that the resident eats enough food. Adequate protein, vitamins, and minerals are needed for healthy skin. Report any change in the resident's weight or how much food they eat. Make sure the resident drinks enough fluid. Adequate fluid intake helps all body systems and keeps the skin moist.
Observation	Inspect the resident's skin daily, especially if they cannot move or use the toilet independently. Check under all skin folds daily. Keep the area clean and dry.
Range-of-motion (ROM) exercise	Exercise is important for maintaining strength and muscle tone. It also increases the blood supply to an area.
Toileting	Help the resident with toileting as needed. Monitor them frequently for incontinence. If the resident is incontinent, clean their skin after each incident. Make sure the resident is never left in wet clothes or in any product used for incontinence that is wet.
Bathing and moisturizing	Keep the resident's skin clean and dry. Moisturize their skin daily. Use the resident's own products; if they do not usually use such products and you notice their skin is dry, ask the charge nurse what to use (Fig. 19-3). 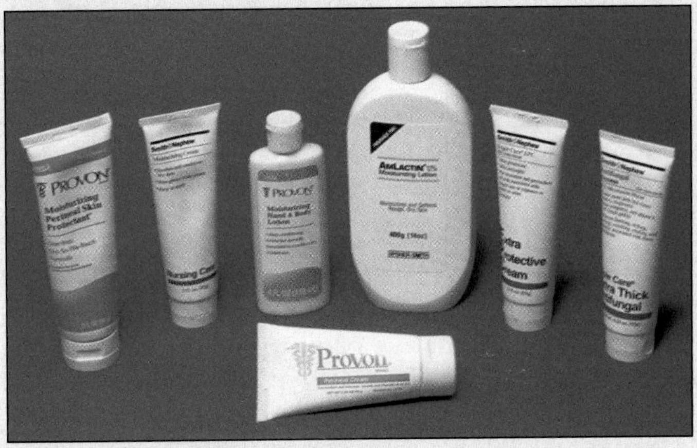 Fig. 19-3 – Skin care products help keep the resident's skin moisturized so that the skin does not crack from dryness.
Reporting	Immediately report any change in the condition of the resident's skin.

PRESSURE ULCERS

If a resident's skin health is not maintained, they may develop a pressure ulcer. This is also called a decubitus ulcer or bedsore.

Pressure ulcers are a breakdown of the skin. They are caused by pressure, including pressure from rubbing, friction or shearing. Pressure ulcers form when a resident cannot or does not change positions often enough. Think about how you sleep: you may fall asleep on your back but wake up on your side. While you sleep, and during the day, your brain tells your body when there is too much pressure on a body area. Then you automatically change position to relieve the pressure. Residents with a serious disease or condition, however, need your help to change position to relieve pressure. Pressure over even short periods of time decreases the flow of blood to the area. This reduces the nourishment and oxygen the skin receives. Skin cells die, blood vessels break, and an open wound forms.

Pressure ulcers occur most often where the skin is thin and you can easily feel bone underneath. Common places are the elbows, shoulder blades, hips, base of the spine ("tailbone" or coccyx), and heels. Other problem areas are the ears, under the breasts, between the buttocks, and other areas experiencing frequent rubbing or friction. Friction and shearing forces occur when skin rubs against an object or another area of skin. For example, the side of a resident's leg may rub against the side of their wheelchair, or the inside of the knee may rub against the other knee. Even rubbing just a few times can cause the skin to tear. Frequent rubbing can damage blood vessels and other tissue along with skin breakdown. This can also happen when the resident is moved or pulled across the bed, such as during positioning.

Moisture can build up in areas such as under a female's breasts, between the buttocks, or in the groin area if a resident is incontinent. Prolonged moisture can cause the skin to weaken or break down. A resident who is incontinent is at greater risk for skin damage. Weakened skin can contribute to the formation of a pressure ulcer.

Early Signs and Symptoms of Pressure Ulcers

- any reddened area of the body that does not return to its original color after repositioning—the area may look bruised
- blistering or breakdown of skin
- increased sensitivity, change in temperature, or pain

Your observations and prompt reporting of these early pressure ulcer symptoms may save your resident from developing a more serious ulcer.

Decubitus ulcer (pressure ulcer) – an opening or wound that appears in pressure areas of skin overlying a bony area in an immobile person

PRESSURE ULCER STAGES

The National Pressure Ulcer Advisory Panel has redefined the stages of pressure ulcers and added two more skin injury categories (unstageable and deep tissue injury).

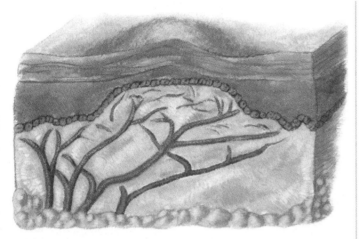

Stage 1
Intact skin with non-blanchable redness (does not become lighter in color when pressed with a finger) of a localized area usually over a bony prominence. Darkly pigmented skin may not have visible blanching; its color may differ from the surrounding area, or the feel and look of the skin may be different from the surrounding tissue.

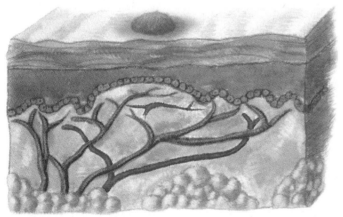

Stage 2
Partial-thickness loss of dermis (layer of skin tissue) seen as a shallow open ulcer with a red or pink wound bed, without slough (dying skin tissue forming a crust). There may also be an intact, open, or ruptured blister.

Unstageable
Full-thickness tissue loss in which the base of the ulcer is covered by slough (yellow, tan, green, or brown) and/or eschar (tan, brown, or black) in the wound bed. (not shown)

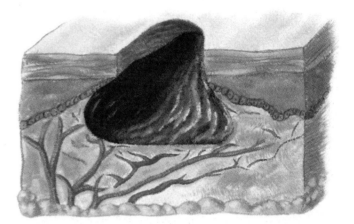

Stage 3
Full-thickness loss of skin tissue. Fat tissue fat may be visible under the skin, but bone, tendon, and muscle tissue are not exposed. Slough may be present but does not obscure the depth of tissue loss. The wound may include undermining and tunneling (skin tissue dying below the surface).

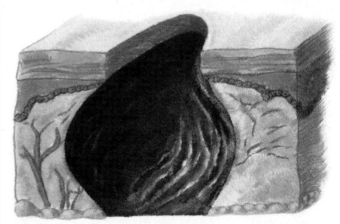

Stage 4
Full-thickness tissue loss with bone, tendon, or muscle tissue showing through the wound. Slough or eschar (a thick crust) may be present on some parts of the wound bed. Often undermining and tunneling are present.

Deep Tissue Injury
Purple localized area of discolored intact skin or a blood-filled blister due to damage of underlying soft tissue. (not shown)

Source: National Pressure Ulcer Advisory Panel, 2007 www.npuap.org

Treatment of Pressure Ulcers

Preventing pressure ulcers is one of the most important jobs you do as a nursing assistant. Treatment and healing are difficult, painful, and costly for the resident, family, and facility staff. Your primary role in treatment is to report information to the nurse. Even when an ulcer first looks "healed," the skin area is still damaged and can more easily become an ulcer again.

Be sure to always use the strategies outlined in Table 19-1. These strategies help prevent pressure ulcers. These strategies are particularly important for residents at risk, but you should often monitor the condition of all residents' skin. If the resident is at risk, inspect their skin at least every two hours and whenever providing personal care.

The following guidelines are important for prevention, treatment, and healing of skin problems:

• To promote resident's circulation
  – change the resident's position and inspect bony skin areas at least every two hours (see Chapter 15, Learning to Position and Move Correctly).

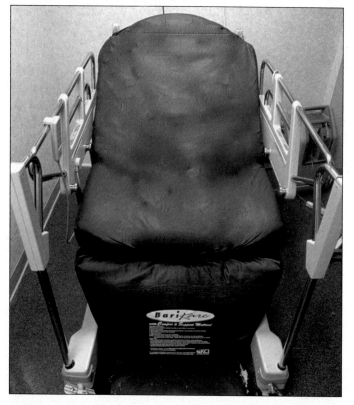

Fig. 19-4 – Special mattresses help distribute the resident's weight evenly to prevent pressure in some areas.

  – perform passive ROM exercises as directed in the resident's care plan.
• To relieve pressure
  – use a special pressure-reducing device, such as an air mattress, a circulating air mattress, or a mattress containing water or gel. These help distribute the resident's weight evenly to reduce pressure on certain areas (Fig. 19-4).
  – for residents on bed rest, use devices that totally relieve pressure on their heels. This can be done by raising their heels off the bed (Fig 19-5).

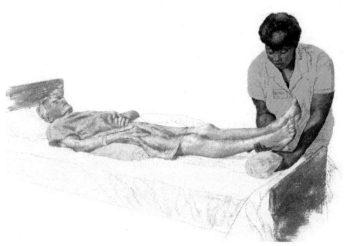

Fig. 19-5 – Elevate the resident's heels off the bed to prevent pressure on the heels.

  – inspect the heels when repositioning the resident and during bathing
  – minimize skin-to-skin contact by using positioning devices like pillows between the resident's knees or under their elbows and forearms (Fig 19-6, next page).
  – be sure that residents who wear shoes also wear socks; check their heels and toes to be sure the shoes fit properly and do not rub.
• To prevent injury
  – keep the resident's skin clean and dry.
  – prevent friction on the resident's skin. For example, lift the resident in bed from underneath instead of pulling them up. Use padding on wheelchair arms and legs.
  – keep the bed clean and free of objects like crumbs, combs, and glasses, and keep the bedding free of wrinkles.
  – use cornstarch on the bedpan or commode seat to prevent the resident's skin from sticking to it.

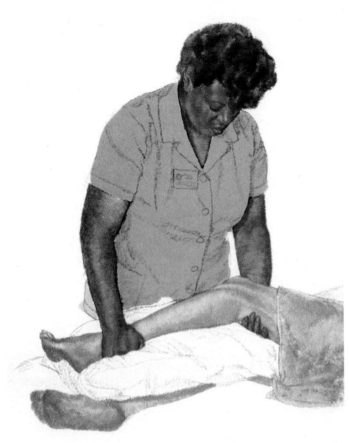

Fig. 19-6 – Pillows or other devices help prevent skin from touching skin.

- keep skinfold areas clean and dry. Constant moist contact leads to skin breakdown.
- do not elevate the head of the bed higher than 30 degrees. This prevents the resident from sliding down, causing friction and shearing forces on their skin.
• To promote nutrition
- closely monitor the resident's fluid and food intake. Encourage good nutrition and drinking enough fluids. Offer snacks or nutritional supplements between meals as ordered. Notify the nurse if the resident has poor food or fluid intake.
- weigh the resident often and report any change immediately.

These steps along with specific treatments help promote healing. The health care team will use different treatments in each stage, but you must always continue the preventive strategies. Your primary role is to prevent and observe pressure ulcers and report any skin changes right away.

Many facilities now have an interdisciplinary team (led by a physician) that examines the ulcer and assesses the need for any treatment change each week. The nurse usually performs treatments for the ulcer and assesses the area to help the physician decide if the treatment is working. You may be asked to help the nurse with positioning the resident or gathering supplies. All health care professionals should keep up to date about new, effective ulcer treatments and approaches for prevention. Different treatments may be used depending on the stage of the ulcer. Box 19-1 outlines treatment of pressure ulcers in each stage.

BOX 19-1.
TREATMENT OF PRESSURE ULCERS

STAGE I: PRE-ULCER FORMATION
• Notify the charge nurse immediately about any change. Ask them to inspect the area.
• Focus on preventing pressure on the area. Use all prevention methods.

STAGE II: BREAKDOWN OR BLISTERING OF THE TOP LAYERS OF SKIN
• The nurse cleans the area, and covers it with a dry sterile dressing or a protective dressing.

Note: *The key is prevention. All members of the team are responsible for preventing any skin breakdown.*

STAGE III: BREAKDOWN INTO DEEP TISSUE
• The nurse cleans the area and applies medications and dressings ordered by the physician. The wound may require packing or irrigation. Assist the nurse as asked. Observe and report if the dressing becomes saturated or dislodged.
• Closely watch the resident for infections. Watch for any foul smell, discharge, or redness around the area. Report these findings to the nurse.

STAGE IV: INVOLVEMENT OF THE MUSCLE AND BONE
• The nurse cleans the area and applies medications and dressings as ordered by the physician. The wound may require packing or irrigation. In some instances a "wound vac" (which promotes healing by removing excess drainage from the wound) may be used. Assist the nurse as asked. Observe and report if the dressing becomes saturated or moves, or if the "wound vac" moves.
• Surgery may be needed to remove dead tissue or provide a new top skin layer (a "flap").

OTHER TYPES OF WOUNDS

Remember that a wound is a break in the continuity of the skin. Wound healing involves restoring the skin to its intact state.

One way to classify wounds is by the type of injury to the skin. These are common types of wounds:

1. **Incision** – made by a sharp instrument, such as a surgical scalpel
2. **Contusion** – made by blunt force causing a break in small blood vessels (bruising) and swelling
3. **Laceration** – made by some object causing an irregular, jagged wound
4. **Puncture** wounds – made by something pointed
5. **Lesions or skin breakdown** – caused by from a disease, such as cancer, HIV, or poor circulation

WOUND CARE

The type of wound affects what care is needed. Your role in caring for a resident's wound may include helping the nurse with dressing changes. Also report any changes such as signs of infection. If a wound becomes red or swollen, or has a foul smell and discharge, this means infection is likely. You must report this immediately to the nurse.

To promote wound healing, be sure the resident has good nutrition, the wound is kept clean and protected from further injury, and the resident gets enough rest. Different types of dressings are commonly used on wounds (Box 19-2).

Dressings are not used on all wounds. For example, a day after surgery, the wound may be dry and skin edges intact, and a dressing may not be used. Not covering a wound with a dressing has two benefits:

- Allows watching for healing
- Helps prevent conditions that may cause infection, like warmth, too much moisture, and darkness

BOX 19-2. COMMON TYPES OF DRESSINGS

DRY DRESSING
This type of dressing is primarily used for surgical incisions. A dry dressing protects the wound and absorbs drainage.

WET-TO-DRY DRESSING
This type of dressing is rarely used because it pulls away good tissue as well as bad tissue. It is only used for infected wounds or wounds that contain dead or poor tissue. Gauze soaked with a sterile saline or antiseptic solution is first packed into the wound. This is covered by a dry dressing.

WET-TO-WET DRESSINGS
This type of dressing is used on clean open wounds. Sterile saline or antiseptic solution is put on the dressing. This wet dressing is placed on the wound. A moist wound generally heals more naturally.

PROTECTIVE AND ABSORPTIVE DRESSINGS
These dressings protect as well as absorb drainage from a shallow wound. They are changed every two or three days. These are called hydrocolloid dressings and include Duoderm® and Tegasorb® dressings. The dressing provides a moist environment for more natural wound healing.

PROTECTIVE OR 2ND SKIN® DRESSINGS
These dressings cover and protect a superficial wound. Because the dressing is transparent, the nurse can observe how the wound is healing.

The primary purposes of any dressing are to protect the wound and absorb excess drainage.

If you are responsible for changing a resident's dressing, follow Procedures 19-1 to 19-3.

Contusion – a type of wound made by blunt force, causing bruising and swelling but usually the skin is not broken

Incision – a type of wound with straight edges, made by a sharp instrument or object, including surgical incisions

Laceration – a type of wound made by an object causing an irregular, jagged wound

Puncture – a type of wound down into the skin, made by something pointed

PROCEDURE 19-1. REMOVING A WOUND DRESSING

 REMEMBER: BE AWARE

Items Needed
- disposable gloves
- disposable bag

1. Put on disposable gloves. You do not need sterile gloves to remove the dressing.

2. Gently loosen the tape on the dressing, and pull the tape ends toward the wound. Holding the skin at the same time helps to prevent damage to the skin.

3. Remove the old dressing and place it in an appropriate disposable bag.

 REMEMBER: UNDERSTAND

PROCEDURE 19-2. CLEANING A WOUND

 REMEMBER: BE AWARE

Items Needed
- sterile gloves
- cotton-tipped applicator or gauze
- cleaning solution
- disposable bag

1. Open the sterile gloves and the sterile cleaning supplies.

2. Put on gloves.

3. Clean along the wound edges. Be sure to clean each side of the wound separately. Repeat using another moistened gauze or swab, until the entire wound is clean.

4. Dispose of used cleaning supplies in an appropriate disposable bag.

5. Pat the wound site dry with a sterile dressing sponge.

 REMEMBER: UNDERSTAND

PROCEDURE 19-3. DRESSING A WOUND

 REMEMBER: BE AWARE

Items Needed
- sterile gloves
- dressing pad
- tape or other adherent dressing or 2nd Skin® dressing

1. Maintain sterile technique with the use of sterile gloves.

2. Apply the appropriate dressing based on the care plan.

3. Secure the dressing, using only the amount of tape (or other method) required to secure the dressing.

 REMEMBER: UNDERSTAND

IN THIS CHAPTER YOU LEARNED:

• Factors that influence skin health
• Why maintaining skin integrity can be a problem for people in any health care setting
• Strategies for keeping residents' skin healthy
• What can happen when a resident's skin integrity is not maintained
• How to prevent pressure ulcers
• How to care for other types of wounds

SUMMARY

This chapter discusses many factors that influence skin health. This knowledge will help you care for all residents. You learned strategies to use in the daily care of residents to help maintain their skin integrity. Without these strategies, the resident may develop a pressure ulcer. You also learned about other types of wounds, how to care for them, and how to use dressings.

PULLING IT ALL TOGETHER

Most residents are admitted to long term care facilities because they can no longer care for themselves. Often this is a result of a medical condition. This condition can be temporary or permanent. Because of their condition, the resident may be at high risk for developing pressure ulcers. An example is a resident who falls at home and fractures his hip, has hip replacement surgery in the hospital, and is admitted to the facility for rehabilitation. In this unfamiliar setting, the resident may become depressed, have a decreased appetite, and may not progress with mobility as fast as the resident and caregivers hoped. Can you identify the risk factors this resident has for problems with skin integrity?

Another example of a resident at risk is someone with congestive heart failure. This person may be admitted because they have shortness of breath and cannot care for themselves. This resident may have mobility and nutritional problems that put them at high risk for pressure ulcers.

As you begin your work as a nurse assistant, you will find that most of the residents you care for are at some risk for developing pressure ulcers. They may be at risk for different reasons, but if prevention strategies are not used from the beginning, the outcome could be the same for all. Therefore you must use these preventive strategies and immediately report any change in the resident. Only in this way can you carry out your important role of ensuring that the resident's skin integrity is maintained.

In addition, your residents may have other types of wounds due to surgery or an injury. You need to help ensure a wound does not become infected. Keep it clean, and make sure the resident gets good nutrition and fluid intake and enough rest. If you see any sign of infection, report it to the nurse.

1. **When is a resident most at risk for skin breakdown?**
   - A. When they are hungry.
   - B. When they are immobile.
   - C. When they do not bathe each day.
   - D. When they are coughing or sneezing because they have a cold.

2. **What is the cause of a decubitus ulcer?**
   - A. Uncomfortable clothing.
   - B. Dirty pajamas.
   - C. Pressure on the skin.
   - D. Stress caused by family arguments.

3. **How can you help keep a resident's skin healthy?**
   - A. Encourage them to spend time everyday sitting in the sun.
   - B. Rub their skin vigorously after they bathe.
   - C. Rub cocoa butter on their skin at bedtime.
   - D. Help them maintain good circulation.

4. **Who performs the assessment of a resident's risk for skin breakdown?**
   - A. The interdisciplinary team.
   - B. The charge nurse.
   - C. The nurse assistant.
   - D. The resident.

5. **What daily preventive care is needed for a resident's skinfold areas?**
   - A. Apply an antiperspirant daily.
   - B. Apply ointment to lubricate and moisten the skin.
   - C. Check for growth of tumors.
   - D. Keep the area clean and dry.

6. **What is an early sign of a pressure ulcer?**
   - A. Pain at a joint.
   - B. Tingling sensations like the hand or foot "fell asleep."
   - C. Swelling around a joint.
   - D. Redness that does not go away.

7. **To prevent a stage one pressure ulcer from getting worse, you should:**
   - A. Frequently give the resident ice chips to suck on.
   - B. Give the resident three vitamin pills daily.
   - C. Follow the charge nurse's instructions.
   - D. Cover the area with a warm, moist cloth at all times.

8. **What is a sign of a stage II pressure ulcer?**
   - A. Redness that goes away quickly when the pressure is relieved.
   - B. Shallow open ulcer.
   - C. Breakdown of the skin exposing the bone beneath.
   - D. Breakdown of the skin to a deep crater accompanied by bleeding.

9. **What kind of bedding may be used for a resident with pressure ulcers?**
   - A. A large flat ice pad.
   - B. A firm hotel-style mattress.
   - C. A mattress that is filled with air, water, or gel.
   - D. A board placed on top of the mattress to provide a smooth, hard surface.

10. **To help prevent pressure ulcers in a bedridden resident, you should:**
    - A. Keep the resident awake as much as possible.
    - B. Change the resident's position every two hours.
    - C. Let the resident sleep only in the prone position.
    - D. Maximize skin-to-skin contact.

(Answers to "Check What You've Learned" are in the Instructor's Manual.)

Chapter 20

EMERGENCY CARE

In Chapter 11 you learned about diseases and medical conditions a resident may experience. You learned the difference between acute and chronic episodes. Some diseases and conditions can be treated and go away, but others cannot, so a resident must learn to adjust their life to them.

Residents may have various diseases and conditions for which they are being treated. In some cases, their condition may suddenly worsen and cause a medical emergency. In other cases, a resident may be injured unexpectedly or develop a life-threatening condition. These situations are medical emergencies. The initial first aid given to a resident in a medical emergency—before a physician or emergency medical professionals arrive—can prevent a serious problem for the resident. It may even save their life. In a long term care facility the nursing department has the most staff members. As a nurse assistant, you spend more time with residents than anyone else. You are the most likely staff member to observe an emergency. You are most likely the first to respond to it. This chapter describes what to do in the most common emergencies. You can use this information not only as a nurse assistant but also with your family and friends. In this chapter you will learn your responsibilities in an emergency as well as guidelines to follow in all emergencies. You will also learn specific steps to take in emergencies such as cardiac arrest, choking, seizure, shock, burns, and bleeding.

OBJECTIVES

- Define emergency first aid
- Explain your role and responsibilities in an emergency
- State general guidelines to follow in an emergency
- Identify five signs and symptoms of a heart attack and the care to give a resident having a heart attack
- Explain how to give cardiopulmonary resuscitation
- Identify the signs of choking and explain the Heimlich maneuver
- Identify the signs of a seizure and how to care for a resident who is experiencing seizures
- Explain what care to give a resident who has a burn
- Explain what care to give a resident who is bleeding
- Identify the signs and symptoms of shock and the care for a resident in shock

MEDICAL TERMS

- **Aura** – a subtle sensation that often precedes a seizure
- **Cardiopulmonary resuscitation (CPR)** – procedure to maintain breathing and circulation in a person experiencing cardiac arrest
- **Cholesterol** – a substance present in animal cells and body fluids
- **Hemorrhage** – excessive loss of blood in a short period of time
- **Palpitations** – strong, rapid heartbeats
- **Plaque** – fatty deposits on blood vessel walls
- **Protein** – combination of amino acids that are essential for all living cells
- **Seizure** – a condition resulting from an abnormality in the brain
- **Shock** – a condition in which vital organs in the body are not getting enough blood and oxygen to maintain good function
- **Sternum** – breastbone

"You are my lifeline.

I know that I can count on you

to act quickly in an emergency."

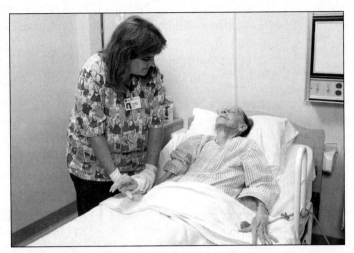

Fig. 20-1 – First aid for bleeding involves covering the wound with your gloved hand and putting pressure on it.

Have you ever been involved in an emergency? How did you feel? What went through your mind? What was the first thing you did? Did you panic and run, or scream for help, or calmly take action? Your reaction in an emergency often depends on who the victim is and your confidence in knowing how to respond.

Emergencies can happen anytime, anywhere. As a nurse assistant, you must be prepared for emergencies and know how to respond. Being prepared helps prevent or at least control the chaos that often surrounds emergencies and can prevent the potential death of a resident. Keeping calm and knowing exactly what to do in these situations is crucial.

FIRST AID

First aid is the treatment immediately given to a person in an emergency. The goal of this treatment is to save the resident's life, prevent disability, and prevent an injury or sudden illness from getting worse. You give first aid to a resident only until health care personnel with more training arrive and give additional care. For example, if a resident cuts their wrist and is bleeding heavily, first aid involves covering the wound with a pad and putting pressure on it to stop the bleeding (Fig. 20-1). This is the initial care, the first aid to give. When the nurse arrives, the wound is bandaged. If necessary, the resident is transported to the hospital for stitches to close the wound.

If you had not given first aid by covering the wound and putting pressure on it to stop the bleeding, the resident would have lost blood. They might require a transfusion. The wound might be infected. Using your first aid knowledge can make a huge difference.

There is no better feeling than helping another or even saving a life. Imagine how wonderful you would feel if you saved the life of a resident, family member, friend, or stranger on the street.

YOUR ROLE AND RESPONSIBILITIES IN AN EMERGENCY

As a nurse assistant, you are expected to know what to do in an emergency. You are expected to stay with the resident, call for help, and begin first aid. When help arrives, you are expected to assist as needed. Your facility should periodically review their policy and procedures manual and tell you your role in emergencies. Study this information so that you are ready to do what is expected of you.

When you first realize an emergency is happening, before you begin to do anything, ask yourself these questions:
• What exactly is the emergency?
• Do I know what to do?
• What should I do first?

Here are general guidelines to follow in any emergency:
• If possible, use standard precautions (see Chapter 9, Prevention and Control of Infection).
• Remain calm at all times.
• Let the resident know you are there to help them.
• Know your facility's policies and procedures.

- Do not move the resident unless you must remove them from a dangerous situation. Moving a resident if you are not properly trained could cause further injury. The charge nurse and emergency medical personnel are trained to move residents.
- Know where emergency equipment is located on the floor or unit where you work (Fig. 20-2). You should become familiar with emergency equipment such as oxygen and oxygen supplies because the charge nurse may ask you to get these supplies in an emergency.

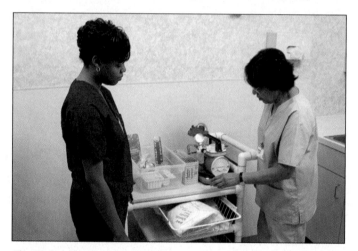

Fig. 20-2 – Always know where the emergency equipment is kept.

- When your facility holds emergency drills, treat the practice situation as you would a real emergency. When you are completely prepared and know what to do in an emergency, the steps to take will be natural to you during a real crisis
- Know the codes your facility uses to identify emergencies. When a code is called, all staff must know what is happening so that valuable time is not lost.
- Always answer call lights promptly. This is necessary both for quality care and to promptly discover emergency situations. Most resident calls are not emergencies, but you never know until you check. A fire might have started in a trash can, someone might be choking, or a resident could be having severe chest pain.
- Keep an injured or suddenly ill resident warm by covering them with a blanket. If it is very hot, lightly cover them with a sheet.
- After the charge nurse arrives, you may be asked to call 911 or your local emergency number. Give the operator this information:

- the name and address of the facility
- the telephone number
- the nature of the emergency
- what first aid has already been given

HEART ATTACK AND CARDIAC ARREST

Heart Attack

The heart is a muscular, hollow organ with four chambers (Fig. 20-3). The heart pumps blood containing oxygen and nutrients to the entire body. The heart muscle has its own blood supply. The coronary arteries bring it blood, nutrients, and oxygen. When this blood supply is interrupted due to a blockage, a heart attack occurs. The blockage can be due to **plaque** or **protein** along with **cholesterol** in the inner lining of the arteries that breaks off and forms a clot. This clot can then interrupt or block the flow of blood. Another name for a heart attack is coronary or myocardial infarction (MI).

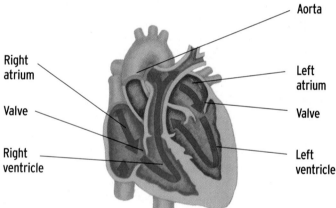

Fig. 20-3 – The major structure of the heart.

You must report chest pain right away. If a resident tells you they are having chest pain, this is very serious. Chest pain is always considered a sign of a heart attack until the medical team that responds makes a decision. Chest pain can also be caused by gastrointestinal problems, but neither you nor the resident can be sure of the cause.

Some residents with known heart problems carry nitro-

Cholesterol – a substance present in animal cells and body fluids
Plaque – fatty deposits on blood vessel walls
Protein – combination of amino acids that are essential for all living cells

glycerin tablets with them. The tablet is placed under the tongue, never swallowed. The resident may feel side effects like a headache or dizziness after taking the nitroglycerin tablet. Be sure to report these side effects to the charge nurse.

If the resident cannot administer their own medication, the nurse will give them the nitroglycerin tablet to see if it relieves their chest pain. If the resident's chest pain is not relieved after three nitroglycerin tablets, or if the resident's pulse or blood pressure changes, the resident is usually sent to the hospital. The charge nurse may ask you to monitor the resident's pulse and blood pressure during the episode. You should immediately report any change in the resident's vital signs.

Many people having a heart attack do not feel they have chest pain. They think they are feeling "stomach pain" or "upset stomach." They often experience shortness of breath and pain in the arm. Other signs and symptoms include dizziness, nausea, anxiety, chest **palpitations**, and sweating.

Often, residents downplay their symptoms because they do not want to believe that something could be wrong with their heart. If a resident has any of these signs and symptoms, report them to the charge nurse immediately. Report them even if the resident says something like "I'm fine—it will go away." Early treatment of a heart attack improves the resident's chance of survival and can minimize damage to the heart muscle. Delayed treatment puts the resident at risk for more heart muscle death.

Residents are more likely to tell you how they are feeling if they have a good relationship with you. You are the one who can notice even subtle changes in them. Remember these heart attack signs and symptoms and report any of them to the charge nurse immediately:
• chest pain, which may spread to the shoulder, neck, or arms
• difficulty breathing, shortness of breath
• palpitations
• nausea
• anxiety
• stomach upset or pain
• weakness, fatigue
• pale coloring of the skin
• cold, clammy skin
• rapid, weak, irregular pulse

Time is critical when a resident is having a heart attack, so you must immediately notify the charge nurse. Take the resident's vital signs, and help them to a comfortable position. Loosen tight clothes. Stay with them. Often the resident is frightened, so stay calm yourself and try to reassure them that help is on the way.

The key to medical treatment is to dissolve the clot or open the blocked artery, so that the blood supply, with its oxygen and nutrients, can get back to the heart before more damage occurs or the heart stops altogether. This is why the resident needs immediate medical attention and will be taken to the hospital.

Cardiac Arrest

Cardiac arrest means the heartbeat and circulation have stopped. Cardiac arrest may result from various causes, including a heart attack. The signs of cardiac arrest include:
• no pulse
• lack of normal breathing
• cool, pale, gray color of the skin and blue lips
• loss of consciousness

The treatment for cardiac arrest is **cardiopulmonary resuscitation (CPR)**. Each facility has its own protocol for treating a resident who is experiencing cardiac arrest. Know the procedure where you work.

Not all residents receive CPR. Some residents have signed a living will or advance medical directive stating that they do not wish to be resuscitated if their heart stops. Sometimes, depending on a state's laws, the family and physician may decide for a resident who cannot make their wishes known. If you find a resident who is not breathing and has no pulse, call for help immediately. Every second counts. The nurse knows who should receive CPR and who should not.

You may assist with CPR, depending on your facility's policy. To give CPR, you need special training and certification. Talk with the charge nurse, head nurse, or staff development nurse for more information. If your facility does not offer CPR training, you can take a CPR course from the local American Red Cross, American Heart Association, or community hospital.

Cardiopulmonary resuscitation is performed when a resident has cardiac arrest (except in the case of a living will or advance medical directive, as mentioned earlier). The key is to maintain some blood flow to the brain and other vital organs. Three basic skills are used in CPR:
• Give chest compressions to circulate the blood.
• Open the airway to allow your rescue breaths to reach the lungs.
• Give rescue breaths (mouth to mouth).

Cardiopulmonary resuscitation (CPR) – procedure to maintain breathing and circulation in a person experiencing cardiac arrest
Palpitations – strong, rapid heartbeats

Chest compressions. Begin CPR with chest compressions as described below. Chest compressions provide artificial circulation of the blood and oxygen to vital organs such as the brain and heart. Start chest compressions as soon as you determine the person is unresponsive, is not breathing normally, and lacks a pulse. Be sure to call for help from the charge nurse or others as you begin CPR.

1. Position the resident flat on their back. Kneel next to the resident.

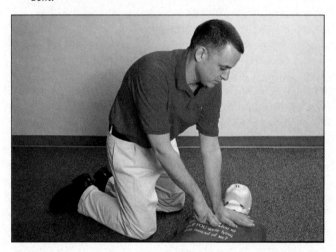

2. Place the heel of one hand on the resident's **sternum** in the middle of the resident's chest. Place your other hand directly on top of it and interlock your fingers.

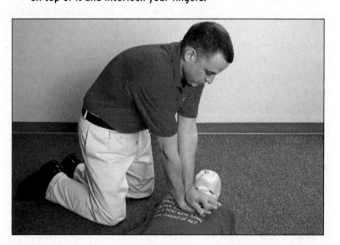

3. Pump the chest by pushing down at least 2 inches in a hard and fast rhythm. Keep your elbows straight with the weight of your shoulders directly over your hands. Push each compression down hard, then release the pressure and let the chest come back up (keeping your hands on the chest). Give 30 compressions, counting aloud at a fast rate (at least 100 compressions per minute).

Open the airway. After giving 30 chest compressions, you must first open the airway before you can give rescue breaths. Follow these steps:

4. With one hand on the resident's forehead and your other on the chin, tilt the resident's head back while lifting the chin ("head-tilt, chin-lift").

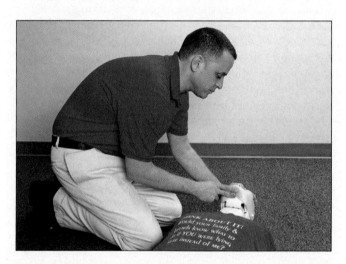

5. Do not use time now looking for breathing, but if you see that the resident is now obviously breathing normally, you do not need to give rescue breaths. Otherwise, proceed directly to give breaths.

Give two rescue breaths. This is sometimes called artificial respiration or mouth-to-mouth resuscitation. The air you blow into the resident's lungs puts oxygen in the blood that you are helping circulate with chest compressions. Follow these steps:

6. While maintaining the head-tilt, chin-lift position, pinch the resident's nose closed.

7. Put your mouth completely over the resident's mouth with a tight seal.

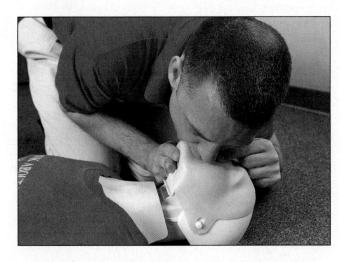

8. Give two quick breaths, each lasting only 1 second, watching the resident's chest rise while you blow in and fall when you remove your mouth. Do not blow too hard or keep blowing after the chest has risen.

Note: *In your CPR training course you will learn other methods of giving rescue breaths, such as breathing into a resident's stoma or nose. You will also learn to use a barrier device such as a face shield.*

Continue cycles of CPR.   Immediately after giving two breaths, give chest compressions again. Give 30 compressions, then two breaths, then 30 compressions, and continue this cycle until another staff person arrives to help or take over.

Note: *CPR can be more effective when given by two people. One is positioned by the resident's head to give the rescue breaths, and the other gives the chest compressions. Follow the same pattern of 30 compressions followed by two breaths.*

Additional information about CPR:
- CPR performed immediately doubles the resident's chances for survival.
- CPR is practiced on mannequins in training courses.
- Do not be afraid of disease from mouth-to-mouth rescue breaths. There has never been a case of HIV being transmitted during CPR.
- A resident's rib may crack during chest compressions, but this is better than dying. Be sure your compressions are at least 2 inches deep.
- If the resident starts moving and is breathing normally, stop CPR. If the resident is still unresponsive but breathing normally, you may need to hold the airway open to support breathing.

CHOKING

Many people die each year by choking. Choking usually happens when food or another object gets stuck in the throat. Residents are at risk of choking when:
- Their bites of meat or other food are too large or poorly chewed.
- They talk or laugh too much while eating (Fig. 20-4).

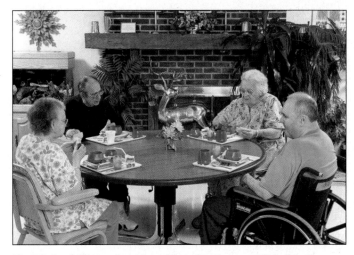

Fig. 20-4 – Talking or laughing while eating increases the risk of choking.

- Their dentures do not fit well.
- They have a chronic illness or stroke, which is causing weakness and difficulty with swallowing.

Sternum – breastbone

When a resident is choking, you should:

1. Ask the resident, "Are you choking?" The resident will not be able to answer you if their airway is completely blocked.

2. Call for help.

3. Never leave the resident. This is a life-threatening situation.

4. Give the treatment called the Heimlich maneuver. When performed properly, this procedure will dislodge the object from the resident's throat.

If the throat is completely blocked, this is called an airway obstruction. You must act quickly. You have only 4 to 8 minutes to save the resident's life. A choking victim who is still conscious will usually grab or gesture at their throat (Fig. 20-5). The resident may already have become unconscious before you find them.

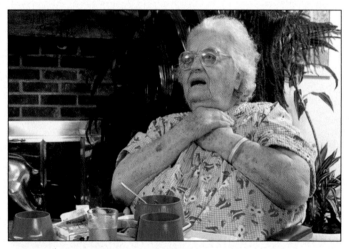

Fig. 20-5 — Residents who are choking will grab at their throats.

Other possible signs of a complete airway obstruction are:
• The resident's skin, lips, and nails look bluish.
• The resident has difficult, noisy breathing or is not breathing at all.
• The resident cannot speak.
• The resident may become unconscious.
• The resident cannot cough with force.

A resident may have only a partial airway obstruction, however. This resident can speak, breathe, and cough but may have difficulty breathing and may not be getting enough oxygen.

If the resident cannot eject the object from their throat by forceful coughing, the charge nurse may seek assistance from an emergency medical team. The charge nurse may ask you to call 911 for help. It is important that you are familiar with the emergency equipment used in your facility because the charge nurse may also ask you to get things like oxygen or suction equipment.

You can learn the Heimlich maneuver in a CPR or first aid course, or from a certified CPR or first aid instructor in your facility. Here is a basic explanation of how to perform it.

First Aid for Choking

If the resident is sitting or standing, use the Heimlich manuever:

1. Stand behind the resident.

2. Wrap your arms around the resident's waist. Try to lean the resident slightly forward.

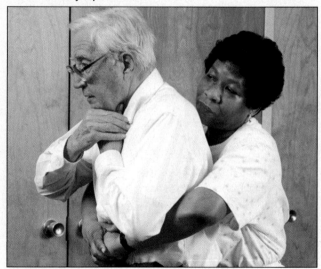

3. Make a fist with one hand and put it on the resident's stomach below the rib cage and a little above the navel. Keep your thumb on their stomach and place your other hand over your fist.

4. Sharply thrust your fist inward and upward. This causes a burst of air from the lungs to dislodge the food or object.

5. Repeat the thrusts until the blockage is dislodged .

If the resident is standing when they become unconscious, gently lower them to the floor and shout for help if you have not already. Once they are on the floor:

1. Place the resident on their back.

2. Kneel down at the resident's side.

3. Place the heel of one hand on the lower part of the resident's sternum, located midline on the resident's chest. Place your other hand directly on top of it and interlock your fingers.

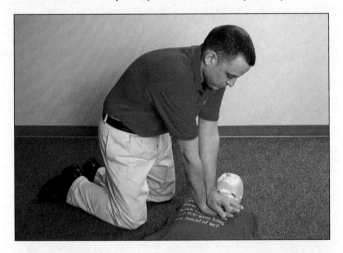

4. Push down approximately two inches on the sternum, keeping your arms straight and your shoulders directly over the middle of the resident's body (the training mannequin in the photo).

5. Begin CPR. Remember the ratio is 30 compressions to two quick breaths.

6. Continue until help arrives or the object is visible in the resident's mouth and can be removed.

SEIZURE

A seizure can be caused by several different things, such as a brain tumor, an infection in the brain or spinal cord, a head injury, medications, poisoning, or a seizure disorder such as epilepsy. Often, residents with a seizure disorder are on medication. In all seizures there is a change in behavior due to an abnormal electrical activity in the brain.

Seizures may be classified as simple or complex. With a simple seizure, there is usually no loss of consciousness. With a complex seizure, there is usually a change in the level of consciousness. Seizures are also classified as generalized and partial seizures. The type of seizure depends on how much of the brain and body is affected. With generalized seizures, the entire brain is affected, and the resident may:
• lose consciousness
• fall
• have massive muscle spasms
• be incontinent of urine or stool

Follow these steps to help a resident having a generalized seizure:

1. Call for help.

2. Remain calm.

3. Do not leave the resident alone.

4. Reassure the resident that you are there to protect them.

5. To prevent a fall, help the resident to the floor.

6. Place something soft under the resident's head.

7. Remove any objects in the resident's way that could cause injury.

8. Try to turn the resident on their side to prevent aspiration and allow for drainage of saliva and vomit.

9. Do not put anything in the resident's mouth.

10. Do not try to hold the resident down, or to stop the convulsions. The resident is not aware and cannot control the seizure activity.

11. Remove any tight jewelry, especially from around the resident's neck.

12. Loosen any tight clothes (such as a belt or tie) to help the resident breathe better.

13. Do not give CPR unless the resident does not have a pulse or respirations after the seizure.

Seizure – a condition resulting from an abnormality in the brain

14. Do not give the resident anything by mouth until the seizure has stopped and they are fully awake and oriented.

15. Remain with the resident until the seizure is over. Reassure and comfort the resident as best you can. The resident may be confused, disoriented, frightened, and even embarrassed.

16. Record the time the seizure began, the parts of the body involved, the strength of the activity, whether the resident lost bowel and bladder control, the resident's mental status, and how long the seizure lasted.

In a partial seizure, the abnormal activity happens in only part of the brain. This resident has symptoms specific to the part of the brain, and only one side or part of the body is involved. A resident having a partial seizure may have:
- a dazed, blank look
- jerking movements of a specific body part

First aid may not be needed for this type of seizure, but you should remain with the resident and observe, report, and record what you see during the seizure.

Before any seizure a resident may tell you they feel an **aura**. An aura may occur just before or hours before the seizure. Often the aura involves one of the senses. For example, the resident may tell you they smell a certain smell, have an odd taste in their mouth, see spots before their eyes, or hear a particular sound. If the resident recognizes an aura from a past seizure, you can take measures to protect them from injury during the coming seizure.

📖
Aura – a subtle sensation that often precedes a seizure

BURNS

Burns may be caused by many different things such as a hot object, fire, hot water, too much sun, electricity, or chemicals. The first aid for all burns is the same, except for electrical burns.

The immediate treatment for a burn other than an electrical burn is:

1. Remove the resident from the fire or the source of heat.

2. Call for help. The charge nurse may ask you to call 911 for assistance.

3. Depending on the size and degree of the burn, the charge nurse may ask you to run cool water over the burn.

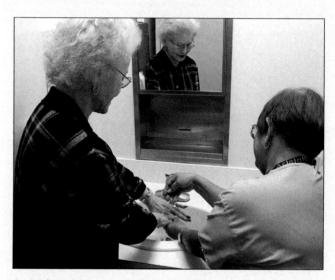

4. Apply a clean cotton cloth over the burn.

5. Do not put soap, ointment, butter, oil, or margarine on the burn.

Note: *Try to remove any jewelry or clothing that has not adhered to the burn.*

6. Keep the resident warm.

The charge nurse will determine if the resident needs emergency help.

If the resident has an electrical burn, you should:

1. Make sure the resident is no longer in contact with the power source, because the electricity can travel to you if the power is still on. If the resident is in contact with the electricity, the power source must be turned off first.

2. Call for help. The charge nurse may ask you to call 911 for assistance.

3. Lay the resident down. Raise the lower portion of the resident's body to reduce shock, if possible.

4. Check for breathing and circulation. Perform CPR if the resident has no pulse and respiration.

5. Once the charge nurse has determined that the resident is stable, you may be asked to run cool water over the burn.

6. Cover the burn with a clean cotton material. Do not use a towel or blanket, because loose fibers may stick to the burn.

7. Do not put soap, ointment, butter, oil, or margarine on the burn.

Note: *Try to remove any jewelry or clothing that has not adhered to the burn.*

8. Keep the resident warm.

The charge nurse will determine additional steps to take.

HEMORRHAGING
The human body normally circulates 5 to 6 quarts of blood. Losing a small amount of blood from a cut usually causes no harm. But if 1 to 2 quarts or more of blood is lost, the situation is life threatening. This is called **hemorrhaging**. A resident who loses this much blood may go into shock and even die.

Bleeding can be internal or external. Although you do not see internal bleeding, the resident may vomit blood, cough up blood, or have blood in the urine or stool. They may complain of pain, lose consciousness, and go into shock.

Follow these steps to help a resident who is hemorrhaging internally:

1. Call for help.

2. Remain calm.

3. Reassure the resident that help is on the way.

4. Keep the resident warm.

5. Do not try to move the resident unless the resident is vomiting. But if they are vomiting, place them on their side to prevent aspiration and maintain an open airway.

6. Elevate the resident's legs about a foot high if they are on their back and there is no injury to the their neck, back, or legs.

7. Do not give the resident anything to eat or drink.

8. The charge nurse will determine what other steps to take.

Follow these steps to help a resident who has external hemorrhage:

1. Call for help, but do not leave the resident alone.

2. If possible, use standard precautions (see Chapter 9).

3. Place a clean cloth over the bleeding wound.

4. Put pressure on the wound with the palm of your hand until the bleeding stops.

5. If you can, elevate the wound above the level of the resident's heart to slow the bleeding.

6. Do not apply a tourniquet to stop the bleeding. Applying a tourniquet may cause unnecessary tissue death or even loss of a limb.

The charge nurse will determine what additional steps to take.

Hemorrhage – excessive loss of blood in a short period of time

SHOCK

Shock results when not enough blood and oxygen reach the vital organs in a resident's body. There are many causes of shock, including:
- an allergic reaction
- an injury or wound
- a heart problem or heart attack
- a severe infection
- serious internal bleeding
- serious external bleeding

A resident who goes into shock may have these signs and symptoms:
- pale bluish skin color
- skin cool to the touch
- vomiting
- unusually great thirst
- weak, rapid pulse
- decreased blood pressure
- increased respirations
- periods of unconsciousness

Shock is an emergency that requires immediate medical attention. Follow these steps to help the resident until medical help arrives:

1. Call for help. The charge nurse may ask you to call 911.

2. Remain calm.

3. Reassure the resident.

4. Do not try to move the resident unless they are vomiting. But if they are vomiting, place them on their side to prevent aspiration and maintain an open airway.

5. If they are on their back and there is no injury to their neck, back, or legs, then elevate their legs about a foot high.

6. If the resident is bleeding externally, place a clean cloth over the wound, put pressure on it, and elevate the wound above the level of the resident's heart if you can.

7. Keep the resident warm.

8. Do not give the resident anything to eat or drink unless instructed to by the charge nurse.

MANAGING YOUR OWN FEELINGS IN AN EMERGENCY

When an emergency happens, it is natural to be nervous. You may feel your own body reacting with increased pulse and respiration. You may feel light-headed and scared, especially at the sight of a wound that is bleeding. You may begin to sweat or have a sudden burst of energy. Whatever you feel, know that this is normal. The most important thing is to remain calm. Take a deep breath and a moment to steady yourself, if needed, as you prepare to give first aid.

Never let the resident know that you are nervous. Reassure them. Comforting and reassuring the resident helps them feel confident that you are doing everything possible to assist them through this very frightening episode.

📖

Shock — a condition in which vital organs in the body are not getting enough blood and oxygen to maintain good function

IN THIS CHAPTER YOU LEARNED:

- What emergency first aid is
- Your role and responsibilities in an emergency
- General guidelines to follow in an emergency
- The signs and symptoms of a heart attack and the care for heart attack
- How to give cardiopulmonary resuscitation
- The signs of choking and how to perform the Heimlich maneuver
- Identify the signs of a seizure and how to care for a resident who is experiencing seizures
- Care for a resident who has a burn
- Care for a resident who is bleeding
- The signs and symptoms of shock and the care for a resident in shock

SUMMARY

This chapter covers first aid and your role and responsibilities in an emergency. You learned basic information about common emergencies and what steps to take in these emergencies, such as the use of cardiopulmonary resuscitation and the Heimlich maneuver. This chapter is just the beginning for learning first aid and CPR, however. Depending on your facility's policy, you may want to take a certificate program in first aid and CPR, and renew it yearly.

PULLING IT ALL TOGETHER

Imagine you are working the night shift on a weekend with one nurse. This particular night, two staff members have called in sick at the last minute. You and the charge nurse will be the only staff for 30 residents.

In reporting at the beginning of your shift, you learn that all of the residents are stable except one resident. Staff on the 3-11 shift report that Mr. Kane has not been feeling well all evening. He complained of pain in his lower abdomen, but no other changes were reported. As you begin your rounds, you first go to Mr. Kane to take his vital signs and see how he is feeling. Mr. Kane tells you the pain in his abdomen is getting worse. He says that when he went to the bathroom, he noticed bright red blood in his urine. His blood pressure is 90/50, his pulse 110 and weak, his respirations 32, and his oral temperature 98.6 F. This is a significant change in his blood pressure, pulse, and respirations. He also says that he is very thirsty. You notice that his skin is cool to your touch.

Immediately you put on the call light for the charge nurse. You update the nurse about Mr. Kane's condition. The charge nurse evaluates your findings and calls 911. The nurse tells you to remain with Mr. Kane, to reassure him that help is on the way, and to monitor his vital signs every 10 minutes.

Emergency medical services (EMS) personnel arrive within 15 minutes and take Mr. Kane to the emergency room at the local hospital. A telephone call from the emergency room staff later in the shift informs you that Mr. Kane was bleeding internally. He is receiving emergency surgery. They say they will keep you updated about his progress. The next day the director of nursing tells you that Mr. Kane did well with the surgery and that she believes your actions during the emergency contributed to his favorable outcome.

1. **In any emergency involving a resident you should:**
    A. Try not to move the resident unless you must remove them from a dangerous situation.
    B. Scream as loud as you can so that everyone knows there's an emergency.
    C. Pull the fire alarm to summon help.
    D. Remove the resident's clothing so that they do not become too warm.

2. **If a resident is experiencing a heart attack, what symptom are they likely to experience?**
    A. Hunger.
    B. Chest pain.
    C. Swollen wrists.
    D. A rash or hives.

3. **When performing CPR, what ratio of breaths to compressions should you use?**
    A. One deep slow breath per 15 compressions.
    B. Two deep slow breaths per 5 compressions.
    C. Two deep slow breaths per 20 compressions.
    D. Two quick slow breaths per 30 compressions.

4. **Mr. Krulsky may be having a heart attack. He has chest pains, looks very pale, and has a rapid, weak, irregular pulse. You've called the charge nurse, who is on the way. Your first aid for Mr. Krulsky should include:**
    A. Helping him into a comfortable position.
    B. Encouraging him to drink as much fluid as possible.
    C. Wrapping blankets very tightly around him.
    D. Starting CPR immediately.

5. **The Heimlich maneuver is used with a resident who is:**
    A. Vomiting.
    B. Having a seizure.
    C. Choking.
    D. Feeling nauseous.

6. **Mr. Nathanson is experiencing a seizure and you have called for help. What else should you do for him?**
    A. Put a toothbrush or something firm between his teeth for him to bite on.
    B. Help him to the floor to prevent a fall.
    C. Ask other residents to help you hold him down firmly.
    D. Pour water into his mouth.

7. **One of your residents has burned his hand on a hot light bulb. What is the correct step to take?**
    A. Ask the resident to wave his hand around in the air.
    B. Run cool water over the burn.
    C. Put butter on the burn.
    D. Rub soap into the burn until it lathers.

8. **A person who is bleeding heavily is:**
    A. Hypertensive.
    B. Hallucinating.
    C. Hemorrhaging.
    D. Hyperventilating.

9. **Mrs. Colson is in shock. While waiting for help you should:**
    A. Keep her on her feet and walking.
    B. Give her as much water as she can drink.
    C. Vigorously rub her arms, legs, and back.
    D. Keep her warm.

10. **If a resident is hemorrhaging externally from a leg wound, what should you do to control the bleeding?**
    A. Apply a tourniquet around the thigh.
    B. Immerse the resident in cold bath water.
    C. Put pressure on the wound with your gloved hand.
    D. Start CPR immediately.

(Answers to "Check What You've Learned" are in the Instructor's Manual.)

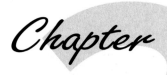

Chapter 21

PAIN MANAGEMENT, SLEEP, AND COMFORT

To feel good, we need to get enough sleep, be physically comfortable, and be free from pain. Health care is now focusing more on these three factors. If a resident is in pain, they are not comfortable. Their sleep and activities will be disrupted. This will affect the quality of their life. In many health care settings, including long term care facilities, pain is thought of as the fifth vital sign. This means that residents are asked about pain when they are admitted and then routinely. Their pain is assessed at least weekly and whenever their condition changes. Thinking of pain as a vital sign—along with temperature, pulse, respiration, and blood pressure—reminds staff to ask residents often about their pain. This is important because residents do not always mention their pain if they are not asked.

How residents perceive and respond to pain is influenced by their cultural or religious background and beliefs. Your own beliefs also affect how you think residents should respond to pain. As a nurse assistant caring for residents who are in pain, you must evaluate your own attitudes about pain. How you react to a resident when they report pain may affect the quality of their life. Your reporting of a resident's pain may make the difference in whether it is managed or not.

Pain management is a key part of your residents' care. Studies show that unrelieved pain can affect healing and rehabilitation. Pain also affects socialization, ambulation, length of stay in a nursing home, and overall well-being. In addition, pain can create problems with the resident's immune system and other body systems. This means pain can affect how the body fights infection. This can cause further deterioration in the resident's health.

In this chapter you will learn about pain management. You have an important role in communicating information about the resident's pain. You will learn what you can do to help a resident with chronic pain. You will learn about different measures to relieve pain, increase the resident's comfort, and promote sleep (Fig. 21-1).

OBJECTIVES
- Describe your responsibility for reporting pain
- Describe what you might see when a resident is in pain
- List five side effects of pain medications
- Describe five complementary or alternative measures to help manage pain
- List ways to promote comfort and sleep

MEDICAL TERMS
- **Acupuncture** – a medical therapy that originated in ancient China
- **Endorphins** – natural morphine-like substances released by the brain during exercise, which can alter one's feeling of pain

"The hot compress really relieved my joint pain, and I was able to sleep so much better."

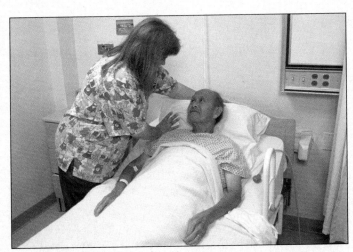

Fig. 21-1 – Comfort measures such as fluffing pillows help relieve pain, increase the resident's comfort, and promote sleep.

Have you ever thought that someone did not believe what you were saying? Did you try to convince the person to believe you? Imagine that you are in pain and are trying to convince your caregivers—who have the capability to relieve your pain—that you are feeling pain. What if they do not believe you? How would that make you feel? Would you be able to trust them? Could you have a positive relationship with them? What would your quality of life be like?

PAIN

In the past, pain was often viewed as a symptom of something else, another condition or disease. Health care professionals often ignored the pain and focused only on treating the underlying cause. But in today's health care, pain should never be ignored. Pain is recognized as a devastating health problem. Health care professionals today focus on finding better ways to treat pain. More research is also being done today to find new ways to help manage pain and bring relief.

Pain cannot be measured like temperature or pulse. Pain is whatever the resident says it is. Pain is what the resident feels. You must accept what a resident says about the pain they feel and its severity. Report their pain the same way as they tell you it makes them feel. You cannot interpret someone else's pain yourself. Believe what the resident says.

Consider this: You see a resident walking down the hall laughing. Because they are laughing, you do not believe they really are in pain, so you do not report their complaint of pain. Now consider a different resident who reports to you that they experience pain when they walk.

You see this resident crying and holding onto the railing in the hall as they walk.

Would you think differently about these two residents' pain? Can you be sure one is in pain and the other is not? Would one of them receive pain treatment because you reported it, while the other would not because you did not report their pain? What you report can determine whether residents are treated properly. You must not try to judge their pain. Remember: you cannot know what they actually feel inside. It is your responsibility to report whatever the resident states, regardless of whether you believe them or not.

Sometimes residents need pain medications around the clock. That means they must receive the medication on schedule. This is the best way to treat their pain even if the nurse must wake them up in the middle of the night. You may think that waking the resident is not a good thing. But if the resident's pain increases because they missed a dose of medication, it may then become difficult to control their pain.

Screening for Pain

Most facilities have pain assessment tools that residents can use to rate their pain. A number scale is often used for adults. You ask the resident, "If zero is no pain and 10 is the worst pain possible, what is your pain right now?" It may be easier for some residents, especially residents who do not speak English, to use a visual pain scale like the one shown in Figure 21-2, next page. Other scales may be used for residents with impaired cognitive ability. A resident's pain should be assessed at least weekly and whenever their condition changes. Let the charge nurse know how much pain the resident is experiencing so that a more detailed pain assessment can be performed.

The charge nurse, along with other members of the interdisciplinary team, may assess the resident's pain. Residents are asked about the following pain qualities:

- The location of their pain
- What their pain feels like, using terms such as:
  - "achy"
  - "throbbing"
  - "sore"
  - "burning"

Pain – bodily sensation that causes suffering and distress

- "pins and needles"
- "knife-like"
- "shooting"
- "crampy"
- "pressure"
- "discomfort"
- When the pain started
- Whether the pain is always there or if it comes and goes
- What makes the pain worse or better
- How the pain affects their walking, eating, sleeping, and mood

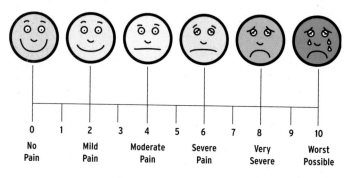

Fig. 21-2 – Example of a tool a resident can use to rate their pain.

Used with permission, University of Colorado Health Sciences Center, Denver, Colorado.

The interdisciplinary team uses all this information to create a plan to help relieve the resident's pain.

Pain management is the responsibility of the whole team. The charge nurse may ask you to report when the resident complains of pain or to observe how the resident responds after being given a pain medication. The physician or another member of the interdisciplinary team may prescribe complementary (nonmedical) or alternative therapies for pain relief. These may include the application of heat or cold. The charge nurse will explain your responsibilities with these therapies. Later in this chapter you will learn strategies for pain relief that can be administered along with medications or instead of them.

You have a key role helping the interdisciplinary team assess a resident's pain. Listen carefully to how the resident defines their pain. The charge nurse or other health care professional evaluates the resident's pain, but you should report any other signs or nonverbal cues to pain that you see in the resident or that they tell you about. Encourage residents to talk openly about their pain. They

should understand that pain is not a normal part of aging. They should never be made to feel they should hide their pain. Pain can be managed, and they have the right to pain treatment.

In some situations, a resident may try to hide their pain because their culture or religion encourages that. Always respect the resident's cultural and religious views while you work with the team to address the pain. Remember that it is crucial to report their pain so that it can be treated appropriately.

Understanding Pain

The severe pain from some forms of cancer has led health care professionals to improve our understanding of pain and how to manage it. Pain used to be defined in three categories: (1) acute pain, such as caused by a sprain, strain, infection, inflammation, or surgical procedure; (2) chronic pain, such as caused by arthritis; and (3) malignant pain, such as in cancer.

More recently, pain research defines pain in relation to different forms of nervous system damage. This approach helps the interdisciplinary team more effectively treat residents' pain. Certain medications or alternative strategies for comfort and pain relief work better with one kind of pain than with another. In this way, the team can use the best pain management strategies for the resident's specific kind of pain.

Your role in pain management is to always report information about the resident accurately and in a timely manner, and to perform other strategies as directed.

Common Resident Concerns About Pain

Some residents have certain beliefs about pain and its treatment. These beliefs may interfere with reporting their pain and good pain management. Table 21-1 lists common misconceptions or beliefs about pain as well as the facts. Be aware of these misconceptions and beliefs. When appropriate, talk about them with your residents.

Reporting Pain Accurately

Pain is very subjective. In Chapter 8, Documentation Principles and Procedures, you learned that subjective information is what the resident tells you. For example, a resident may tell you that they could not sleep all night because they had pain in their hip. You must report this subjective information exactly as the resident stated it. In

TABLE 21-1
MISCONCEPTIONS ABOUT PAIN AND ITS TREATMENT

MISCONCEPTIONS ABOUT PAIN	FACTS ABOUT PAIN
"If I take too much pain medicine I will get addicted."	The risk of addiction is rare (less than one in 10,000 people) when pain medications are taken for pain.
"Pain is inevitable as you get older—I just have to live with it."	As you age, conditions that cause pain become more common. But pain is not normal. Good pain relief is possible for all types of pain.
"The nurses and nurse assistants are so busy—I don't want to bother them by asking for pain medication."	The nurses and nurse assistants want to know about your pain. The staff want to provide the best treatment possible.
"If my pain medicine doesn't work as well as it used to, it means I am getting immune or addicted to it."	Sometimes people get used to a medicine. This is called tolerance—*not* addiction. If tolerance happens, staff can increase the dose or change to a different pain medicine.
"It is better to save pain medicine for when the pain gets really bad."	If a resident waits too long to take pain medicine, they may actually need a stronger medicine or higher dose. Taking pain medicine on a regular schedule may help prevent pain.
"It's easier to cope with the pain than with the side effects of pain medication, especially constipation."	Pain medicine, particularly narcotics, can cause constipation. But constipation can be prevented and treated with stool softeners and laxatives. Worries about side effects should not stop the resident from taking pain medicine for their pain.

Used with permission, University of Colorado Health Sciences Center, Denver, Colorado. Development of pamphlet was supported by AHRQ grant U18-HS11093-3.

TABLE 21-2
SIGNS OF PAIN

OBSERVATION	SIGNS OF PAIN
The resident's facial expression	• Frown, wrinkled forehead • Furrowed brow • Grimace • Expression of fear • Expression of sadness • Tense muscles around the mouth and eyes (Fig. 21-3)

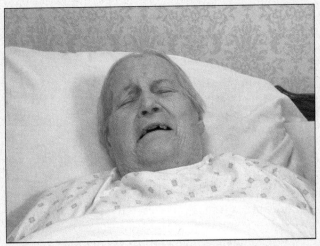

Fig. 21-3 – A resident with a facial expression such as a frown, grimace, or expression of sadness may be in pain.

OBSERVATION	SIGNS OF PAIN
The resident's physical movements	• Restlessness, fidgeting, agitation • Absence of movement, slow movements • Cautious movements, guarding, or bracing • Rigidity, generalized tension • Rubbing a body part
What you might hear	• Groaning, moaning • Crying • Noisy breathing • Saying things like "Ouch!" or "Don't touch me"

this case you would tell the charge nurse that the resident said they could not sleep all night because they had pain in their hip. The charge nurse may ask you questions such as: "Is the resident up now? Did they say they felt pain when you helped them with their ADLs? Do they show any other signs of pain?" Then you would tell the nurse what you observed, being careful to identify subjective and objective information.

Table 21-2, previous page, describes some common signs of pain you may observe. But always remember that regardless of what you observe or do not observe, pain is what the resident says it is.

Pain That Is Left Untreated

Each resident feels pain differently and responds in their own way. You may hear someone say that one resident has a "high pain threshold" while another has a "low threshold." The reasons for such differences are very complex and not fully understood. Researchers believe that cultural influences, the brain's release of **endorphins**, and previous experiences with pain all may play a role in pain sensation, along with other individual factors.

Regardless of differences among residents, pain that is not relieved can lead to terrible problems. As mentioned earlier, the resident's immune system is compromised by unrelieved pain. Pain also affects other body systems. Because of the constant effect of pain on the nervous system, even the lightest touch can cause a resident more pain. The charge nurse can give you more information about how the body is affected by unrelieved pain.

A resident in pain is not happy. They cannot get comfortable and relax. They do not sleep well. They may feel that the quality of their life is poor. If a resident's pain is not managed, the resident may experience some or all of the following feelings:
• Fear
• Depression
• Anxiety
• Helplessness
• Hopelessness
• Distress
• Decreased will to live

Pain Treatment

The most common treatment of pain is medication. Many drugs are available today to treat residents' pain. Typically, a combination of drugs is used to manage pain caused by cancer or chronic illness. The physician and other members of the team select what drugs to use. Your input about the resident's experience is a key part of this decision. The team must clearly understand what type of pain the resident is experiencing and other information about the resident's pain. In addition to communicating your knowledge about the resident's pain, you also are responsible for reporting any side effects, or undesired effects, of the pain medication on the resident. Box 21-1 lists some possible side effects.

BOX 21-1.
POSSIBLE SIDE EFFECTS OF PAIN MEDICATION

• Constipation
• Diarrhea
• Nausea and vomiting
• Sleeping too much
• Complaints of stomach pains
• Rash
• Confusion
• Slowed respiratory rate
• Dizziness when standing or changing position

In addition to pain medication, other therapies are used to help manage residents' pain (Fig. 21-4, next page). These therapies also help the resident be more comfortable and sleep better. Complementary or alternative therapies often help the resident feel more in control. It is difficult to feel in control when in pain. The choice of other treatments or therapies depends in part on the resident's preferences and cultural beliefs. The choice also depends on their ability to tolerate certain body positions, the experience of the health care team, and other factors. Box 21-2 describes some nondrug therapies that may be used to help relieve residents' pain.

Endorphins – natural morphine-like substances released by the brain during exercise, which can alter one's feeling of pain

Your role with nondrug therapies depends on your experience. The charge nurse or the physical therapist will train you in techniques used in your facility. The charge nurse and other team members decide what alternative or complementary therapies to use for each resident. You may be asked to report how effective the treatment is in comforting the resident or relieving pain.

If the physician prescribes heat or cold application, follow the guidelines on the use of heat or cold therapy in Chapter 24.

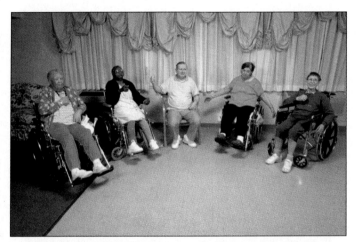

Fig. 21-4 – Exercise like stretching helps residents manage their pain.

PROMOTING COMFORT AND SLEEP

Research has shown that frequent sleep disturbances, such as getting up to go to the bathroom, may affect the body's natural pain inhibitors and cause more pain. This is especially so with women. You are responsible for helping all residents to feel comfortable and get enough sleep. The techniques listed in Box 21-2 can be used with all residents to help promote comfort and sleep in addition to relieving pain. You can also help control the resident's environment in the following ways to help make them comfortable and to promote sleep:

• Ask the resident about their room temperature. Be sure the room it is not too hot or too cold. Remember that what you consider a comfortable temperature yourself may be different from what the resident finds comfortable. Be sure the resident has enough blankets nearby so that they can pull up more covers if they get cold during the night. If residents cannot do this by themselves, be sure to check on them throughout the night.

• Limit noise at night. Do not not talk to others in the resident's room or outside their door.

• Lower the lights in the hallways. Close the resident's door if appropriate. Be sure to pull window shades and close curtains so that outside lights do not shine in the resident's window.

• Pay attention to any odors. Make every effort to empty bedpans, change soiled linens, and manage incontinence in a timely manner.

• Encourage residents to use the bathroom before going to bed at night.

In addition to these guidelines, encourage the resident to rest during the day. This can simply mean quiet time reading or listening to music. Understanding how the resident likes to relax and to prepare for sleep will help you know what to do for the resident.

BOX 21-2.
NONDRUG THERAPIES
FOR PAIN

- **Heat/cold application** involves using dry or moist heat or cold on a specific area to relieve pain or increase the resident's comfort.
- **Vibration** can be used to promote comfort or help relieve pain. This form of electrical massage is applied lightly or with pressure on various body areas. Different types of vibrating devices are available for different parts of the body.
- **Massage** is a method of relaxation that can be used to help residents relax both physically and mentally. A three-minute backrub using slow, rhythmic strokes is a safe and effective way to decrease pain and promote relaxation.
- **Acupuncture** is an ancient Chinese healing method. The acupuncturist inserts very thin needles in specific body sites. Acupuncture is said to allow energy to flow to or from areas that do not have enough energy or have too much energy. Acupuncture is believed to help restore and regulate the body's energy balance.
- **Distraction** is a technique used to direct a resident's attention away from pain. With distraction, the resident deliberately focuses on something other than the pain and thus responds less to it (Fig. 21-5). Talking, books, movies, and social activities are all distractions.

- **Humor** is an enjoyable and often effective form of distraction that can be used to get the resident's mind off their pain.
- **Relaxation** techniques are methods that help reduce anxiety, muscle tension, and pain. Such techniques include meditation, music, massage, and deep breathing (Fig. 21-6).

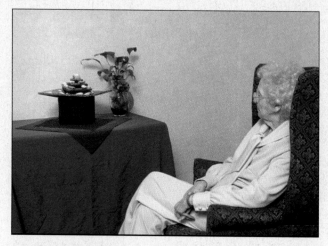

Fig. 21-6 — Meditation can help residents relax and reduces their pain.

- **Guided imagery** is a healing technique that uses words and sometimes music to bring the body and mind to a relaxed and focused state.
- **Animals** provide relaxation and companionship and help distract a resident's attention from pain.

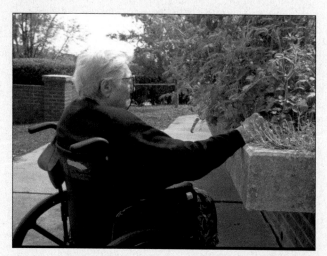

Fig. 21-5 — Encouraging residents to participate in activities they enjoy can help distract them from their pain.

IN THIS CHAPTER YOU LEARNED:
- Your responsibility for reporting pain
- Signs you might see when a resident is in pain
- Common side effects of pain medications
- Complementary or alternative measures to help manage pain
- That hot and cold applications are used to decrease pain
- Ways to promote comfort and sleep

SUMMARY
In this chapter you learned how important it is for a resident to sleep well, be comfortable, and be free from pain. Your role of reporting the resident's pain is critical, so that treatments can be given to relieve their pain. In addition to drug therapy, many alternative measures can help promote sleep, make the resident comfortable, and relieve pain.

PULLING IT ALL TOGETHER
Your responsibility to report information can make the difference in how residents are treated. Consider these examples:

Example 1. Mrs. Bailey is a resident newly admitted to your facility. She has Alzheimer's disease and can no longer safely care for herself. At the end of your shift you report to the charge nurse that she seemed irritable and stubborn. You do not report that she was hugging her knees and resisted releasing them when you tried to help her go to the bathroom, dining room, and her arts and crafts group.

Example 2. At the end of your shift you report to the charge nurse that Mrs. Bailey was rocking in the bed and holding her knees when you tried to help her with activities of daily living.

In example 1 you reported your opinion.
In example 2 you reported the facts.
Now think about what could happen in each situation. In the first example, your opinion could result in the resident being labeled as difficult. In the second example, reporting the facts would prompt the charge nurse to assess the resident. This assessment is preferable, because it might discover that Mrs. Bailey has pain in her knees from an old injury.

CHECK WHAT YOU'VE LEARNED

1. **What is considered the fifth vital sign?**
   A. Pain.
   B. Anxiety.
   C. Hearing.
   D. Mental status.

2. **How residents perceive and respond to pain is influenced by:**
   A. Their nutritional status.
   B. Sunlight.
   C. The clothing they are wearing at the time.
   D. Their cultural or religious background and beliefs.

3. **How can you help a resident manage their pain?**
   A. Make the lights in their room as bright as possible.
   B. Report any signs or symptoms of pain to the charge nurse.
   C. Offer them plenty of snacks and beverages between meals.
   D. Turn the television up loud.

4. **Why is it important to manage a resident's pain?**
   A. Untreated pain makes residents sleepy.
   B. Untreated pain can cause Alzheimer's disease.
   C. Untreated pain can lead to hypothermia.
   D. Untreated pain can put a resident at increased risk of illness.

5. **Mrs. Samuelle doesn't ask for pain medication, even though she has chronic pain from arthritis in her hip. What is a possible reason for why she tolerates her pain?**
   A. Her roommate never asks for pain medication.
   B. In her family, complaining about pain is a sign of weakness.
   C. Staff in long term care facilities cannot administer pain medication.
   D. Pain will make her immune system stronger.

6. **If a resident tells you their knee hurts, but they don't show any signs of pain, you should think they are:**
   A. Disoriented.
   B. Telling you the truth.
   C. Addicted to pain medication.
   D. Just trying to get your attention.

7. **A possible side effect of pain medication is:**
   A. Sleeplessness.
   B. Constipation.
   C. Acute sensitivity to light.
   D. Increased respiratory rate.

8. **The technique of distraction may include:**
   A. Sneaking up on a resident to startle them.
   B. Watching a movie.
   C. Acupuncture.
   D. Taking a Sitz bath.

9. **Which of these nondrug therapies can help reduce painful swelling?**
   A. Exercise.
   B. Vibration.
   C. Music therapy.
   D. Cold application.

10. **How can you help residents sleep well at night?**
    A. Give each resident a sleeping pill.
    B. Limit noise and conversations in the hallway.
    C. Give each resident a glass of warm milk before bed.
    D. Never go into a resident's room during the night.

(Answers to "Check What You've Learned" are in the Instructor's Manual.)

Chapter 22

END OF LIFE

Do you ever think about dying? Do you wonder what it would be like and when it will happen? Have you ever shared your thoughts, fears, and feelings with anyone, or are you too afraid to think or talk about it? You are not alone. In general people are afraid to talk about death and dying. Many people seem to feel that if they do not think or talk about death, maybe it will not happen. But knowing when and how is the only mystery. As individuals, we all have different experiences with the dying and death of friends and loved ones, just as our own will be different. Death is not something you get used to.

You may think the residents you care for have dealt with the thought of dying because they have lived many years and have entered a long term care facility. Although they may be aware of their future dying, this does not mean that they have dealt with it. When death approaches, many residents and family members feel they suddenly have to deal with the reality of end of life.

Some residents in long term care facilities are admitted for end of life care. Others are admitted with a chronic illness that later becomes terminal, resulting in the need for end-of-life care. Others simply reach the natural end of life. What happens to someone when they approach the end of their life? This is a very difficult time. You can help the dying resident deal with common physical changes at the end of life as well as psychosocial issues that they may need to address.

This chapter is about what you need to know to care for residents at the end of their life. Your role includes helping to relieve symptoms that distract a resident from dealing with issues they feel they must deal with. You will learn about the stages of dying and your role in this process. Your role also includes interacting with family members and friends of terminally ill residents.

OBJECTIVES
- Describe a living will
- Describe different feelings about death
- Describe end-of-life care
- List the stages of dying
- List specific things you can do to help residents and family members during the dying process
- Describe the care of the body after death

MEDICAL TERMS
- **Hospice** – program with a specially trained inter-disciplinary team that cares for a terminally ill resident who is expected to die within six months
- **Palliative** – care focused on comfort and symptom relief rather than cure
- **Postmortem** – after death

"Stay with me and hold my hand. Your being with me is such a comfort."

Death is a natural stage in life, but most people do not like to talk about it. When we face the death of another person, we are reminded that we, too, will die someday. Many people fear death because they are afraid of the unknown. The dying person realizes they will have no more chances to do things they wanted to do.

Often at this time people ask themselves many questions. These may include "What is the meaning of life?" or "What have I done that has made a difference or will be remembered after I'm gone?" These fears and thoughts lead to issues that you as a nurse assistant can help residents with.

LIVING WILLS

A **living will** or **advance directive** is a legal document communicating a resident's wishes about lifesaving care or death. The federal Patient Self-Determination Act requires all health care facilities to inform residents of their right to make such a directive and of the form they need to complete. Different states use different forms, but all are similar in meaning. The most powerful type of advance directive is the durable power of attorney for health care.

A durable power of attorney for health care may also apply if the resident cannot later make decisions for themselves. This often happens when a resident has a serious disease or terminal illness. It designates someone, usually a family member or an attorney, to make health care decisions for the person if they become incapacitated.

A living will must be written while the individual is mentally competent. The resident can revoke it at any time by giving verbal notice or simply tearing up the document. A living will states the resident's wishes about withdrawing or withholding life-sustaining procedures if the person becomes terminally ill. The document also spells out which treatments the person accepts or rejects.

Not all advance directives are living wills, and there are some important legal differences. You do not need to know all the legal issues. Your facility will handle the legal issues. You should know your facility's general policy about living wills and advance directives, however. You should also know which residents in your care have them.

FEELINGS ABOUT DYING

Although most residents do not come to facilities intending to die, many are older and debilitated and thus more likely to die sooner than younger, healthier persons. Elderly people often have experienced the death of their own loved ones. Because of this they may think more about life and death. Their spiritual needs often become more important as they review their lives.

A person's feelings about their approaching death vary greatly. A resident's feelings depend in part on their life experiences and spiritual beliefs. Cultural background also plays a role in what a person believes and how they respond to dying. Some welcome death as a release from pain and suffering. Many have positive expectations based on their religious beliefs. Following are some common beliefs:

- There is a life after death that is free of pain and hardship.
- One will be reunited with loved ones who have already died.
- One will be **reincarnated** into another body or form.

To support a resident throughout the dying process, you need to understand their beliefs about death. For example, some dying residents fear dying alone, even though they may accept death as positive or freeing. If a resident seems fearful about being alone, develop a plan to be with them as needed. Give them a bell to ring when they are afraid, and be sure to respond. Many also fear that dying will be painful. Ask the charge nurse to discuss pain management with the resident. Residents may also have fears related to how they have lived their lives. For example:

- The resident may feel they have unfinished business. For example, they may still be planning for a disabled child who needs lifelong care or resolving a dispute with a family member.
- The resident may not feel good about how they lived their lives. They may feel they failed to achieve all they wanted.
- The resident may feel guilty about something they did or did not do. For example, they may feel they were not supportive enough of a family member.

The process of life review is very important. Be supportive, open, and nonjudgmental. Always listen to the resident (Fig. 22-1, next page). Think about basic human needs as you care for a dying resident, and try to meet as many of their needs as possible. Be sure to report to the charge nurse any information the resident communicates to you so that other members of the team can also provide support.

Living will/advance directive – a legal document used by a resident to communicate their wishes about the care they want if they become incapacitated and cannot make decisions

Reincarnation - rebirth in another form of life

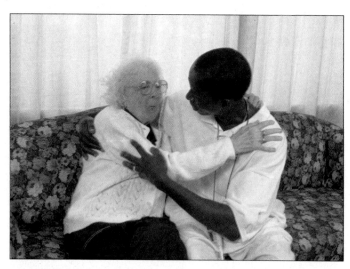
Fig. 22-1 – Listening and being supportive is very important during this difficult time.

STAGES OF DYING

Regardless of individual differences in attitudes and spiritual beliefs, most dying people go through the same feelings in the same stages. Dr. Elisabeth Kubler-Ross, a psychiatrist who worked with many dying patients, described five stages of dying. These stages also apply to experiencing other kinds of loss, such as the loss of a loved one. These stages of feelings are also called the stages of grief:

1. When most people first learn that they are dying, they experience denial, a "not me" reaction. This is the first stage. They may refuse to talk about death or to acknowledge physical evidence that they are dying.

2. The second stage is anger. The person asks, "Why me?" They may lash out at family members, caregivers, or even God. Often they are looking for someone to blame.

3. The third stage is called bargaining. The individual seems to be saying, "OK, maybe it's going to happen soon, but before it does I want to...." The person often tries to bargain to gain time to complete "unfinished business." For example the resident may say, "I want to live long enough to see the birth of my first great grandchild."

4. The fourth stage is depression. This occurs when the individual acknowledges that death is coming. They are aware of their sadness and are beginning to mourn their loss of self.

5. The fifth and final stage is acceptance. The dying person has worked through most of their earlier feelings and reached a calm state or peacefulness.

Reaching the stage of acceptance does not mean a resident has decided to stop living because they accept dying.

Typically, a person who has reached acceptance focuses on living each day to its fullest. You may even see a dying resident helping friends and family work through their feelings of grief and loss over their approaching death. Residents may even ask you to help their loved ones accept that they are dying. In Chapter 3, Understanding People, you learned about Erikson's stages of psychosocial development. In the stage called maturity, residents evaluate their lives and come to accept both the good and bad aspects. Letting a dying resident talk and being an active listener are key for their success in this stage and the stages of dying.

As with the hierarchy of basic human needs, people seldom go smoothly through the five stages of grief in order. Often a person moves back and forth between different stages. For example, someone who has accepted their death may go back to bargaining, to try for more time "just to see my son graduate." Not everyone goes through all the stages. Someone with a strong spiritual belief in an afterlife, for example, may move quickly to the final stage, acceptance. Someone else may never get beyond the second stage, anger.

Almost everyone who is terminally ill knows their death is inevitable. A resident may ask questions such as, "Am I going to get any better?" You may hear family members or staff say a resident hasn't been told about their approaching death. This does not mean that they do not know. Often it means only that the person is not ready yet to talk with loved ones about their fears and feelings.

You may need to tell family members and other staff about clues you notice about the resident's attitude. Encourage them to listen carefully to what the resident says. Use your communication skills to let a resident know that it is all right to talk to you about their feelings.

END-OF-LIFE CARE

End-of-life care involves a team effort. This includes support for the resident in their decision making, support groups, **bereavement** support, and symptom management. The focus of care is to meet the resident's individual needs. The resident and family make choices about how the resident wants to be cared for as they approach death.

A critical part of end-of-life care is the resident's understanding that they will be treated with dignity. Their choices will be honored and their symptoms relieved. If the

---

Bereavement – period of grief after a loved one dies

resident does not want medical care in an effort to prolong life, it will not be given. End-of-life care focuses on treating the resident's symptoms and providing emotional and spiritual support. This is known as providing **palliative** care.

End-of-life care is typically discussed with residents and family members when the residents are admitted to the facility. Decisions do not have to be made immediately, but thinking about these decisions should be encouraged. The residents need enough time to make choices, discuss their fears, and address any issues. It is better to introduce residents to this subject of end of life not at the end of their lives but as a necessary planning stage. This planning ensures each resident's wishes will be honored when the time comes. Think about what you see in magazines and on television, such as court battles and families torn apart because of disagreements about what the person's wishes were. Planning and documenting the resident's wishes at an early stage will prevent these problems.

Your role in this process is to get to know residents. Know their likes and dislikes. Listen to what they say about their fears. Then tell other members on the team about issues they need to address. Always report changes in residents. Your observations and reports will ensure early intervention for each resident's symptoms. Helping to alleviate symptoms is a key part of your care. Giving comfort and emotional support to residents can make a huge difference in how they experience the end of their lives.

Maintaining or creating a positive relationship with a terminally ill resident is important. Spend time with the resident. Do not rush your care. If you feel you need more time with the resident than your other duties allow, talk about this with the charge nurse.

Hospice

Many people think of **hospice** care simply as end-of-life care, but these terms mean different things. Hospice is a specific program, not just general care for someone who is dying. Medicare includes a hospice benefit to provide hospice services for eligible people. Many people select hospice services in their home. When a person selects hospice care, a specially trained team provides their medical care. Residents in long term care facilities also have this Medicare benefit. Medicare covers hospice care for residents who are terminally ill and expected to die within 6 months. Like end-of-life care, hospice care focuses on palliative services. Pain management is a common service (Fig. 22-2).

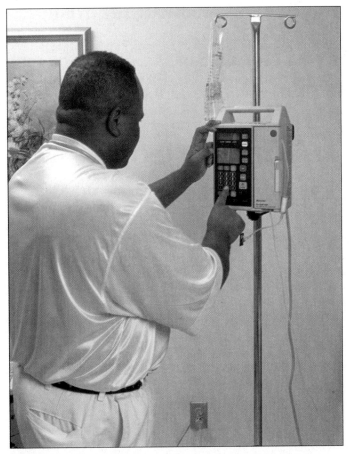

Fig. 22-2 – Medication for pain management is often a key focus of palliative care.

The Medicare benefit applies only when life expectancy is six months or less. This is often a problem in long term care facilities for residents who want palliative care but who have a longer life expectancy. For example, residents with end-stage Alzheimer's disease may live much longer than six months but would benefit greatly from hospice services.

Some facilities have special floors or wings for residents receiving hospice care. Many people are admitted specifically for this service. You will be asked to work with the hospice team. Even with this service, you still follow the resident's care plan.

Hospice – program with a specially trained interdisciplinary team that cares for a terminally ill resident who is expected to die within six months

Palliative – care focused on comfort and symptom relief rather than cure

YOUR ROLE THROUGHOUT THE DYING PROCESS

Your role when a resident is dying includes providing comfort measures. You also help family members and other residents cope with their feelings. Remember that the dying process can be brief or may last a long time. You may also need to deal with your own feelings. The next sections discuss these issues.

Helping Dying Residents Cope With Their Feelings

Death can occur very quickly or be a long process. When death is approaching soon, the resident may need more help coping with their feelings. Often the resident becomes restless because of their fear. Report this to the nurse so that an anti-anxiety medication may be given if appropriate. Use the communication techniques you have already learned to help. Stay calm to avoid adding to the residents' fears.

Listening is the best thing you can do for most people (Fig. 22-3). If you stay calm and listen carefully, you will know what they need. Your physical presence also helps reassure them that they are not dying alone.

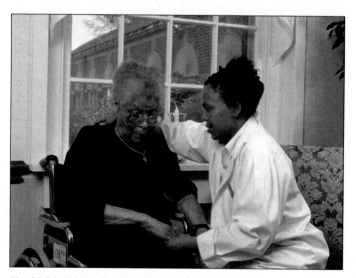

Fig. 22-3 – Residents must feel able to talk about their fears of dying.

Use the communication technique of reflection to encourage residents to talk about their fears and feelings. You may say something like, "It must be hard to talk about these things." Ask open-ended questions such as "What are you most worried about?" If a resident is worried about their care, ask what they would like to have done. Assure them they will be made as comfortable as possible. Tell them they will not be left alone. Take time to sit with a dying resident and hold their hand. Sometimes a simple touch can comfort the resident. Often you do not have to say anything.

If a resident seems to be denying their impending death, do not try to force them to "face reality." The person is not ready to deal with that realization. You can do more harm than good by forcing the issue. Let the resident adjust at their own pace.

Residents in the stage of anger often blame caregivers for not giving them enough treatment or not keeping them comfortable. They may be short-tempered with everyone, including other residents and even devoted family members. Do not take personally any anger they direct your way. Do not try to talk a resident out of being angry by saying things such as, "You shouldn't feel that way" or "You shouldn't talk to your wife that way." Acknowledge the person's feelings. Say things like, "What you're going through is really hard, isn't it?"

A resident in the stage of bargaining may say things such as, "I just want to be able to hold my grandson one more time." Relay their wishes to the family. Help in any way you can to meet their request for "one more...." Often bargaining involves what the resident considers to be "unfinished business." If the person can complete whatever that is, they may be able to move more easily to the stage of acceptance.

The stage of depression may be marked by withdrawal from others, crying, or a lack of interest in anything but themselves. Your role is again to be supportive. Be there, and accept the resident's need to work through these feelings. You might try to express the feelings you see by saying, "You seem very sad" or "You're having a really hard time today." Even if they do not answer, you have communicated your concern and your presence as a listener.

When a resident reaches the stage of acceptance, their attitude is usually much calmer. They can more easily talk about dying. They often want to talk about what they want done with their belongings, how they want to be cared for at death, and even their funeral arrangements.

In our culture people are often uncomfortable talking about these things openly with a dying person. Family members may refuse to talk about death directly with a dying loved one. You and other staff may be the only ones residents can talk to openly if they want to avoid upsetting family members. Keep listening.

Comfort Measures for the Dying Resident

In Chapter 21 you learned how to promote sleep and comfort and about your role in pain management. Apply this knowledge when caring for a dying resident. Show your caring, and do everything you can to ensure the dying resident is comfortable. Continue to incorporate the themes of care in your activities with the resident. Continue to provide for their privacy. Follow these guidelines:

- Keep the room well lighted and well ventilated. To offset noises, ask the resident about playing soothing music or their favorite music. Offer the resident and family privacy as needed. Keep distracting conversations away from the resident's area.
- Identify yourself frequently. Explain everything that you are doing, even if the person is not responsive.
- Offer food and fluids if the resident can tolerate them.
- Change the resident's position frequently. Use pillows for supportive positioning unless ordered not to. Sometimes repositioning is painful, such as with some residents who have bone cancer. Sometimes a catheter is used in a resident with a terminal illness to reduce the need for frequent repositioning.
- Change the resident's clothing and bedding when it is soiled by perspiration, urine, or feces.
- Apply makeup if desired, and keep the resident well groomed. Help the resident live as well as possible while dying.
- Give skin care to prevent or reduce skin breakdown.
- Because the dying resident often breathes through their mouth, give mouth and lip care frequently (Fig. 22-4).
- Take the resident's vital signs as often as the charge nurse directs. Notify the nurse of any change. Also immediately report to the nurse any changes in the resident's pain or other changes in the resident's condition, such as increased restlessness.
- Spend time talking and listening to the person. Listen with understanding. Let the resident know how special you feel to be with them. Share memories and stories from the resident's family and loved ones. Remember that because hearing is the last sense to fade, the resident may be listening even when they do not seem to be fully conscious.

Helping the Family During the Process of Dying

Family members go through the same stages of grief as the dying person. But they may not move through the stages

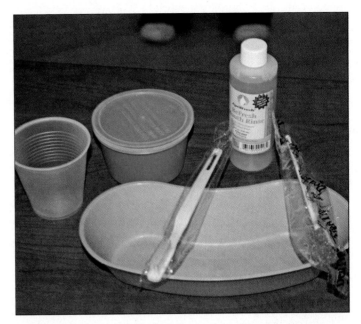

Fig. 22-4 – A dying resident needs frequent mouth and lip care.

at the same time. Then you may have to assist the communication between family members and the resident.

Some family members do not pass beyond the denial stage at all while their loved one is still alive. They may refuse to talk with the person about their wishes for care or funeral arrangements, saying, "No, you're not going to die." If you see this behavior, tell the charge nurse. The charge nurse may need to schedule a meeting with the family to address their fears and the resident's knowledge and wishes.

Some family members express their anger and guilt by insisting on giving all the care to their loved one. Or they may be very critical of the care you give. Other family members may withdraw and not visit the person because they are unable to express their feelings directly to them.

Encourage family members to participate as much as they can in the dying resident's care. You may have to encourage them to take time out for themselves. They need to rest and take care of their own health. Reassure them that their loved one will be well cared for in their absence. Say that you will call them if there is any change in the resident's condition. Do not take personally any criticisms or complaints the family makes during this time. Give them time to talk—and listen, listen, listen. If a family member requests to be notified about any change in the resident's condition, be sure to communicate that to other staff.

When a resident dies, offer the family time alone with the body. Offer to sit with them. Pray with them, if they ask and you feel comfortable doing so. Give them privacy, and offer to call a spiritual counselor.

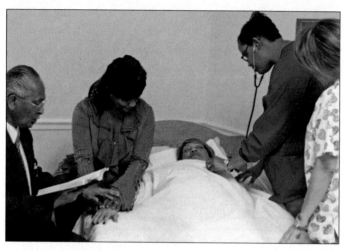

Fig. 22-5 – When a resident is dying, offer to call a spiritual counselor for the resident and their family.

Religious and Cultural Practices

By now you should have had a chance to learn from the resident and family members about their religious beliefs and practices. You will know their wishes for rituals at the time of death (Fig. 22-5). Many residents want to have religious symbols, medals, statues, or pictures with them. You may be asked to read from the Bible or another religious book, or to pray with them. Do this if you are comfortable doing so. If not, maybe you can find another nurse assistant who is.

A rabbi, priest, minister, or other spiritual counselor may visit this resident and family regularly. Their presence is often requested at the time of death. A religious resident may want to talk with their spiritual counselor or make a confession when they know death is near. Be sure to provide privacy for these visits.

Take care to understand the concerns of family members at the time of death. A family member may insist on staying with the body. Although sometimes this shows their difficulty accepting the death, usually it involves their traditional religious or cultural practices of caring for the body after death.

Family members often want assurance the body will be treated with respect. Reassure them. Explain what will

happen with the body. If the family wants to bathe the body or perform another ritual, let them help prepare the body if their request is appropriate and allowed by facility policy. This participation is often important for their emotional healing.

Helping Other Residents Cope With Their Loss

A resident's death affects all residents. For some, it is a reminder that their own death is not far away. For others, the death means the loss of a good friend. Residents should always be informed of another resident's death. Encourage them to talk about their sadness, loss, anger, fear, and other personal feelings. Reminisce with them about the resident who died.

A memorial service held in the facility is a good way to give residents and staff a chance to talk about their feelings of loss and to remember the good things about the person who died (Fig. 22-6).

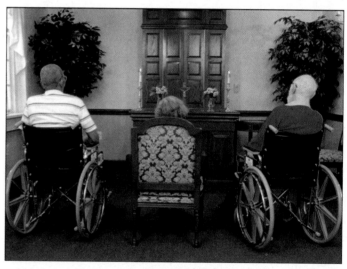

Fig. 22-6 – Attending memorial services gives residents an opportunity to discuss their feelings about the loss of their friend.

Often, other residents want to know about how the person died. Were they in pain? Was someone there when they died? These questions may arise from their concern for how they will be treated "when my time comes." Answer their questions as completely as you can without violating confidentiality.

Managing Your Own Feelings

You will often develop close relationships with residents. Before or after they die, you may experience the same feelings as the family and other residents. You are trying to help the dying resident, the family, and other residents deal with their feelings, but who will help you deal with yours? If you are really listening to the dying resident, however, you can learn much from them. They may be offering support in various ways to everyone involved. If you have helped the person to have a peaceful death, take comfort from that knowledge.

Talking with other staff is another good way to handle your feelings. Identifying your own feelings is the first step in resolving them. Knowing that others feel this way too also helps. You will probably find that other staff members have similar feelings. Also realize it is OK to cry sometimes (Fig. 22-7).

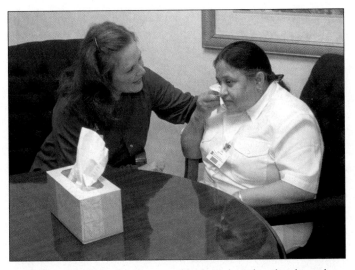

Fig. 22-7 — It is OK to cry when a resident you have loved and cared for dies.

SIGNS OF APPROACHING DEATH

There are usually physical signs that death is approaching. You may see these signs hours or minutes before the person dies:

- Decreased blood circulation causes the resident's hands and feet to feel cold to the touch. Their face becomes pale or gray. The skin looks spotted.
- The resident's eyes may stare blankly into space, with no eye movement, even when you pass your hand in front of their face.
- Breathing becomes irregular, sometimes rapid and shallow, at other times slow and heavy.
- Heavy perspiration is common.
- Loss of muscle tone causes the body to seem limp. The resident's jaw may drop and their mouth stay partly open.
- You will hear what is sometimes called the "death rattle," a gurgling sound when the resident breathes.
- The resident's pulse becomes rapid, weak, and irregular.
- Just before death, respiration and pulse stop.

When you recognize the signs of impending death, notify the nurse immediately. The family should be contacted. If you had advance knowledge of the resident's approaching death, you should already have talked with the resident or the family about their final wishes. Make every effort to meet the resident's and family's requests concerning the last hours of their loved one's life. Surviving family members will remember their last interaction with their loved one for a long time. That will have a lasting effect on their emotional health.

PHYSICAL CARE OF THE BODY

Every facility has specific procedures for caring for the body after death. Typically these are written in a policy titled "Postmortem Care." Box 22-1 lists common practices. In addition to these, your facility may include other procedures in postmortem care. Be sure to read and follow your facility's policy.

BOX 22-1.
CARING FOR THE RESIDENT'S BODY AFTER DEATH

1. Treat the body gently and with respect.
2. If the resident has a roommate who is aware of their surroundings, arrange for the roommate to go somewhere else until the body is removed.
3. Close the door or pull the curtain for privacy.
4. Remove any tubes and dressings
5. Put the resident's body in a flat position with the limbs straight. Place one pillow under the head to prevent their face and neck from becoming discolored.
6. Put their hands on their chest.
7. Put their dentures in their mouth.
8. Wash the body as you would when giving a bed bath. Place a fresh dressing over any open or draining wounds.
9. Comb their hair.
10. Cover their perineal area with a pad to absorb any drainage.
11. Put a clean gown on their body.

IN THIS CHAPTER YOU LEARNED:

- About different feelings about death
- About living wills
- End-of-life care
- The stages of dying
- Specific ways you can help during the dying process
- The care of the body after death

SUMMARY

This chapter discusses your responsibilities at the end of a resident's life. Death is part of a natural process, and there are natural stages in the dying process. You learned what is involved in end-of-life care and what you can do to help the resident during the dying process, as well as the care you will give after a resident has died. Residents are encouraged to document their wishes in a legal form called a living will.

PULLING IT ALL TOGETHER

Throughout this text you have been challenged to get to know residents and at the same time discover things about yourself. For example, if you are young and have never seen what happens to an aging body crippled with arthritis, this may initially shock you. You may feel the pain experienced by a child of a resident with Alzheimer's disease when you hear them cry, "Mom, don't you remember me?"

To successfully care for a dying resident, you must also deal with your feelings. In this case you deal with your feelings about death. Recognize that you will become emotionally attached to some residents but not to others. This fact may cause conflict for you. It may lead you to question what your relationship should be with each resident.

All these feelings are OK. The key is to be sure you treat each resident with the dignity and respect they deserve. Each resident has the right to live and die with dignity and respect and to be free of pain. You have a very important role in ensuring that this will happen.

Postmortem — after death

1. **To support a resident through the dying process, you need to:**
   A. Agree with their beliefs about death.
   B. Understand their beliefs about death.
   C. Assure them that there is life after death.
   D. Share their religious convictions.

2. **People who feel that after death they will be reborn in another life form believe in:**
   A. Reinvention.
   B. Resuscitation.
   C. Reunification.
   D. Reincarnation.

3. **What is the purpose of a living will?**
   A. To settle property and financial issues when a person dies.
   B. To help family members decide how they want their loved one cared for.
   C. To keep family members away from a dying resident.
   D. To guide decisions about a person's care if they become incapacitated.

4. **Bereavement is:**
   A. A normal reaction to the loss of a loved one.
   B. The resident's final stage of acceptance of their coming death.
   C. An abnormal response to anything one cannot control.
   D. A process nurse assistants use to comfort a dying resident.

5. **What is the best way to show your concern for a dying resident?**
   A. Leave them alone to work things out.
   B. Move their roommate out of their room.
   C. Ask the family to provide all their care.
   D. Encourage them to talk about their feelings.

6. **You can help a dying resident cope with their feelings by:**
   A. Discouraging them from talking about painful topics.
   B. Using techniques of reality orientation.
   C. Explaining your own views about death.
   D. Listening to what they have to say.

7. **What is palliative care?**
   A. Care focused on curing a disease.
   B. Care given the family members of a dying resident.
   C. Care focused on comfort and symptom relief.
   D. Care of the body after death.

8. **Hospice care paid for by Medicare may be provided for:**
   A. Anyone with a terminal illness.
   B. Any resident who can no longer afford a long term care facility.
   C. Residents with early-stage Alzheimer's disease.
   D. A person who may not live longer than 6 months.

9. **According to research by Dr. Elizabeth Kubler-Ross, what is the last stage of the dying process?**
   A. Anger.
   B. Bargaining.
   C. Depression.
   D. Acceptance.

10. **Comfort measures for a dying resident may include:**
   A. Keeping their room well lighted and well ventilated.
   B. Asking family members to stay away.
   C. Keeping the resident in the same position in bed.
   D. Celebrating with funny hats and party noise-makers.

(Answers to "Check What You've Learned" are in the Instructor's Manual.)

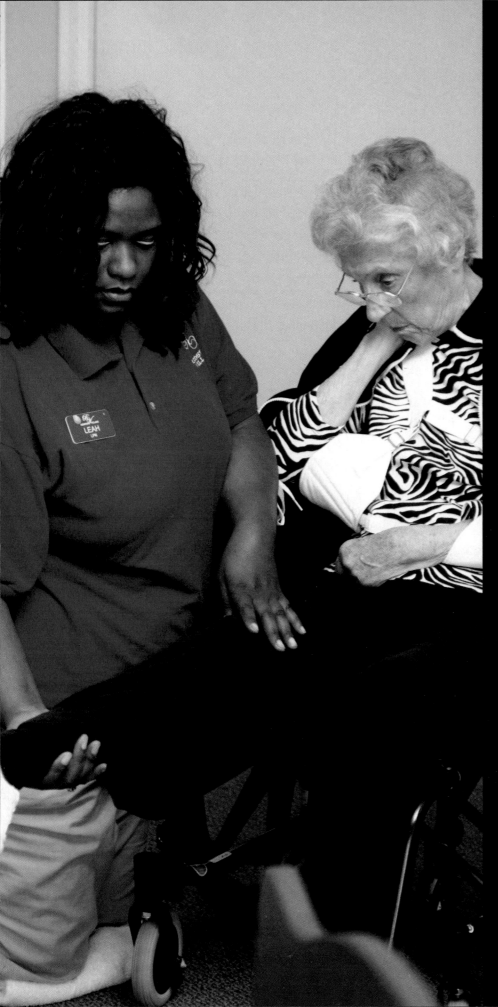

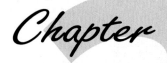

Chapter 23

OTHER WORK ENVIRONMENTS AND RESIDENT POPULATIONS

Previous chapters in this text have focused mostly on the needs of the elderly with various chronic illnesses. Most people are usually admitted to long term care facilities because their poor health leaves them unable to care for themselves.

Nurse assistants also work in different long term care environments with other resident populations. Your knowledge and skills from earlier chapters apply also in other facilities that provide care for other populations. The knowledge you have already gained is the foundation for caring for these other populations too. With other environments and populations, you may have to learn new terms and new approaches to care. But you will find that your knowledge of how to provide quality care while maintaining the resident's quality of life will apply to all settings with all populations.

This chapter will introduce you to other people you will care for in other environments, such as assisted living facilities and subacute care units. You will also learn about how to care for a person with Alzheimer's or one who is intellectually/developmentally disabled with a variety of conditions. This chapter is devoted to the unique needs of these populations.

OBJECTIVES
- Describe the services that are provided in an assisted living facility
- Describe the types of patients admitted to subacute care units
- Define developmental disability
- Describe mental retardation, Down syndrome, autism, cerebral palsy, and epilepsy
- Define the habilitation model used for the care of residents with developmental disabilities
- List the diseases that can cause dementia
- Name five symptoms of each stage of Alzheimer's disease
- Describe six principles guiding your care of residents with Alzheimer's disease
- List general techniques for responding to behavioral symptoms
- Discuss ways to change your care when helping residents with Alzheimer's with the activities of daily living

MEDICAL TERMS
- **Agenda behavior** – tending to follow a certain agenda, often a past routine
- **Agitation** – movements that are irregular, rapid, or violent; state of excitement, often troubled
- **Alzheimer's disease** – a progressive, incurable disease that affects the brain and causes memory loss and eventual death
- **Anxiety** – an uneasiness in the mind
- **Autism** – rare, severe disorder in which the child withdraws from the world; the cause is not known, and there is no cure
- **Behavioral symptoms** – actions that are caused by a disease or condition
- **Cerebral palsy** – condition resulting from damage to the central nervous system before, during, or after birth
- **Cognitive impairment** – disruption in knowledge, memory, awareness, or judgment
- **Delusion** – thinking that one's false thought is real
- **Dementia** – loss of mental functions such as memory, thinking, and reasoning
- **Developmental disability** – chronic, severe condition that a person develops from various causes, which prevents them from living independently without assistance
- **Down syndrome** – condition in which a person is born with an extra chromosome, causing some level of mental retardation, abnormal features, and often other medical problems; also known as mongolism and trisomy 21 syndrome
- **Epilepsy** – disorder of the nervous system that causes seizures and may also cause a developmental disability
- **Hallucination** – seeing or hearing things that are not really there
- **Insomnia** – inability to sleep enough
- **Mental retardation** – condition in which the individual has significantly below-average intelligence and minimal adaptive skills
- **Multi-infarct** – damage to blood vessels that may cause a loss of function in a tissue or organ
- **Sundown syndrome** – situation later in the day when a resident may become irritable or combative, or tearful and withdrawn
- **Wandering** – aimless movement from one place to another

"No matter how much care I need, my nurse assistants always give me the help I need."

Have you ever struggled to learn something new and then discovered it was very similar to something you already know? Or maybe you enjoy realizing how you can solve a new problem by applying something you learned from a totally different problem.

Think for a moment about hand washing. Do you use the technique you learned as a nurse assistant at home and in restaurants? Have you realized that the skill should be done the same way in all environments to prevent the spread of infection? Often people behave one way in one environment and do not realize the same principles hold true in other settings. But quite often they do hold true.

Applying knowledge in different situations involves critical thinking skills. You can learn to draw from your knowledge and experience in one area and apply it to other situations or different environments. In the same way you can learn to apply the skills you have learned for caring for elderly residents with chronic illness in a long term care facility to the care of other resident populations in other kinds of facilities.

DIFFERENT LONG TERM CARE ENVIRONMENTS

Chapter 1 introduced you to the services and types of facilities in the long term care system. You can successfully apply the knowledge you have learned in all the chapters in this book in other environments with different resident populations. As you read this chapter, think about how you would apply what you have learned to the other kinds of facilities described here.

ASSISTED LIVING FACILITIES

The development of assisted living facilities is based on the idea that people should "age in place." This means that as people grow older and become unable to care for themselves, they receive support in their home rather than having to move into a facility.

The National Center for Assisted Living (NCAL) defines assisted living as a group residential setting that provides or coordinates personal care services, 24-hour supervision, scheduled and unscheduled assistance, activities, and health-related services. Assisted living facilities are designed to reduce the resident's potential need to move from their present care setting. They are designed to accommodate individual residents' changing needs and preferences and to maximize residents' dignity, autonomy, privacy, independence, choice, and safety. Assisted living also encourages family and community involvement.

Assisted living facilities provide 24-hour supervision. Most residents can perform all or most of their own activities of daily living. They are able to bathe, get dressed, move in and out of bed, go to the toilet, and eat with little or no assistance.

Assisted living facilities provide a safe living environment along with support services. Services include three meals a day, help with medications, recreational activities, transportation, housekeeping, laundry services, emergency services, 24-hour caregivers, and help with personal care as needed. These services may be provided directly by staff or subcontracted to outside agencies, like a home health agency.

Many assisted living facilities employ nurse assistants. In this role you may be called a personal care attendant or direct care staff. You may work directly for the assisted living facility or for an agency that provides services to the assisted living facility. The focus of care in assisted living facilities is to provide only the care that the resident needs and that they and their families request. This care is outlined in the resident's service plan.

Assisted living facilities are also called residential care, board and care, personal care, or basic care facilities. They may also be referred to as elderly housing with services. Different states use different terms, but assisted living facility is the most common name for this kind of care.

SUBACUTE CARE UNITS

As mentioned earlier, changes have been made in long term care to meet the needs of the growing elderly population. Another factor that has led to changes is the need to manage health care costs. The goal is to minimize the length of hospital stay and thus control the costs of care. In addition, managed care providers and other insurers reevaluated how care is provided, exploring different ways to provide care in order to control costs.

Partly because of these initiatives, it became clear that there was a need for a new kind of service to provide health care to patients after they left the hospital but before they could go home or to a long term care facility. This service is called subacute, short-stay, or postacute care. A subacute facility or unit provides a higher level of care than is typically given in a long term care facility but a lower level of care than a hospital. The resident usually needs this care only for a short period of time, generally less than 30 days. In a subacute unit, residents, or patients, may have intravenous infusions (Fig. 23-1). They may have just had surgery and need postsurgical care, such as wound care and help with deep-breathing exercises. They may have a complication from surgery such as an infected wound. You learned about wound care in Chapter 19. In Chapter 24 you will learn about deep breathing, and Chapter 25 will help you understand postsurgical care.

You learned many of the other skills in other chapters needed to work in a subacute facility or unit. For example, you may take a patient's vital signs every 4 hours. This is the same skill you have already learned, although in this setting you will perform it more often.

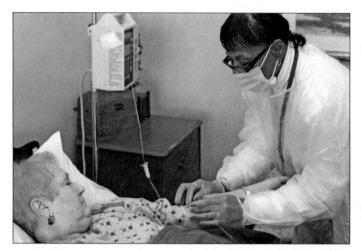

Fig. 23-1 – Residents in subacute settings often have intravenous lines and oxygen.

A typical example of a patient in a subacute care unit is someone who has a broken hip. They may stay in the hospital for three or four days and then be transferred to a subacute care unit for intensive rehabilitation for 10 to 15 days (Fig. 23-2). Once they have improved and can walk independently, they are discharged home.

Subacute care is provided in many different settings. Some are units in hospital wings, others are free-standing rehabilitation centers, and still others are units in long term care facilities (Fig. 23-3, next page). Regardless of the setting, the goal is the same: to care for the resident in transition from the hospital to their home or to a long term care facility.

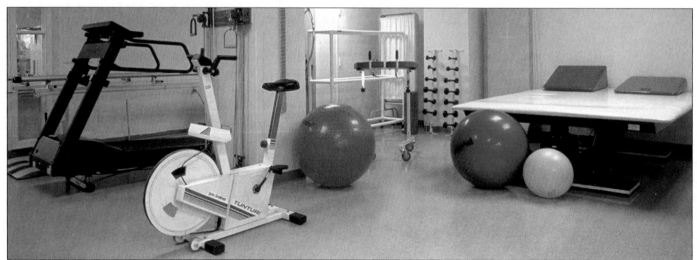

Fig. 23-2 – Residents in a subacute facility receive intensive therapy for a short time.

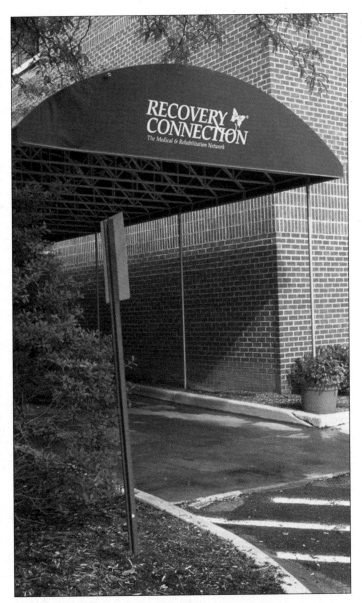

Fig. 23-3 – Subacute care is offered in many different settings.

FACILITIES FOR RESIDENTS WHO ARE INTELLECTUALLY/DEVELOPMENTALLY DISABLED

You may also work as a nurse assistant in a facility that provides service and care for residents who are developmentally disabled. These residents vary in age from the very young to the elderly.

An individual with a developmental disability has a chronic, severe condition that prevents them from living independently without assistance. The legal definition of developmental disability, mandated in 1970 by Congress and revised in 1978, states that the disability:

- is known before the person is 22 years old
- continues, or is likely to continue, indefinitely—no cure is likely
- is caused by a physical or mental impairment or injury, or a combination of both
- limits the person's ability in three or more of the following areas:
  - Learning: the ability to increase one's knowledge or skills
  - Mobility: the ability to move from one place to another without help
  - Independent living: the ability to live independently without assistance
  - Activities of daily living: the ability to care for oneself without assistance
  - Language: the ability to make oneself understood by others and to understand others
  - Self-direction: the ability to make decisions about one's life
  - Economic independence: the ability to support oneself
- requires an individualized, specialized program of developmental services for an extended period or for life

Facilities that provide care to residents with developmental disabilities are called Intermediate Care Facilities/Mental Retardation (ICF/MR) facilities. They are also called ICF/DD—DD for Developmental Disability. Where the person lives depends on their needs and preferences. The goal is for the environment to be as unrestricted as possible. Many residents living in an ICF/MR facility have mental retardation and a lifelong developmental disability. Some of the other conditions that cause developmental disability are Down syndrome, autism, cerebral palsy, and epilepsy. These are described in the following sections.

Today many people with developmental disabilities live in their community. You should understand that some people with developmental disabilities need very little assistance even though others need many services. They may live in their own home or apartment or in a shared

---

📖

Developmental disability – chronic, severe condition that a person develops from various causes, which prevents them from living independently without assistance

living arrangement such as a group home, congregate housing, or an apartment with a roommate. A group home is a house where usually six or fewer individuals live together, usually with 24-hour support. Congregate housing is a managed home environment with some support services. Residents have their own space within the building for sleeping and eating. Congregate housing includes common rooms where residents can meet to watch television, eat, or socialize. Some individuals live and work in the community and need only limited services. Others live in long term care facilities.

Individuals with Intellectual Disability

According to the American Association on Intellectual and Developmental Disabilities (AAIDD), intellectual disability is a disability characterized by significant limitations both in intellectual functioning (reasoning, learning, problem solving) and in adaptive behavior, which covers a range of everyday social and practical skills. This disability originates before the age of 18. **Adaptive behaviors** include communication skills; skills used in the activities of daily living; social skills; and other skills used for leisure activities, health and safety, self-direction, basic literacy (reading, writing, and math), and involvement in the community and work.

There are three major criteria for intellectual disability:
- Significant limitations in intellectual functioning.
- Significant limitations in adaptive behavior.
- The individual's condition was present before the age of 18.

Intellectual disability can be caused by hundreds of things. Any condition that damages the brain before birth, during birth, or during childhood can result in intellectual disability. Some common causes are listed in Box 23-1.

New methods are continually being developed to help prevent some of the causes, such as giving newborn screening tests, prescribing vitamins during pregnancy, using vaccines to prevent childhood illness, removing lead from the environment, using child safety seats and bicycle helmets, participating in early intervention programs for children, and administering other treatments to women before and during pregnancy.

BOX 23-1.
COMMON CAUSES OF INTELLECTUAL DISABILITY

- Down syndrome
- Fetal alcohol syndrome, caused by the mother's alcohol intake during pregnancy
- Fragile X syndrome: a genetic disorder and the most common hereditary cause of intellectual disability
- Problems or maternal habits during pregnancy, such as drug use, smoking, malnutrition, and certain infections such as rubella or syphilis
- Problems after birth, such as certain childhood diseases (whooping cough, measles, or chicken pox, for example), injuries (such as a blow to the head or a near drowning), or lead or mercury poisoning
- Problems resulting from malnutrition, inadequate medical care, or environmental hazards
- Cultural deprivation such as under-stimulation, which can result in irreversible damage

Down Syndrome

In **Down syndrome** the person was born with an extra chromosome. This causes some level of mental retardation, abnormal facial and physical features, and often other medical problems. Other names for Down syndrome are mongolism and trisomy 21 syndrome.

Research shows that Down syndrome occurs in one out of every 800 to 1100 live births. The risk of having a child with Down syndrome increases with the mother's age, especially after 35.

Although the exact causes of Down syndrome are unknown, some professionals believe that maternal factors before or during pregnancy may play a role, including hor-

---

📖

Adaptive behaviors – skills people use every day to live, work, and play

Down syndrome – condition in which a person is born with an extra chromosome, causing some level of mental retardation, abnormal features, and often other medical problems; also known as mongolism and trisomy 21 syndrome

IQ test – test of a person's intelligence (IQ means intelligence quotient)

monal abnormalities, X-rays, viral infections, problems with the immune system, or genetic problems.

Individuals with Down syndrome may have characteristic facial and physical features, but often the person is more like an average person than they are different. One child may have none or few of the characteristic facial and physical features, while another may have most of them. The facial and physical characteristics of Down syndrome may include the following (Fig. 23-4):

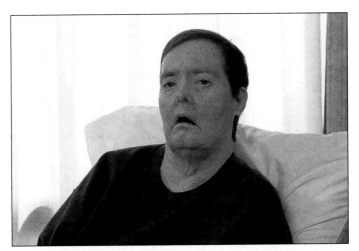

Fig. 23-4 – Residents with Down syndrome have characteristic facial features.

- flattening of the back of the head
- slanting of the eyelids (almond-shaped eyes)
- small skin folds at the inner corners of the eyes
- a flat bridge of the nose
- slightly smaller ears
- a small, open mouth
- a protruding tongue
- a short neck with extra skin
- small hands and feet
- short height

Individuals with Down syndrome need the same kinds of preventive health care and medical care as everyone else. In addition, they generally have problems requiring special attention. These problems include the following:
- hearing problems
- gastrointestinal problems
- eye problems
- obesity
- skeletal problems

In addition, a person with Down syndrome has a greater risk of getting heart disease, thyroid disease, Alzheimer's disease, leukemia, infections, diabetes, seizures, sleep apnea, skin disorders, and other medical problems

Many of these conditions can be successfully treated. Individuals with Down syndrome live longer today than in the past, but there still is no cure for Down syndrome.

Autism

Autism is a rare disorder that is usually diagnosed by the time a child reaches the age of two. Autism can vary greatly in severity from person to person: Some cases are relatively mild, others can be severe. A child with autism withdraws from the world around them. They become unresponsive to people. The autistic child makes their own world and creates rituals. They often have compulsive, uncontrolled behaviors and responses that may seem strange to others. In response to changes in the world around them they may have screaming fits, bang their heads, rock back and forth, or flap their hands. Their language skills and intelligence are significantly underdeveloped. They may be mute.

The causes of autism are still not known. Treatment must begin early and continue for years. It includes the child, parents, caregivers, teachers, and therapists. Treatment includes encouraging the child to adjust to their social world, helping them develop speech and language skills, and discouraging behaviors that might cause injury to the child. Behavioral techniques use food and other rewards to encourage behavioral changes. Most people with autism need special, planned living arrangements for their entire lives.

Autism – rare, severe disorder in which the child withdraws from the world; the cause is not known, and there is no cure

Cerebral Palsy

Cerebral palsy is caused by damage to the central nervous system that occurs before, during, or after birth. This disorder is more common in premature infants and in infants who are small or have a low birth weight. Cerebral palsy is caused by factors that limit the oxygen the brain receives, by hemorrhage, or due to other damage to the central nervous system.

A person with cerebral palsy often has some degree of paralysis. Additional common problems include the following:

- seizure disorders in 25% of those afflicted
- speech, vision, and hearing problems
- language problems
- mental retardation in up to 40% of those afflicted
- dental problems
- respiratory problems such as swallowing and gagging

There is no cure for cerebral palsy, but treatment can help children reach their full potential. The treatment of cerebral palsy includes the use of braces, splints, and special appliances to help children perform activities as independently as possible. Range-of-motion exercises are used to minimize contractures. Sometimes these exercises are not enough to prevent contractures, and orthopedic surgery is then needed.

Epilepsy

Epilepsy is a disorder of the nervous system. An individual with epilepsy has seizures, also called convulsions. Epilepsy may be a developmental disability if the person's condition meets the legal criteria of developmental disability described earlier. In addition, epilepsy may be present along with mental retardation or cerebral palsy. On the other hand, some people with epilepsy do not have a developmental disability.

Although many people with mental retardation have epilepsy, epilepsy does not cause mental retardation. Nor is every individual with epilepsy also mentally retarded.

CARE OF RESIDENTS WITH DEVELOPMENTAL DISABILITIES

The habilitation model of caregiving is used with residents with developmental disabilities. This is based on a principle known as normalization. Normalization involves creating an environment for individuals that is as close as possible to a normal environment. Caregiving emphasizes the resident's positive qualities and strengths rather than negative qualities or weaknesses.

In the habilitation model environment, residents receive the same types of treatment and care as others of their own age. For example, residents are dressed and groomed appropriately for their age and gender. You would never put a child's barrettes and ribbons in the hair of a 65-year-old woman. On the other hand, you would make sure that the resident you are caring for participates in activities that they choose for themselves and that are appropriate for their age.

As a caregiver for a resident with a developmental disability, your main responsibility is to give guidance and support and help them be as self-sufficient as possible. The goal of care is based on a philosophy of "person-centered" planning. An individualized habilitation plan, also called an individual service plan or individual program plan, is developed for each resident. This plan provides for special accommodations and sets the priorities of care for the resident. This approach encourages a resident with a developmental disability to participate as fully as possible in all aspects of their life. This includes their family, community, and social life. Many people with developmental disabilities successfully meet their individual goals with the help of caring people, organizations, and facilities.

📖

Cerebral palsy – condition resulting from damage to the central nervous system before, during, or after birth

Epilepsy – disorder of the nervous system that causes seizures and may also cause a developmental disability

Habilitation plan or model – philosophy of care in which an individual with a developmental disability is educated or trained to participate as fully as possible in all aspects of life, including interaction with their family and community, and to have a satisfying social life

Individual service plan or individual program plan – plan of care that provides special accommodations and sets the priorities of care for the resident; also called an individual habilitation plan

Normalization – the creation of an environment for individuals with developmental disabilities that is as close to normal as possible

The plan is based on an assessment of each individual's abilities. The interdisciplinary team gathers the information for the resident assessment. The resident, along with family members or a guardian, participates in meetings in which the plan is developed and updated. You, too, will be asked to provide information during this process. The plan includes all the resident's activities, from personal care to recreational activities. Your role as caregiver is to follow the plan and give feedback about the plan to the charge nurse.

If you are working with residents with developmental disabilities, you become a coach to help them maximize their potential. Your role is to give them whatever help they need while making sure you let them do as much for themselves as they can.

CARE OF RESIDENTS WITH ALZHEIMER'S DISEASE AND RELATED DISORDERS

"Dementia" is a cognitive impairment or loss of mental functions such as memory, thinking, and reasoning. For such a loss to be considered dementia, it must be so severe that it interferes with the person's daily activities. Dementia is not a disease but a group of symptoms. Changes in personality often occur with dementia. Sometimes dementia can be cured, such as when it is caused by drugs, alcohol, or poor nutrition. In other cases the dementia cannot be cured, such as when it is caused by **Alzheimer's disease**.

The Alzheimer's Association says:
- Half of all nursing facility residents have Alzheimer's disease or a related disorder.
- 14 million Americans will have Alzheimer's disease by the middle of this century unless a cure or prevention is found.
- More than 22 million individuals worldwide will have Alzheimer's disease by 2025.
- One in 10 people over age 65 and nearly half of those over 85 have Alzheimer's disease.

From this you can see that knowing how to care for residents with Alzheimer's disease and related disorders is important.

To successfully care for residents with Alzheimer's disease and related disorders, first think about everything you have learned so far. Know how to change certain procedures before caring for a resident with Alzheimer's disease. For example, you have to change how you approach residents. After months you will know each resident and greet them familiarly. Most residents you work with will recog-

nize you, too, and will know things that happened yesterday or minutes ago. A resident with Alzheimer's disease, however, cannot do this. Your approach to this resident therefore has to be different. For example, you may have to greet the resident each time as if it is your first time meeting them (Fig. 23-5).

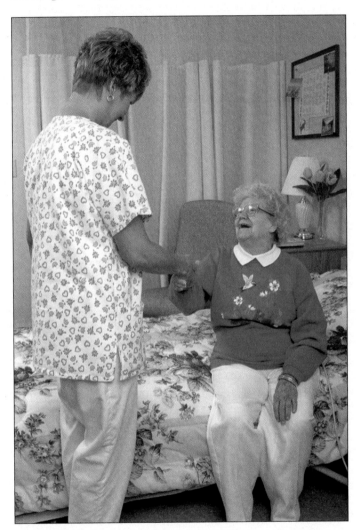

Fig. 23-5 – You may have to introduce yourself to a resident with memory loss each time you approach them.

Alzheimer's disease – a progressive, incurable disease that affects the brain and causes memory loss and eventual death

Think about your first day at a new job. Wasn't it exhausting? You encountered what seemed like a million new things and new people. You tried to handle all of it at once and remember it all. Most of the time you felt overwhelmed and wondered how you'd make it through the day. How long did it take until you felt you knew what to do on the job? How long before you did not have to rely on others to tell you where things were? Can you imagine feeling like that every day—feeling that everything you do is unfamiliar and you don't know the people around you? Would you be angry, frustrated, or frightened? Imagine what it would be like to never remember how to do even the smallest task.

Think about this as you learn about caring for residents with Alzheimer's disease or a related disorder. For many of these residents, each moment is a new experience, like the first day of a new job.

UNDERSTANDING COGNITIVE IMPAIRMENT AND DEMENTIA

Cognitive impairment is a form of temporarily or permanently altered thinking. Normally you can learn and remember things with your cognitive abilities. You can learn how to be a nurse assistant, for example. Your cognitive abilities help you live a productive life. When a person is cognitively impaired, however, they may have more than just memory loss. They may also have impaired language comprehension (both speaking and understanding language) and expression (understanding and speaking to others). They also may have suffered the loss of their attention span, judgment, and recognition and use of common objects.

Cognitive impairment has many causes. Temporary causes include stress, medications, depression, a vitamin deficiency, thyroid disease, alcohol, or head trauma. Permanent causes include severe head trauma, illness, brain disease, or brain damage at birth. In long term care facilities, most cognitive impairment is caused by brain disease. Following are diseases that can cause cognitive impairment or **dementia**:

- degenerative diseases of the nervous system, such as Alzheimer's, Lewy body, Parkinson's, or Huntington's
- diseases that affect blood vessels such as stroke or **multi-infarct** dementia, which is caused by multiple strokes in the brain
- toxic reactions, such as from excessive alcohol or drug use (Fig. 23-6)

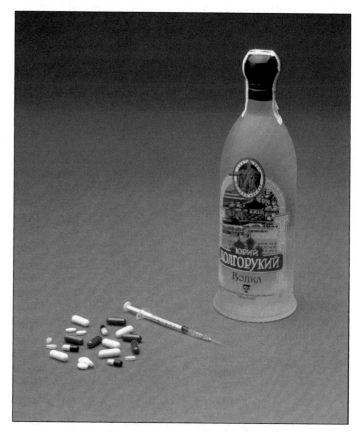

Fig. 23-6 – Misuse of drugs or alcohol can cause brain damage.

- nutritional deficiencies, like vitamin B12 or folic acid deficiency
- infections that affect the central nervous system, such as AIDS dementia complex or Creutzfeldt-Jakob disease
- certain types of hydrocephalus (a buildup of fluid in the brain), infections, injuries, or brain tumors
- head injury—either a single severe head injury or smaller injuries over time, as may happen with boxers
- other illnesses such as kidney, liver, or lung diseases

📖

Cognitive impairment – disruption in knowledge, memory, awareness, or judgment

Dementia – loss of mental functions such as memory, thinking, and reasoning

Multi-infarct – damage to blood vessels that may cause a loss of function in a tissue or organ

Alzheimer's disease is the most common incurable illness that causes dementia. It is one of the top ten leading causes of death in adults over age 65. No one knows exactly what causes brain deterioration with Alzheimer's disease. However, nerve cells in the brain die, causing the symptoms of dementia.

Nurse assistants play an important role in compassionately caring for people with Alzheimer's or other forms of dementia. Your role is to help a resident with a cognitive impairment get through each new day. The following sections focus on residents with Alzheimer's disease and related disorders. The terms "cognitive impairment" and "cognitive loss" are also used to refer to residents' memory, reasoning, or understanding capacities. The term "behavioral symptoms" refers to symptoms associated with personality changes or behaviors associated with the disease process.

STAGES OF ALZHEIMER'S DISEASE

A resident with Alzheimer's disease may have both cognitive and behavioral symptoms. Cognitive symptoms include memory loss, disorientation, confusion, and problems with reasoning and thinking. Behavioral symptoms include agitation, anxiety, delusions, depression, hallucinations, insomnia, and wandering. Alzheimer's disease generally progresses gradually through stages (Box 23-2).

Agitation – movements that are irregular, rapid, or violent; state of excitement, often troubled

Anxiety – an uneasiness in the mind

Behavioral symptoms – actions that are caused by a disease or condition

Delusion – thinking that one's false thought is real

Hallucination – seeing or hearing things that are not really there

Insomnia – inability to sleep enough

Wandering – aimless movement from one place to another

BOX 23-2.
STAGES OF
ALZHEIMER'S DISEASE

EARLY-STAGE (MILD)
- less sparkle
- less initiative and drive
- problems remembering certain words
- short-term memory loss
- person may be aware there is a problem
- increasing inability to handle routine tasks
- appears self-absorbed, insensitive
- difficulty planning or making decisions
- unable to make calculations
- seeks and prefers the familiar, shuns the unfamiliar
- changed ability to show feelings, control temper, handle frustration
- difficulty remembering how to get from one place to another
- confusion
- personality changes
- judgment problems
- difficulties with routine tasks
- gets lost or disoriented in familiar places

MID-STAGE (MODERATE)
- difficulty with personal care activities (bathing, dressing, eating)
- behavioral changes (sleep disturbances, insomnia, wandering, pacing, anxiety, agitation, paranoia)
- disoriented regarding time and place
- problems understanding others and speaking and writing
- problems with judgment
- may not recognize familiar people
- repetitive actions
- great difficulty making decisions
- catastrophic reactions (exaggerated responses for circumstances)
- poor or failing memory of recent past
- memory of distant past astonishingly clear
- lethargic, seems cold to others, indifferent

LATE-STAGE (SEVERE)
- apathetic, unable to communicate
- unable to care for self, complete dependence on caregiver
- poor long-term and recent memory
- assumes fetal position
- loss of speech
- loss of appetite
- loss of bladder and bowel control
- eventual shutdown of mind and body

Adapted from Alzheimer's Association, Massachusetts Chapter, "Alzheimer's Disease: Progressive Stages," 2006.

Understanding the different stages helps you know how to support residents and how to change your care. Note that these stages may overlap.

YOUR ROLE CARING FOR RESIDENTS WITH ALZHEIMER'S DISEASE AND RELATED DISORDERS

Your role in caring for residents with Alzheimer's disease is different from your role with other residents. Instead of focusing the resident on regaining lost function (rehabilitation), you focus on maintaining an ability to meet changing basic needs (habilitation). The problems caused by this brain-damaging disease cannot be reversed. The disease cannot be cured. Your role is to support the person and help them be as productive and happy as possible, and to reduce their agitation and fear. You can help meet many of their needs and work closely with their family to give support.

New approaches to residents with Alzheimer's disease try to **maximize** their functional independence and morale. You should value what the resident can still do instead of focusing only on what they cannot do. Support the resident's capabilities. Work to help them have positive emotions and experiences. Following are six principles for caring for residents with Alzheimer's disease or related disorders.

1. Provide Guidance and Direction

Your first role is to gently guide and direct residents through the day. The amount of guidance and direction needed depends on the resident's stage of the disease. Help them focus on the task they are trying to do. Think again of your first day at a new job, when everything was new and you were trying to manage everything at once. By late afternoon you probably felt you couldn't deal with anything else that day. You were worn out and maybe irritable. This is how many residents feel every day. By late afternoon or early evening, they are less able to cope. You may see a change in their behavior. They may become irritable or combative or tearful and withdrawn. This behavior is called sundowning or **sundown syndrome**. Your gentle direction is needed to help get them through each day.

2. Discover and Use Residents' Abilities

As residents move through the stages of cognitive decline, they lose many abilities. Instead of focusing on what they cannot do, work to discover what they can still do. Try to

involve these abilities in your caregiving. Whenever possible do things with the resident, not for or to them. Involve residents in any way possible in their care, and help them only as needed. For example, encourage a resident to put soap on the washcloth before you wash their body, or ask a resident to hold wash items before you start washing. Always think about the task before you do it. Try to break down your directions into short statements to help the resident more successfully achieve the goal. Think about making changes in the environment. This includes improving the lighting or making more pleasant surroundings with less clutter and more limited choices. Remember that these residents have difficulty making decisions.

As you notice a resident's abilities declining, talk with the charge nurse. Do not assume the resident has lost a capability. Talk with the team about anything you can do differently to help. Try to avoid situations that may cause the resident to fail because of their lost ability. For example, a resident with Alzheimer's disease should not get the same food tray as other residents. They may improperly use silverware and condiments, lick the butter pats, suck the sugar out of sugar packets, and drink the coffee cream. This may frustrate the resident, and you only make your job harder. Instead, make sure these residents' meals are ready to eat as soon as the food is served (Fig. 23-7).

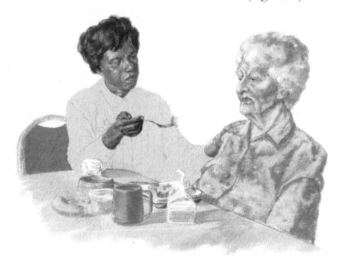

Fig. 23-7 – Always have everything ready for the resident and promote their use of the skills they still have.

Maximize – to increase to the highest degree
Sundown syndrome – situation later in the day when a resident may become irritable or combative, or tearful and withdrawn

The meat should be cut, the cream should already be in the coffee, the butter should be on the roll, etc. Now this resident can succeed using their remaining abilities.

In every situation, think of yourself as the person's champion. You help them succeed by encouraging them to use their abilities.

3. Promote Each Resident's Dignity

Another important role is to promote the resident's dignity. Everyone has their own idea of what dignity means and what is embarrassing or undignified. You can tell if you are respecting a resident's dignity by their reaction to your care. If a resident gets upset when you do something, ask yourself if you are offending their dignity. Be gentle with your assistance and be careful not to offend them.

Be especially careful not to assume that a resident does not understand what is happening or what you are saying. Residents sometimes experience moments of clarity or lucidity, when their brain functions well and they clearly understand what is happening. Always treat residents with respect and dignity.

4. Comfort and Reassure Each Resident

Your role is also to comfort and reassure these residents (Fig. 23-8). They are losing their abilities and often feel distress. Help them find physical, emotional, or spiritual support throughout the day. Anticipate their needs, provide gentle touches, sit with them, read from familiar books, and ask clergy to visit. Be positive, polite, and enthusiastic about them. Compliment their dress or how their hair looks. Mention things you know about their past, like the fact they were a great cook. Try to bring out positive emotions all day.

5. Anticipate Basic Needs

Anticipate the resident's basic needs so that you can meet them. In every situation, and especially if a resident resists care, ask yourself, "Have this resident's basic needs been met?" Think about Maslow's hierarchy of needs (Chapter 3, Understanding People). For example, if a resident does not want to sit down to eat, they may need to go to the bathroom first. When did this person last eat, have a drink of water, or go to the bathroom? Always address these basic needs first when giving care. The hierarchy of needs helps you remember the priorities for meeting a resident's basic needs.

6. Enjoy Residents and Help Them Enjoy Life

Your final role is to enjoy residents and help them enjoy life moment to moment. Residents enjoy life more when they feel successful and secure. Help them feel this way by being gentle and guiding, making the most of their abilities, promoting their dignity, giving them comfort, and satisfying their basic needs. They need to feel that you are looking out for them and that they don't have to worry about their care. Your job will also go more smoothly. You will more fully appreciate and enjoy your residents. When a resident can no longer use their mind, they still respond to emotions. Smiles and sensitive laughter often bring a positive response.

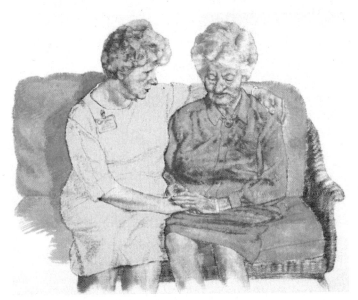

Fig. 23-8 – Since residents with Alzheimer's disease are often distressed, try to comfort and reassure them.

GENERAL TECHNIQUES FOR RESPONDING TO BEHAVIORAL SYMPTOMS

Residents with Alzheimer's disease often misinterpret things around them. They may not understand what you are asking them to do or why. They may become frustrated, upset, defensive, or agitated. Because of this, they may resist your care.

Remember: Behavioral symptoms like outbursts and tearfulness often show the resident is in distress. Finding the cause of this distress or threat is important for providing good care. This also makes your job easier and your time with the resident more enjoyable. Pay close attention to residents. See if you can identify a time of day they get upset. Watch to see what tasks are pleasurable for them and which ones are not. Share information with other staff. Maybe together you can discover what makes a resident happy. Then you can do those things before the resident becomes upset.

Following are **techniques** to help support the resident. Some techniques work only in certain stages of the illness, but others work in all stages. As you get to know the resident and their needs, you learn valuable information. Together with the care team, you can decide which techniques work best and when to use them. These techniques help lessen the intensity of some behavioral symptoms.

Enter a Resident's Reality

Reality orientation is a common practice in long term care facilities. Some residents benefit from knowing their current reality. But reality orientation does not work with residents with dementia because they no longer understand reality. If you try to convince them of something they cannot understand, they will become frustrated, agitated, and resistant to care.

Instead, use the positive practice called **validation** therapy. With this approach you try first to understand the resident's feelings (enter their world). Then you support their feelings (validate their perception of the world). By doing this, you are reassuring and comforting the resident. For example, a resident may tell you she wants to dress up because her husband is coming. Accept this and help her dress up even though you know her husband is dead.

Think about what will happen if you do not validate residents' feelings. For example, if a resident says that she saw her mother but you tell her that her mother is dead, she will begin grieving. Minutes later she may forget that you said her mother died but still feel sad even if she doesn't know why. A better strategy is to use a positive approach:

"I heard your mother was a wonderful lady. Tell me all about her." Use this approach when you can bring about positive emotions for the resident. Residents' statements about negative issues should be handled differently. For example, a resident is frightened or thinks someone is going to kill them. Discuss these situations with the charge nurse.

Remember there is always more than one way to see things. You may feel the resident's behavior is abnormal, but for that resident it is normal. Behaviors of each stage of the illness are normal for that person at that stage. When you understand how they view the world, you can see their behaviors in a whole new light. The world can be viewed in many different ways. Find out how the resident views the world. Then you can enter that world to care for them.

Know Your Resident

To care for residents, you need to know them well. How do they like things done? How did they do things in the past? Gather as much information as you can to help understand them. Ask questions of a resident, other staff members, and family members and friends. Be mindful and discover their routine. Consider these questions:
• What did they do for a living?
• What is their religion? (Fig. 23-9)

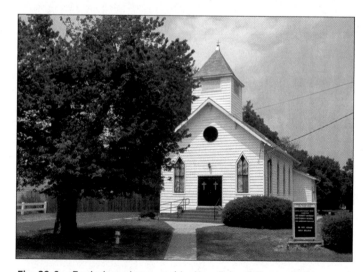

Fig. 23-9 – Try to learn how a resident's religion influenced who they are.

📖

Technique – a method for reaching a desired goal
Validation – confirmation of something

• Did they have any hobbies (Fig. 23-10)?

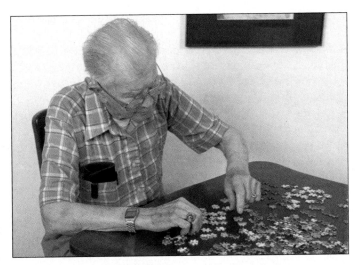

Fig. 23-10 – Try to discover things the resident likes to do.

• What is their social background?
• What were they proud of?
• What made them feel sad?
• Did they experience major losses?
• What were they afraid of?
• How did they handle stress?
• What was a typical day like for them before their illness?
• What behavioral symptoms do they have?
• What stage of illness are they in?

This information helps you enter their reality and makes your care giving easier. Residents often act with **agenda behaviors**. They want to follow a certain agenda during the day. Often a resident still tries to follow a past routine. Disrupting this routine causes stress. Knowing their agenda and honoring it when you can helps the resident feel positive.

Know Your Resources

In addition to knowing your residents, know what resources can help you give care. Consider equipment in the facility and department resources. Can the nursing or dietary department suggest procedures that can make your job easier? Have you read the resident's latest care plan? Does the activities department have special things the resident enjoys? Can you offer sweets to the resident to make a bath more pleasant? Be aware of all your resources. They will make your job easier.

Communicate With the Resident

The most important skill you can learn is how to communicate with residents. This includes learning how the resident communicates. As their disease progresses, they do not always communicate their needs directly. Eventually they lose the ability to speak and understand you. Watch for signals that show their needs. Be aware of signals you send them. Chapter 7 describes the basic principles of communication for all residents. Following are communication techniques to use with residents with cognitive loss.

Body Language.   Understanding residents' body language helps you anticipate their needs. For example, if a resident wraps their arms around their chest and rocks back and forth, they are having trouble accepting something. This resident needs comfort and reassurance, so you should not insist on giving care at that moment. Be careful of your own body language, too. Try to send positive messages to residents.

Facial Expressions.   As their illness progresses you will see residents "mirror" or copy your facial expressions, tone of voice, and sometimes body language. A smiling, welcoming face is much more appealing than a frown (Fig. 23-11). Residents take their cues from you about how to

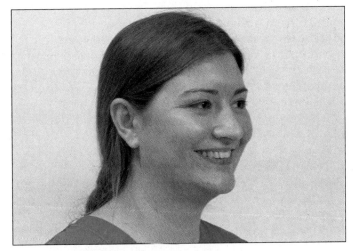

Fig. 23-11 – Residents with Alzheimer's disease often copy your facial expressions and body language.

📖

Agenda behavior – tending to follow a certain agenda, often a past routine

respond. Your facial expression affects your communication with a resident who has Alzheimer's disease.

Tone of Voice.   Tone of voice often communicates more than words. Your gentle, patient tone tells residents they can feel safe with you and trust you. The resident's tone also helps you understand their needs even when their words do not make sense. Is their tone angry or desperate? Is it lighthearted or happy?

Communication Techniques.   As their disease progresses, you need to change how you communicate with the resident. Watch the resident for cues. Adapt your communication to make positive experiences for the resident.

In the moderate stage of illness, residents can communicate fairly well and generally understand simple, one-step commands. They state their needs simply, such as saying "My lips are dry" instead of asking outright for help. They commonly have problems finding the right word, especially the names of things. (This is called "tip of the tongue" syndrome.) They may use the wrong words, ramble, or talk around the point. They may also stutter mildly.

As the disease progresses, residents have problems forming full sentences and understanding simple sentences. They may stop speaking except when spoken to. They have more trouble finding the right word. They may speak in only a few words, and they have difficulty staying on the topic. Residents who speak English as a second language often return to their first language.

In the late, severe stage of illness, residents have only the most basic verbal skills. They cannot comprehend or feel much. They communicate mainly through body language. They may also moan or scream.

Depending on the disease progression and the resident's reactions, choose the best communication techniques. Following are some suggestions:

- Speak slowly and clearly, using simple one-step commands. Give residents time to respond. You may have to give a resident 5 or 10 minutes; you can go away and come back. Limit choices you offer residents to two things. State each choice simply. Give them time to respond to the first choice before offering the second. If the resident cannot make choices, do not give them choices. For example, do not say, "What would you like to drink?" but say instead, "Would you like me to bring you some orange juice? I made it just for you." With late-stage residents, use only the simplest words and communicate through pleasant tones of voice, facial expressions, and a gentle touch. Meet residents' needs with

simple instructions without treating them like children. Remember they are adults and they still have feelings.
- Listen for a resident's verbal "cues" (simple statements like "Do me" or "My mouth is dry").
- Validate a resident's perception of reality whenever possible. Try to distract them from any troubling thoughts. Do not try to force a resident to do something that upsets them.
- Do not test a resident, which may set them up for failure. For example, do not ask questions that make them use nouns or names, such as "Who came to visit today?" or "What is my name?" or "What is this called?" Try to ask simple questions the person can answer with a "yes" or "no." Say things like, "How nice, your wife came today" or "Did you have a nice visit with your wife?"
- When giving directions, use only one or two words. Include nonverbal cues whenever you can (Fig. 23-12).

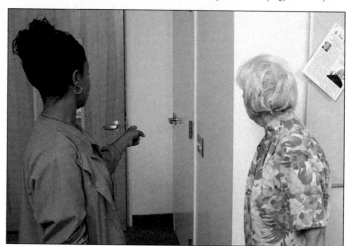

Fig. 23-12 – Giving nonverbal cues when you speak will help the resident understand what you want them to do.

As a resident's communication skills decline, you will need to send them nonverbal cues that will use their other senses. For example, at bath time, first show them the towel and then the soap, then run water in the sink and let them feel the wet washcloth. While doing this, never stop talking: "Time for a bath." "Here is the towel." "Here is the soap." "I am turning on the water." The person will understand your tone, if not the words.
- Watch the resident's body language for signs of physical discomfort or needs. Try to meet basic needs before continuing with care.

Motivate the Resident

People do only what they want to do. When someone asks you to do something, you consider why you should do what the person wants or what you will gain by doing it. Residents are motivated the same way. Learning what motivates them helps you avoid unpleasant behavior and difficult caregiving.

What motivates this resident? Residents want to do things that feel physically and emotionally good. A warm washcloth is more inviting than a cold one. Strange people and unfamiliar places and equipment make people feel threatened. When you insist that the resident do more than they can, that is also emotionally threatening. Even residents with Alzheimer's disease like to feel successful.

Residents with Alzheimer's are often motivated by something funny (a silly hat or clown nose) or anything new, interesting, or unexpected (Fig. 23-13). Curiosity is a big motivator. These techniques are also **distractions** that let you give care.

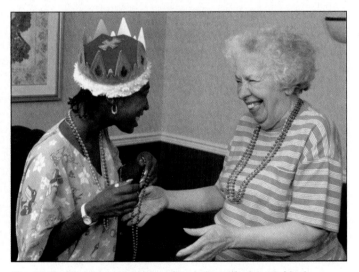

Fig. 23-13 – Humor and laughter often help motivate a resident.

Motivation also involves catching someone at the right time. Is the person ready to do something? Does it meet their needs at this time? For example, residents who are hungry and thirsty focus only on those needs until they are met. If you are trying to change their clothes at this moment, they are not very motivated to do this. Meet their basic needs first and other motivators will be easier.

Residents, like everyone else, are motivated by pleasant and inviting things and people. Is the environment inviting and pleasant? Be inviting to the resident, be pleasant, smell good, be clean and neat. Does the person like you, feel safe and secure with you, and find comfort being with you?

Finally, almost no one is motivated by something that seems like work. So don't make it work—make it fun! For example, if you are about to bathe, groom, and dress Mrs. Mancino, tell her she's "Queen for the Day" and your job is to pamper, bathe, groom, dress, and spoil her all day long.

Stop When a Resident Resists Your Care

As you communicate with the resident and offer motivators, constantly check to see how well your approach is working. If you accomplish your task and the resident is happy, your technique is successful. Look for verbal and nonverbal signs that the resident either is enjoying the activity or is becoming tired or agitated. When a resident resists your care, this signals that they are becoming distressed.

Resisting care tells you the resident is stressed or feeling threatened. When **confronted** with this situation, stop caregiving immediately! A resident cannot resist if you do not insist. Then consider the person and situation to understand the cause of the resistance, and then try to continue care. If you avoid confrontation, you are successful. Box 23-3 (next page) describes common factors that may cause resistance to care.

Finally, sometimes you must give routine care to a resident who resists care. In this case validate the person's distress and try to provide comfort during and after the care. Offering a drink of juice when you complete the care may help.

Specific Behavioral Symptoms

The following sections describe behavioral symptoms along with suggestions to help residents having them. Behavioral symptoms common in residents with Alzheimer's disease are agitation, anxiety, delusions, depression, wandering, insomnia, and hallucinations. You can do many things to help residents with these. Remember that any change in a resident may mean something is physically wrong—it may not be just a symptom of the disease. Report all changes in the resident to the charge nurse.

Confront – to face with a challenge

Distraction – something that directs the resident's attention away from something or eases mental confusion

BOX 23-3.
FACTORS THAT CAUSE RESISTANCE TO CARE

MEDICAL/EMOTIONAL FACTORS

A resident may have an unmet basic need such as pain, hunger, thirst, or need for elimination. (Do not try time-consuming care like bathing and dressing before a meal because hunger will keep a resident from cooperating.)

COMMUNICATION FACTORS

A resident may be responding to your negative body language, tone of voice, or facial expressions.

ENVIRONMENTAL FACTORS

The room may be uncomfortable or upsetting to a resident (too cold, too large, too much equipment, etc.).

NATURE OF THE TASK

A resident may not understand the care procedure. They may not know what is expected of them, what is being done, why the care is being given or when it will end, or who you are. Giving care too quickly or not giving short, simple directions and cues may also create resistance. Sometimes giving residents something sweet to eat or something to hold during care helps. You may need to try an alternative care procedure. For example, a resident who is frightened of a tub bath can have a bed bath or shower.

STAGE OF DISEASE

A resident's needs and abilities change as the disease progresses, and you must simplify your care to match their new needs and abilities.

Agitation. Agitation involves movements by the resident that are irregular, rapid, or violent.

Things you may see:
- appears very restless, uncomfortable, distressed
- repeats behavior, like calling a name over and over or asking the same question over and over
- paces back and forth
- swings an arm or leg repeatedly
- rubs or picks at their skin repeatedly
- fingers tap a table top repeatedly
- may be up all night and want to sleep all day
- bites, spits, or hits others
- resists care
- sensitive to noise

Things you can do to help an agitated resident:
- Make sure there is no physical problem causing the resident to be restless, uncomfortable, or distressed. Often residents become agitated because they need to go to the bathroom or have a pain they cannot describe. Ask questions so that you understand what the resident needs.
- Try to divert the resident's attention when they are repeating a behavior. Play soft music. Take them for a walk or bring them back to their room for some quiet time. Spend time sitting quietly with them. Use a gentle, soft tone when speaking to them.
- Give the resident something to do, such as knitting, folding towels, or sweeping.
- Try to reduce the noise level around the resident.
- Be kind and loving.
- Offer a nutritious snack like a piece of fruit to help divert the resident's attention (Fig. 23-14).

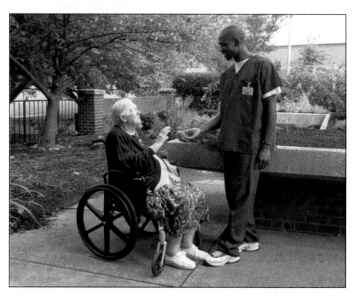

Fig. 23-14 – Food can be used as a distraction to help change a resident's behavior.

- Make sure the resident is eating enough nutritious foods.
- Limit caffeine in the resident's diet by not offering coffee, tea, or chocolate.
- Allow the person to sleep.

Anxiety. A resident who is anxious has an uneasy mind.
Things you may see:
- fearfulness
- tension
- increased pulse
- increased blood pressure
- sweating

Things you can do to help a resident who is anxious:
- Be supportive, kind, and gentle.
- Assure the resident that they are safe.
- Keep things simple for the resident. Give them simple choices, because many choices can be very frustrating and cause more anxiety.
- Provide quiet rest periods throughout the day.
- Watch for anything that triggers the resident's anxiety. Replace these triggers with a more pleasant, quiet activity.
- Observe the resident's nutritional intake and report any changes to the charge nurse.

Delusion. A resident with delusions has false thoughts or beliefs about themselves, someone else, or an object.
Things you may see:
- accusatory remarks made to staff
- fearfulness
- hiding
- suspicious looks

Things you can do to help a resident who is having delusions:
- Reassure the resident constantly, even if the resident seems distracted.
- Be kind. Do not argue with the resident about their thoughts and beliefs, which are very real to them.
- Help them feel loved and supported.
- Observe the resident's nutritional intake.
- Participate in the resident's reality.

Depression. A resident who is depressed feels sad (Fig. 23-15). Depression can usually be treated with success
Things you may see:
- reduced activity level
- difficulty concentrating or thinking
- trouble sleeping
- fatigue
- appetite changes
- agitation

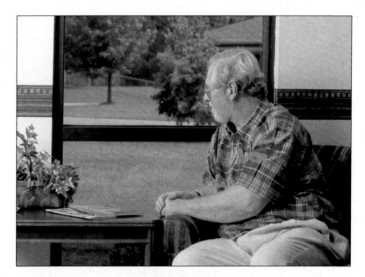
Fig. 23-15 – Depression can usually be treated successfully.

Things you can do to help a resident who is depressed:
- Let the resident talk about how they feel.
- Encourage the resident to participate in activities, which will help boost their morale.
- Keep things simple, and give only limited choices.
- Have rest periods often throughout the day.
- Encourage good nutritional intake. Offer frequent nutritious snacks. Talk with the dietary staff about nutritious snacks the resident would enjoy, especially if they have a decreased appetite.

Wandering. Allowing a resident to wander can be unsafe. Most residents who wander do not know where they are going or remember how they got there (Fig. 23-16, next page).

Residents wander for different reasons. As you get to know a resident you will learn why they wander. Residents wander with some agenda. For example, the resident may tell you they are going to work; this is called a "reminiscent wanderer." The resident may also wander because of other past habits.
Things you may see:
- walking with purpose (hat and coat on)
- opening and closing doors
- walking as if frightened
- walking up and down long hallways
- looking for something or someone

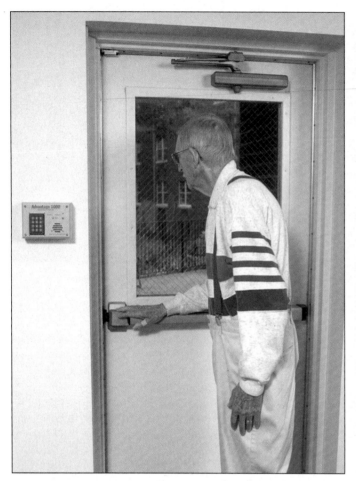

Fig. 23-16 – A resident with Alzheimer's disease may wander.

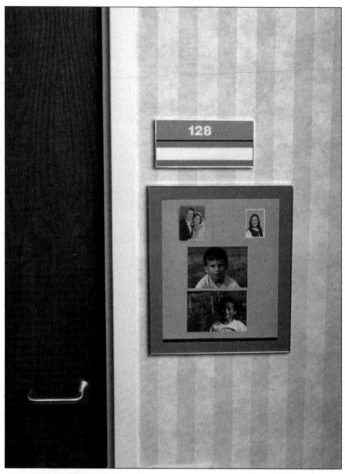

Fig. 23-17 – Visual cues often help a resident recognize their room or the bathroom.

Things you can do to help a resident who wanders:
- Put signs on doors, walls, and hallways that help the resident know where they are (Fig 23-17).
- Divert the resident's attention by offering meaningful activities. Speak with the facility's activities director for tips on what activities would be good for the resident.
- Help the resident to get daily exercise, such as walking or dancing.
- Make sure the resident has identification on them.
- Keep the resident's room and hallways free of clutter.
- Offer frequent rest periods.
- Provide proper nutrition, which is important for residents who are often moving.
- Do not argue with a resident who wanders. They may tell you they are going to work or school and cannot be late. In such a situation you can say that today is Saturday or a holiday and they don't have to work today.

Ask them to go for a walk with you or get something to eat. Activities that are similar to what the resident did in their job can also be helpful.

Insomnia.   Insomnia involves prolonged episodes of sleeplessness.
Things you may see:
- awake at night
- restless in bed

Things you can do to help a resident who has insomnia:
- Offer frequent rest periods throughout the day.
- Help the resident with a regular exercise program.
- Be sure the resident is getting proper nutrition.
- Give back rubs.
- Play soft, soothing music.

Hallucinations.   A resident with hallucinations has false perceptions. These false perceptions feel very real to the resident and can be distressing or frightening. Residents may hear or see things that are not there.

Things you may see o hear:
- Resident says, "Did you hear that?"
- Resident speaks as if talking to someone.

Things you can do to help a resident having hallucinations:
- Do not argue with the resident.
- Listen to the resident.
- Be kind and supportive.
- Be sure the resident is getting proper nutrition.

SPECIFIC TECHNIQUES FOR ACTIVITIES OF DAILY LIVING

Residents with Alzheimer's and related disorders have unique needs that you must meet to give routine care and to help them with the activities of daily living. You will be challenged to give care in ways that do not cause distress. Tailor your methods to the individual resident to help them do daily activities easier and with dignity.

Remember the stage of the resident's disease as you plan care. Always individualize your care based on each resident's needs. The goal is to help the resident have a positive experience with the activities of daily living. Whenever you give care, the resident should feel as though they are participating as fully as their ability allows.

Toileting

Residents with Alzheimer's eventually lose control of their bladder and bowels. Because of their cognitive loss they cannot identify the feeling of needing to go to the bathroom. They lose the ability to find the bathroom, to undress, to use the toilet, and to clean themselves. They may reach this stage sooner if they have difficulty locating restrooms or communicating their need to go. Their verbal and nonverbal cues may show you when they need to go to the bathroom. For example, Mrs. Morgan may not ask you directly where the bathroom is or may not say, "I need to use the restroom." Instead she may pace and look agitated. She may try to take off her skirt. Be aware of these cues. You can prevent residents from becoming incontinent at an early stage and maintain their dignity and independence longer if you recognize their cues.

As a resident's disease progresses, you will see changes in their independence in toileting. For example, some resi-

dents can control their bowel and bladder if you help them find bathrooms and remind them to toilet. Then they will need your help in the mechanics of toileting, such as wiping, flushing, and pulling their underwear down and up. Eventually they become completely incontinent. They may not hear or understand reminders to use the toilet and may resist your help and your offer of incontinence products.

Follow these guidelines to help a resident remain continent as long as possible. This will make toileting easier for both of you.
- Always be ready to help residents find bathrooms, and help as needed with toileting.
- Know residents' individual toileting schedules to predict when they may need your help. This also helps you recognize cues that a resident needs to use the bathroom. Residents often need to use the bathroom in the morning, 1/2 to 1 hour after meals or snacks, and before bed.
- Help a resident with incontinence products when they need them. You can ease the transition into using incontinence products by placing underwear over them.
- Communicate slowly and gently with residents while toileting. Give them extra time to respond.

Providing a distraction may help when a resident resists your help with toileting. A pleasant distraction is to give them something sweet to eat.

Finally, remember that toileting is personal. Wearing incontinence products can be embarrassing and upsetting. Put yourself in the person's position and think how you would like to be treated. Remember respect and dignity.

Hydration

The body has a basic need for fluids. This is called hydration. Water is the primary source of hydration. You may not understand how a resident can be thirsty when a water pitcher or water fountain is within easy reach. But think for a moment: Do you have a water fountain in your home or a water pitcher by your bed? Neither did most residents. These objects become unfamiliar to them and they do not notice or recognize them. The resident may go thirsty without your help in locating or providing water.

Because these residents have difficulty telling you what they need, watch for verbal and nonverbal cues that show you their needs. For example, a person may say, "My mouth is so dry" or act in ways that suggest being thirsty, including acting agitated or searching for something aimlessly.

As the disease progresses, residents needs change. Residents may not be able to find water fountains or a water pitcher. They may not ask you for something to drink when they are thirsty. Eventually they may not give you any cue at all. Follow these basic techniques to meet residents' hydration needs:

• Offer residents fluids according to their individual needs. Offer fluids more often and in smaller amounts, especially to residents who have difficulty swallowing. If a resident has trouble swallowing, tell the nurse immediately.

• Offer fluids when a resident gives verbal cues (like "My mouth is so dry"). Offer fluids when a resident shows nonverbal signs of thirst (dry mouth, agitation, tongue hanging out, or seemingly aimless rummaging or searching behavior).

• Don't ask if the resident is thirsty; just bring a drink and let them drink.

Eating

Residents with Alzheimer's disease and related disorders need help finding the dining area and then eating. Tell the nurse about any changes in their abilities so that dietary trays are set up and the food choices are appropriate for each resident's abilities.

In the early stage of illness residents can eat by themselves, but watch that they can still use their knife properly. They eventually lose eating skills and the ability to use knives, forks, and straws. They may have problems with positioning and swallowing. Try these techniques:

• Prompt them and give cues to keep eating, chewing, and swallowing as needed.

• Give them time to eat.

• Cut, season, and de-bone their food for them. Their food should be ready to eat when the tray is put before them.

• Watch for any trouble using utensils. Give a fork and spoon to residents who cannot use a knife properly. Then give only a spoon when the fork is no longer manageable. When a spoon is no longer manageable, give the resident only finger foods.

It is OK for residents to use their fingers when they eat. Watch for problems like the person ignoring one side of their plate (which may result from a visual problem), not being able to handle food and drinks served together, not eating other food if dessert is served with the meal, or having trouble swallowing.

Follow these guidelines, too, for supporting the resident:

• Ensure proper body positioning.

• Peel fruit for them.

• Watch for a resident pouring their drink in their plate. If a resident does this, do not give food and drink at the same time.

• Add a sweetener to give food more appeal if needed.

• If a resident will not sit long enough to eat, offer nutritious finger foods like a sandwich, cookie, breakfast bar, etc.

Dressing

Like other activities of daily living, a resident's ability to dress and undress will change as the disease progresses. At first these residents can get dressed by themselves with limited supervision. You may only have to choose clothing appropriate for the season or occasion. Some residents may need coaxing to change their clothes or take off their clothes at night. Others may try to change their clothes repeatedly throughout the day.

Some residents need help putting their clothes on properly, like putting shoes on the right feet and tying their shoelaces. They may have problems wearing their glasses, dentures, and hearing aids all day. They may resist your help in dressing or undressing.

Eventually they need total assistance with dressing and cannot wear supportive appliances. They may take their shoes and socks off or clothes that fasten in front. They may fiddle constantly with buttons, zippers, or hems. They may resist changing their clothes and wearing underclothes.

Try to make dressing simpler and more enjoyable for you and the resident. Be ready to help whenever you see your help is needed. Simplify the process according to the person's individual needs. Use these tips for dressing residents as the disease progresses:

• Offer only two outfits and ask the person to choose one.

• Select clothing for the person to wear.

• Simplify dressing by laying clothes out in the order they are put on.

You may also have to help them place their arms, legs, and head in clothing openings and fasten buttons, snaps, etc. Dress residents in clothing that is easy to put on and take off. For example, use over-the-head dresses and shirts, slacks and skirts with elastic waistbands, and clothing with no front closures (such as buttons and snaps). Avoid using belts and ties. If a resident resists your efforts to dress or undress them, they may need friendly coaxing. If that is not enough, take these steps:

- If they resist in the morning, wait until after breakfast.
- If they resist at night, encourage the family to bring in clothing they can wear day or night, like jogging suits, housecoats, or muu-muus. Then you can change their clothing only once a day, in the morning.
- If a resident resists wearing nonessential clothing like bras, slips, or nylons, do not force them to wear them.
- Always make sure that the resident's shoes are on the correct feet.

Remember: Always be gentle and patient. Use words and gestures to communicate, move slowly, and give the resident time to understand what is happening. If the resident resists, leave and come back later. Try again with a big smile and a slow, patient manner.

Residents who begin wearing only one shoe may need to be assessed for a foot problem, or their shoes should be checked for fit and condition. If no problem is found, they might wear slipper socks with non-slip soles instead of shoes. Talk to the nurse about this.

Bathing

Bathing is often a traumatic experience for these residents, but it need not be. With your help, bathing can be done smoothly and in a manner that does not upset the resident. Consider each resident's needs and past routine.

Residents may rely completely on you to tell them when to bathe. They may need help finding the bathroom and supplies like soap, washcloth, towel, and shampoo. They may need help getting into and out of the shower or bath, adjusting the water, and washing and drying themselves. Help a resident in these ways:

- Help them get ready for bathing, such as getting undressed, finding the bathroom, etc. You do not always have to help, but you should be ready to help if the resident is struggling.
- Help with shampooing if the resident needs help.
- Give directions for washing and drying to make sure a resident does a good job. Talk the resident through it or show them with body language.

As a resident experiences more physical and cognitive difficulties, their ability to bathe may become limited to washing and drying their hands and face. Encourage any action a resident can do independently, even if it seems very small. Residents may develop a fear of water in a shower or tub. They may resist your efforts to help them bathe. Help in these ways:

- Help the resident undress, get into and out of the shower or bath, and wash and dry.
- Encourage residents to bathe themselves in easily reached areas like their face, chest, and thighs.
- Good communication makes helping easier. Use simple one-step commands ("Rinse your arm ... now rinse your shoulder"). Place your hand over the resident's hand to show them how to wash their arms, dry their legs, etc.
- Avoid things that may make residents afraid of bathing. Do not wet a resident's face or hair directly with the shower spray. Give a sponge bath as needed instead of putting a resident completely in the water. Think about what you would not want someone to do to you if you were afraid of water. Experiment to see what time of the day works best—not everyone needs to be bathed in the morning. Use a hand-held shower nozzle. Do not wash the person's hair in the shower. Wash hair at the sink and make sure the person's face does not get wet. Spend time planning the activity and you will have less trouble with it. This is called the "spend five minutes to save 20" principle.

A resident who needs total assistance may resist your efforts because they no longer understand bathing and may have a fear of water. Often it is better to give a sponge bath or bed bath. Help in these ways:

- Communicate gently while bathing them. Remember to use both verbal and nonverbal communication.
- Move slowly and give the person more time to understand what you are communicating or doing.

When a resident resists, you can distract them with something sweet to eat or offer a drink after bathing. Make bathing more comfortable by warming the bathroom ahead of time. Make bathing less fearsome by wetting their feet first in the tub or shower before immersing them in the water or just give them a sponge bath. Help residents be less afraid. Remember you are trying to coax someone into doing something they do not want to do.

Grooming

Good grooming helps preserve a resident's dignity. Poor or incomplete grooming often causes the family to complain. Grooming includes combing the hair, washing the face, brushing the teeth, removing and reinserting dentures, shaving, and applying makeup and cologne or lotion. Meeting the grooming needs of residents is not difficult.

Some residents can groom themselves with your encouragement and supervision. As their skills decline, they will need more help from you. Residents may resist having their hair washed. They may stop using their glasses, hearing aids, or dentures. They may resist shaving and stop using supportive appliances. Eventually they completely depend on you for their grooming.

Use these techniques to make grooming easier and a more pleasant activity for both you and residents:

- Be ready to help with any part of grooming.
- Simplify the tasks of grooming as needed to encourage self-grooming. Help them get started with each activity. For example, put the toothpaste on the resident's toothbrush.
- Encourage a resident to attend the facility's morning grooming program (if offered) and apply any "finishing touches" like cologne and makeup. This promotes a positive self-image and good self-esteem.
- When a resident stops using supportive appliances all day, give them to the resident only at beneficial times. For example, dentures are needed at meals but are not necessary at other times. Make sure you retrieve the resident's dentures after each meal.
- Gently communicate with residents during grooming. Use sensory cues to encourage grooming, like putting a warm washcloth on their face or applying warm shaving cream with a shaving brush. As always, move slowly to give them more time to understand what you are doing.
- If a resident resists shaving, check for pain, such as a razor burn, dry skin, oral problem, earache, or discomfort from other unmet needs. If they keep resisting, do not force the shaving at this time. Try later using more sensory cues. If they still resist, try every day but do not force your care on them. Advise family members that this is a normal behavior and that you will resume shaving them when they stop resisting.

To help a resident with the activities of daily living, consider their individual needs and adapt your care accordingly.

Keep in mind the general principles to prepare yourself, to use good communication and motivation skills, and to create a positive experience that enables the resident to do as much as they can for themselves. Consider the cause of any resistance. Remember that if you simplify your requests of the resident, you will get more cooperation.

Talk with the charge nurse about any concern you have about caring for the resident. Share your ideas for adapting care with other team members. Always have a philosophy of mindful caregiving and remember the themes of care (see Chapter 12).

A resident with cognitive impairment will challenge you, but your successful caregiving will be rewarding (Fig. 23-18).

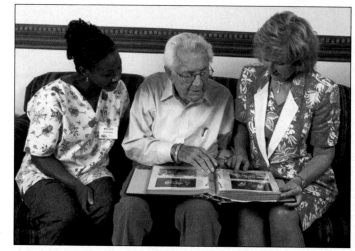

Fig. 23-18 — Often you will develop positive relationships with both the resident and their family members.

IN THIS CHAPTER YOU LEARNED:

- How to change your care when helping with the activities of daily living
- The services that are provided in an assisted living facility
- The types of patients who are admitted to subacute care units
- What a developmental disability is
- About mental retardation, Down syndrome, autism, cerebral palsy, and epilepsy
- The habilitation model used for the care of residents with developmental disabilities
- The diseases that cause dementia
- The symptoms of each stage of Alzheimer's disease
- Six principles guiding your care of residents with Alzheimer's disease
- General techniques for responding to behavioral symptoms

SUMMARY

In this chapter you learned about other long term care environments where you might work as a nurse assistant. In these environments you may care for residents with various developmental/intellectual disabilities or Alzheimer's. For all populations of residents in all long term care environments, you use the same basic skills and themes of care you have learned throughout this text.

PULLING IT ALL TOGETHER

Nurse assistants have many opportunities for working with residents in different environments. For residents in these other settings you might make only minor modifications in the skills and themes of care you have learned to use when caring for residents in long term care facilities. Let's look, for example, at your care for residents with a similar need in four different settings:

In a long term care facility you may be assigned to a resident with a weak left arm who has physical therapy three times a week. This weakness resulted from a stroke the resident had two years ago. You are responsible for helping the resident get ready and helping them to the physical therapy (PT) room at the scheduled time.

Working in a subacute unit, you might care for a similar resident who has just been discharged from the hospital after a stroke. Here, the physical therapist comes to the resident's room to give therapy until the resident is strong enough to go to the PT department. Your role here is to help the resident get ready for the appointment and to assist the physical therapist as needed.

In an assisted living setting, your role with a similar resident is to help them get ready and to get to the main entrance on schedule. A taxi may pick up the resident, who goes independently to a local outpatient PT department.

In a community setting for residents who have developmental disabilities, your role with a similar resident is to help them get ready and to go with them on public transportation to their PT appointment, ensuring that they arrive safely and on time.

In each of the above settings, your role is to help the resident get ready and to ensure that they arrive at their appointment safely and on time.

Let's look at another example of how a nurse assistant's basic skills and themes can be transferred to other settings. A frequent task is helping a resident get out of bed and into a chair. The goal when moving a resident is to make sure they are moved safely, without injury to either you or the resident. In long term care facilities, subacute care units, and rehabilitation units, you have the help of other staff and mechanical lifts. In assisted living and group homes mechanical devices may not be available, but you can still meet the same goal of safety. For example, you may have to place the resident's bed against a wall and secure the chair to prevent them from moving during the transfer.

Think about the many skills you have learned throughout this text. Now think about each of the different populations and settings described in this chapter. Can you see that what you have already learned will help you to be successful wherever you work?

1. **Which statement describes a resident in a subacute care unit?**
   A. They have a chronic illness.
   B. They have a mental disability requiring permanent assistance.
   C. They need their vital signs taken only once a week.
   D. They may have just had surgery and need short-term postsurgical care.

2. **What are adaptive skills?**
   A. Skills used to cure disease.
   B. Skills used to score high on an IQ test.
   C. Skills used every day to live, work, and play.
   D. Skills used to communicate with health care personnel.

3. **What is the goal of the habilitation model of caregiving?**
   A. To train a mentally retarded person for a job.
   B. To help a person with HIV live a normal life without transmitting the infection to others.
   C. To encourage someone with a developmental disability to participate as fully as possible in all aspects of their life.
   D. To enable someone with Down syndrome to earn a college degree.

4. **A child with autism:**
   A. Withdraws from the world around them.
   B. Needs special treatment to prevent seizures.
   C. Often has respiratory problems and problems swallowing and gagging.
   D. Generally outgrows the condition by age 12.

5. **Which of these statements about Alzheimer's disease is true?**
   A. Alzheimer's disease is incurable.
   B. Alzheimer's disease causes death within a few weeks.
   C. In Alzheimer's disease nerve cells in the brain multiply uncontrollably.
   D. Residents with Alzheimer's disease must be isolated from all other residents.

6. **Which of the following symptoms is typical of mid-stage dementia?**
   A. Loss of appetite.
   B. Tendency to feel cold most of the time.
   C. Great difficulty making decisions.
   D. Improved recent memory.

7. **Mr. Walker has dementia and thinks she is living at home and you are her cousin Hilda. What should you do?**
   A. Show her your ID badge to prove to her who you really are.
   B. Ask another nurse assistant to take over for you.
   C. Use reality orientation techniques to demonstrate to her that she is in a long term care facility.
   D. Try to understand her reality and use validation techniques.

8. **Mrs. Henry has moderate dementia and is resisting your attempts to help her with care. What may be the reason she won't cooperate?**
   A. She can care for herself.
   B. She may be thirsty, hungry, or in pain.
   C. She expects you to give her candy first.
   D. She no longer understands English.

9. **Which of the following techniques is helpful when you are dealing with an agitated resident?**
   A. Yelling.
   B. Distraction.
   C. Reality orientation.
   D. Clapping your hands and stomping your foot.

10. **How can you help to prevent a resident from wandering?**
    A. Divert the resident's attention by offering meaningful activities.
    B. Constantly remind the resident that they must remain seated.
    C. Lock the main doors of the building.
    D. Use a restraint to keep them in their bed.

(Answers to "Check What You've Learned" are in the Instructor's Manual.)

Chapter 24

SPECIALTY SKILLS FOR SUBACUTE ENVIRONMENTS

As medical care improves, people are living longer and often need more types of health services. The responsibilities and opportunities for nurse assistants are also growing. Certain common tasks, in the past performed only in hospitals, are now being done in long term care settings. Common tasks only performed by nurses are now being done by nurse assistants. The skills in this chapter affect the quality of care residents receive. Depending on the state in which you will work, you may need a special certificate or training course to perform such skills. Advanced training in these skills may provide you with great personal reward. In this chapter you will learn about glucose testing and foot care for residents and patients with diabetes. You will learn about the person receiving dialysis and those receiving enteral nutrition. You will also learn about oxygen therapy and the use of heat and cold applications in subacute settings.

As explained in Chapter 23, in a subacute setting patients receive health care after leaving the hospital before going home or to a long term care facility. Subacute settings give a higher level of care than most long term care facilities but a lower level of care than hospitals. The person usually needs this care only for a short period of time, usually less than 30 days.

OBJECTIVES

- Describe a subacute setting
- Demonstrate how to obtain a blood glucose sample by fingerstick
- Demonstrate how to provide diabetic foot care
- Describe your role in oxygen administration
- Demonstrate how to assist with diaphragmatic breathing, deep breathing and coughing, and an incentive spirometer
- List safety rules during oxygen therapy
- Demonstrate how to assist with administering oxygen by nasal cannula and by simple face mask
- Describe the three common types of artificial airways, and mechanical ventilation
- List the types of heat applications and explain guidelines to follow when applying heat
- List the types of cold applications and explain guidelines to follow when applying cold
- Describe dialysis and your role in caring for a person receiving peritoneal dialysis
- State the signs and symptoms to observe and report when a person is receiving hemodialysis
- State the reasons for enteral nutrition and describe your role in caring for a person receiving enteral feedings or total parenteral nutrition

MEDICAL TERMS

- **Artificial airway** – a tube placed into the trachea of a person's respiratory system, through the nose, mouth, or surgically through a stoma in the neck, to assist in breathing
- **Blood sugar** – measures the amount of one type of sugar (glucose) in the blood
- **Dialysis** – a method used to artificially remove waste from the blood when the kidneys are not functioning well
- **Diaphragmatic breathing** – deep breathing that uses muscles of the abdomen
- **Dry cold** – dry cold application
- **Dry heat** – dry warm application
- **Endotracheal tube** – a tube placed through the mouth or nose into the trachea for breathing
- **Enteral nutrition** – providing liquid nourishment through a tube passed into the nose and down to the stomach (a nasogastric tube, or NGT) or a tube surgically inserted through the abdominal wall into the stomach (a gastrostomy tube, or G-tube)
- **Fasting blood sugar (FBS)** – test of blood glucose level using a blood sample (from a prick in a finger or ear or through a needle from a vein) taken at least eight hours after last eating
- **Hemodialysis** – a process for removing waste and fluid directly from the person's blood through a tube that has been surgically implanted; the tube is connected to an artificial kidney machine that filters and returns the blood to the person
- **Hyperglycemia** – blood sugar level that is too high

- **Hypoglycemia** – blood sugar level that is too low
- **Hypoxia** – a state in which the blood oxygen level shows that the body is not getting enough oxygen
- **Incentive spirometer** – a device that measures and shows how deeply a person breathes; seeing the result helps to encourage deep breathing
- **Mechanical ventilator** – a machine used to assist or replace spontaneous breathing when a person cannot breathe on their own
- **Moist cold** – moist cold application
- **Moist heat** – moist warm application
- **Nasal cannula** – two-pronged tube inserted into the nostrils to deliver oxygen
- **Oropharyngeal tube** – a tube placed through the mouth into the pharynx for breathing

- **Oxygen** – an odorless, tasteless, and colorless gas
- **Peritoneal dialysis** – process used for removing waste and fluid from the blood through a surgically placed catheter in the abdominal (peritoneal) cavity
- **Sitz bath** – a bath in a tub or special basin in which only the perineum and buttocks are immersed
- **Total parenteral nutrition (TPN)** – nutrition administered intravenously
- **Tracheostomy or tracheotomy** – a stoma through the trachea into the respiratory airway
- **Tracheostomy tube** – a breathing tube placed directly into the trachea through a surgical opening (stoma) in the person's neck
- **Ureterostomy** – a stoma through the skin into the kidney ureter

"The staff at this facility are always so attentive to my needs. They have the newest equipment and they make my glucose testing painless and easy."

PROCEDURE 24-1
Blood Glucose Monitoring by Finger Prick

PROCEDURE 24-2
Diabetic Foot Care

PROCEDURE 24-3
Assisting With Diaphragmatic Breathing

PROCEDURE 24-4
Assisting With Deep Breathing and Coughing

PROCEDURE 24-5
Assisting With Incentive Spirometer

PROCEDURE 24-6
Administering Oxygen by Nasal Cannula

PROCEDURE 24-7
Administering Oxygen by Simple Face Mask

As explained in Chapter 23, patients in a subacute setting receive health care services after leaving the hospital before going home or to live in a long term care facility. Subacute settings give a higher level of care than residents receive who live permanently in a long term care facility, but a lower level of care than hospitals. The term "level of care" refers to the type, frequency, and complexity of care or services provided. The person usually needs this care only for a short period of time, usually less than 30 days.

As a nurse assistant you may be working on a subacute floor that cares for people with serious complications from diabetes, kidney disease, or gastroenteral problems. It is important for you to understand the impact of the disease on the person physically, psychologically, and socially.

Imagine what the person must be going through as they patiently wait for their kidney transplant or know they may lose a limb or cannot chew their food anymore. Just imagine what changes are taking place in this person's life.

CARE OF RESIDENTS WITH DIABETES IN A SUBACUTE SETTING

Chapter 11 describes the endocrine system and residents with diabetes. Remember, with diabetes, either the pancreas does not produce enough insulin or the body does not use the insulin well enough. Insulin controls how the body uses carbohydrates, which include sugar and starches. When insulin cannot do its job correctly, the person's blood sugar level may become either too low (hypoglycemia) or too high (hyperglycemia). Table 24-1 shows the American Diabetes Association (ADA) recommendations for blood sugar levels depending on the type of test and time it is performed. The most common way to test a person's blood sugar level is to do a finger prick test.

TABLE 24-1 RECOMMENDED BLOOD SUGAR LEVELS		
BLOOD SAMPLE SOURCE	**TIME OF TESTING**	**RECOMMENDED LEVEL**
Vein	Before meal	80-120 mg/dl
Vein	1-2 hours after meal	< 160mg/dl
Fingertip	Before meal	90-130 mg/dl
Fingertip	1-2 hours after meal	< 180mg/dl

A fasting blood sugar (FBS) blood sample is taken after a person has not eaten for at least eight hours. A blood glucose test may also be performed two hours after eating a meal or at a random time. You may assist in these ways:
- Make sure the person does not eat during the time prescribed before the test. Sips of water are allowed.
- Encourage the person not to smoke. Smoking may affect the test results.
- For a random blood glucose test, note the time and content of the last meal.
- Listen to and talk with the person about any concerns they have.

A person with diabetes is at risk for problems with their feet. Problems may include pressure ulcers due to already poor circulation, an inability to feel ulcer pain due to peripheral neuropathy (when the person's nerve endings are damaged), and susceptibility to infection. When giving foot care, be sure to inspect, wash, and dry them thoroughly. Apply moisturizing lotion, but not between the toes. Trim the nails only after soaking.

Blood sugar – measures the amount of one type of sugar (glucose) in the blood

Fasting blood sugar (FBS) – test of blood glucose level using a blood sample (from a prick in a finger or ear or through a needle from a vein) taken at least 8 hours after last eating

Hyperglycemia – blood sugar level that is too high

Hypoglycemia – blood sugar level that is too low

PROCEDURE 24-1.   BLOOD GLUCOSE MONITORING BY FINGER PRICK

Note: Many patients and health care settings now use other locations on the body or other methods to get blood samples for measuring blood glucose levels. However, the finger prick or finger stick method has proved the most reliable.

 REMEMBER: BE AWARE

Items Needed
- soap and water or alcohol swab
- gloves
- disposable bag
- sharps container
- glucometer
- test strips
- lancet
- gauze pad
- adhesive bandage (Band-aid)

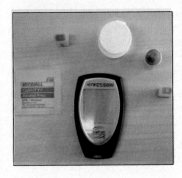

1. Have the person wash their hands in warm water and soap or use an alcohol wipe to cleanse the fingertip. Dry thoroughly.

2. Put on disposable gloves. Turn on the glucose meter. Some meters require that the glucose test strip be inserted at this time.

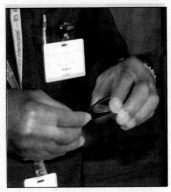

3. Squeeze/milk the end of the person's finger toward the fingertip. Quickly and confidently prick the person's finger using a lancing device. Continue to squeeze or "milk" the fingertip until you see a large drop of blood.

4. Place the blood on the strip test area. Follow the guidelines for the specific glucose meter.

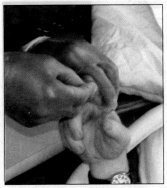

5. Read and record the results. With some meters, the blood must remain on the strip as the meter times and processes the result. With other meters, the blood must be wiped off the test strip; then the strip is inserted into the meter for the final result and reading.

6. Cover/clean the prick site with alcohol pad, gauze, or a tissue until the bleeding stops. If needed, then apply a Band-aid.

Note: *The better you are able to squeeze or "milk" the fingertip, the less deeply do you need to "prick" the skin. Remember: the person will have many finger pricks/sticks during their stay, and each one should be as painless, yet effective, as possible.*

 REMEMBER: UNDERSTAND

PROCEDURE 24-2.   DIABETIC FOOT CARE

> **REMEMBER: BE AWARE**

Items Needed
- basin of warm water
- nondrying soap
- towel

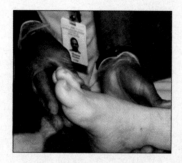

1. Inspect the feet daily. Report to the nurse any calluses, corns, blisters, abrasions, redness, and nail abnormalities.

2. Wash the feet daily in warm water, using nondrying soap.

3. Dry thoroughly between the toes to prevent skin breakdown.

4. Be sure the person wears well-fitting shoes and socks to prevent any pressure on the feet.

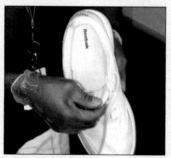

5. Inspect the inside of shoes for foreign objects or areas of roughness.

6. Report any injury to the nurse immediately.

> **REMEMBER: UNDERSTAND**

CARE OF RESIDENTS AND PATIENTS NEEDING OXYGEN THERAPY

Remember that the major function of the respiratory system is to deliver **oxygen** into the body (with inhalation) and remove carbon dioxide (CO_2) (on exhalation). Many residents and patients need oxygen therapy. This involves giving them higher concentrations of oxygen than exist in the air. Your role may include assisting with the setup and providing psychosocial support to the patient or resident who is receiving oxygen therapy.

Oxygen is an odorless, tasteless, and colorless gas. It exists in the air all around us but in a low concentration, about 21%. In higher concentrations, oxygen is used to treat or prevent symptoms of respiratory distress. These symptoms can be caused by:
- the inability to inhale enough oxygen into the body
- an inability of the lungs or circulatory system to use oxygen
- an inability of the lungs to exhale or remove enough carbon dioxide

If our lungs or circulatory system cannot provide enough oxygen to our body cells, this condition is called **hypoxia**. A person experiencing hypoxia may have any of these signs and symptoms:
- rapid breathing
- fatigue
- anxiety
- restlessness
- dizziness
- confusion
- cyanosis (an abnormal bluish tint of lips, nailbeds, tongue or other parts of the body)
- unconsciousness

Hypoxia – a state in which the blood oxygen level shows that the body is not getting enough oxygen

Oxygen – an odorless, tasteless, and colorless gas

Unless treated, continuing severe hypoxia will lead to death. A person may have a temporary or permanent condition that causes respiratory distress and/or hypoxia. Temporary conditions may include:

- broken rib(s)
- recent surgery to nose, mouth, neck, chest, back, or abdominal area
- pneumonia or another respiratory condition
- severe anemia
- unconscious state
- acute heart attack

Permanent conditions may include:
- chronic obstructive pulmonary disease (COPD)
- congestive heart failure in an acute state
- asthma in an acute attack

Administering Oxygen Therapy

Oxygen therapy in a facility usually is given from a piped-in system or oxygen concentrator. In emergency situations oxygen may also be given from a cylinder (tank). In home care or transport situations oxygen may also be supplied from liquid oxygen in a cylinder. Oxygen can be administered by many methods. These include a **nasal cannula**, face mask, or an **airway**. Oxygen delivery devices are described in Table 24-2 and illustrated in Fig. 24-1.

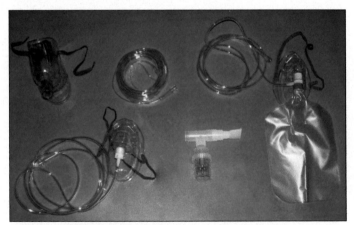

Fig. 24-1 - Oxygen delivery devices

📖

Airway – a tube placed into the trachea of a person's respiratory system, through the nose, mouth, or surgically through a stoma in the neck, to assist in breathing

Nasal cannula – two-pronged tube inserted into the nostrils to deliver oxygen

TABLE 24-2
OXYGEN DELIVERY DEVICES

DEVICE	DESCRIPTION
Nasal cannula	A two-pronged tube. The prongs are carefully inserted into the person's nostrils and secured in place by wrapping the tubing around the ears and adjusting the tubing under the chin. This method can be used only if the person is able to, and does, breathe through his/her nose. It cannot be used if the person is a "mouth breather." It delivers a low oxygen concentration. **Note:** observe the nostrils and ears often and carefully for signs of pressure. Remove and reapply or reposition the cannula and ear tubing every two hours.
Face mask	This mask covers the person's entire nose and mouth. Holes in the mask allow exhaled carbon dioxide to escape. It can deliver a higher oxygen concentration.
Venturi mask (or venti-mask)	This mask allows an exact amount of oxygen to be delivered, using color-coded adaptors
Partial rebreather mask	This face mask traps part of the exhaled carbon dioxide in a bag attached to the mask. It has valves that allow a mix of exhaled carbon dioxide and oxygen to be inhaled to stimulate normal breathing. **Note:** always be sure that the bag is inflated
Nonrebreather mask	This face mask allows only administered oxygen to be inhaled. Valves in the mask prevent room air from mixing with the oxygen. This mask also has a bag. **Note:** Always be sure that the mask fits securely to the person's face. Always be sure that the bag is inflated.

A patient who is on a mechanical ventilator may also receive oxygen directly. The method of oxygen administration depends on the physician's orders.

In addition to oxygen, positioning the person with head elevated or in a less painful position can also help them breathe more easily and get more oxygen. Other health care team members may perform other techniques to help drain lung secretions such as postural drainage with percussion (clapping on the lung/rib area). You may also assist the person with deep-breathing exercises using an incentive spirometer (Fig. 24-2).

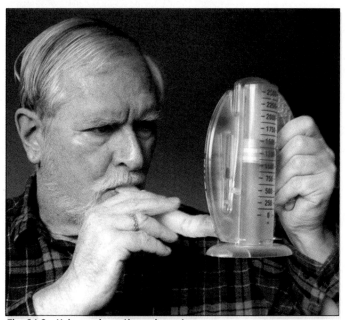

Fig. 24-2 - Using an incentive spirometer.

POSITIONING FOR EASIER BREATHING

Many people who are having difficulty breathing are more comfortable sitting in a semi-Fowler's or Fowler's position. In Chapter 15 you learned how to place residents in those positions. Some residents may also feel better sitting up with their head resting over the bed table. Place a pillow under the head for comfort. Encourage the person to change position frequently to help prevent secretions from pooling in any one area of the lungs. Pooled secretions can cause an infection.

Some residents may breathe easier if positioned on one side or another. The care plan should indicate the correct positioning for easier and more effective breathing (Fig. 24-3).

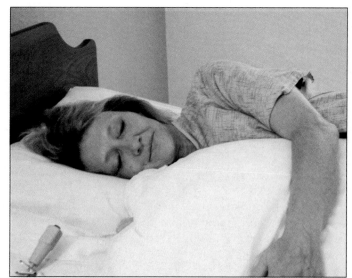

Fig. 24-3 - Correct position for easier and more effective breathing.

Postural Drainage

Postural drainage involves putting the person into a position so that gravity helps move bronchial secretions so that they may be coughed up or suctioned out. The correct position(s) to use are described in the person's care plan. Typically, each position is held 3 to 15 minutes. Always ask the nurse if you have any questions about a position (Fig. 24-4).

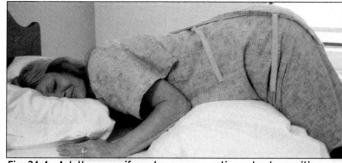

Fig. 24-4 - Ask the nurse if you have any questions about a position.

📖

Diaphragmatic breathing – deep breathing that uses muscles of the abdomen

Incentive spirometer – a device that measures and shows how deeply a person breathes; seeing the result helps to encourage deep breathing

Mechanical ventilator – a machine used to assist or replace spontaneous breathing when a person cannot breathe on their own

Deep Breathing Exercises

Diaphragmatic breathing is deep breathing that uses the muscles of the abdomen rather than the chest muscles (Fig. 24-5). Deep breathing exercises serve many purposes. The exercises:

- help the person relax
- reduce anxiety
- slow the breathing rate
- strengthen respiratory muscles
- help with oxygenation when exercising
- prevent infection in the lungs after surgery

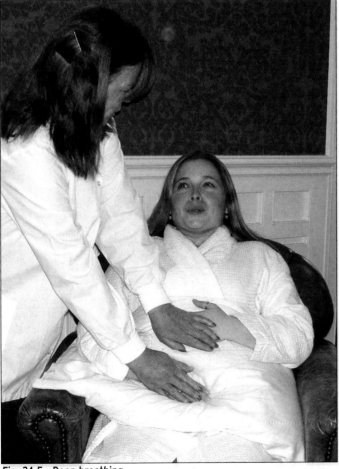

Fig. 24-5 - Deep breathing.

Your role in administering oxygen therapy is to gather the equipment needed, assist the nurse as requested, be sure the person is comfortable, and report any changes. With oxygen therapy you must follow the guidelines for fire and patient safety in Box 24-1.

BOX 24-1.
SAFETY DURING OXYGEN THERAPY

FIRE SAFETY
- Post a no-smoking sign on the person's door and in their room (Fig 24-6).

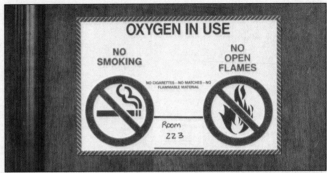

Fig. 24-6 - Oxygen in use—No smoking sign.

- Be sure no smoking materials or other flammable substances such as alcohol are present in the room. Read labels on all products to ensure none are flammable.
- Before unplugging any electrical device, be sure it is off. This prevents electrical sparks.
- Be sure all electrical items are approved and in good working order.

ADDITIONAL SAFETY GUIDELINES
- Be sure that the tubing is always connected to the oxygen supply source and that there are no kinks in the oxygen tubing.
- Check that the oxygen flow is on. If using oxygen humidification equipment, ensure that there are bubbles in the container.
- For nasal cannula use, be sure that the prongs are actually in the person's nostrils. Check for skin irritation under the person's nose and around the ears.
- For face masks, be sure that the face mask fits snugly against the patient's face. Check their face for irritation around the mask and the elastic band. Be sure the band is not too tight or loose. Reposition the band and mask periodically.
- Report any unusual signs immediately to the nurse. These signs or problems may include:
  - increased or decreased respiratory rate
  - change in mental status; if the person cannot communicate, these signs may include thrashing of arms or legs, pulling at bedclothes, or lack of consciousness
  - any equipment malfunction

PROCEDURE 24-3.   ASSISTING WITH DIAPHRAGMATIC BREATHING

Note: most persons do not normally breathe using the diaphragm or abdominal muscles. It may take several sessions for a person to successfully and consistently perform diaphragmatic breathing. A person with cognitive impairment may require slow and repetitive instruction, or may never be able to perform this type of breathing.

 REMEMBER: BE AWARE

Items Needed
- pillow for splinting (support for a painful site) if needed

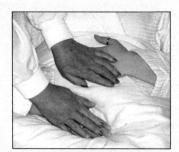

1. If able, have the person place one hand on the abdomen and the other hand on the middle of the chest. If the person is not able, ask the person if you can place your own hand on the abdomen to see and feel movement.

2. Have the person breathe in slowly and deeply through the nose, while pushing out the abdomen as far as they can. You should be able to see, and the person should be able to feel, the abdomen push out the hand.

3. Then have the person breathe out through pursed (partially closed or "puckered") lips while tightening their abdominal muscles. The person inhales in through the nose for a count of two and exhales through pursued lips for a count of four. You can help by counting this out for the person: 1, 2... 1, 2, 3, 4. You should be able to see, and the person should be able to feel, the abdomen move inward.

4. With this type of breathing, you should be able to see, and the person should be able to feel, no chest movement—only movement in the abdomen.

REMEMBER: UNDERSTAND

PROCEDURE 24-4.   ASSISTING WITH DEEP BREATHING AND COUGHING

REMEMBER: BE AWARE

Items Needed
- pillow or splint
- tissue
- emesis basin
- gloves

1. Explain that after surgery a person needs to take deep breaths and cough. This helps to remove anesthesia and prevent the accumulation of lung secretions. Coughing and deep breathing are also important for someone who has been on bed rest for a period of time.

2. When ready, ask them to take at least four diaphragmatic breaths as described in Procedure 24-3.

3. Put on gloves.

4. Elevate the head of the bed as much as the person can tolerate.

5. Tell the person how to hold a pillow or splint over the surgical site.

6. While holding the pillow, ask the person to take a deep breath, hold it for 3 seconds,

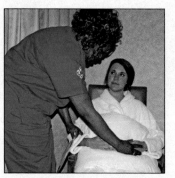

and then exhale. Repeat this at least five times if the person can tolerate it. With the last two deep breaths, encourage the person to take a deep breath and cough as hard as possible while you hold the emesis basin to catch any sputum secretions.

7. Clean up any secretions using tissues and the emesis basin. Note the color and consistency of any respiratory secretions. Report your findings to the heath care team.

8. Instruct the person to continue the deep breathing and coughing exercises once an hour.

REMEMBER: UNDERSTAND

PROCEDURE 24-5. ASSISTING WITH AN INCENTIVE SPIROMETER

Items Needed
- pillow for splinting if needed
- incentive spirometer

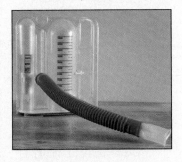

1. Clean mouthpiece using disposable alcohol wipe.

2. Place the patient in a comfortable sitting or semi-Fowler's position.

Note: If the person has had surgery, this procedure should be done approximately 30 minutes after the patient has had pain medication. You and the nurse should coordinate and communicate medication times with this procedure.

Also, have the person place the pillow on top of the incision to "splint" it if necessary.

3. Set the incentive spirometer as communicated to you by the nurse or noted in the orders or care plan. Instruct the person to exhale fully.

4. Then the person should
   a. Place mouthpiece into the mouth—hold lips tightly around the mouthpiece.

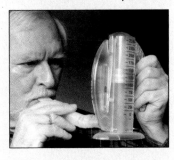

   b. Take in a slow, easy, deep breath through the mouthpiece, trying to reach the goal by watching the ball move up in the spirometer tube

   c. When the goal is reached, or if the ball will move upward no further, hold breath for three seconds
   d. Remove the mouthpiece, relax and exhale.

5. Encourage the person to cough.

6. Praise the person's results.

7. Notify the nurse if the person was not able to reach their spirometer goals.

PROCEDURE 24-6. ADMINISTERING OXYGEN BY NASAL CANNULA

Items Needed
- no-smoking signs
- humidification container
- distilled water
- nasal cannula tubing
- flow meter if not already present

1. Post no-smoking signs.

2. If ordered, fill the humidifier to the appropriate level.

3. Attach the connecting tube from the nasal cannula to the humidifier.

4. The nurse will set the flow rate at the prescribed liters per minute.

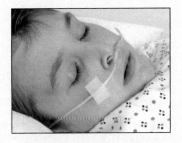

5. Assist the nurse to place the tips of the cannula in the person's nose and adjust the straps around ears for a snug, comfortable fit.

PROCEDURE 24-7.   ADMINISTERING OXYGEN BY SIMPLE FACE MASK

Items Needed
- no-smoking signs
- humidification container
- distilled water
- ordered face mask and tubing
- flow meter for the wall if not already available

1. Post no-smoking signs.

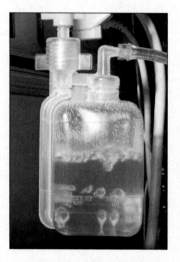

2. Make sure the humidifier is filled to the appropriate level.

3. The nurse will adjust the flow meter.

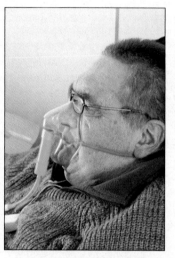

4. Assist the nurse to apply the mask on the person's face and adjust the straps so the mask fits securely.

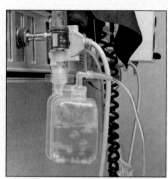

5. If the tubing fills with water, drain the tubing by emptying the water. Do not drain it back into the humidifier.

6. If a heating element is used, check the temperature. The humidifier bottle should be warm, not hot, to the touch.

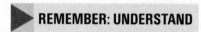

Artificial Airway and Mechanical Ventilation

You may at some time care for a patient with an artificial airway or someone who requires assistance in breathing and is on a mechanical ventilator. An artificial airway is a tube that enters the person's respiratory system. Some patients may have an artificial airway but not require a mechanical ventilator or oxygen therapy. In other situations, the artificial airway allows the mechanical ventilator to deliver needed oxygen directly to the person's respiratory system. A person may need mechanical ventilation assistance because of a temporary or permanent condition such as:
- acute respiratory failure
- central nervous system depression with lack of consciousness, or an inability for the body to trigger normal respiration
- neuromuscular disease
- pulmonary disease

- upper airway obstruction caused by a tumor, inflammation, or foreign body
- trauma to the respiratory system

The most common types of artificial airways are:

Oropharyngeal tube – A tube placed through the mouth into the pharynx

Endotracheal tube – A tube placed through the mouth or nose into the trachea

Tracheostomy tube – A tube placed directly into the trachea through a surgical opening (**stoma**) in the person's neck—**tracheostomy** or **tracheotomy**

Stoma – a surgically created opening, hole, or connection from outside the body into a body part; the name of each kind of stoma depends on the body part

Tracheostomy or **Tracheotomy** – a stoma through the trachea into the respiratory airway

You will not be responsible for the direct care of an artificial airway, but you must report to the nurse any abnormal or unusual situations, such as:

- The tube falls out, is pulled out, or is disconnected, or an alarm sounds.
- You hear gurgling sounds, indicating the need for suctioning.
- Any redness or discharge is present around the tube.
- The person seems restless or acts or moves differently. For example, you may see thrashing of limbs, attempts to pull out the tube, rapid eye movements, chest movements not associated with the normal mechanical ventilation pattern, or other actions. The person may attempt to communicate the problem to you (verbally or in writing).

The presence of a tracheostomy or the need for mechanical ventilator assistance does not always mean that the person cannot understand others or does not have a need to communicate. Many persons who need mechanical ventilator assistance are alert and oriented. They want to know and communicate about "normal" things. They may be frightened, in pain, or unclear about what you are doing. They also may want to know the score of a recent baseball game. Always do your job as if the person understands everything, helping the person communicate with you. Offer pen and paper, a communication board with pictures, flashcards with common needs on them, a chalk or dry eraser board—anything to help the person communicate their needs, problems, or concerns.

Although a person with an artificial airway cannot talk normally, many people with tracheostomies have learned how to "plug" the tracheostomy and speak. Others learn to use ancillary muscles to speak with an amplifying device.

HOT AND COLD APPLICATIONS

Hot and cold applications are used for treating specific conditions when ordered by the person's physician. Heat or cold may be applied to the entire body for a general effect. Usually the application is ordered for a specific body area. Heat and cold may be applied either dry or moist, depending on the situation and the physician's orders.

Hot Applications

Heat speeds up tissue healing. The application of heat causes the blood vessels to dilate (get larger), which increases the blood flow to the area to promote healing.

Heat also eases pain for some residents who have specific areas of pain. For example, if someone hurts their ankle, hot applications after the initial 24 hours help reduce swelling and promote healing by increasing blood flow to the area. When blood vessels are dilated, the increased blood flow often absorbs and carries fluids away from the area of the swelling. This is why warm-water exercise is so beneficial for some residents with arthritis. Heat also helps to reduce painful muscle spasms because it helps muscles relax.

Types of heat applications include (Fig. 24-7):

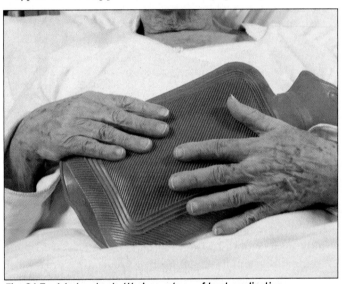

Fig. 24-7 - A hot water bottle is one type of heat application.

- **Moist heat.** Warm moisture is in direct contact with the person's skin. Moist heat works faster than dry heat.
  - Sitz baths provide moist heat to the genitals or anal area.
  - Tub baths provide moist heat to the whole body.
  - Hot, moist compresses using a cloth or disposable pack provide moist heat to a specific area.
  - Soaks provide moist heat to a specific area.
- **Dry heat:**
  - Rubber hot-water bottles provide dry heat to a specific area.
  - Electric pads (heat pads) provide heat to a specific area.

Dry heat – dry warm application
Moist heat – moist warm application
Sitz bath – a bath in a tub or special basin in which only the perineum and buttocks are immersed

Consider the following questions before applying heat to a person. Always follow the care plan for the use of heat.
- What method should be used? What equipment do you need?
- Where exactly should heat be applied to the person? Is it a specific or generalized area?
- How long should the heat be applied?
- What safety rules should be followed?

Before using a heat application, follow these guidelines:
- Know how to use the heat equipment. Check with the nurse about the correct temperature and the type of heat to use.
- Ask the nurse to show you exactly where the heat should be applied.
- Apply heat for 20 minutes or less, as directed by the nurse or the care plan.
- Expose only the part of the body where you are applying heat.
- When using a soak, be sure the person is positioned correctly to prevent spilling the solution.
- Always double-check the temperature of the heating device to make sure it is not too hot. Check with the nurse if you are unsure. Ask the person if it feels too hot. Check the person every 5 to 10 minutes. Look for any area that seems red, discolored, or blistered. This may indicate that the person is being burned. If so, stop the treatment immediately and call the nurse. It is critical to carefully evaluate residents with paralysis or limited feeling in the area being treated with heat. Residents who cannot feel if the heat becomes too hot are at a higher risk for burns. Also closely check residents who cannot express themselves.

Note: *Never place an electric heating device over a wet dressing or compress. This could cause a burn because the moist heat may become too hot and intense. Using an electric device around moisture also increases the risk of a shock.*

Heat application should remain at the correct temperature the whole time. If the application becomes too cool, it cannot have the desired effect. After applying a hot compress, cover it with plastic to help prevent heat loss. Cover the plastic with a towel or other dry material. You may use a hot water bottle along with the compress to preserve the heat, but first check with the nurse and be sure that it is not too hot.

Cold Applications

Like hot applications, cold applications can be used on a specific area or generalized. Cold applications are used for a several reasons, including:
- To reduce painful swelling in an area. Cold causes the blood vessels to constrict (become smaller), which decreases the blood flow to the area. This helps if used within the first 48 hours after a bruise or sprain.
- To help control bleeding. Bleeding is reduced or stopped because the cold constricts the blood vessels. Cold applications are used immediately after some surgeries.
- To lessen pain sensitivity. Cold does this by numbing the area.
- To help reduce a high body temperature.

An example of a cold application is Fig. 24-8:

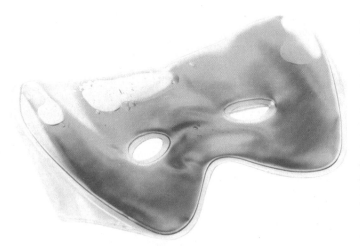

Fig. 24-8 - One type of cold application is a cold compress.

- Moist cold:
  - cold compresses
  - disposable packs:
    cooling solutions
    alcohol sponge baths
- Dry cold:
  - ice cubes in bags or collars (special rubber collars that can be filled with ice)
  - ice packs

Dry cold – dry cold application
Moist cold – moist cold application

Consider these questions before applying cold:
- What method should be used? What equipment do you need?
- Where exactly should the cold be applied to the person? Is it a specific or generalized area?
- How long should the cold be applied?
- What safety rules should be followed?

Before using a cold application, follow these guidelines:
- Know how to use the cold equipment. Check with the nurse about the type of cold application to use.
- Ask the nurse to show you exactly where the cold should be applied.
- Apply the cold for 20 minutes, or as directed by the charge nurse or care plan.
- Use ice cubes, not crushed ice. Crushed ice melts quickly and changes the temperature of the solution. Place the ice in a container made for ice, such as an ice bag.
- Take the person's temperature before and after the application of cold, and report it to the nurse. If the cold is being applied for a fever, their body may not have cooled down enough after the allotted time. If so, the treatment may need to be repeated.

Note: *If a person begins to shiver during the application, remove the cold pack and notify the nurse immediately. The nurse will give you further instructions.*

When a generalized cold application is used, there is a risk of shock developing. Shock is caused by a large drop in blood flow in the body. One sign of shock is a change in a person's vital signs. Before applying cold, take the person's vital signs for later comparisons. Observe the person frequently for:
- gasping or labored breathing, often at a faster than normal rate
- fast, possibly irregular pulse
- bluish or darker color (cyanosis) in such areas as the lips, fingernails, and eyelids

If you observe any of these signs, stop the cold application treatment immediately. Inform the nurse. Shock is a life-threatening condition that needs immediate treatment.

CARING FOR THE PERSON RECEIVING DIALYSIS

Look back at Chapter 11 and think again about the anatomy and physiology of the kidneys. If a person develops chronic kidney disease or acute renal failure, their kidneys are not working properly or at all. One of the many problems that occurs is the kidneys cannot filter and remove extra fluid and waste from the body. This person then needs dialysis. Dialysis is a method used to artificially remove waste from the blood in someone with kidney failure. Dialysis is a form of artificial filtration of the blood. The purpose of dialysis is to maintain the person's life. Without dialysis the person could become seriously ill and die due to the build-up of waste in the blood. Dialysis is a temporary solution while the person waits either for kidney function to return or for a transplant. The two methods are called peritoneal dialysis and hemodialysis. The physician decide which method is best for the person.

Peritoneal Dialysis

Peritoneal dialysis is a process for removing waste and fluid from the body. A fluid called dialysate (about 2 liters) is instilled into a catheter that was surgically placed through the wall of the abdomen into the abdominal cavity (peritoneal cavity). This dialysate stays in the peritoneal cavity for a few hours. As blood flows through vessels in the cavity, the extra fluid and waste is filtered into the dialysate fluid. After a few hours the fluid is drained out. Peritoneal dialysis is less expensive than hemodialysis.
There are three types of peritoneal dialysis:
- continuous ambulatory peritoneal dialysis (CAPD)
- continuous cycling peritoneal dialysis (CCPD)
- intermittent peritoneal dialysis (IPD)

📖

Dialysis – a method used to artificially remove waste from the blood when the kidneys are not functioning well

Hemodialysis – a process for removing waste and fluid directly from the person's blood through a tube that has been surgically implanted; the tube is connected to an artificial kidney machine that filters and returns the blood to the person

Peritoneal dialysis – process used for removing waste and fluid from the blood through a surgically placed catheter in the abdominal (peritoneal) cavity

Continuous ambulatory peritoneal dialysis is the most common type. The dialysate is instilled into the peritoneal cavity for four to six hours and then drained. The procedure is repeated four or five times daily. The person can learn to do the procedure at home, allowing more independence and freedom.

Continuous cycling peritoneal dialysis takes about 10-12 hours and is usually done at night when the person sleeps. A machine automatically fills and drains the dialysate from the catheter in the peritoneal cavity.

Intermittent peritoneal dialysis is rarely used today. The process is much like CAPD but is done intermittently.

Nurse Assistant Role in Caring for a Person Receiving Peritoneal Dialysis

The most common problems or complications that occur with peritoneal dialysis are infection around the catheter site or inside the peritoneal cavity. This is called peritonitis. It is important for you to watch for signs of infection and report them immediately to the team. You will be responsible for monitoring the person for any changes along with the rest of the health care team. Your responsibilities will include measuring the person's weight before and after the dialysis and taking and recording vital signs as ordered by the physician. Vital signs are often taken every 15 minutes for the first two hours and then once every two hours. You must notify the team immediately if there are any changes. Some of the other important signs and symptoms to observe and report are:

• redness, bleeding, or drainage (pus) around the catheter site
• leaking fluid around the catheter site
• catheter tubing that is twisted, kinked, or disconnected
• catheter site pain or complaints of abdominal pain
• blood in the drainage fluid
• fluid not draining properly
• complaints of feeling dizzy or lightheaded
• abnormal abdominal distention
• shortness of breath and/or chest pain
• the person is withdrawn, won't talk, or seems depressed

Hemodialysis

Hemodialysis is another method used to filter waste products and extra fluid from the body. During hemodialysis the person is connected to a filter machine (sometimes referred to as an artificial kidney machine) by tubes attached to the person's blood vessels. The blood is pumped from the body into the machine. There it is fil-

tered using the solution dialysate. Once the blood is clean and all the waste products removed, the blood is pumped back into the person's body. The physician determines what type of access site is created for removing and replacing the blood once it is clean. Figure 24-9 shows a person receiving hemodialysis.

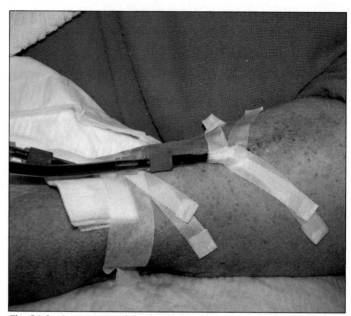

Fig. 24-9 - A person receiving hemodialysis.

Three access methods are used for hemodialysis:
• A venous catheter is a tube placed in the neck, chest, or groin. This type of catheter is usually used until a permanent access is placed.
• A fistula is the most common and most durable access site. The fistula is created by making a surgical connection of an artery to a vein in the lower forearm. It can take 6 to 12 weeks for the fistula to form.
• A graft is a tube implanted under the skin of the arm. The tube becomes an artificial vein that can be accessed within a week for hemodialysis.

Nurse Assistant Role in Caring for a Person Receiving Hemodialysis

You may care for a person in a subacute setting who is receiving hemodialysis. Your role may be to assist the person to and from the dialysis center and care for them between sessions. The sessions are often scheduled three or four times a week. Each session may take three to five hours. You are not expected to perform the dialysis or care for the access site, but you do need to know how to care for the person on hemodialysis. The most common problems with hemodialysis are:
- low blood pressure
- muscle cramps
- nausea, vomiting
- infection at the surgical site
- blood clots

A person on hemodialysis will be restricted for fluids and foods. Restrictions involve proteins, sodium, potassium, calcium, and phosphorus. The physician will determine how much fluid can be taken in a 24-hour period. You will take vital signs and weight measurements before and after treatments and monitor for changes. Blood pressure must never be taken in the person's arm used for dialysis. You must also monitor, measure, and record the person's fluid and food intake and output. Some of the other important signs and symptoms to observe and report are:
- redness, bleeding, or drainage (pus) around the surgical site
- complaints of pain at the fistula or graft site
- fluid intake and output changes
- food intake changes
- complaints of feeling dizzy, lightheaded, or unsteady when walking
- swelling in the feet, legs, or other areas of the body
- complaints of nausea, vomiting, muscle cramps
- shortness of breath or chest pain
- the person is withdrawn, won't talk, or seems depressed

ALTERNATIVE NUTRITION

If a person cannot or should not eat food, there are other ways to supply the body with essential nutrients needed to maintain health or to heal. A person may be unable to eat normally due to:
- swallowing difficulties
- choking problems
- persistent vomiting

- confusion
- anorexia (eating disorder)
- bowel infection or disease
- a state of semi-consciousness or unconsciousness
- recent surgery of the mouth, throat, or digestive tract

The physician will decide the best way to provide nourishment to the person. The most common alternative routes are enteral feedings or intravenous total parenteral nutrition (TPN).

Enteral Nutrition

Enteral nutrition or feeding is liquid nourishment passed through a tube through the nose to the stomach. This is called a nasogastric tube (NGT) (Fig. 24-10). Or the tube may be inserted surgically through the abdomen into the stomach. This is called a gastrostomy tube (G-tube). People receiving enteral feedings may or may not be restricted from eating food and drinking liquid (NPO).

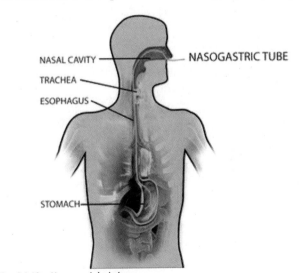

NASAL CAVITY — NASOGASTRIC TUBE
TRACHEA
ESOPHAGUS
STOMACH

Fig. 24-10 - Nasogastric tube.

Enteral nutrition – providing liquid nourishment through a tube passed into the nose and down to the stomach (a nasogastric tube, or NGT) or a tube surgically inserted through the abdominal wall into the stomach (a gastrostomy tube, or G-tube)

Total parenteral nutrition (TPN) – nutrition administered intravenously

It is important for you to know why the person has the enteral tube for feedings. You must follow the physician's orders. The NGT or G-tube must be checked by x-ray to make sure it is in the correct place. After placement is confirmed, the physician will order the type of nutrition that meets the person's needs.

To begin a feeding, the nurse will elevate the head of the bed. The head of the bed must be elevated at all times during and for at least an hour after the feeding. The nurse will check the x-ray. Even if the x-ray indicates proper placement into the stomach, the nurse will check its placement before each feeding. The bell of the stethoscope is placed over the stomach area, and the nurse will listen for air being injected into the stomach from a syringe injected through the tubing. The nurse also gently pulls back on the plunger of the syringe until a small amount of stomach contents comes into the syringe. If air is heard entering the stomach and stomach contents are obtained, the nurse will know that the tube is in the correct place.

The nutrition bottle is connected to a pump that is hooked to the NGT or G-tube. The pump helps control the amount of nutrition the physician ordered over the correct period of time.

Nurse Assistant Role in Caring for a Person Receiving Enteral Feedings

Your role is to monitor the person during the feeding process. You must always be sure the head of the bed is elevated during and after feedings to prevent aspiration of liquid nutrition into the person's lungs (Fig. 24-11).

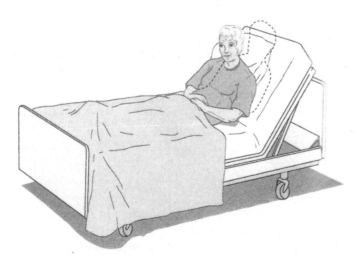

Fig. 24-11 - Elevate the head of the bed during and after feedings.

You can position the person carefully from side to side slightly, while the head of the bed is elevated, to prevent skin breakdown. Other key factors involved in caring for a person receiving enteral feedings include:

- Monitor the skin at the insertion site of the G-tube for signs of infection, such as redness, swelling, and drainage (pus). Keep the skin clean and dry.
- Monitor and report any respiratory problems such as shortness of breath, choking, gurgling sounds, or skin color changes, especially a blue tint around the lips and mouth (cyanosis).
- Prevent the tubing from becoming dislodged. Always check the tubing to make sure it is not kinked or twisted. Tubing should be taped and secured. The pump alarm will go off if there are any problems with the tubing or the infusion. Call the nurse immediately if the alarm sounds.
- Provide comfort measures such as back rubs to increase circulation and prevent skin breakdown. Always provide good mouth care for a person who is NPO, especially if an NGT is in place. Often a person with an NGT will mouth-breathe, which causes the mouth to become dry and the lips to crack. Inspect the nose area for any sores or signs of infection.
- Monitor the person's intake and output. Note any loose watery stools. Always report and record the amount, color, and consistency of bowel movements. The physician may change the strength or rate of the feeding if diarrhea persists. Be sure to assist with cleaning the area after voiding or bowel movements.
- Monitor the person's weight everyday for any gain or loss. Weights should be taken each day at the same time, preferably wearing the same amount of clothing, to obtain the most accurate reading.
- Maintain infection control with proper handwashing and wearing gloves when appropriate.
- Take vital signs as ordered, and record and report changes.
- Listen to the person's concerns. The person may feel depressed or anxious about their health. It is important to listen and be supportive.

Total Parenteral Nutrition

Total parenteral nutrition (TPN), sometimes called hyperalimentation, is providing nutrients through a vein. The goal is to provide all needed nutrients for the body to function. TPN is used when a person cannot tolerate enteral nutrition or digestion must stop to allow the bowel to rest and heal. The nutrients in TPN include carbohydrates for energy, protein for muscle strength, lipids for essential fats, necessary electrolytes, and trace minerals for the body to function. It is administered intravenous through a large central vein. The IV line is connected to a pump machine programmed to administer the amount ordered by the physician for the specified time (Fig. 24-12).

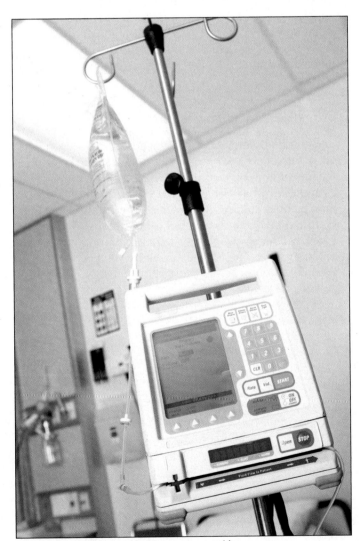

Fig. 24-12 - IV line connected to a pump machine.

Your Role in Caring for a Person With Total Parenteral Nutrition

A person receiving TPN must be weighed everyday at the same time wearing the same amount of clothing to obtain an accurate weight. Ensure that the tubing does not get dislodged. A Kelly clamp must be placed in a visible location at all times in case the tubing is dislodged. If the tubing is dislodged, it is extremely important to clamp the tubing close to the person's body so no air can enter the tubing. If air gets into the line, it could be fatal for the person. Other key factors involved with caring for a person on TPN nutrition include:

- Monitor the skin at the IV insertion site for signs of infection such as redness, swelling, and drainage (pus). Watch for swelling or redness near the collarbone area. The nurse will use sterile technique to change the dressings. It is important to keep the skin clean and dry around the infusion site.
- Always check the tubing to make sure it is not kinked or twisted. Tubing should be taped and secured. The pump alarm will go off if there are any problems with the tubing or the infusion. Call the nurse immediately if the alarm sounds.
- Provide comfort measures such as back rubs to increase circulation and prevent skin breakdown. Always provide good mouth care for a person who is NPO.
- Monitor the person's intake and output. Note any issues with loose watery stools. Always report and record the amount, color, and consistency of bowel movements. Assist with cleaning the area after voiding or bowel movements.
- Maintain infection control with proper handwashing and wearing gloves when appropriate.
- Observe for pain in the neck or chest area, recording and reporting any changes immediately.
- Take vital signs as ordered, recording and reporting changes.
- Listen to the person's concerns. The person may feel depressed or anxious about their health. It is important to listen and be supportive.

IN THIS CHAPTER YOU LEARNED:

- About nurse assistant roles in subacute care environments
- The importance of reporting information about the resident, even if you think it may be minor
- The importance of always checking equipment for accuracy and not using equipment that may be faulty
- Never to do a procedure you are not comfortable with
- How to monitor a person's blood glucose level
- How to provide diabetic foot care
- How to assist with diaphragmatic breathing
- How to assist with deep breathing and coughing
- How to assist with incentive spirometer
- How to administer oxygen by nasal cannula
- How to administer oxygen by simple face mask

SUMMARY

This chapter outlines some of the specialty skills nurse assistants use in subacute environments. If you decide to work in such a setting, you will need to learn these advanced skills. Some facilities offer inservice education classes in these skills. Other facilities have a formal, advanced training course. In some states special certification is needed to work in subacute care. When working in a subacute environment, always ask questions if you are unsure how to care for a person who requires care that you have never learned.

PULLING IT ALL TOGETHER

Imagine what could happen if you did not communicate and work closely with the health care team. What if you did not provide valuable information for proper decisions about care to be given? As you study these skills, think of what could happen if you did not actually check a person's blood glucose level or did not report a blood glucose level that was too low or high. The person could become unconscious. Amputation can become necessary for a diabetic with cuts or pressure ulcers on their feet that are not treated. The person may not realize that there is a problem because they have no feeling in their feet. Not reporting a change in the mental status of someone with kidney failure could lead to devastating results. If adequate nutrition was not provided to a frail woman, they could develop pressure ulcers and potentially die. Reporting any change is critical because even the slightest change can have serious medical consequences.

Not being careful with the application of heat or cold can cause a burn, tissue damage, or even shock. Any change in the person, any problem with faulty oxygen equipment, or the loss of an intact airway can make the difference between life and death in someone needing oxygen support. These are just a few examples of what can happen if you do not observe the person and the situation or do not communicate information to others on the health care team.

Remember always that you are very important part of the team. As you learn more skills, you become even more important in the quality of care for all the persons we care for.

1. **When a person needs a fasting blood sugar, how many hours must the person fast?**
   A. At least eight hours.
   B. At least two hours.
   C. At least six hours.
   D. At least 12 hours.

2. **What is a diabetic person at risk for developing?**
   A. Facial nerve tics.
   B. Poor circulation, peripheral neuropathy.
   C. Low blood pressure.
   D. Hearing issues.

3. **What is a major function of the respiratory system?**
   A. To improve a person's life.
   B. To artificially deliver oxygen.
   C. To deliver oxygen into the body and remove carbon dioxide.
   D. To deliver carbon dioxide into the body and remove oxygen.

4. **What term describes if the lungs or circulatory system are not able to provide enough oxygen to body cells?**
   A. Fatigue.
   B. Hyperglycemic.
   C. Dizziness.
   D. Hypoxia.

5. **What position is best to help a person who is having difficulty breathing?**
   A. Head of bed flat.
   B. Head of bed elevated.
   C. Head of bed flat with foot of bed slightly elevated.
   D. Head of bed lowered with foot of bed elevated.

6. **What is diaphragmatic breathing?**
   A. Deep breathing that uses the muscles of the abdomen.
   B. Deep breathing that uses the muscles of the chest.
   C. An increase in inhalation and exhalation.
   D. A decrease in inhalation and exhalation.

7. **Which is a safety guideline to follow when a person is receiving oxygen?**
   A. Post a sign indicating smoking is allowed in a small corner of the person's room.
   B. Be sure the oxygen tubing is kept damp.
   C. Report any unusual signs to the change nurse.
   D. Remove the oxygen if the person states they have had enough.

8. **What is a common type of artificial airway?**
   A. An NGT.
   B. A G–tube.
   C. An oropharyngeal tube.
   D. A colostomy.

9. **What is your role in caring for a person receiving hemodialysis?**
   A. To assist in surgically implanting the catheter.
   B. To assist by hooking the catheter to the dialysis machine.
   C. To observe and report any signs such as redness, bleeding, or drainage around the surgical site.
   D. To schedule the next hemodialysis treatment.

10. **What is your role in caring for a person receiving enteral nutrition?**
    A. To insert the NGT tube.
    B. To evaluate the position of the person in bed during a feeding.
    C. To check for placement of the tube.
    D. To apply moist heat to the intravenous site during total parenteral nutrition.

(Answers to "Check What You've Learned" are in the Instructor's Manual.)

Chapter 25

CARE OF THE PERSON HAVING SURGERY

Nurse assistants work in many different areas within the health care system. You can use the skills you are learning now in those different areas. Your role as a nurse assistant can be an interesting and rewarding experience as well as a career. If you choose to work in long term care, you can gain valuable skills and experience in different areas. For example, you might work on a subacute floor, an Alzheimer's unit, or a rehabilitation floor. Your experience may also lead to working in exciting areas in acute care, such as with surgical patients (Fig. 25-1, next page). In this chapter you will learn new knowledge and skills for working with the surgical team. The next chapter then includes additional health care areas such as the care of the mother and newborn, children, adolescents, or young adults.

OBJECTIVES

- Explain how you can help reduce a person's fear and anxiety about having surgery
- State what information is given to the person during preoperative teaching
- Explain your role in preoperative phase of surgery
- Describe how you can support family members during surgery
- Name at least five items on the preoperative checklist
- Explain your role in postoperative care

MEDICAL TERMS

- **Anesthesia** – state of being unaware or unable to feel; anesthesia can be general (whole body) or local (a specific body part or region)
- **Anesthetic** – the medication given to a person before surgery to induce anesthesia; administered in different ways depending on whether general or local
- **Anti-embolism stockings** – elastic stockings often worn after surgery to help prevent blood clots
- **Incentive spirometer** – device that measures how deeply a person inhales, to encourage deep breathing
- **Postoperative** – time after surgery
- **Preoperative** – time before surgery
- **Prosthesis** – a device that substitutes and functions in the place of a missing body part, such as dentures

PROCEDURE 25-1
Shaving the Surgical Site

PROCEDURE 25-2
Assisting with Deep Breathing and Coughing

"I believe it was the wonderful care I received after my surgery that helped me recover so quickly."

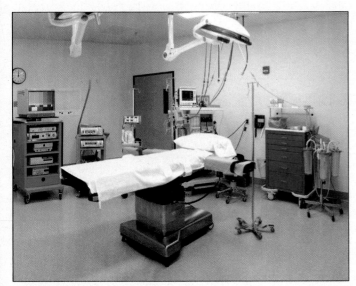
Fig. 25-1 - Operating room suite.

R Remember how you learned in Chapter 11 that the body systems work together to support life. You also learned that for the body as a whole to be healthy, each part of each body system must work by itself. Each system must also work with other systems. With illness or injury, however, a system or body part is not working fully. Sometimes surgery is needed to repair, remove, or replace the injured or ill body part.

COMMON FEARS ABOUT SURGERY

Have you ever had surgery? What do you remember? Did you feel afraid or anxious? Did you feel excited and eager? How long did it take to feel like yourself again after the operation? Having surgery is usually a very difficult time for everyone. Some people are afraid and feel a lot of anxiety before surgery. People deal with their fear and anxiety in different ways. Some people become quiet and withdrawn. Others want to talk about it. Some people may talk about why they need surgery and may ask you whether you think it is a good idea. Some people even like to talk about unpleasant events they have heard about—like a neighbor's story about a wrong kidney being removed.

Common fears before surgery include questions like these:
• Do I have cancer?
• Will I have a lot of pain?
• Who will take care of me, my house, my family?

• What if I don't wake up from anesthesia?
• What complications might I have?
• Will I look different?

Help the Person Understand and Reduce Fear and Anxiety

Your role is to listen to the person (Fig. 25-2). Never give your own opinion. Be respectful and kind during this difficult time. Report any signs of fear or anxiety to the health care team so that everyone is aware of the person's feelings. An appropriate team member can help the person talk about and understand their fears and anxiety. For the surgery to be successful, the person needs to feel prepared.

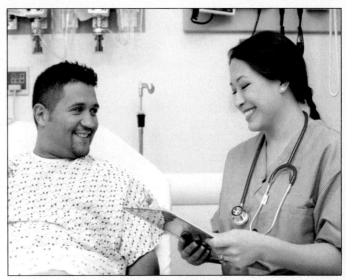
Fig. 25-2 - Listen to the person.

If the person asks you about the actual procedure, refer these questions to the nurse or surgeon. The surgeon who will perform the surgery will always explain things to the person, such as:
• why the surgery is needed
• the risks of surgery
• any complications that may occur
• how long the surgery will take
• what happens during the recovery process

There is a lot of new and sometimes complicated information the person must hear, understand, and remember. Whenever possible, other people, such as a family member or nurse, should join the surgeon and surgical patient in this discussion. The family member or nurse can help the patient ask the surgeon questions. If the patient does not speak English, either the family member or another person must interpret to ensure communication is good between the surgeon and the patient.

Each person may have different feelings about surgery. Some may be excited or feel relieved. For others, this can be a very fearful and trying time. The person may not be able to carefully listen or understand all the information. Fear and anxiety can also make it difficult to remember things that are said. Sometimes the person might ask you about something the surgeon just explained, if they were not able to listen closely or did not understand. Remember that your role is to report this so that the right member of the health care team can answer all the person's questions.

BEFORE THE SURGERY

The time before the surgery is called the **preoperative** phase. Members of the health care team often call this pre-op. This phase may last a short or long time. With surgery that is not urgently needed, the person may have days, weeks, or even months to wait. In an emergency the pre-operative time may be very short. If time allows, the person having surgery should be taught everything about the surgery to be prepared.

It is important to know what the person is like before surgery. If time allows, the health care team must pay particular attention to the person's mental status. If there is no time to get to know the patient, as in an emergency surgery, staff should try to talk to family, friends, or others about the patient. Knowing the person's baseline mental status before surgery is important. The trauma of surgery, medications, and **anesthesia** can have side effects that may alter a person's mental status. Knowing the patient's baseline status helps the health care team understand if abnormal changes happen after surgery.

Preoperative Teaching

In the preoperative phase, your role is to reinforce the pre-op teaching. Preoperative teaching involves information about what will happen before, during, and after the surgery. The nurse and surgeon do this teaching.

The nurse will explain the purpose of pre-op blood tests and other tests such as an EKG. Usually the patient cannot have anything to eat or drink after midnight before surgery. This is called NPO (nothing per oral, or nothing by mouth) (Fig. 25-3). This helps ensure the person does not vomit during or after the operation. This is especially important if the person has general anesthesia.

NPO
after midnight

Fig. 25-3 - Sign placed over patient's bed.

In addition, the nurse will explain the different areas the person will experience, including the different areas of the hospital involved. The patient will be moved first to the pre-op room for final preparation (Fig. 25-4, next page). The surgery will then be performed in the operating room, sometimes called the O.R. or surgical suite. Afterwards, the patient is moved to the recovery room until they wake from the anesthesia and are stable. The person is taught what to expect in each room and which staff they will meet there. For example, in the pre-op room the person may have more blood tests, and vital signs will be taken. The person will have an intravenous tube and surgical cap in place and the person will be started on intravenous fluid.

The surgeon and nurse will explain the actual surgery itself and any other tests that must be performed. They will explain if any other tubes or catheters will be inserted. The patient meets the anesthesiologist and learns about the anesthesia before surgery. The anesthesiologist will explain information like this:
- how they will be put to sleep
- what they will feel like when they wake up
- what medications they will get before, during, and after the surgery
- what type of anesthesia they will be given and its effect

Anesthesia − state of being unaware or unable to feel; anesthesia can be general (whole body) or local (a specific body part or region)
Preoperative − time before surgery

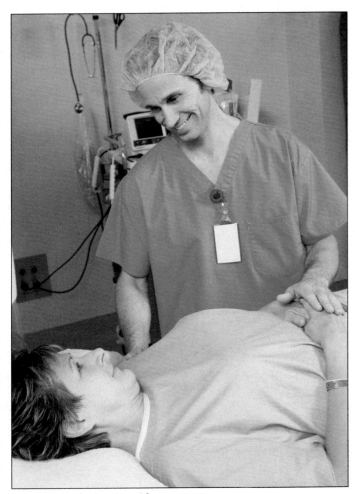

Fig. 25-4 - Patient prepared for surgery.

• why deep breathing and coughing are important to prevent postoperative complications in the lungs
• when and why changing positions is important to prevent pneumonia, skin breakdown, and blood clots
• when and why moving out of bed and walking are important to increase the blood flow to all body parts and prevent complications
• the care for the surgical wound
• when the wound staples, stitches, or Steri-Strips™ will be removed (Fig. 25-5)

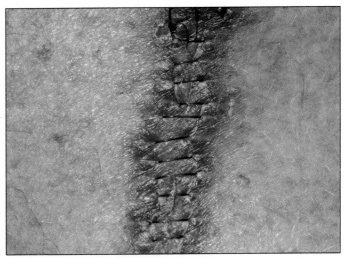

Fig. 25-5 - Wound with stitches.

• what to watch for as the would heals
• how often dressings will be changed
• why it is important to eat nutritional food to repair and build new tissue after the operation
• any special restrictions, instructions, or information because of the specific surgery

Your Role in the Preoperative Phase

Your role in the preoperative phase includes listening to any concerns the person has. Direct any questions about the surgery to the nurse. Reinforce the nurse's pre-op and post-op teaching. The person has a lot to remember and often looks to you for added support.

A local **anesthetic** is a medication usually given with a needle. It causes a loss of feeling in a specific area of the body. General anesthesia, on the other hand, puts the person into a temporary state of unconsciousness for the surgery.

The nurse also explains what happens after the surgery. The patient is moved into the recovery room. The nurse explains what this room looks like, what equipment will be there, and what to expect. Once the patient is awake and stable, they may be moved to a regular hospital room. There they receive **postoperative** care. The surgeon orders the care that should be given. The nurse explains the postoperative care to the person. This may include:

• why it is important to tell staff when they are feeling pain
• the pain medication they will be given
• when intravenous and other tubes will be removed

Anesthetic – the medication given to a person before surgery to induce anesthesia; administered in different ways depending on whether general or local
Postoperative – time after surgery

Your role may also include:
- helping with lab work ordered by the surgeon before or after the surgery
- making sure the person does not eat any food or drink anything after the specified time
- assisting with personal care including:
  - bathing
  - removing jewelry, nail polish, makeup
  - removing and taking care of false teeth (dentures), hearing aids, eyeglasses, hair care items, and any prosthesis.
- assisting in pre-op preparations, such as:
  - giving an enema before bowel surgery
  - cleansing the body area with a special soap to help remove bacteria
  - shaving the surgical area
- offering to call the person's clergy for spiritual support
- helping the person feel safe and comfortable
- assisting the nurse with checking that all the tasks on the preoperative checklist have been completed (See page 455 for an example)
- assisting the nurse with checking that all information is present in the person's chart before surgery
- documenting and reporting the person's mental status so the surgical team will be alert for any changes after the surgery

In addition, you must follow your facility's policy to protect the person's personal belongings while they are in surgery. Some people may be unable or unwilling to remove their wedding ring. In this case, ask the nurse if the ring should be left on and wrapped with clear tape.

The Importance of a Preoperative Checklist

The preoperative checklist is used just before the person is taken into the operating room. The checklist is a standard form listing everything to be done before surgery. The list is usually put on the outside of the person's medical record where operating room staff can see it. Every item on this checklist must be checked off before surgery by the nurse. If you are assisting and obtaining any item on the preoperative check list it must be double checked by the nurse. The preoperative check list is an important communication tool. It helps to ensure all staff are being mindful of what is needed for the patient and to be sure the safest surgery occurs. The list communicates information to all staff involved in the surgery. It is a quick indicator to the surgical team that specific tests were done,

results are posted, procedures were carried out, and forms filled out and signed by the appropriate people. The surgical team performing the actual surgery would be most interested in making sure some of the following items are present and accounted for in the patients chart:
- The surgical consent form is present, has been reviewed with the patient and signed by the surgeon as well as the patient.
- Any consultation sheets that makes recommendations pertinent to the patient and the surgery.
- The patient's history and physical indicating the patients past medical history and recent physical findings.
- Lab test, x-rays, vital signs results are present in the chart.

The anesthesiologist would be especially interested in some of the following standard preoperative check list items:
- ID bracelet is on the patient's wrist with the correct information.
- All the patient's jewelry is removed or taped, prosthetic devices, artificial limbs, dentures, make up, nail polish, wigs, hair pins glasses, contacts and hearing aids are removed.
- Any preoperative medications were administered with a signature.

Standard items on the preoperative checklist are listed in Box 25-1, page 454.

Supporting Family Members

If family members are present during the preoperative phase, they also may be fearful and anxious. It is important to support them at this time. If they will remain in the hospital during the surgery, let them know where they can wait. Reassure them the surgeon will come to speak with them as soon as the surgery is over. You may want to check in on the family periodically to reassure them or make sure they are comfortable. If the person having surgery does not speak English but a family member does, it is important to involve that family member in the preoperative, operative, and postoperative phases. The family member can translate for the person so that they have the needed information and do not feel isolated and scared. If

Prosthesis – a device that substitutes and functions in the place of a missing body part, such as dentures

PROCEDURE 25-1.   SHAVING THE SURGICAL SITE

 REMEMBER: BE AWARE

Items Needed
- gloves
- wash cloth
- towel
- wash basin filled with warm water
- soap
- plastic-covered pad
- prep kit or disposable razor
- bath blanket

1. Raise the bed to a good working height.

2. Assist the person to a comfortable position.

3. Cover the person with the bath blanket. Fold the bed linens to the bottom of the bed.

4. Place the plastic-covered pad under the person. Remove any clothing to expose only the surgical prep area.

5. Put on gloves.

6. Wash and lather the surgical prep site with warm water and soap, or use the surgical prep cleansing solution to clean the skin.

7. Hold the skin taut with one hand. With the other hand hold the razor at a 45 degree angle to shave the hair in the area of the surgical site. Shave in the direction of hair growth using short strokes. Be careful not to cut the skin or remove moles on the skin. If using an electric razor, gently move it over the area. If using a depilatory cream, check with the nurse and read the directions on the package before applying it to the skin. Always ask for help if you are unsure how to shave a surgical site.

8. Be sure to clean any excess lather and dry the person's skin when finished.

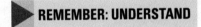 **REMEMBER: UNDERSTAND**

there is no English-speaking family member to translate, call for an interpreter. It is important for a patient having surgery to understand all aspects of the process.

Shaving the Surgical Site

The surgical site is not shaved before surgery as often as in the past, but some surgeons order the area to be shaved for certain surgeries. Shaving is often done right before surgery. Some surgeons may order an electric razor or depilatory cream to be used. Before shaving the surgical site, make sure you understand where the site is located and the exact area to shave. Note any skin redness, moles, cuts, or any other skin issues at the prep site. Always put on gloves for shaving the surgical site.

AFTER THE SURGERY

The time after the operation or surgery is called the post-operative, or post-op, phase.

Operating Room to Recovery Room

After the surgery, the patient will be transported to the recovery room. In some hospitals this is called the post-anesthesia care unit (PACU). The person stays here until they are stable and awake. The person arrives here with operating room staff.

A full report is given to the health care team, including:
- what surgery was done
- how the person is doing
- any complications or anything unusual that happened during surgery

BOX 25-1.
PREOPERATIVE CHECKLIST

- The surgical consent form. The surgeon reviews every detail of the surgical consent form with the person before surgery. This form states the type of surgery to be performed and the risks involved. The person signs their name and the date. Make sure this form has been signed and is present in the person's chart. This is considered informed consent.
- A surgical admission sheet. This form has personal information about the person, such as the family's telephone numbers.
- Any consultation sheets. This is information from other members of the health care team who helped make the diagnosis or recommended the surgery.
- History and physical examination. This includes the person's past medical history and recent physical exam findings.
- Lab reports. These may include blood test results, the person's blood type and crossmatch in case a blood transfusion is needed during surgery, urinalysis results, and sometimes a pregnancy test.
- Chest x-ray results. This is a written report about the admission chest x-ray.
- Preoperative vital signs.
- Any known allergies.
- Surgical preparation information, such as:
  - ID bracelet with the correct information put on the person's wrist
  - All jewelry removed or taped
  - All prostheses removed, such as artificial parts or dentures
  - Other items removed, including items such as wigs, hair clips, glasses or contacts, hearing aids, nail polish, and make up
- The time the person last voided.
- Other ordered surgical prep performed.
- Preoperative medications given and documented. The nurse who gives the medications records the name of the medication, the dose, the route, and the time administered. Medications given before surgery may include
  - sedatives to help the person relax and help the anesthesia take effect
  - antibiotics to decrease the chance of infection
  - a medication to reduce respiratory secretions
- Signature of the member of the health care team responsible that
  - all the information is present in the person's chart
  - all procedures have been completed and checked off on the list

- the medications used for anesthesia
- the use of any tubes or drains
- dressings present
- the need for oxygen
- the person's vital signs and urine output
- the administration of intravenous fluids
- any other pertinent information

The member of the health care team in charge explains the postoperative orders from the surgeon. During this phase, the person is "waking up" from the anesthesia and is constantly monitored. Vital signs, breathing status, alertness, reflexes, and responsiveness are all checked often. If a local anesthetic was used, the person's sensation in that area is checked. If there are complications, or if a breathing tube needs to remain in place, the surgeon may send the person to a surgical intensive care unit. The person stays there until they become stable or can breathe without the tube. If there are no complications, the person is transported back to the surgical floor where they were admitted. Or they may go to the surgical day room if the surgery was a day surgical procedure. Once the person leaves the recovery room or PACU, the next phase of postop recovery begins.

The recovery room staff calls ahead to alert staff that the person is ready to be moved from the recovery room. The recovery room staff escort the person to their destination and give a full report on the surgery and the person's time in the recovery room. This information is similar to what the operating room staff reported to the recovery room staff, as described earlier. The most recent information about the person's status in the recovery room is also reported. It is very important for the recovery room staff to compare the person's mental status now with the person's status before the surgery, to assess for complications such as postoperative confusion.

PRE-OP CHECK LIST
DEPARTMENT OF NURSING

Check List

This list must accompany each patient

Nurse preparing the patient must complete and sign checklist form

Nurse releasing the patient must verify the patient's id and sign form

List to be kept with patient's record until discharged then destroyed

Identification Bands	**Clinical data in chart** ( )
A) Arm ( )	CBC EKG if ordered
B) Leg ( )	Urinalysis Blood set up as ordered
C) Allergy ( )	Chest X-ray

Skin Preparations ( )	Medication charted ( )
Note abnormalities	Medication sheet sent w/patient ( )

Vital signs recorded ( )	**Record assembled** ( )
Height and weight ( )	Current record Medication sheet
Catheterized ( )	Old records Vital signs sheets
Voided ( )	X-ray Doctor's order sheet
Time _____	Other
Amount _____	

Dress	Pre op orders reviewed ( )
A) Hospital gown ( )	Procedure consent ( )
B) Hair pins, wigs removed ( )	Anesthesia consent ( )
C) Nail polish removed ( )	

Valuable checklist	none	removed	not removed
1. Dentures upper	( )	( )	( )
lower	( )	( )	( )
2. Glasses	( )	( )	( )
3. Contacts	( )	( )	( )
4. Prosthetic-devises	( )	( )	( )
5. Jewelry/earrings	( )	( )	( )
6. Hearing aids	( )	( )	( )
7. Other	( )	( )	( )

_____

Signature of Nurse Preparing Patient

_____

Signature of Nurse Releasing Patient

Your Role in Postoperative Care

The information you will hear from the recovery room nurse is important for you to provide the best possible postoperative care. Your role is to assist the nurse with post-op care. Postoperative care involves the following:
- Take vital signs as ordered and report any changes immediately to the nurse.
- Help the person to a comfortable position and change positions often if allowed.
- Observe for mental status changes.
- Be aware of common conditions that often occur after surgery, such as nausea, vomiting, gas pains, constipation, dry mouth, and postoperative pain.
- Help prevent nausea and vomiting by eliminating odors from the person's room, offering small sips of fluid if ordered, and encouraging deep breathing to help rid the effects of anesthesia. If the person vomits, offer an emesis basin, provide mouth care, change the sheets quickly to get the odor out of the room, and report the vomiting to the nurse.
- Help decrease gas and constipation by encouraging the person to move in bed and walk as soon as ordered by the surgeon. Often a person is helped to walk a few steps just hours after surgery. Early ambulation helps gas move out, prevents constipation, and increases circulation.
- Offer sips of water or ice chips if ordered, and provide mouth care to reduce dry mouth. When ordered by the surgeon, encourage the person to drink fluids to prevent dry mouth, to stay well hydrated, and to prevent constipation.
- To reduce pain, it is important for the person to tell staff when pain begins so that the proper medications can be given. You can help by reporting any signs of pain immediately, helping the person to a comfortable position, reducing noise around the person, and encouraging the person to take deep breaths often. Ask the person to think about the medication working and the pain slipping away.
- Help the person with their ordered rehabilitation program.
- Help the person with their personal care. Often the person needs help with bathing and grooming after surgery. Since many surgical patients did not need this help previously, respect their feelings and provide privacy.
- Encourage good nutrition, following the surgeon's orders, to help in wound healing and for good health.
- Always use standard precautions when handling any dressing or providing care.

- Observe for any signs of infection like redness, swelling, drainage, and odor at the wound site. Report your observations to the nurse.
- Provide measures to prevent complications. A common preventive measure a surgeon may order is elastic stockings. These are also called TED stockings or anti-embolism stockings. The next section describes the use of elastic stockings.
- Encourage deep breathing and coughing often to prevent any complications. Teach the person to splint the wound when coughing or moving. A later section describes how to assist with deep breathing and coughing.

Elastic Stockings
Elastic stockings are used to prevent thrombophlebitis (inflammation of the veins). When applied to the person's legs, the elastic in the stockings causes pressure that promotes venous blood flow. Elastic stockings are often ordered by the surgeon to prevent the postoperative complication of a blood clot formation if the person will be on bed rest for a time. Elastic stockings must be put on while the person is in bed. They should be removed and reapplied every 8 hours or as ordered by the surgeon. Be sure the elastic stockings are the correct size and length before applying them. It is best to order two pairs of elastic stockings. To clean the stockings, read the manufacturer's guidelines. Usually you soak them in warm water and mild soap for a few minutes and hang them to dry. See Chapter 11 for the procedure for applying elastic stockings.

Sequential Compression Devices
Like elastic stockings, sequential compression devices are used postoperatively to increase blood flow and decrease the risk of blood clot formation. These devices can be used alone or with elastic stockings. There are many different types from different manufacturers, so it is important always to read the directions for using them. Always follow the health care professional's orders for their use and the length of sleeve to use. The health care professional also orders the inflation/deflation sequence settings.

Anti-embolism stockings – elastic stockings often worn after surgery to help prevent blood clots

Emesis basin – a special basin used to catch vomit or secretions coughed up ("emesis" is the medical term for vomiting)

Splint – to hold or keep an area from moving

PROCEDURE 25-2. ASSISTING WITH DEEP BREATHING AND COUGHING

▶ **REMEMBER: BE AWARE**

Items Needed
- pillow or splint
- tissue
- emesis basin
- gloves

1. Explain that after surgery a person needs to take deep breaths and cough. This helps to remove anesthesia and prevent the accumulation of lung secretions. Coughing and deep breathing are also important for someone who has been on bed rest for a period of time.

2. When ready, ask them to take at least four diaphragmatic breaths as described in Procedure 24-3.

3. Put on gloves.

4. Elevate the head of the bed as much as the person can tolerate.

5. Tell the person how to hold a pillow or splint over the surgical site.

6. While holding the pillow, ask the person to take a deep breath, hold it for 3 seconds, and then exhale. Repeat this at least five times if the person can tolerate it. With the last two deep breaths, encourage the person to take a deep breath and cough as hard as possible while you hold the emesis basin to catch any sputum secretions.

7. Clean up any secretions using tissues and the emesis basin. Note the color and consistency of any respiratory secretions. Report your findings to the heath care team.

8. Instruct the person to continue the deep breathing and coughing exercises once an hour.

▶ **REMEMBER: UNDERSTAND**

The sleeves come in small, medium and large. The sleeve is attached to a pump that inflates and deflates the sleeve in a sequential motion. It is important the sleeve is not too tight on the person's leg. You should be able to put two fingers between the sleeve and the person's leg. When the device is running, frequently check the person's toes for color, sensation, mobility, and warmth.

Deep Breathing and Coughing

Encourage deep breathing and coughing often to prevent post-op complications. The nurse teaches the person to splint the wound with a pillow when coughing or moving. The surgeon often has the respiratory therapy department teach the person to use a respiratory breathing exercise device such as an incentive spirometer to prevent postoperative breathing complications. The respiratory therapist teaches the person how to use the device. You may assist and remind the person to perform the exercises. Although the nurse teaches these exercises, you should know the proper procedure so you can assist.

📖
Incentive spirometer – device that measures how deeply a person inhales, to encourage deep breathing

IN THIS CHAPTER YOU LEARNED:

- How to reduce a person's fears and anxiety when going for surgery
- What is involved in the preoperative phase of surgery
- What is included in preoperative teaching
- What tasks are on a preoperative checklist
- What to do if the person having surgery does not speak English
- Your role in the postoperative phase

SUMMARY

In this chapter you learned how to care for a person having surgery. You learned what you can do to help reduce a person's fears and anxieties. Most important, listen to what the person is feeling. You learned about the preoperative phase, what is included in preoperative teaching, and what tasks and information are recorded on the preoperative checklist. For the surgery to be a success for someone who does not speak English, an English-speaking family member or interpreter is needed. This person helps by exchanging information about the surgery. You also learned your role in the postoperative phase after the person is stable.

PULLING IT ALL TOGETHER

Imagine you have been working in a long term care facility for three years, and now you are thinking about going to nursing school. One of the nurses you work with tells you about a position open at the local hospital and encourages you to apply. The nurse feels you should work in an acute care setting before starting nursing school. You apply and get the job working on a surgical floor. At first you feel overwhelmed. Soon you find the skills you used in long term care also apply in this setting, and you become more comfortable. You enjoy learning new information about surgery and the process a person goes through with surgery. You are especially interested in the immediate post-op phase when the person is in the PACU awakening from anesthesia. You decide this is where you would like to work after finishing nursing school. But imagine if you had not taken the nurse's advice and applied for the surgical floor position—you might never have discovered your true interest. As a nurse assistant, keep your mind open and try working in different areas. Until you try, you can never know how far you might advance in the field of your choice.

CHECK WHAT YOU'VE LEARNED

1. **Early this morning Mrs. Stanovitch was admitted to the surgical floor where you are working. She is having surgery for removal of two toes on her right foot because of diabetes . She is an 82-year-old and speaks only Russian. What can you do so that the health care team can learn as much as possible about Mrs. Stanovitch in this short period of time?**

   A. Call her family and friends and ask them questions about her.

   B. Get a Russian/English interpreter to assist in the entire preoperative phase.

   C. Let other staff members handle her preoperative needs since you do not speak Russian.

   D. Tell the nurse you could not obtain any information because you cannot communicate with her.

2. **As a team member caring for Mrs. Stanovitch, what information is most important for you to learn before surgery so that staff can provide the best possible post-op care?**

   A. Who she lives with.

   B. Her nutritional likes and dislikes.

   C. Her baseline mental status.

   D. How much assistance she needs with the activities of daily living.

3. **How can you help reduce a person's fear and anxiety before surgery?**

   A. Tell the person it is ridiculous to feel fearful or have anxiety.

   B. Be honest and tell them stories about your own personal surgery experiences.

   C. Listen to the person and always be kind and respectful.

   D. Advise the person to cancel the surgery.

4. **Before surgery, the surgeon will tell which of the following to the patient?**
   A. The risks involved in the surgery.
   B. That there will be no complications.
   C. The person will never need surgery again.
   D. The person will not die.

5. **Before surgery, the health care professional and surgeon will do the preoperative teaching. What is your role in preoperative teaching?**
   A. Discuss with the person the medication you will be administering during the surgery.
   B. Explain postoperative care to the person.
   C. Discuss with the person the type of anesthesia being used during the surgery.
   D. Assist the health care professional in documenting and reporting the person's mental status as the baseline.

6. **What is your role in caring for a post-op surgical patient immediately after returning from the recovery room?**
   A. Report the post-operative orders.
   B. Administer pain medications.
   C. Take the person's vital signs as ordered and report any changes immediately to the nurse.
   D. Assist in removing the breathing tube.

7. **As a nurse assistant working with Mr. Smith less than 24 hours after surgery, which of the following would you report immediately to the health care team?**
   A. "I took care of Mr. Smith for three days when he was admitted to the surgical floor. He was alert, and he knew his name, the date, where he was, and why he was having the surgery. But today he doesn't recognize me and doesn't remember his name or why he is here at the hospital."
   B. "Mr. Smith's vital signs are T 98.6 oral, P68, R16, and B/P 122/78."
   C. "Mr. Smith was able to ambulate with assistance today up and down the hall. Tomorrow the plan is to see how he does on stairs."
   D. "The rehabilitation facility called to say they have accepted Mr. Smith. The admission nurse would like a full report on his postoperative care before he arrives next week."

8. **To help reduce pain after surgery, what measures can you take?**
   A. Tell the person to wait a while after the pain starts, because it may go away.
   B. Check the dose of pain medication because it must not be enough.
   C. Report the pain immediately to the health care professional and provide comfort measures. Making sure the person is in a comfortable position, reduce any outside noise, and encourage deep breaths until the health care professional returns with the pain medication.
   D. Check the person's vital signs, because you know vital signs are elevated when a person is in pain, and report your findings.

9. **When caring for a person after surgery, which of the following is your responsibility?**
   A. Administer post-op pain medications.
   B. Review the pathology report about the tumor cells removed during surgery.
   C. Assist the person with personal care while always respecting their feelings and privacy.
   D. Order post-op blood tests.

10. **Which of these would you report immediately to the health care professional when caring for Mrs. Jones after surgery?**
    A. "Today Mrs. Jones was having difficulty moving from her bed to the chair. It took two nurse assistants to help her out of bed."
    B. "Today Mrs. Jones's pulse and respirations were slightly elevated when she was having pain."
    C. "After more than 24 hours, Mrs. Jones is still not easy to arouse. She seemed very confused when I asked her questions about things we talked about before her surgery."
    D. "Mrs. Jones sat in her chair for only 10 minutes this morning."

(Answers to "Check What You've Learned" are in the Instructor's Manual.)

Chapter 26

SPECIAL SKILLS FOR SPECIAL TIMES

The primary focus of this text is learning to care for residents in long term care facilities. In Chapter 25 you learned skills that can be transferred from one health care setting to another. For example, when caring for someone having surgery, you perform skills such as bathing, positioning, moving, denture care, and/or bed making. You use the same principles for all persons in all health care settings. Your other skills such as listening to, communicating with, and respecting residents and patients are also very important in any area where you may work. But you will also need some new skills to work in other health care settings or with persons who have different health needs. In this way you are like an athlete. Most athletes use similar basic workout skills, but they also learn new skills to improve their performance and be more competitive. In this chapter you will understand how you can transfer skills you have already learned to other people and other places. You will also learn new special skills to care for a new mother and newborn, children, adolescents, and young adults. This chapter previews some of the new and constantly expanding opportunities for nurse assistants.

OBJECTIVES
- Explain your role in prenatal care
- Identify signs and symptoms during pregnancy to report to the health care team immediately
- State two normal signs and symptoms of pregnancy for each of the three trimesters
- Explain the reason for childbirth classes
- Explain two signs that labor is about to begin
- Identify the five physical characteristics of the newborn evaluated at one and five minutes after birth
- Explain the immediate care of the neonate
- Name at least one reason why a woman might need a cesarean birth
- Explain what care is given to the mother during the postpartum period and how to promote postpartum health
- Demonstrate how to assist a postpartum mother with a Sitz bath
- Identify standard care given to the newborn in the first 24 to 48 hours after birth
- Name two questions parents frequently ask about caring for their newborn
- Demonstrate how to diaper a newborn, how to bathe a newborn, and how to care for a circumcision
- Explain how to assist a mother and newborn with breastfeeding and bottle feeding
- Give four examples when parents should call the health care team about their infant
- Name two standard procedures followed before mother and newborn are discharged from the hospital
- Describe pediatric areas in which nurse assistants may work
- Explain why evaluating a child's growth and development is important
- Name two standard procedures followed when a child is admitted to a pediatric floor, and describe your role in caring for a hospitalized child
- Identify two safety tips to teach parents, and describe the importance of immunizations
- Name two universal good health habits for all age groups, two specific good health habits for adolescents, and at least five behavior risks for youths today

MEDICAL TERMS
- **Amniotic sac** – membrane that encloses the fetus inside the uterus; it contains amniotic fluid that cushions and supports the fetus during development
- **Apgar scale** – a tool for assessing the health status of a newborn
- **Cervix** – the opening of the uterus into the vagina
- **Cesarean section** – giving birth through a surgical incision made through the abdomen into the uterus
- **Circumcision** – surgical removal of the foreskin at the head of the penis
- **Colostrum** – the watery "first milk" that appears from a newborn mother's breasts
- **Delivery** – the act of giving birth
- **Epidural** – a type of anesthetic given by injection to minimize the pain of childbirth
- **Episiotomy** – a surgical incision made to enlarge the vaginal opening for childbirth
- **Labor** – stages of expulsion of the fetus from the uterus through the vagina, beginning with contractions and the release of amniotic fluid and ending with delivery
- **Lactation** – the production of breast milk
- **Neonate** – the newborn infant up to one month of age
- **Placenta** – a temporary organ that develops in the uterus during pregnancy to transfer oxygen and nutrients to the fetus and remove carbon dioxide and some waste products; commonly called "the afterbirth"
- **Postpartum** – the period after childbirth
- **Prenatal** – the period of pregnancy before childbirth
- **Trimester** – one third of the normal period of pregnancy, which is divided into three trimesters
- **Umbilical cord** – a tube connecting the fetus to the mother's placenta.

"I can't wait to bring the baby to see the staff at my first clinic visit. They are going to be so surprised at how big and beautiful he is!"

Have you ever been pregnant or had a wife, friend, or significant other who was pregnant? What do you remember? Do you remember the day the baby was born? Was it a vaginal or a cesarean birth? Were you anxious and excited? Experiencing pregnancy and having a baby can bring out many emotions. Different people have different—and often changing—emotions during pregnancy, birth, and afterwards. Your role is to provide support during this time.

For a mother to have a healthy pregnancy and a healthy baby, it is very important for her to receive prenatal care. Prenatal care begins when the woman first learns she is pregnant and lasts until the baby is born. A normal pregnancy lasts for about 280 days or 40 weeks (nine calendar months), counting from with the first day of the last menstrual period. Often you will hear the health care team refer to a pregnancy in terms of the first, second, or third trimester. The first trimester consist of weeks 1-12, the second trimester is weeks 13-27, and the third trimester is weeks 28 to 40. The woman's estimated due date, an estimate of when the baby will be born, is calculated by adding seven days to the first day of the woman's last menstrual period and subtracting three months. As a nurse assistant, you may work in an obstetrical clinic or other settings where the mother receives prenatal care (Fig. 26-1).

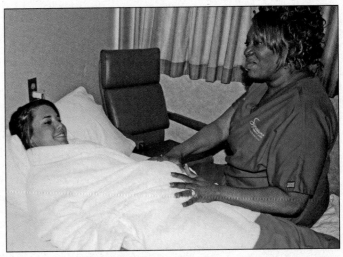

Fig. 26-1 - The mother receives prenatal care.

Prenatal - the period of pregnancy before childbirth
Trimester - one third of the normal period of pregnancy, which is divided into three trimesters

YOUR ROLE IN PRENATAL CARE

The goal of prenatal care is to ensure the health of the mother and the birth of a healthy baby. Changes take place in the woman and the fetus (the term for an unborn baby) during the pregnancy that indicate it is a healthy pregnancy. At the pregnant woman's first visit, early in the first trimester, a thorough history is taken and a physical examination performed. Chapter 13 describes how you assist with the physical exam. Your role is to assist in the prenatal physical exam in the same way. In the prenatal physical exam additional information will be gathered to assess the health of the mother and fetus. This information includes a history of the mother's menstruation and other pregnancies, the mother's nutritional status, and a detailed history of drug, alcohol, and caffeine use. After the first physical exam, routine prenatal visits should occur at least monthly for the first three months, twice a month until the middle of the last trimester, and then weekly until the baby is born. In each routine visit, the health care professional assesses the woman and fetus. You will assist with gathering information, which may include:

- Weight—to assess if her weight gain is appropriate for the trimester. Weight gain is normal as the fetus grows and the circulatory system produces and circulates more blood to the fetus.
- Blood pressure—to assess if her circulatory system is adjusting normally or abnormally to the increased burden on her system from the fetus.
- Urine glucose test—to assess if her kidneys are handling the increased circulatory burden (Fig. 26-2).

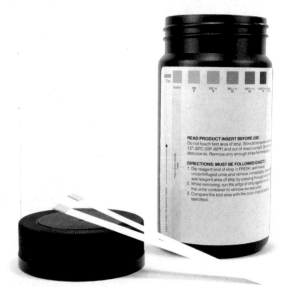

Fig. 26-2 - Test strips for urine glucose test.

The health care professional will teach the pregnant woman signs and symptoms of a healthy pregnancy and birth. It is very important for her to understand what is happening to her body and to understand how the fetus is growing. She will be given specific information about eating nutritious food and exercising everyday. She will also learn what to do if she experiences any unusual signs and symptoms and to report them to the health care team immediately. These include:

- vaginal bleeding
- elevations in blood pressure
- increased swelling in hands and feet—rings or shoes "just don't fit"
- shortness of breath
- headaches
- inability to eat because of nausea and vomiting
- dizziness or blurred vision
- abdominal pain or contractions

At any time in the pregnancy the health care team may order certain common tests. An ultrasound is a test that uses sound waves to look at how the fetus is developing and moving and to determine the age of the fetus (Fig. 26-3).

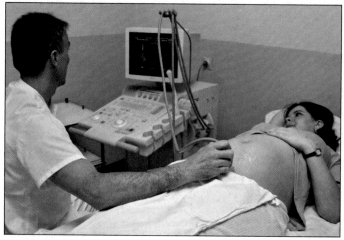

Fig. 26-3 - Ultrasound uses sound waves to see how the fetus is developing.

Throughout prenatal care, it is important to establish and maintain an open relationship with the mother. This helps her to express her emotions, which may be conflicting and troublesome. If her emotions seem troublesome, report this immediately to the health care professional. Additional professional support may be needed to help the mother understand and more comfortably handle her feelings.

Normal Signs and Symptoms of Pregnancy

Signs and symptoms of a normal first trimester:

- Menstrual period is absent, and pregnancy test is positive
- Tender and swollen breasts
- Frequent urination that continues as the fetus grows
- Nausea and/or vomiting, called "morning sickness" because it often occurs in the morning.
- Fear and anxiety about the pregnancy and all that it means
- May begin to feel fatigue

Some of the signs and symptoms of a normal second trimester:

- Weight gain
- Abdomen becomes enlarged as the fetus grows
- May develop stretch marks on the abdomen
- May feel the fetus move at approximately 20 weeks (Fig. 26-4)

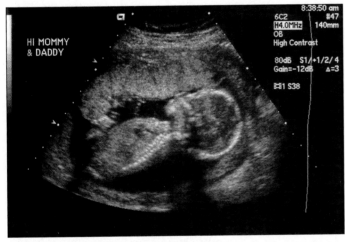

Fig. 26-4 - Ultrasound of a fetus at 20 weeks.

Some signs and symptoms of a normal third trimester:

- Abdomen enlarges more as the fetus grows
- Mother may develop back pain, swollen feet, indigestion, and shortness of breath
- Mother may feel contractions as the uterus prepares for the delivery (Fig. 26-5)

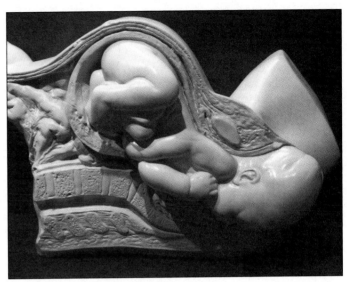

Fig. 26-5 - Uterus prepares for delivery.

Preparing for Birth

In addition to the scheduled prenatal physical exams, the pregnant woman has special training for childbirth. This is often done with her husband or another person who will be the coach during the delivery. This training is called "birthing class" or "childbirth class." Different methods are used, but the goal of all birthing classes is to help the mother and significant others prepare for birth by teaching them what to expect during labor and delivery. This is a good time for everyone to ask questions and resolve any concerns. Often they will see a video of a normal vaginal delivery and a cesarean birth. In a vaginal birth, the fetus is born through the birth canal and out through the vagina. A cesarean section is another form of delivery in which a surgical incision is made in the abdomen and into the uterus. The baby is removed through the incision. All the reasons for both types of delivery, and their risks, are discussed.

Cesarean section – giving birth through a surgical incision made through the abdomen into the uterus

Delivery – the act of giving birth

Labor – stages of expulsion of the fetus from the uterus through the vagina, beginning with contractions and the release of amniotic fluid and ending with delivery

Many childbirth classes include a tour of the birthing facility. This helps to reduce anxieties about the staff, equipment, and physical surroundings before the actual birth. The mother and her coach learn breathing and relaxation techniques that will help during labor and delivery. They will also learn some comfort measures and positions used during labor to help lessen pain or pressure or aid in the delivery of the baby. Common procedures performed in labor and delivery are discussed. The mother and/or significant others can also attend other classes about breastfeeding, caring for a newborn, and parenting.

LABOR AND DELIVERY

At the end of the pregnancy, at about 40 weeks, the woman normally shows signs that labor is about to begin. These include:

- The fetus "drops" (moves downward into the birth canal).
- The cervical mucus plug becomes loose and dislodges.
- The amniotic sac may rupture and release the fluid (the "water) that surrounds the fetus.
- The uterus begins to contract.

The health care team will have already given the mother and coach instructions about when to go to the hospital or birthing facility. The mother and coach are admitted to the labor room until she is ready for delivery. Some hospitals have a special combination labor and delivery room called the birthing room. During labor and delivery, you may assist in:

- providing a safe, healthy environment
- preventing infection
- minimizing labor pain
- providing comfort
- reducing the mother's and coach's fears and anxiety (Fig. 26-6)

As labor progresses, contractions become strong, regular, and closer together. The health care professional assesses the mother's cervix to make sure it gradually becomes effaced (thin) and dilated (opened). The health care professional periodically examines the mother to determine the degree of dilation as labor progresses. If this is her first childbirth, labor could last from 18 to 24 hours. Labor and delivery are often shorter if she has already given birth.

As labor progresses and the mother's cervix continues to dilate, medications may be given to reduce her pain and to assist in relaxation. Anesthetics may be used to block pain during labor and delivery. The most common is an epidural.

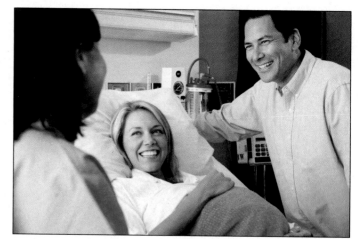
Fig. 26-6 - Talking to a nurse can reduce anxiety.

The anesthetic is placed into the epidural space around the spinal cord. Its effects are limited to the reproductive organs and other nearby areas. Other drugs may also be given to help the labor and cervix dilation progress if needed. If the mother is in the hospital during labor, a fetal monitor is placed either on the fetus's head or on the mother's abdomen. This monitor measures the fetal heart rate. A rapid drop or increase in fetal heart rate must be interpreted by the health care professional.

When the cervix is fully dilated and the baby has moved down the birth canal, the health care professional usually encourages the mother to bear down and begin to push with each contraction. The mother may need to push as long as one to two hours. As the baby is being delivered, the health care professional may perform an episiotomy to make the vaginal opening larger so that the baby can pass through without tearing the vagina (Fig. 26-7, next page).

During delivery a number of health care team members usually perform specific tasks in the care of the mother and baby. As the baby's head is being delivered, the baby's face is cleaned and mucus is aspirated from the mouth and nose. When the baby's body is fully delivered, the umbili-

Amniotic sac – membrane that encloses the fetus inside the uterus; it contains amniotic fluid that cushions and supports the fetus during development

Cervix – the opening of the uterus into the vagina

Epidural – a type of anesthetic given by injection to minimize the pain of childbirth

Episiotomy – a surgical incision made to enlarge the vaginal opening

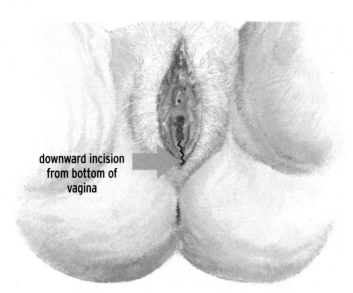

downward incision
from bottom of
vagina

Fig. 26-7 - Episiotomy.

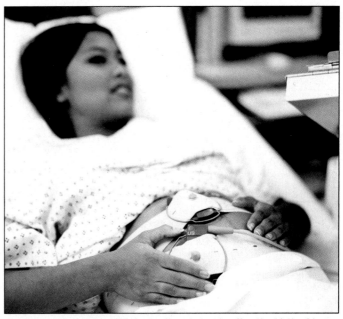

Fig. 26-8 - The new mother is monitored closely after the birth of her baby.

cal cord (attached to the placenta, which is attached to the uterine wall) is cut and clamped. The baby is placed either on the mother's abdomen or in a warmer for assessment. A health care professional observes and records the Apgar assessment score just after birth and again at 5 minutes. The "best" Apgar score is 10, the lowest is 0. The tool measures the newborn's (A) activity – for muscle tone, (P) pulse, (G) grimace—for reflex irritability, (A) appearance of skin color, and (R) respiration. This system evaluates five physical characteristics:

• heart rate
• respiratory effort
• muscle tone
• reflexes
• color

Both the mother and baby receive identification bracelets. A footprint is taken of the newborn. This provides a memento for the mother and helps reduce the risk of misidentification, a nursery mix-up, or illegal removal of the newborn from the nursery or home.

Not long after the baby is born, the placenta is delivered and is evaluated. The episiotomy is sutured. The first hour after the delivery of the placenta is critical because postpartum bleeding is most likely to happen then. Staff will massage her fundus to help the uterus return to its normal size. The mother is evaluated closely during this time (Fig. 26-8).

Immediate Care of the Neonate

The new baby is called a neonate. The neonate's condition is evaluated by a health care professional at one and five minutes after birth using the Apgar scoring system. To promote body warmth, the health care team cleans and dries the neonate's body. The newborn's axillary temperature is measured. The baby may be placed in a warmer for a few minutes. The head is covered with a cap and a warm blanket wrapped around the entire body. Depending on the mother's wishes and the delivery setting, the mother and baby may remain together for the next few hours or days. In other settings, the mother and newborn are separated for a time so that the individual needs of each can be met (Fig. 26-9, next page).

Fundus – the top of the uterus
Neonate – the newborn infant up to one month of age
Placenta – a temporary organ that develops in the uterus during pregnancy to transfer oxygen and nutrients to the fetus and remove carbon dioxide and some waste products; commonly called "the afterbirth"
Postpartum – the period after childbirth
Umbilical cord – a tube connecting the fetus to the mother's placenta

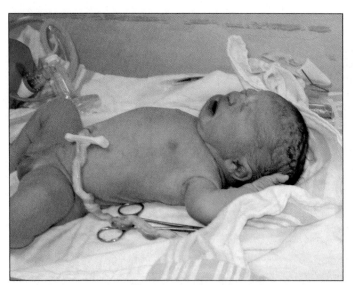

Fig. 26-9 - Mother and newborn are separated for a short time to take care of their individual needs.

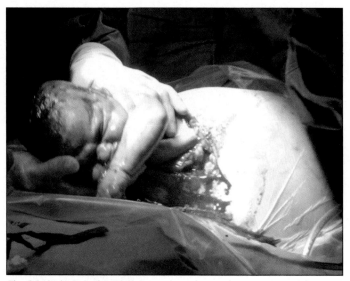

Fig. 26-10 - A Cesarian birth.

Additional standard procedures done in the delivery room within the first hour after birth include measuring the neonate's height and weight and administering Vitamin K. The blood type of the fetus may be determined from cord blood or sometimes from a heel-prick. Once the mother and neonate are stable, they may be transferred individually to the postpartum floor and newborn nursery or together to another setting.

Cesarean Section Births

About a fourth of all infants are born by cesarean section in the United States today. In a cesarean birth, the fetus is removed through a surgical incision in the abdomen and into the uterus. The mother is given a spinal or epidural anesthetic to block feeling from her upper abdomen to her toes. A cesarean section may be performed for many reasons, including:

• The mother had a previous cesarean birth (Fig. 26-10).
• The fetus is in distress.
• The labor fails to progress.

CARE OF MOTHER DURING THE POSTPARTUM PERIOD

Imagine giving birth for the first time. You are now a parent and will be totally responsible for the care of your newborn baby. Just think for a moment about how new parents must feel. The postpartum period can be a very exciting but often anxious and confusing time for a new mother and family.

Immediately postpartum you may assist the health care team in transferring the new mother to the postpartum floor. In some hospitals, labor, delivery, and postpartum care occur in the same room. Often the newborn spends as much time in the room as possible with the mother. The key is to provide a safe and healthy beginning for the mother and new baby. Always follow standard precautions when caring for the postpartum mother because you may come in contact with blood and other body fluids. If the mother was given an anesthetic, follow the postpartum orders written by the heath care professional. Remember that the mother is at risk for infection and bleeding. Vital signs are taken and recorded at least every four hours during the first 24 hours, then every eight hours or when ordered by the health care professional. Your role will be to take vital signs and report any changes.

When caring for the mother in the postpartum period, the health care professional must pay attention to the following care:

Take and record the mother's vital signs and observe for bleeding:

- A decrease in blood pressure of 15 to 20 mm Hg below the mother's baseline blood pressures may indicate a problem with fluid volume or blood loss.
- An increase in the mother's temperature may indicate infection.
- An increase in the mother's pulse rate greater than 100 beats per minute may indicate blood loss, fever, or pain.
- An increase in the mother's respiratory rate greater than 24 breaths per minute may indicate more serious blood loss or a blood clot in the lung. A decrease in the mother's respiratory rate below 12 breaths per minute may result from the medications used for pain during labor.
- Immediately after delivery of the placenta, the health care team pays attention to the size and firmness of the mother's uterus. A uterus that is soft and enlarging may indicate excessive bleeding. The health care team will massage and measure the top of the uterus (the fundus). The fundus should remain firm as the uterus slowly returns to normal size. The fundus is measured at the umbilicus or two fingers' width below it for the first day after delivery.
- Report if the mother feels light-headed or dizzy when sitting upright or before walking the first time. If the mother feels these symptoms, have her lie back in the bed, take her vital signs, and report your findings to the health care team. Explain to the mother the importance of asking for help when getting out of bed, especially the first time.
- Check the mother's pad for blood clots and for the amount of bleeding. The vaginal discharge that occurs for the first three weeks after birth is called lochia. The mother normally has a moderate amount of red lochia the first three days. Then the amount should lessen, and the color should become pink to pinkish brown to yellowish brown before it stops. If the pad is saturated with blood within an hour, this is excessive and needs to be reported immediately.
- Report any changes immediately.

Check for effects of anesthesia:

- Check the mother for sensation (feeling) and motor ability (able to move) her lower legs if a regional anesthetic (such as a spinal) was used in labor and delivery.
- Expose one leg at a time, and ask the mother to wiggle her toes and move her legs. Check for sensation by using gentle touch, moving down the mother's leg and asking if she feels the touch.

- If a regional anesthetic was used, check the mother's lower legs to the toes for sensation and motor ability before she gets out of bed. The health care member orders how long the mother must remain in bed. Call the health care team if the mother does not have any feeling in her legs after the time ordered.

Encourage food and drink as tolerated:

- During labor and delivery the mother expends a large amount of energy and loses a large amount of blood and other body fluids. When the health care member orders the postpartum diet, encourage the mother to eat and drink as tolerated to increase her energy and replace the fluids.
- If the mother is breastfeeding, she must understand proper nutrition during this time for her and her baby. A nutritionist can help the mother with a diet plan.

Minimize pain:

- Help the mother apply ice packs to her perineal area for the first 24 hours to decrease swelling and pain. Then help apply heat to the area. Always place a thin barrier between the ice pack and the skin. Take breaks between applications to prevent tissue damage. When the mother can sit on the toilet for a period of time after the first 24 hours, encourage her to use a warm Sitz bath (Procedure 26-1, page 470) three times a day for 15 to 20 minutes for perineal discomfort.
- Explain other methods for relieving perineal pain and discomfort. Teach the mother to contract her buttocks before sitting down, and to use positioning cushions and pillows while sitting. She may also use a perineal bottle to squirt warm water over her perineum during and after voiding. The health care professional may also order pain medication or a topical cream for the mother to apply.

Check the mother's breasts:

- Check the mother's breasts for signs of engorgement (swollen, tender, tense, shiny breast tissue).
- If a mother who is breastfeeding experiences painful engorgement, help her take a warm or hot shower

---

Engorgement – a postpartum mother's breasts being swollen with milk, which may be uncomfortable or painful

Lochia – vaginal discharge that occurs after childbirth

Sitz bath – a bath in a tub or special basin in which only the genital area and buttocks are immersed, used to relieve pain and swelling

allowing the water to flow over her breasts. Or you may help to apply warm compresses. Also encourage her to nurse the newborn or express some milk manually or with a breast pump. A "lactation specialist" (a nurse or other health care professional) may visit and teach the mother successful breastfeeding guidelines.

• If a mother who is bottle-feeding experiences painful engorgement, tell her to avoid handing her breasts because this action stimulates more milk production. She may wear a snug, supportive bra night and day. She should avoid warm water on her breasts during showers because the heat stimulates milk production. She may also use ice bags on her breasts for comfort.

Observe urinary elimination:

• The mother normally urinates the first time within six to eight hours after delivery. If the mother is unable to urinate, report this to the health care team.
• If the mother urinates frequently in small amounts, this may be a sign that she has urinary retention and is only urinating the overflow. Report this.
• Instruct the mother to void every several hours to keep her bladder empty. This may help decrease the uterine cramping that occurs after delivery.

Promote normal bowel movements:

• Explain to the mother that she may experience sluggish bowel movements for several reasons. Her abdominal muscle tone is decreased. The anesthetic used in labor and delivery may have this effect. She has had less solid food intake during labor. This may also result from hormones released during labor and childbirth.
• Explain that she may feel pain with her first bowel movement due to the episiotomy, hemorrhoids, or lacerations in the perineal area during delivery.
• To avoid pain during bowel movements, encourage her to get adequate amounts of fresh fruit, vegetables, fiber, and at least eight glasses of water daily.
• Encourage walking and other forms of exercise when the mother feels better.

Prevent infection

• Observe and report an elevated temperature above 100.4 F. (38 C).
• Observe the mother's episiotomy and perineum for redness, swelling, and discharge (note color, amount, and odor). Report any unusual findings to the health care team.
• Observe and report frequency or urination and any pain or burning the mother feels.

Reduce fatigue:

• Encourage the mother to sleep while the baby is sleeping and to rest whenever possible.
• Provide a quiet environment.
• Encourage the mother to have visits with family or friends after she has time to rest.

The usual length of stay in the hospital for mother and newborn is now two days if there are no complications. As soon as the effects of anesthesia and labor have subsided, the mother is encouraged to do as much as possible for herself and her newborn. Encourage the parents to invite family or friends to join any classes to learn about helping in the newborn's care. Explain to the mother what to expect and how to maintain her health in the six weeks before her first postpartum visit (Fig. 26-11. next page).

Promoting Postpartum Health

The mother needs to understand the changes taking place in her body as it begins to return to her pre-pregnant state. Knowing what to look for and what to expect will help her focus on adjusting to her new role as mother. Following are ways to help the mother maintain her health:

• Perform perineal care to promote comfort, cleanliness, and healing. Using a perineal bottle, pour warm water over the perineum after each void and after each bowel movement.
• Give Sitz baths to promote comfort, cleanliness, and healing (Procedure 26-1, page 470).
• When applying perineal pads, touch the outside only. Always keep the portion that will touch her perineum clean.
• Breastfeeding, or using breast milk to feed the neonate, provides the newborn with the best natural defense to many diseases. The mother's milk contains antibodies that help protect the newborn. The first watery milk that appears in about 12 hours after delivery is called colostrum. On about the second day, the flow of normal milk begins, called lactation. The mother should wash her hands and breasts before breastfeeding or express-

---

Colostrum – watery "first milk" that appears from a newborn mother's breasts

Express – technique used by breastfeeding mother to remove breast milk to a container to be used later for bottle feeding

Lactation – the production of breast milk

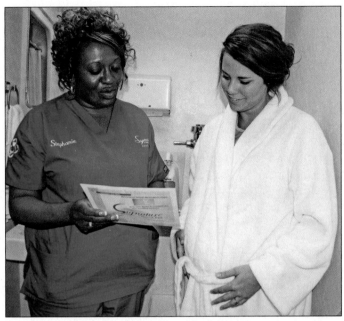

Fig. 26-11 - Teaching about postpartum health topics like perineal care can begin even before childbirth.

ing milk to feed the newborn. When washing, use a circular motion and wash from the nipples outward. Between feedings, she should wear a good fitting bra and breast pads to absorb leaking milk.

- Inspect the nipples for redness and any abnormal appearance. Reddened areas may be improved by air-drying for 15 minutes. The health care professional may order an ointment to be applied on the nipples. Instruct the mother to remove any ointment before breastfeeding the newborn.
- When bathing, use warm water and no soap, because soap would remove protective skin oils.
- During the night and day the mother should wear a supportive bra specially constructed for breastfeeding mothers.
- A mother who is breastfeeding has extra nutritional and fluid needs. She is usually advised to drink additional liquids each day and to eat more calories and protein-rich foods. Vitamin and mineral supplements may be prescribed by the health care professional. The health care professional gives each mother individual instructions based on her request and needs.
- If prescribed by the health care professional, the mother is taught how to perform postpartum exercises. Immediate postpartum exercises can be performed in bed. Some exercises may be not be advised for certain mothers.

- To tighten perineal muscles, do exercises to strengthen the pelvic floor. Contract your buttocks for a count of five, and relax. Contract your buttocks and press your thighs together for a count of seven, and relax. Contract your buttocks, press your thighs together, and draw in your anus for a count of 10, and relax.
- To tighten calf muscles, do toe stretches while lying on your back. Keep your legs straight and point your toes away from you, then pull your legs toward you and point your toes toward your chest. Repeat 10 times.
- To tighten vaginal muscles and muscles in the bladder, do Kegel exercises. Contract the vaginal and bladder muscles as if stopping stream of urine. Do 15 per day, increasing by adding five more each week to a maximum of 40 per day.
- To increase cardiovascular health and overall mental state, walk every day. Wear good walking shoes. Begin by walking slowly for five to 10 minutes, and increase the speed and time by five minutes per day or as tolerated (Fig. 26-12).

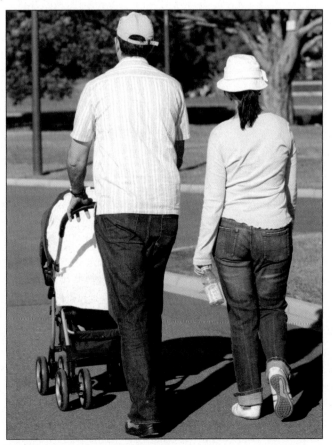

Fig. 26-12 - Go for a walk every day.

PROCEDURE 26-1. ASSISTING WITH A SITZ BATH

Items Needed
- disposable Sitz bath
- cover
- wash cloth
- towel
- gloves
- bath blanket

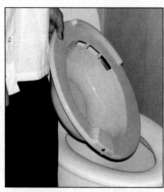

1. Fill the Sitz bath two thirds full with warm water. Check the water temperature with a thermometer. Place the disposable Sitz bath on the toilet. You may only need to set the Sitz bath up, or to demonstrate how to fill the bath with water and place it on the toilet so that the mother can do it on her own at home.

2. Put on gloves if you will be assisting with the Sitz bath.

3. Assist the mother if needed, to the bathroom. Help her remove clothing and the peripad, and then help her onto the toilet.

4. Cover her with a bath blanket.

5. If she complains of dizziness or feeling light-headed, stay with her until she feels better and then assist her back to bed.

6. Allow for privacy. Give her the call light.

7. Check on her every five minutes. Allow 15 to 20 minutes total for the bath, or stop when the water becomes too cold or the mother has had enough.

8. Assist her with washing, drying, and dressing. Help her safely return to her bed or chair if needed.

Note: *Most mothers will be able to take a Sitz bath alone.*

Being a new mother can be very overwhelming and stressful. Encourage the mother to take some time to exercise and to do things she enjoys. Encourage her to allow family members or others some special time with the newborn so she can have time off for herself. Siblings and family pets also need time and help to adjust to the newborn.

NEONATAL CARE
Think for a moment about how much work is involved in a fetus being born. After hours and hours of labor and delivery, expending enormous energy passing through the birth canal, the neonate's work is not over. Think about what needs to happen for the neonate to survive in the outside world.

After the immediate care in the delivery room, the neonate may spend time bonding with the mother, father, and other involved persons. Then the infant is transported to the newborn nursery. More procedures are done in the nursery. The health care team reports what procedures were done in the delivery room so the everyone knows what procedures still need to be carried out. The first 24 hours are critical for the newborn to adjust to the surroundings outside the mother's uterus. The key is to provide a safe and healthy beginning for the mother and new baby. The health care professionals are responsible for the care and health care teaching needed to care for the newborn (Fig. 26-13, next page).

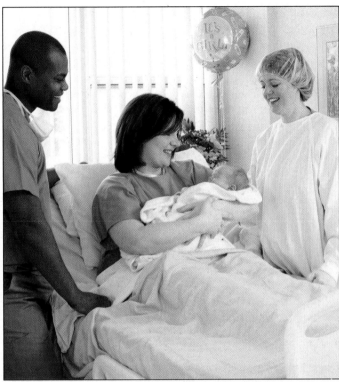

Fig. 26-13 - Health care professionals help the new mother care for the newborn.

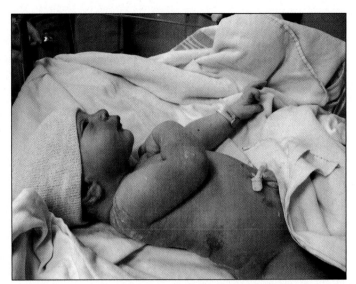

Fig. 26-14 - Clean the area around the umbilical cord with an antiseptic solution.

Standard precautions must be used when caring for the newborn. Following are some standard care activities:

• The newborn's vital signs are taken and recorded. Axillary temperature is taken every 30 to 60 minutes until it is normal, and then usually every four hours or when ordered. Take the axillary temperature by placing a thermometer in the axilla and pressing infant's arm gently but firmly against it for 10 minutes. Do not take a rectal temperature because this could irritate the rectal lining.

• When and how the newborn is bathed depend on the facility's policy. In some facilities a bath is given on admission to the nursery using a special antiseptic solution of oil or soap. Other facilities wait for 24 hours before giving the newborn a bath. Always follow your facility's policy.

• The area around the umbilical cord is cleaned with an antiseptic solution (Fig. 26-14).

• The height and weight are measured and recorded upon admission to the nursery and before discharge. The health care professional needs to know if the newborn has any weight loss.

• The newborn is wrapped in a warm blanket to keep the body warm. A cotton stockinet cap is placed on the newborn's head to prevent heat loss from the top of the head.

• Silver nitrate is sometimes administered to the newborn's eyes by a health care member to reduce the risk of infection from the birthing process.

• Feeding usually begins five to six hours after birth. Sometimes the mother is not sure if she wants to try breastfeeding and may have many questions. The health care team can answer the mother's questions and help her get started. Help teach the mother the benefits of breastfeeding or using expressed breast milk to feed the newborn. If the mother decides to bottle-feed, however, do not try to change her mind.

• If the newborn is a boy, the parents may want him circumcised before discharge from the hospital. In a **circumcision** the skin surrounding the penis (foreskin) is removed. The circumcision choice may be based on personal, religious, or cultural reasons. In some religions, circumcision is performed by a trained person in a special ceremony after discharge (Fig. 26-15, next page).

Circumcision – surgical removal of the foreskin at the head of the penis

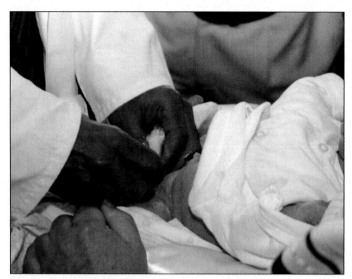
Fig. 26-15 - Performing a circumcision.

It is very important to help the new mother and others involved learn how to care for their new baby. Often there is much to learn in a very short period of time. Sometimes the amount of information can be overwhelming, especially for new parents. Be sensitive for signs of overload. Sometimes informational, "how to" literature is given. Common questions involve how to care for the newborn. You may want to review some of the more important frequently asked questions about bathing, diapering, proper lifting, holding and positioning, bonding, breastfeeding, care of a circumcision, and proper use of an infant car seat.

Promoting Neonatal Health

The mother, father, and involved others need to know what to look for and what to expect as they adjust to their new roles. The health care professional will review the following guidelines to help them maintain the health of the newborn:

- Encourage them to attend baby care and parenting classes.
- Encourage them to participate in the daily care of the infant, such as diapering and bathing the infant, while in the hospital (Procedures 26-2 and 26-3, pages 473-475).
- If the male newborn has a circumcision while in the hospital, teach them to perform circumcision care (Procedure 26-4, page 475).

Feeding an Infant

Assist the mother and infant in the breastfeeding process, following these guidelines:

- Have the mother wash her hands before feeding to help prevent infection.
- Have the mother get into a comfortable position.
- The mother should hold the baby close (to prevent muscle strain) with the infant facing the mother.
- To begin breastfeeding, the mother should cup the breast with her hand in a C position, with bottom of the breast in the palm of her hand and the thumb on top. Then place the nipple against the side of the infant's mouth. When the mouth opens, guide the nipple and the areola into the mouth. The infant should latch on so that as much of the areola as possible is in the infant's mouth. If the infant latches onto only the nipple, have the mother take the baby off the breast by putting the tip of her finger in the corner of the infant's mouth to break the suction (to prevent trauma and pain to the breast). Then reposition the infant on the breast (Fig. 26-16).

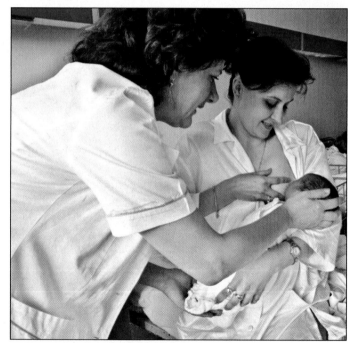
Fig. 26-16 - Breastfeeding the newborn.

(Text continued on p. 476)

PROCEDURE 26-2.   DIAPERING A NEWBORN

Items Needed
- clean diaper
- gloves
- plastic trash bag
- wash cloth or commercial baby wipe
- basin with warm water
- baby soap
- baby cream, lotion, or petroleum jelly if used
- antiseptic wipe, if used
- towel
- disposable or cloth changing pad
- supplies needed for cleaning around the umbilical cord or care of the circumcision

1. Put on gloves.

2. Remove the diaper by lifting the plastic tabs attached to the sides of the disposable diaper, or remove the diaper pins from a cloth diaper.

3. Wash, rinse, and dry the infant's genital area, using the same principles you learned for bathing a resident, or clean the genital area with the disposable wipe using the same principles for bathing the genital area.

4. Clean the area around the umbilical cord with an antiseptic wipe or as ordered, if applicable.

5. For newly circumcised male newborns only, clean and apply petroleum jelly to the head of the penis using a cotton-tipped applicator, if it was ordered. Then wrap it with a small piece of gauze.

6. Apply a small amount of cream or lotion to the genital area and buttocks to prevent diaper rash, if used.

7. With the clean diaper in one hand, gently grasp the infant's legs with your other hand. Raise them up enough to slide the diaper under the infant's buttocks. If using a cloth diaper, make a fold in the diaper in the front for a male infant and a fold in the back for a female; this adds extra protection where it is needed. Bring the diaper between the infant's legs.

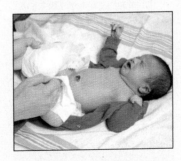

8. Hold the diaper snug around one hip and the abdomen, and fasten the tab snugly. Do the same for the other side. If using a cloth diaper, hold the cloth snugly with one hand while positioning the pin on each side carefully so the opening faces the infant's back. Do not pinch the infant's skin.

9. If the infant still has the umbilical cord stump, fold down the top of the diaper.

10. If using a cloth diaper, add a rubber pant over the diaper so the infant's clothes are not soiled. With a disposable diaper rubber pants are not needed.

Note the color and consistency of the infant's stool. Transitional stools change from tarry black to greenish black, to greenish brown, to brownish yellow, to greenish yellow.

PROCEDURE 26-3. BATHING A NEWBORN

▶ **REMEMBER: BE AWARE**

Items Needed

- three soft wash cloths or cotton balls
- basin filled with warm water or plastic disposable tub
- bath thermometer
- mild baby soap
- mild baby shampoo
- small disposable cup
- two towels
- clothes
- receiving blanket
- clean diaper
- two pairs of gloves
- plastic trash bag

1. Put on gloves. Undress the newborn, and remove the diaper. If using disposable diapers, dispose of the diaper in the plastic trash bag; if using a cloth diaper, dispose of the diaper into the container. Take off your gloves, and discard them in the plastic trash bag. You may want to place a wash cloth over the infant's genital area in case the infant voids during bathing.

Note: *Put on gloves if this is the infant's first bath. If not, use standard precautions as they apply to bathing. Put gloves on at the beginning of the bathing procedure if you are giving the infant a tub bath, because you use one hand to always hold the infant secure in the tub.*

2. Check the temperature of the water. It should be at 100 to 101 degrees F. If you do not

have a thermometer, use the inside of your wrist to test the water temperature. The water should be warm to the touch but not hot.

3. Begin by bathing the infant's eyes. With the wash cloth, make a mitt as you learned in Chapter 16. Using no soap, wash one eye at a time. Be sure to wash from inside corner of the eye outward toward the infant's ear, never using the same corner of the wash cloth twice. Rinse and dry the eyes.

4. Wash, rinse, and dry the infant's face, ears, and neck.

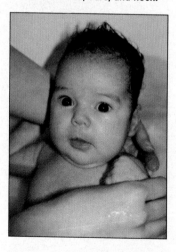

5. Pick up and hold the infant as though you were holding a football in one hand. Support the infant's head in your hand and rest the body on your forearm.

6. Holding the infant over the basin, wash the infant's head by pouring a small amount of warm water from the disposable cup over the infant's head. Do not let the water go into the infant's eyes. Place a small amount of shampoo (approximately the size of a dime) on the infant's head. Using gentle circular motions, wash the infant's head and hair. Rinse thoroughly by pouring more warm water from the cup over the infant's head. Pat dry.

7. If you are using a tub (after the umbilical cord stump has fallen off), gently place the infant into the tub filled with warm water feet first, using both your hands with one hand supporting the upper part of the infant including the head and neck, and one hand supporting the lower part of the infant's body. Once you have placed the infant into the tub, always keep one hand securely under the infant's upper back and shoulders to keep the infant safe. If you are not using a tub, the best way to bathe the rest of the infant's body is to lay the infant down on a clean surface.

8. Wash using baby soap. If the skin is dry, use only water because the soap may dry the infant's skin more. Rinse and dry the front of the infant

including the arms and hands. Clean around the umbilical cord stump, but do not get it wet.

9. Wash, rinse, and dry the legs and feet.

10. Carefully turn the infant over to a prone position. Wash, rinse, and dry the infant's back and buttocks. If bathing the infant in a tub, reverse the hold with your other hand holding the infant as you wash, rinse, and dry the infant's back and buttocks.

11. If you are not bathing the infant in a tub, put on gloves and with a new clean wash cloth, wash, rinse, and dry the perineal area of a female by gently spreading the labia, using a different corner of the wash cloth for each downward stroke. Move from the front of the genital area back toward the rear anal area. For a male infant, wash using a new clean wash cloth from the tip of the penis down the shaft toward the scrotum. Then wash the scrotum, groin, and anal area last. Be sure to clean between the skin folds. If the male has been circumcised, follow the procedure for caring for a circumcision. If bathing the infant in the tub, using a new clean wash cloth wash and rinse the genital are using the same principles described above for male and female infants.

PROCEDURE 26-3. BATHING A NEWBORN (CONTINUED)

12. With both hands lift the infant out of the tub, or place the infant after a sponge bath, onto a bath towel covering the infant's head.

13. Put on a clean diaper.

14. Dress the infant. Wrap the infant in the receiving blanket for warmth.

Note: *While bathing the infant, observe the skin and report any unusual findings. When bathing, move as quickly as possible so the infant does not loose unnecessary body heat.*

▶ **REMEMBER: UNDERSTAND**

PROCEDURE 26-4. CARE OF A CIRCUMCISION

▶ **REMEMBER: BE AWARE**

Items Needed
- gloves
- cotton-tipped applicator
- clean diaper
- basin with warm water
- wash cloth or commercially prepared wipes
- towel
- mild soap
- plastic trash bag
- petroleum jelly or gauze prepared with petroleum jelly

1. Put on gloves.

2. Place the infant on the back.

3. Remove the soiled diaper and dressing surrounding the tip of the penis, if one is present. Dispose of the soiled diaper and dressing in a plastic bag.

4. With each diaper change, gently clean the tip of the penis with warm water and mild soap. Rinse and dry this area. Then wash and dry the rest of the perineal area.

5. Put some petroleum jelly on a cotton-tipped applicator and place it on the tip of the penis. The health care professional may order a petroleum jelly gauze to be gently wrapped around the tip of the infant's penis for the first 24 to 48 hours after the procedure.

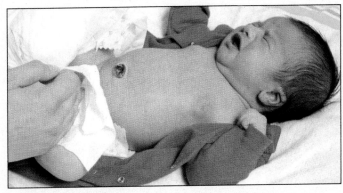

6. Put on a clean diaper.

▶ **REMEMBER: UNDERSTAND**

(text continued from p. 472)

- Tell the mother to alternate breasts. At the beginning, feedings generally take about 20 minutes, with 10 minutes on each breast. In time the mother can increase the time at each breast, allowing the infant to suck until the infant stops sucking.
- The mother should breastfeed frequently to maintain a good milk supply.
- The infant should be burped after feeding to help release the air in the stomach.
- The mother should air-dry her nipples for about 15 minutes after feeding to help prevent nipple trauma.
- Breastfeeding mothers must not take any medications except on the health care member's orders, because many substances pass into breast milk and may harm the milk production and/or the infant.

Bottle-fed infants are given baby formula. Formulas are ordered by the heath care team according to the infant's needs. The three types of formula are ready-to-feed, powder that is mixed with water, and liquid concentrate that is diluted with water (Fig. 26-17).

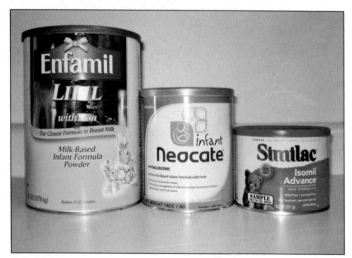

Fig. 26-17 - Types of formula to bottle feed an infant.

Follow these guidelines:
- With the powder and concentrate, the mother must follow the directions for how much water to mix.
- Bottles, nipples, and caps must be washed thoroughly in hot soapy water or in a dishwasher, then rinsed well.
- Bottles can be made up in advance but must be used within 24 hours and must be kept in a refrigerator. Teach the mother to first remove the bottle from the refrigerator and warm it under warm running water or in a container of warm water. Always test the temperature of the formula by squirting some on the inside of the wrist to make sure it is not too hot.
- Never microwave a bottle because this can heat the formula unevenly and burn the infant's mouth.
- When feeding the infant, the mother or father should make sure the nipple is filled with formula to prevent any excess air from entering the infant's stomach. Air can cause gas pain and discomfort (Fig. 26-18).

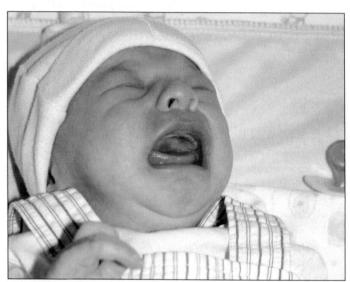

Fig. 26-18 - Air can cause gas pain and discomfort.

- The mother or father should always burp the infant after feedings to release any trapped air. To burp the infant, the person places a towel over their shoulder and gently lifts the baby up to their shoulder. Then gently pat or rub the infant's back for a few minutes or until the infant burps. The person can also hold the infant on their lap in a sitting position with one hand holding and supporting the infant's head and neck. Then burp the baby in the same manner as on the shoulder.
- The health care team will explain how much formula the infant should get at home. Generally, bottle-fed infants feed every three to four hours.

Additional Infant Care
- Explain the importance of bonding with the newborn by holding, touching, having eye contact, and talking to the infant.

- Teach the parents when to contact the infant's health care team. Parents should call for any of the following:
  - Vomiting all or some of feedings
  - Loss of appetite for two consecutive feedings
  - Diarrhea – three watery stools
  - Fever above 100 F (37.8 C) taken axillary for 10 minutes
  - Inability to awaken the baby to its usual state
  - Inconsolable crying or extreme irritability
- Explain the car seat law in your state. Infants and young children who ride in cars are required to be in a special safety seat. The seat must be put in the back seat facing the back of the seat, depending on the child's age. If needed, show the parents the correct way to install a car seat before the infant is discharged (Fig. 26-19).

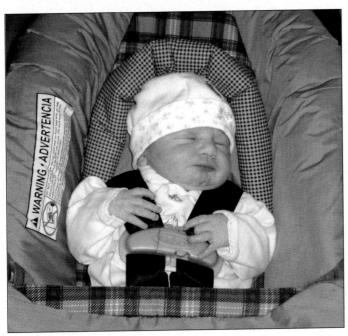

Fig. 26-19 - Infant in a car seat.

Certain standard procedures are followed before the mother and infant are discharged from the hospital. Follow your facility's procedures. Most discharge procedures include these steps:
- Make sure the identifications match for the mother and infant.
- Review all discharge orders with the mother and father.
- Ensure an appointment has been made for follow-up of the mother and infant.
- Give the mother literature to read on child care subjects she had asked about.

- Give the family the immediate supplies needed to care for the infant.
- Transport the mother and infant out of the hospital in a wheelchair by a health care team member.
- Document all discharge information.

WORKING WITH CHILDREN

As a nurse assistant, you may work in a pediatric clinic, office, or pediatric floor in a hospital. When you care for children, you must also include the child's family. The family does not always mean a mother, father, and siblings. Today, "family" is defined as the people the child lives with. The family may be made up of a variety of people. Many children live with grandparents, one parent only, stepparents, or foster parents. The person named as the child's legal guardian has the right to consent for care and hospitalization. In every pediatric environment you and the health care team need to know the legal guardian for every child treated (Fig. 26-20).

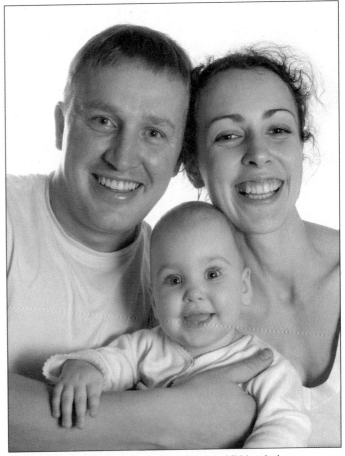

Fig. 26-20 - Know the legal guardian of every child treated.

Certain standard procedures are done when a child comes to the clinic, office, or hospital. One of the first procedures is for the health care team to obtain a health and social history. You may assist in obtaining some information such as the child's name, nickname, age, family information, the child's likes and dislikes, how well they eat, and their sleeping patterns. Someone on the health care team performs a physical exam. You may assist in gathering data, collecting specimens, taking vital signs, measuring the child's height and weight, and assisting the child with dressing and undressing. One area that is different in the physical exam of a child is the focus on the child's growth and development (Fig. 26-21).

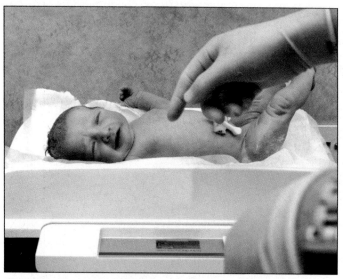

Fig. 26-21 - The physical exam of a child focuses on the child's growth and development.

GROWTH AND DEVELOPMENT

Do you have any children? How old are they now? Have you often wondered where the time went or said to yourself, "My kids grew so fast." You are not alone—many parents feel and say the same about their children. Children grow and develop through many stages. Growth and development begin with birth. As infants and children grow and mature, they go through predictable stages of development. Understanding growth and development helps the health care team and other professionals involved with children screen for physical and emotional problems. Knowledge about growth and development can help guide parents and other caregivers as well (Fig. 26-22).

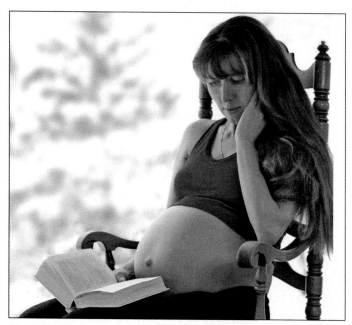

Fig. 26-22 - Knowledge of growth and development can help caregivers and parents.

Different screening methods are used to help the health care team and parents know if the infant or child is growing and developing normally. These screening guides closely evaluate the child according to usual milestones for the child's age. Most guides include charts separated by different ages, beginning at birth to four weeks up to young adulthood. For each stage, areas such as motor development are subdivided into lists of skills that a normal infant or child should be displaying or should have mastered by the specific age. Growth and development charts also assess social, emotional, and psychosocial development.

Growth and development should always be considered carefully when working with infants and children. You will learn firsthand how important your role is in assisting and encouraging a child's growth and development, especially in a hospitalized child. The history and physical exam include questions for the child and parent to see if the child is growing and developing at a normal rate for their age.

Developmental Milestones

Table 26-1 (next page) shows one example of a guide the health care team may use to evaluate a child's development. A parent or guardian is interviewed during the physical exam. Questions are asked about milestones in achievements that most parents can remember. After the interview, the health care member can determine the child's developmental quotient according to the parent's answers. A developmental quotient less than 70% means there may be a developmental delay. The health care team would then order further testing.

After the physical exam, the pediatrician determine whether the child needs further tests. The child's visit may be for an annual physical exam and any needed immunizations.

Your Role in Caring for Hospitalized Children

Most children who are hospitalized are first seen in the emergency department for an acute problem, then sent to a pediatric floor. Most pediatric floors try to keep age groups together. If you are working with children in a specific age group, you should understand their developmental level. Knowing what is considered normal can help you encourage the child during their hospital stay. Children often regress to an earlier stage of development when hospitalized (Fig. 26-23).

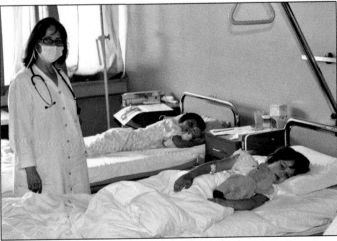

Fig. 26-23 - Children in a hospital can regress to an earlier stage of development.

When a child is admitted to a pediatric floor, often a parent stays with the child. Standard procedures that must be followed when a child is admitted include:

- Wash your hands.
- Introduce yourself to the child and parent(s).
- Explain what you will be doing.
- Assist the child in taking off his/her clothes if necessary (the child may want only the parent to help).
- If the child does not have an identification bracelet from the emergency department, put one on.
- Take and record the child's vital signs. (Remember children have smaller arms than adults, and use an appropriate size cuff to take the blood pressure.)
- Measure and record the child's height and weight.
- Give the child and parent an orientation to the floor (such as call lights and bathroom) and facility policies (if applicable). Explain routine events such as meals and visiting hours.
- Let the parents know they should tell a team member when they will be leaving the floor.
- Tell parents it is a good idea to allow siblings to visit the child.
- Make parents and family feel welcome. Have them participate in care if possible, because they help minimize the child's separation anxiety.

The leading cause of death in the United States for children is injury. As a health care team member caring for a hospitalized child, you need to provide a safe environment. Therefore you should:

- Provide age-appropriate toys. Never allow small children to play with small objects that could potentially cause choking.
- Keep bed side rails up and crib side rails up for safety (Fig. 26-24, page 482).
- Line the crib with soft bumpers or rolled blankets to avoid injury.
- Never allow pacifiers to be tied around the infant or child's neck or taped to the child's mouth.
- Remove any jewelry from around the child's neck and give it to parents for safe keeping.
- Never tie balloons to or near beds or cribs.
- Never leave an infant or child alone with the side rails down.
- Never prop bottles up for infants to feed on their own.
- Remove all sharp items from the child's reach. Use a sharps container to dispose of needles.

(Text continued on p. 482)

Immunization – protected against a disease by vaccination

TABLE 26-1
DEVELOPMENTAL MILESTONES

AGE	PHYSICAL CHANGES AND ABILITIES	SENSE AND MENTAL ABILITIES	SOCIAL ABILITIES
2 months	• Newborn reflexes (like grasping reflex) disappear • Able to hold head still without moving it too much • Able to lift head 45 degrees when on stomach • Less flexing of arms and legs while on stomach	• Head turns side to side with sound at level of ear • Begins to look at close objects • Crying becomes differentiated (different kinds of crying) • Coos (makes soft sounds) • Vocal response to familiar voices	• Recognizes faces • Recognizes parents • Smiles
4 months	• Slower weight gain • Better able to hold head still while in sitting position • Able to sit up straight with help • Can raise head 90 degrees when on stomach • Able to roll from front to back • Tries to reach objects with hands • Able to hold rattle with both hands • Able to place objects in mouth	• Well-established close vision • Begins hand-eye coordination • Able to babble and coo • Able to laugh out loud • Begins to show memory • Recognizes parent's voice or touch	• Reaches for familiar objects • Reaches for people • Anticipates feedings when able to see bottle • Enjoys looking around environment • Demands attention by fussing
6 months	• Doubled birth weight • Able to lift chest and head while on stomach • Able to support weight on hands • Able to sit in a high chair with a straight back • Able to support almost all weight when supported in a standing position • Able to roll from back to stomach • Able to hold own bottle • Able to pick up dropped object	• Has 20/60 to 20/40 vision • Can locate sounds not made at ear level • Starts to imitate sounds • Can make sounds that sound like one-syllable words • Begins to imitate actions	• Recognizes strangers • Begins to fear strangers
9 months	• Gains weight more slowly (approximately 15 grams per day) • Shows parachute reflex to protect self from falling • Able to crawl • Able to sit for a long time • Able to pull self to standing position • Can hold objects between thumb and index finger • Throws or shakes objects	• Develops depth perception • Responds to simple commands • Responds to name • Imitates speech sounds • May be afraid of being left alone	• Feeds self with fingers • Starts to explore environment; • Plays gesture games (e.g., pat-a-cake) • Understands the meaning of "no"
12 months	• Tripled birth weight • Circumference of head and chest are equal • Soft spot at top of head nearly closed • Able to pull self to standing position and walk with help or alone • Able to sit down with help • Can hold an object exactly between thumb and index finger	• Follows fast-moving object with eyes • Has control over response to sounds • Understands several words • Can say "mama," "papa," and at least 1-2 other words • Understands simple commands • Tries to imitate animal sounds • Associates names with objects • Points to objects with index finger • Waves "bye-bye" • Is anxious if separated from parent • Explores away from parents in familiar settings	• Imitates actions • Comes when called • Cooperates with dressing

TABLE 26-1
DEVELOPMENTAL MILESTONES (*CONTINUED*)

AGE	PHYSICAL CHANGES AND ABILITIES	SENSE AND MENTAL ABILITIES	SOCIAL ABILITIES
18 months	• Soft spot at top of head completely closed • Able to control sphincter muscles • Able to run, but without coordination • Able to jump in same place • Able to walk up stairs while holding on with one hand • Able to use spoon and cup with help • Imitates scribbling	• Shows affection • Listens to a story or looks at pictures • Can say 10 or more words • Identifies parts of the body • Frequently imitates others • Feeds self • Able to take off some clothing items • Begins to feel sense of ownership by saying "my"	• Uses spoon and cup without help (15-18 months) • Imitates parent's actions (sweeping, dusting) • Plays with other children
2 years	• Psychologically ready for toilet training • Can run with better coordination • Can kick ball without losing balance • Can browse through book one page at a time • Able to turn a door knob • Can pick up objects while standing without losing balance	• Vision fully developed • Vocabulary increased to 50 to 300 words • Can organize phrases of 2 or 3 words • Able to communicate needs such as thirst and hunger • Increased attention span • Able to dress self in simple clothes	• Asks for food • Asks to go to the toilet • Plays with others (but beside them, not with them)
3 years	• Gains weight at rate of 4 to 5 pounds a year • Has improved balance • Has improved vision • Daytime control over bowel and bladder functions • Can briefly balance on one foot • May walk up stairs with alternating feet • Can easily place small objects in a small opening • Can copy a circle • Can pedal a tricycle	• Has a vocabulary of hundreds of words • Composes sentences of 3 to 4 words • Counts up to 3 objects • Uses plural and pronouns (he/she) • Frequently asks questions • Can dress self without much help • Has longer attention span • Feeds self without difficulty • Acts out social situations through play activities • Less anxious if separated from parent • Fears imaginary things • Knows own name, age, and gender (boy/girl)	• Says first and last name when asked • Gets self drink without help • Plays in a group • Shares toys • Takes turns • Plays well with others • Knows full name, age, and sex
4 years	• Gains weight at rate of 6 grams per day • Has improved balance • Can hop on one foot without losing balance • Can throw a ball overhand with coordination • Can cut out pictures using scissors	• Has vocabulary over 1500 words • Easily makes sentences of 4 or 5 words • Can use past tense • Can count to 4 • Will ask more questions than at any other age • Learns and sings simple songs • Tries to be independent • Understands time better • Able to tell the difference between two objects based on size and weight	• Tells imaginary stories • Plays cooperatively with a group of children • Often has imaginary playmates

TABLE 26-1
DEVELOPMENTAL MILESTONES (*CONTINUED*)

AGE	PHYSICAL CHANGES AND ABILITIES	SENSE AND MENTAL ABILITIES	SOCIAL ABILITIES
5 years	• Developing increased coordination • Skipping, jumping, and hopping with good balance • Can keep balance while standing on one foot with eyes closed • Can tie own shoelaces • Increases skill with simple tools and writing utensils • Can copy a triangle • Can spread butter, peanut butter, etc. with a knife	• Has vocabulary of over 2100 words • Composes sentences of 6 to 8 words • Identifies coins • Counts to 10 and names colors • Answers "why" questions • Behaves more responsibly and apologizes for mistakes • Has fewer childhood fears • Show increased skill in math • Questions others • Identifies with the parent of the same sex • Has a group of friends • Uses imagination when playing	• Plays competitive games • Obeys rules • Likes to help with household jobs

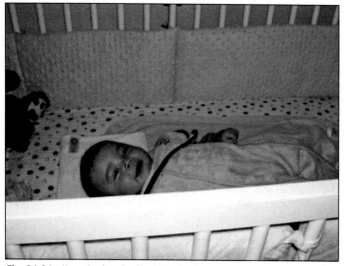

Fig. 26-24 - Keep bed and crib side rails up.

(text continued from p. 479)

Safety Tips To Teach Parents

In addition to providing a safe environment, teach parents, children, and siblings about safety measures to prevent injuries. Remember that every health care team member involved with children is responsible for safety. Share this information with children and parents:

• About 90% of all accidents could have been prevented.
• The type of injury likely to occur is directly related to the child's age and developmental level. Parents who know how their child usually behaves may be able to prevent an injury.
• All children are naturally impulsive and curious. They can be very impatient and may not wait even when told to do so. They love to investigate things such as animals or electric plugs by touching and feeling them. Parents and health care team members must help children learn to play in safe environments.
• Children often copy their parents' and siblings' behavior. Everyone should be a good role model and always be safe.

Preventing injury is the key goal for everyone involved with children. It is your job to help the team educate the parents and others about safety. Following are common areas for parent education:

Emergency situations
• Teach children their name, address, and telephone number.
• Keep emergency telephone numbers by the telephone. Teach children who and how to call in an emergency (Fig. 26-25, next page).
• Have a first aid kit for minor cuts and burns.

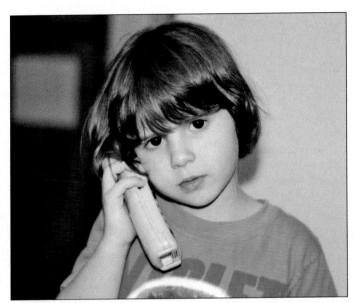

Fig. 26-25 - Teach children who and how to call in an emergency.

Safety around electricity
- Keep radios, transportable heaters, and hair dryers out of bathrooms and away from water.
- Keep garden equipment and machinery in a restricted area.
- Do not allow children to play in area where power tools are used.

Motor vehicle safety
- Use properly installed car seats and seat belts. Know the guidelines for car restraints depending on the child's weight and age.
- Infants riding in a rear-facing car seat should never be placed in a front seat equipped with an air bag.
- The center rear seat is the safest seat in the car for a child.
- Never leave young children in a car alone.
- Always look when backing out of a driveway. Remove all toys from the driveway so that a child is not tempted to run into the driveway when you are pulling out.

Prevent falls
- Keep stairs well lighted and free from toys and clutter.
- Use rubber mats in the bathtub and shower.

Prevent poisonings
- Keep the Poison Control Center number by the telephone for everyone to see.
- Label and keep poisonous household cleaners and chemicals out of children's reach.

Sports and recreation safety
- Always wear a helmet during activities like riding a bike, skate boarding, and skiing.
- Wear appropriate clothing and safety equipment for the activity (Fig. 26-26).

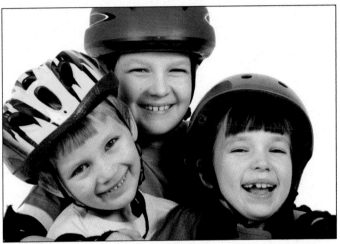

Fig. 26-26 - Wear appropriate clothing and safety equipment for the activity.

- Keep guns, weapons, and ammunition locked up.

Fire prevention and safety
- Teach children fire escape routes as soon as they are old enough.
- Have all children wear flame-retardant sleepwear.
- Mark children's rooms so they are obvious to firefighters.
- Teach children to stop, drop, and roll if their clothing catches fire.
- Store gasoline and other flammable liquids in tightly covered containers that are labeled and stored away from heat and children.
- Keep all smoke detectors in working order.

Swimming pool safety
- Instruct children about safety rules.
- Enclose the pool with a fence that meets regulations (Fig. 26-27, next page).
- Install at least one ladder with handrails at each end of the pool.
- Have proper lighting and label water depths in and around the pool.

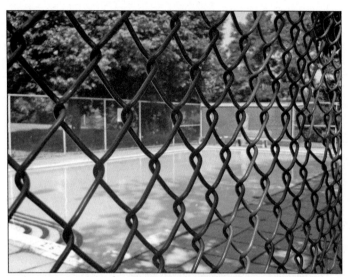

Fig. 26-27 - Enclose the pool with a fence that meets regulations.

In addition to helping the health care team educate parents and children about safety issues, you may also be responsible for routine hospital procedures. These include taking and recording vital signs, weights, and intake and output, as well as bathing, feeding, and changing diapers. Always follow standard precautions when caring for children. Promoting play time is another important part of caring for children. Provide comfort, affection, and love to the children you care for. If the child feels secure and trusts the health care team, healing may occur sooner and may be less traumatic for the child.

Preventing Illness in Children

Children are hospitalized for many different reasons. Regardless of whether the child is in a hospital or just coming for a clinic or office visit, preventing illness and injury are especially important for children. Childhood morbidity has decreased in recent years, but childhood deaths from injuries remain the same. The only way for us to improve this situation is to educate everyone involved. The more we teach parents about safety and health, the fewer deaths will occur.

One common illness we can help prevent is lead poisoning. About one million U.S. children have elevated blood levels of lead. Lead poisoning results from some form of lead ingestion. Elevated blood lead levels can affect a child's mental functions. Houses built before 1950 have the highest surface soil level and internal household dust contaminated with lead. Millions of children live in these houses today. A child can ingest house dust containing lead during normal hand-to-mouth activities. Children with pica who ingest nonfood items such as lead paint chips have more dangerous lead levels in their blood. Children can ingest lead particles in many other ways because lead is used in many things. U.S. laws prohibit painting the inside of homes with lead paint, but the problem still exists in older homes where deeper levels of paint and plaster contaminated with lead are still present. Education, screening, and prevention are needed. An educated parent will be more alert and much more cautious.

Preventing lead poisoning is not the only focus of health care teams. Pediatric health care also focuses on health promotion and disease prevention. Early interventions can positively affect the well being of children and their families. The goal of pediatric health care teams is to achieve physical, emotional, and developmental health for all children. Primary prevention through immunizations, proper nutrition, and safety counseling are key parts of pediatric health care.

Immunizations Prevent Illness

Immunizations have significantly reduced childhood illness and death caused by infectious diseases. However, despite effective immunizations, diseases that can be prevented with vaccines are still present in the United States and pose public health problems. As a nurse assistant, you play a vital role in promoting a child's health by educating family members about immunizations. At every visit to the health care team, the child's immunizations record should be reviewed. Any needed vaccines should be given to keep the child up to date. Every parent or legal guardian must receive a thorough explanation about needed immunizations. In addition, every parent should know the requirements of the National Childhood Vaccine Injury Act (1988). This law says that every parent should know all about vaccines their child receives. The law also says what information must be documented and how. Routine immunizations are started in infants but can be started at any age if the child missed them earlier. The schedule of immunizations depends on the child's age and specific diseases common at the time (Fig. 26-28, next page).

Pica – having an appetite for nonfood items of no nutritional value

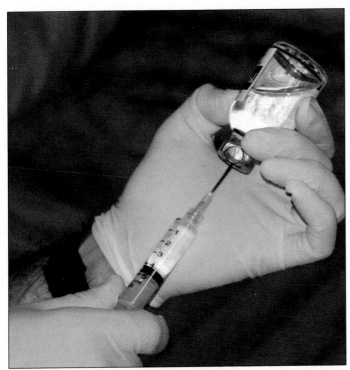

Fig. 26-28 - Schedule of immunizations depends on the child's age and specific diseases common at the time.

Preventing Childhood and Communicable Diseases

In the United States, immunizations have greatly decreased many childhood diseases. On the other hand, many communicable diseases still cause significant illness in children.

Not all diseases have vaccines. Contagious diseases are a great concern for health care teams, communities, schools, and parents. These diseases include:

• Strep throat
• Rubella (German measles)
• Roseola
• Measles
• Mumps
• Erythema infectiosum (fifth disease or slapped cheek)
• Pertusis (whopping cough)
• Staph infections

When caring for children with communicable diseases, always use standard precautions. Teach family members the importance of hand washing and how to prevent the spread of germs. To prevent these diseases, every health care team should continue to educate and promote good living habits.

PROMOTING HEALTH FROM INFANCY INTO YOUNG ADULTHOOD

Good health habits are a key for developing into a healthy adult. Good habits can begin as early as infancy. As infants grow into toddlers, they can learn good health habits like hand washing. This is especially important for toddlers during potty training. While progressing from preschool years to school age and then into adolescence and young adulthood, the person should learn both universal and age-appropriate habits. Universal good health habits for all age groups include:

• infection control measures
• safety
• proper nutrition (Fig. 26-29)
• immunizations
• proper exercise
• proper rest
• regular check-ups

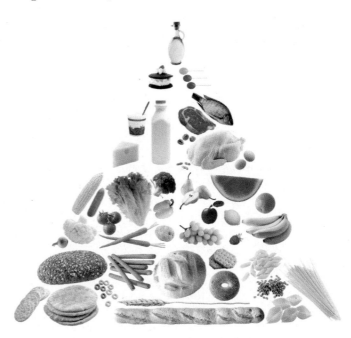

Fig. 26-29 - Proper nutrition is necessary for good health.

In addition, promote good health habits for specific age groups:

Newborn to 1 year

• Promote security, love, warmth, and affection.
• Promote regular check-ups to evaluate the infant's development.

Toddler – 1 to 3 years
- Promote an environment that allows toddlers to safely gain independence.
- Promote regular check-ups to evaluate the child's development. This includes speech and language skills, and bowel and bladder training.
- Promote play (note that toddlers play alongside other children but not with them).

Preschool – 3 to 6 years
- Promote regular check-ups to evaluate the child's development. This includes increasing ability to communicate, performing self-care, knowing right from wrong, and using imagination in play.

School age – 6 to 9 years
- Promote regular check-ups to evaluate the child's development. This includes developing age-appropriate social and physical skills, developing a conscience and morals, striving to achieve, and interest in bodily functions.

Adolescence – 9 to 18 years
- Promote regular check-ups to evaluate the child's development into adulthood. This is a time when numerous body changes occur.
- Promote adolescents' understanding of how to care for their body as it changes. This is a time of rapid physical and social growth. Adolescents enter puberty in this stage. During puberty the reproductive organs begin to function and secondary sex characteristics develop.
- Promote acceptance of the changing body, developing relationships in one's own age group, developing sound morals and values, accepting rules while also developing independence. Provide guidance.
- Promote sex education and good hygiene.
- Promote good social and nutritional choices. At this time learning social skills and making healthy choices is very important. Adolescents strive to fit in. Healthy eating habits are very important. Often adolescents are very conscious of changes in their body. Be careful of adolescents going on a diet because they are not happy with how they look or want to look like someone they know.

Young adulthood – age 18 into early 20s
- Promote making good social choices. This is a time when there is enormous pressure to experiment with drugs, alcohol, and sex. The young adult needs the facts around all the risks involved.
- Promote making good health habits. Bad habits may carry into adulthood when being a good role model for their own children is important.
- Provide guidance for living a productive life. This includes developing skills for problem solving, love, selecting a partner, developing open honest relationships, deciding about a career, and raising children.

Understanding the stages of child development will help you care for children of all ages. You are part of a large team of professionals made up of teachers, health care workers, social workers, local and government agencies, and parents and family. Together, all are responsible for promoting good health habits so children can grow to become healthy, happy adults.

Today, more attention being paid to risk behaviors. These behaviors often cause death, disability, and social problems in children through young adulthood. Federal agencies like the Department of Health and Human Services Center for Disease Control and Prevention (CDC) work with state and local governments, schools, health care teams, and parents to develop strategies to address risky behaviors. These agencies also focus on common diseases such as asthma. Asthma is the leading chronic illness among children and adolescents in the United States. Their goal is to decrease deaths, emergency room visits, hospitalizations, and missed school days. Education programs help youths and schools manage the disease as well.

These agencies also have programs to educate youths about behavior risks. Targeted risk behaviors include:
- physical activity and obesity
- tobacco use
- alcohol (including binge drinking), drug, and other substance abuse
- sexual behavior (abstinence, birth control, and use of condoms)
- pregnancy in adolescent girls
- sexually transmitted diseases such as Chlamydia and HIV
- suicide attempts
- seat belt use
- injuries, violence, and homicides

For the greatest impact, everyone involved with adolescents and young adults should promote healthy habits and work to change these risky behaviors.

IN THIS CHAPTER YOU LEARNED:

- The importance of prenatal care
- What normal pregnancy is like
- The importance of childbirth classes
- What occurs during labor and delivery and standard procedures for newborns
- How to provide postpartum care to a mother
- How to assist with a Sitz bath
- How to diaper a newborn, bathe a newborn, and care for a circumcision
- When parents should call the health care team for their newborn
- What standard procedures are followed before mother and newborn are discharged from the hospital
- What pediatric areas you can work in
- Why evaluating growth and development is important
- What standard procedures must be followed when a child is admitted to a pediatric floor
- Safety tips to teach parents and children
- How important immunizations are for all children
- Universal health habits for all ages and behavior risks for youths today

SUMMARY

This chapter briefly introduces the fields of obstetrics and pediatrics. Obstetrics focuses on labor and delivery and postpartum care of the mother and newborn. Pediatrics focuses on children from infancy to young adulthood. A nurse assistant may work in any of these areas. Although there is much to learn in each area beyond this chapter, many basic skills are universal. These skills are used in any health care setting. Every individual deserves to be treated in a respectful, safe manner.

Care in all these areas focuses on promoting health and preventing disease. As a nurse assistant, you are in a unique position to assist the health care team in educating new mothers, children, adolescents, and young adults to maintain their health. Remember that the basic principles you have learned in earlier chapters can be adapted for these exciting health care fields. For example, the principles for giving a bed bath to a resident in a long term care facility are the same as for bathing a newborn.

PULLING IT ALL TOGETHER

Imagine you are working in a family clinic that provides many different services. You may care for a woman early in her pregnancy, and follow her through the three trimesters until the birth of her baby. The labor, delivery, and initial postpartum care likely take place in a hospital or home setting. In the first follow-up visit for the mother and newborn, you finally meet the new baby. The focus of your care is to assist the health care team to help the mother and newborn get a healthy start. After reviewing the labor and delivery details, the team teaches the mother about postpartum changes she can expect as she returns to her pre-pregnant state. A physical exam is performed to make sure the healing process is coming along well. It is also important to gather facts about how mother and newborn are doing. While gathering this information, you write down any questions the mother may have about her condition and the care of the newborn. You give this to the health care team. The mother may have so many questions about breastfeeding, for example, that the team offers to have a nurse breastfeeding specialist visit the mother at home.

In addition to caring for the mother, you may also care for the newborn. In a family clinic, pediatric care begins just after birth. The mother makes an appointment for newborn care before leaving the hospital or as soon as she gets home. If you continue to work in the same family clinic, you may keep caring for the growing child. Imagine watching the newborn grow through the toddler years, into school age years, and on into adolescence and young adulthood. Many health care teams have the honor of getting to know generations of family members.

1. **Which of these is a nurse assistant's responsibility in a prenatal physical exam?**
   A. Measuring the pregnant woman's height and weight and recording the results.
   B. Prenatal teaching about what unusual signs and symptoms to report immediately, such as vaginal bleeding, elevated blood pressure, or swelling in the hands and feet.
   C. Obtaining a blood sugar sample.
   D. Instructing the pregnant woman when to come to the hospital during labor.

2. **What signs and symptoms are normal in the first trimester of pregnancy?**
   A. Menstrual period absent and positive pregnancy test.
   B. Back pain, swollen feet, indigestion, and short of breath.
   C. Feeling contractions as the uterus gets ready for birth.
   D. May feel the fetus moving.

3. **To prepare for birth, the pregnant woman and significant other(s) should attend childbirth classes. What will they learn?**
   A. They will learn what to expect when labor begins, as labor progresses, and about birth.
   B. They will learn techniques to prevent pregnancy.
   C. They will view a film about high-risk births.
   D. They will learn that birthing centers close at 5 p.m. everyday, so if labor begins they must arrive before 5 p.m.

4. **At the end of pregnancy, at approximately 40 weeks, the woman normally shows signs that labor is about to begin. These signs include which of the following?**
   A. The amniotic sac remains intact.
   B. The fetus "drops" (moves down into the birth canal).
   C. The uterus does not begin to contract.
   D. The mucous plug stays in place during labor.

5. **Approximately how long can a pregnant woman expect to be in labor the first time?**
   A. 18-24 hours.
   B. 6-10 hours.
   C. 48-72 hours.
   D. 24-48 hours.

6. **The health care professional will observe and record the neonate's status using the Apgar assessment. What is observe and recorded with this assessment?**
   A. Respiratory rate, heart rate, and color.
   B. Color, heart rate, and reflexes.
   C. Vital signs, color, reflexes, and muscle tone.
   D. Heart rate, respiratory effort, muscle tone, reflexes, and color.

7. **What is a mother at risk for developing during the first hour after delivering a newborn?**
   A. Hemorrhaging.
   B. Losing too much weight.
   C. Elevation of vital signs.
   D. Infection at the episiotomy site.

8. **Why might a pregnant woman need a Cesarean section?**
   A. The fetus is in distress during birth.
   B. The mother had a previous cesarean section birth.
   C. Labor fails to progress.
   D. All of the above.

9. **What is the leading cause of death for children in the U.S.?**
   A. Cancer.
   B. Lead poison.
   C. Communicable disease.
   D. Injury.

10. **What is a major risk factor for young adults today?**
    A. Being too shy.
    B. Sports injuries.
    C. Sexually transmitted diseases.
    D. Cancer.

(Answers to "Check What You've Learned" are in the Instructor's Manual.)

Chapter 27

RESTORATIVE ACTIVITIES

Rehabilitation (rehab) and restorative activities are used to help residents improve their abilities such as walking, getting up, moving, dressing, and bathing. Rehabilitative care focuses on restoring, improving, or maintaining these abilities. Residents in rehabilitation develop new skills or work on existing skills to live as independently as they can. The goal is to help the residents become as independent as possible, for as long as possible. Restorative activities have great benefits for residents. They involve teaching, prompting, and encouraging residents to care for themselves. You can help residents in rehabilitation by using restorative activities as often as possible in your caregiving.

This chapter is about you as a teacher helping residents learn or relearn information and skills to regain or maintain independent functioning. You will learn how to work with residents in restorative activities. You will learn how to help residents use special equipment and devices to function independently and safely. With your thoughtful attention to residents' physical and emotional needs, you can help improve their quality of life.

CMS guidelines state that all nursing facilities must ensure that a resident's ability to perform the activities of daily living do not diminish unless the resident's health deteriorates. It is part of your job to help them retain their skills and improve whenever they can.

Restorative activities help residents function as independently as possible at whatever level they are able to perform. "Function" means how well particular parts of the body work and how well the whole person accomplishes activities. The more residents can do for themselves—safely—the more functional they are.

OBJECTIVES
- Describe your role in promoting independence
- List different kinds of equipment that promote independence
- Demonstrate range-of-motion exercises and assisted walking

MEDICAL TERMS
- **Brace** – device that supports and strengthens a body part
- **Extremity** – a limb of the body
- **Orthotic device** – supportive equipment made for a resident, such as a brace or splint
- **Prosthetic device** – device made to replace a missing body part or function
- **Rehabilitation** – the process of restoring to a former state
- **Restorative** – activities that help a person be as independent and functional as possible
- **Splint** – device to use to support or immobilize a body part
- **Trapeze** – a short horizontal bar suspended by two parallel ropes, used to pull oneself up in bed

PROCEDURE 27-1
Range-of-Motion Exercises

PROCEDURE 27-2
Assisting With Walking

"Every day I get stronger. I couldn't have done it without you."

Think of activities in your daily life that you take for granted. You get out of bed in the morning. You sit down and then get up off the chair, sofa, or toilet. You walk to the bathroom. You brush your teeth, shower, get dressed. You do hundreds of things everyday. We take for granted that we can get to the bathroom, lift the toothbrush to our mouth, and so on. But many residents do not have these abilities because illness or disability limits their capability for movement. A resident may not be able to reach their feet to put on socks. A resident may not be able to get out of bed and into the wheelchair by themselves. Instead, they will look to you for assistance.

Imagine what it must feel like, after taking these actions for granted most of your life, to be unable to do these things by yourself or to have to learn to do them in a different way. Imagine how frustrating it must be to have to ask someone else to help you all the time (Fig. 27-1). As a nurse assistant, you need to help the resident learn to adapt to their status with respect and patience.

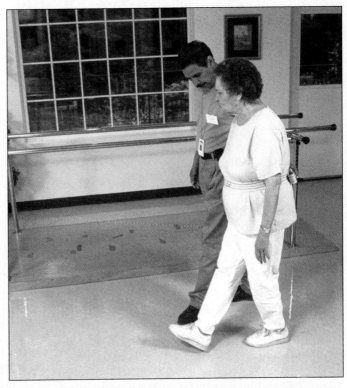

Fig. 27-2 – Restorative activities are designed to help residents regain or maintain their ability to take care of themselves.

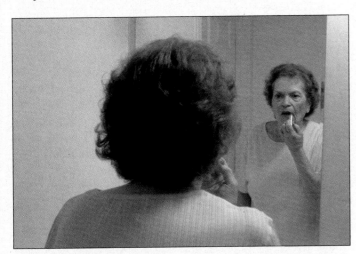

Fig. 27-1 – Imagine how you would feel if you were unable to do things by yourself.

WHAT ARE RESTORATIVE ACTIVITIES?

Restorative activities are ways you can help residents regain or maintain their ability to care for themselves (Fig. 27-2). Everything you do with a resident should involve such activities. Whenever you are helping a resident, ask yourself, "What can I do to help this person regain or maintain their independence?"

Restorative activities promote a person's independence in daily activities. These include eating, bathing, dressing, toileting, and transferring (mobility). These are called the activities of daily living, or ADLs. The goal is to help the resident achieve their optimal, or best, level of functioning with their ADLs.

Restorative activities can be anything done in a way that helps restore function. Sometimes it may seem easier and faster for you to do something for the resident yourself, but this would not be the best care for them. How you interact with a resident can help optimize their function or make them feel more dependent and helpless.

Make sure you ask the resident to perform activities in a clear, respectful way. Keep in mind their capabilities. Encourage them to participate as fully as they can. Give them enough time to complete the task. Prompt, teach, and cue them with patience as needed. How you ask residents to do something, how patient you are with their capabilities, and how you encourage and prompt them make a big difference in their ability to do a task.

Capability – being able to do something
Restorative – activities that help a person be as independent and functional as possible

They may need you to teach them simple everyday activities. These may include how to get out of bed, get dressed, and use a walker or wheel themselves in a wheelchair. Restorative activities also include special activities like exercise. As you support residents in their daily routine, be sure not to do for a resident what they can do themselves. Following are some examples:

1. Mr. Ellis can sit up by himself. It is better for him if you ask him to sit up and give him the time to do so, while you stand by to help if needed, than to lift him to a sitting position.
2. Mrs. Weiss uses a walker to walk to the dining room with help. It is better for her if you help her walk to the dining room using her walker than to wheel her in a wheelchair to the dining room.
3. Mr. White cannot move at all by himself but is **alert** and can converse. It is better for him if you do his range-of-motion (ROM) exercises and talk to him about what you are doing and why, asking how he feels or if anything hurts during the exercise, than to move his arms and legs for him without involving him at all in what you are doing.
4. Mr. West is hard of hearing and sometimes confused. He can walk by himself but forgets to at times. It is better for him if you face him and ask him to get up and walk to the bathroom than to speak with your back to him to remind him to walk to the bathroom by himself (Fig. 27-3).

What do you notice in each example? Why is one technique more helpful to the resident than the other? In each case, it is important to promote the resident's independence. The resident's own success is the primary focus, instead of you just getting the task done.

HELPING RESIDENTS IN THE RESTORATIVE PROCESS

Restorative programs have these key elements:
- short- and long-term goals
- teaching, **prompting**, and encouraging
- assistive devices
- exercise and mobility

The following sections discuss each of these. Design the care you provide around these key elements. If you do not understand how any activity in the care plan will help the resident, talk about it with the charge nurse or the physical therapist.

SHORT- AND LONG-TERM GOALS

We often set goals for what we want to accomplish. Goals help us plan specific ways to make improvements. To help residents optimize their independence, the interdisciplinary team and resident set goals. You should help set these goals because you spend the most time with residents each day. Once you know a resident's goals, desires, and preferences, be creative to find ways to help them meet their goals and to feel good about their progress.

For example, a resident's short-term goal is to learn to safely use a walker to transfer to a chair. Their long-term goal is to walk short distances. Work closely with the resident and discuss their goals as you begin. Next, determine their current ability to use the walker by observing and learning their capabilities. Now you are ready to help them reach their goals. For example, they may be able to get out of bed with some prompting from you. They may need only a little help to stand up. Maybe they are afraid of falling and don't want to let go of your arm to use the walker. Your short-term goal may be to help them feel comfortable and less fearful while using the walker to stand and transfer to the chair. You begin by demonstrat-

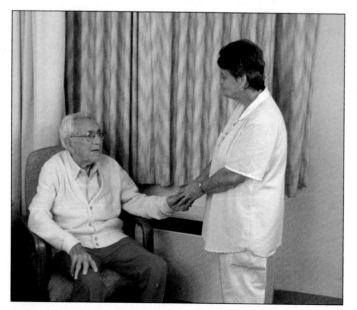

Fig. 27-3 – If a resident has difficulty hearing, it is best to stand directly in front of them when talking to them.

📖
Alert – quick to perceive and act
Prompting – moving a person to action, helping a person remember something

ing how to use the walker when trying to stand up (Fig. 27-4). Show the resident where to place the walker and where to place their hands to help them stand.

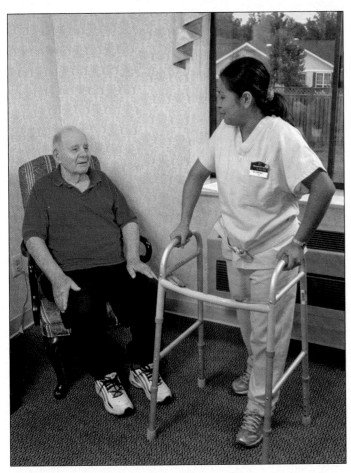

Fig. 27-4 – You can help residents achieve their short- and long-term restorative goals.

- Reinforce the idea that the walker is safe. Show how the rubber stoppers on the bottom prevent slipping.
- Tell the resident you will stay close by to ease their fears. Ask them where you should stand. If they have a weaker side, stand on that side.
- Encourage and support their efforts.

When the resident meets the short-term goal, move on to the next short-term goal until you reach the long-term goal. Keep the long-term goal in mind as you work on each short-term goal. Goals can be changed if the resident shows improvement. Revise the goals as often as needed.

Your ideas to help a resident achieve their goals should fit with the care plan and should be realistic for the resident. Discuss your ideas with the nurse or therapist before trying them with a resident.

CUING, PROMPTING, AND ENCOURAGING

In your role as the daily caregiver, use restorative activities throughout a resident's care. Take the time to cue and encourage residents to help them to do tasks more independently. Cuing means that you prompt a resident to get them started. You do this by telling, teaching, or showing them part or all of the steps to take.

When helping a resident, use common sense and your knowledge of how to do the skill to teach them in clear, simple steps. Here are some ways to teach residents while doing activities with them:

- Explain what you want to help them do. If they do not understand at first what you are saying, say it in a different way. If a resident is hard of hearing, try to speak more clearly while facing them. Try speaking on the side of a resident's better ear. Write things down if needed.
- Always give a resident time to respond to your request. They may be trying to move but just have trouble getting started, or they may move slowly
- If a resident looks puzzled or you think they might be confused by what you said, break down the activity into simple steps. For example, if you want a resident to get out of bed but they do not respond, say, "I would like you to get out of bed now. First, please roll toward me. Good. Now bring your legs over the edge of the bed. Good. Now push your upper body up to sitting." Even more simply, you can say, "Please sit up. Now stand up. Now let me help you get into the chair."
- If a resident still has trouble, you may need to show them what to do or even start each step for them. For example, if you want a resident to brush their teeth but they are having trouble getting started, you could place the toothbrush in their dominant hand and give them the toothpaste. If they still do not respond, put the toothpaste on the toothbrush and help them hold the toothbrush while brushing (Fig. 27-5, next page). If a resident does not want to participate at all, try gently encouraging them to participate before you do it for them. Explain in terms they can understand how important it is for them to do as much for themselves as possible.

Cuing – telling or showing a resident the steps in a task
Reinforce – to strengthen something

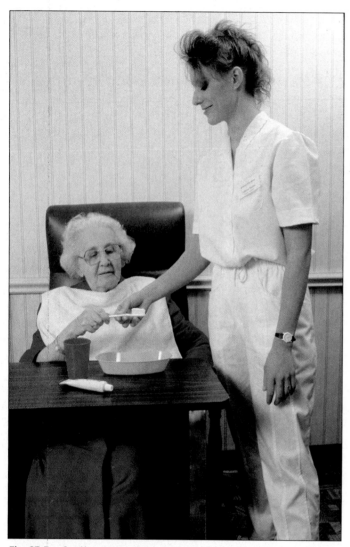

Fig. 27-5 – Gentle encouragement may be necessary to get residents to participate in their own care.

ASSISTIVE DEVICES

Many kinds of devices are used to improve a resident's ability to function. These include braces, walking devices, splints (Fig. 27-6), a trapeze (Fig. 27-7, next page), and dressing aids. Often the therapist assigns this equipment to the resident during their rehabilitation to help them function safely. You must become familiar with each piece of equipment Understand how and why it is used so you can help the resident through the restorative process. Residents may forget to use the equipment or resist using it even if it helps keep them safe from injury. Talk with the charge nurse or therapist about a resident's abilities. Help

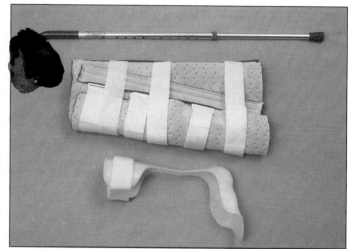

Fig. 27-6 – There are many kinds of devices that can be used to improve a resident's function.

identify equipment they can use to improve their functioning. For example, you may observe a problem, such as a resident having difficulty using a fork. You tell the charge nurse, and together with the therapist, you find an assistive device that will help this resident. A simple change in eating utensils can dramatically improve a resident's nutritional status (Fig. 27-8, next page).

Types of Assistive Devices

Some assistive devices help a resident transfer or walk more independently and safely. These devices give the resident support or assistance, depending on what help they need. Keep the assistive device next to the resident. Always use it when transferring or walking. The device is essential for optimizing the resident's functional independence. Your daily use of it will reinforce the resident's understanding of its use and familiarity with it. It also sets a good example to your co-workers for consistent restorative care.

Walkers and canes are commonly used assistive devices. A walker is used when a resident needs the most support. The person moves the walker first, then the weaker leg, then the stronger leg. If a resident's legs are equally strong,

Brace – device that supports and strengthens a body part
Rehabilitation – the process of restoring to a former state
Splint – device to use to support or immobilize a body part
Trapeze – a short horizontal bar suspended by two parallel ropes, used to pull oneself up in bed

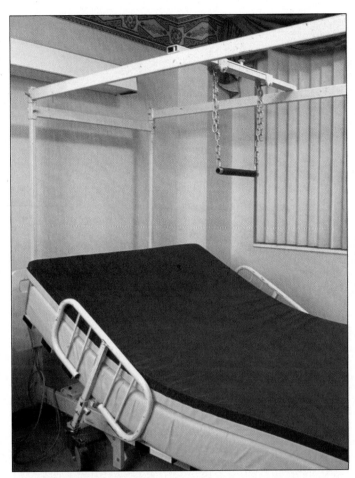

Fig. 27-7 – A trapeze can be placed over the resident's bed to help them reposition themselves.

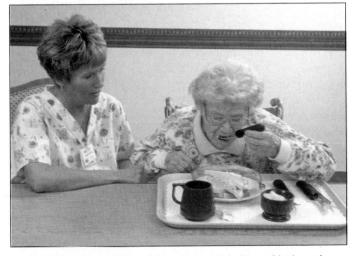

Fig. 27-8 – Assistive devices for eating can help the resident regain or maintain their independence.

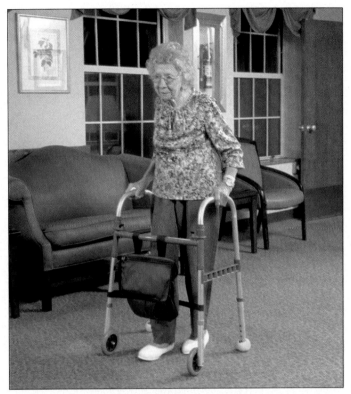

Fig. 27-9 – Walkers help the resident with ambulation.

the person just moves the walker forward, steps with one leg, and then the other (Fig. 27-9). A rolling walker provides a good amount of support. With its two wheels in front, a resident can push it instead of lifting it while walking. This is the most commonly used walker. It is used by residents who may lose their balance lifting a walker off the floor, and by those with less upper body strength. A rolling walker also allows the resident to walk with a more normal gait (walking pattern) at a more normal speed. The walker should be positioned in front of their body with the top of the walker about at the resident's hips. The resident should not have to bend forward much or move the walker too far in front of them while walking. When making a turn, both of their feet should remain between the walker's legs for safety.

A resident may use a cane when they need less support than a walker. A cane is used to support a weaker leg or by a resident with a slight balance problem (Fig. 27-10, next page). When used to support a weak leg, the resident should hold the cane in the hand opposite the weak leg. When used for balance, the resident can hold the cane in either hand. A right-handed person usually prefers the right hand, and a left-handed person the left. The top of the cane should be at the level of the person's wrist so

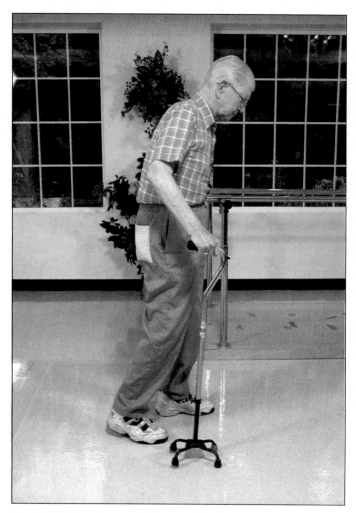

Fig. 27-10 – Canes are used when a resident has one side that is weaker than the other.

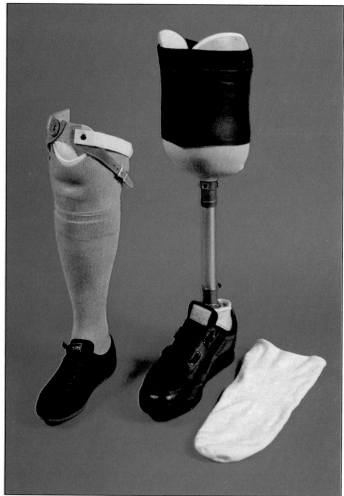

Fig. 27-11 – Prosthetic devices are made specifically for each resident.

that they do not have to bend forward when using it. The physical therapist usually chooses this equipment for the resident and instructs them in its use.

There are two types of canes:

• A quad cane has a large or small base, usually with three or four prongs. The handle faces backward, and the flat side of the base is at the person's side.
• A straight cane is also called just a "cane" or "J cane." This is the typical cane made of wood or metal. Metal canes can be adjusted to the proper height.

Prosthetic and Orthotic Devices

Prosthetic devices are sometimes called prostheses. They are specially made for residents to help improve the func-

tion of a body part that is missing or not fully functioning. Artificial limbs and artificial eyes are common prosthetic devices (Fig. 27-11).

Orthotic devices are are things like braces, splints, and shoe inserts. They improve or help restore the function of a limb or body part. Most often they are specially made for a resident. An orthotic device is sometimes called an orthosis (Fig. 27-12 A/B, next page).

Artificial limb – human-made leg or arm
Orthotic device – supportive equipment made for a resident, such as a brace or splint
Prosthetic device – device made to replace a missing body part or function

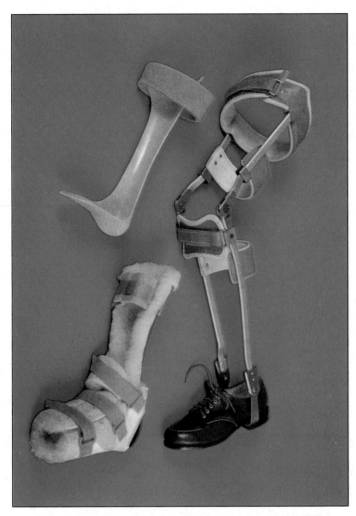

Fig. 27-12 A — Orthotic devices are used to support resident's limbs.

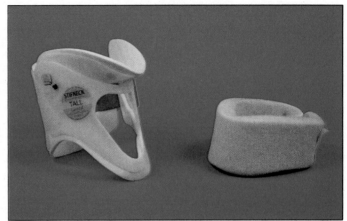

Fig. 27-12 B — Soft and hard neck collars are a type of brace used to support the neck.

Residents should use their prosthetic or orthotic devices in all activities as intended. Always check with the charge nurse if you have any questions about when or how a resident should use their device. Before helping a resident with a prosthetic or orthotic device, you should be instructed by the therapist or nurse. Make sure you understand the proper application and care for such devices. Inspect them daily for any damage or wear and tear.

The most common artificial limbs are artificial legs. A resident may need your help in putting their artificial leg onto the leg **stump**. Use stump socks and prosthesis liners to protect the resident's skin. Inspect their skin daily during application and removal of the prosthesis. If the stump's skin is red or bruised, report this promptly to the charge nurse.

Many long term care residents use leg, neck, or back braces. Braces do what the name implies: they brace a body part if that part of the body is not strong enough to support the body by itself. They are often used during transfers and walking. Some residents use braces permanently for an injured, chronically painful, or weak joint. Other residents use braces temporarily during recovery from a stroke, injury, or surgery. Firm brace material is used for weaker or more severely injured body parts. Some braces are worn only out of bed, and others are worn all the time. You must learn how to put each brace on correctly and know when the resident should wear it.

A knee brace may be made of elastic, which provides less support, or a firmer material. The brace may have metal strips on both sides of the knee for support.

An ankle foot orthosis (AFO) provides support for a weak ankle or to correct foot drop. Foot drop is an inability to flex or bend the ankle without assistance. One type is a shoe with metal uprights that are attached to a calf band. Another type is a plastic shoe insert extending from the back of the calf to the bottom of the foot. Residents who have lost use of their leg above the knee may use a knee-ankle foot orthosis (KAFO), which supports both the knee and the ankle.

A common type of back brace is an elastic brace like a corset that closes in front with Velcro or straps. Firmer materials may be used to support any part of the back.

Stump – the amount of an extremity remaining after the rest is removed

Usually the brace supports only the lower back. After surgery or a spinal cord injury, a resident may have a body jacket brace extending from the lower back to the armpits. A resident wearing this type of brace generally has a very severe back problem.

Residents may wear soft or hard neck collars to support their neck. Some residents use these devices only when in bed, some only when out of bed, and others all the time.

Splints are used to immobilize a joint or body part or restrict its motion in a certain way. Splints are commonly used on the hand, wrist, knee, or foot. The therapist will tell you when and how the resident should wear it. To be safe and effective, you must understand the use and care of each of these devices.

Positioning and Seating Devices

These devices include a variety of cushions, supportive chairs, pillows, towel rolls, splints, and heel and elbow protectors. They are used to position a resident with limited independent movement in the best functional position while lying or sitting (Fig. 27-13). These devices also help prevent problems such as skin breakdown and contractures. With a contracture, the resident's arm or leg joint becomes stuck in a certain position and cannot move through its full range of motion (ROM). Heel and elbow protectors are cloth sleeves that cover the elbows and heels to protect the skin from pressure sores.

Splints keep joints in a good position or restrict undesir-

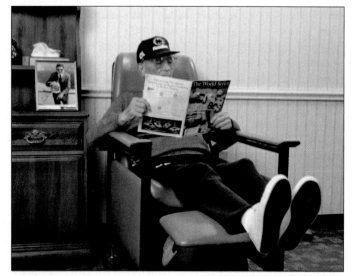

Fig. 27-13 – Seating devices support a resident's position while in a chair.

able motions that may cause tightness, pain, or injury. Splints are used on a finger, hand, wrist, knee, or ankle (Fig. 27-14). A resting splint keeps a body part at rest in

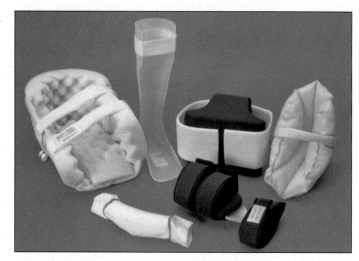

Fig. 27-14 Here are some examples of limb protectors.

the splint. A dynamic splint allows some motion of the joint but restricts undesirable motions.

Reclining chairs are also called recliners or geri-chairs. These are generally larger chairs with more padding on the seat and back. They can be positioned for sitting upright or reclined at different angles. They are used for residents who are unable to move or sit comfortably upright, who sit for long periods throughout the day, or who may tip over a regular wheelchair.

There are many types of wheelchairs (Fig. 27-15, next page). Wheelchairs vary in several ways:
- standard, narrow, or wide width
- high back or regular back
- lightweight or regular weight
- reclining or standard upright position
- removable, stationary, or swing-away arm and leg rests

Most residents who sit in a wheelchair daily have one assigned to them. The physical therapist adjusts it for proper positioning. A special cushion may be used for pressure relief, comfort, or seat height. Each chair should have leg rests. Leg rests should be adjusted to the correct length for proper positioning of the resident's ankle, knee, and hip joints. There are several types of leg rests. All have

📖

Immobilize – to prevent freedom of movement

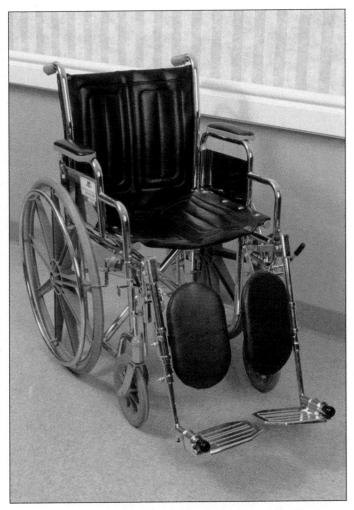

Fig. 27-15 – Wheelchairs can be different. Be sure you are familiar with the type the resident uses.

Get to know the different parts of wheelchairs and how to adjust them. You can help the resident learn about their wheelchair and its use as part of your restorative care. Show them the brakes, located below the armrests in front of each wheel. Teach them to lock the chair at all times when it is not being moved. Make sure the wheelchair brakes are locked securely before starting any transfer. The armrests may or may not be removable or swing out of the way. You might want to remove them or swing them out of the way when transferring a resident to or from the chair. Inspect the wheelchair daily. Report any broken, loose, or non-functioning mechanical parts, especially brakes, to the maintenance department or the charge nurse. Remember that residents who can safely move themselves in a wheelchair will have more independence, which can lead to an improved quality of life. Help the resident to maintain their highest level of independence as long as safely possible.

Aids for the Activities of Daily Living

Many types of assistive equipment are available to help with the activities of daily living (ADLs). These include bathing, dressing, transferring, toileting, and eating. Talk to the therapist if you notice that a resident has difficulty doing something. When you know what devices are available, you may be able to suggest one for a resident. This would be a valuable contribution to their care. Many commonly used devices are described below. If you have any questions about how to use this equipment, ask the therapist for more information or a demonstration.

Some assistive devices help residents dress and bathe without having to bend down as far (Fig. 27-16). These

footplates that either swing away or remain stationary. Some elevate with calf pads for support. Elevating leg rests are usually used for residents with significant edema (swelling) in their legs or feet. The physical therapist or charge nurse will instruct you when and how to elevate the leg rests. Remove or swing leg rests out of the way (if possible) during all transfers for safety and convenience. Learn how to remove and elevate them quickly and easily.

Correct positioning of a resident in a wheelchair is very important for their overall health and well-being. It helps protect skin integrity, promote good upright posture and comfort, and limit or prevent contractures in some joints. If a resident does not use the same wheelchair every day, try to pick the type of wheelchair that is best for that resident's needs.

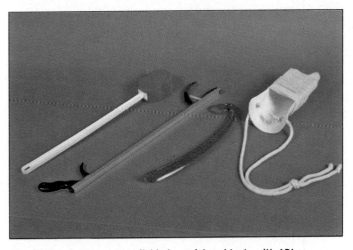

Fig. 27-16 – Devices are available to assist residents with ADLs.

include dressing sticks, long-handled shoehorns, long-handled sponges, sock donners, elastic shoelaces, and reachers. Many residents should not try to bend down because of hip surgery, because they become dizzy or lose their balance, or simply because they cannot bend over very far.

A higher than usual toilet seat is used by residents who have difficulty bending down to sit on a toilet or difficulty getting off a toilet of regular height. It is also used by people after hip replacement surgery to prevent them from sitting too low, which could cause a problem. A raised toilet seat may be attached to the floor or temporarily placed over the toilet.

Grab bars on the walls of bathrooms, tubs, and showers are used for safety and convenience. They give residents something to hold onto when moving onto a toilet, moving into a tub or shower, or standing during bathing (Fig. 27-17).

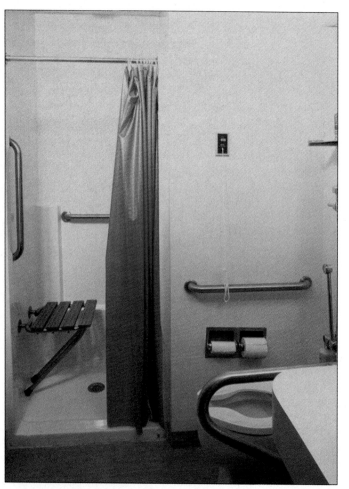

Fig. 27-17 – Grab bars are available to help residents in the bathroom.

Built-up grips on any item or device help a resident with a weak grip hold it better. For example, raised grips may be added to eating or writing utensils or even a toothbrush. The grip may include a strap that wraps around the hand for more support.

Most of this equipment is given to residents by the therapist or nurse to give them more independence. Make sure the equipment is available for residents for their ADLs. Most important, pay attention to residents and report what you notice. If a resident has trouble with a certain activity, tell the therapist. Together you can often find a solution that helps the resident function better. Once again, always make sure all assigned equipment is readily available for the resident's daily use.

Preventing Injury to Residents During Functional Activities

Most injuries that happen during a resident's activities are caused by improper use of equipment or faulty equipment. You can help prevent these injuries by being observant and talking with other staff about what you observe.

Improper Use of Equipment. You can help prevent injuries to residents by following these guidelines:
- Notice if a resident is using a piece of equipment improperly. For example, you see a resident pushing a walker too far in front of them. Show them how to better use the walker. Then observe them to see if they follow your suggestions. You should tell your supervisor and the therapist about the problem as well.
- Help the resident take a safe position until the problem is solved. For example, you notice that a resident is using a walker that is too short, causing them to bend too far forward. First, check to see if they are using their own walker. If not, help them sit safely in the nearest chair, and then try to locate their correct walker. If they are using their assigned walker and the height still seems incorrect, notify the therapist so that it can be properly adjusted.
- Report any problem to your supervisor or notify the therapist. For example, you know a resident is not supposed to put weight on one leg. You see that person using a cane or a rolling walker, which still puts weight on the leg. You explain this to the resident, and tell your supervisor or the therapist as soon as possible. This is important because if the resident is not supposed to put weight on a leg, their injury will not heal well if they bear weight on it too soon.

Faulty Equipment. Another way to help prevent injury is to watch for broken or faulty equipment. If you notice that any equipment has broken, missing, or wobbly parts, ask the therapy or maintenance department to fix or replace it. All staff must try to correct even minor equipment problems quickly before a resident is injured.

EXERCISE

Exercise is an important restorative activity and should be part of a resident's routine. All residents benefit from exercise. You can help a resident's rehabilitation by including exercise in your nursing care activities. An exercise program can greatly increase muscle strength and flexibility and is a key factor for a resident to regain mobility. Many facilities offer regular group exercise programs for residents. Encourage residents to participate in such programs.

Range-of-Motion Exercises

Range-of-motion (ROM) exercises are one of the most common restorative programs used in long term care. Each joint in the body is moved through the resident's full range of motion. The resident's physician, along with the physical therapist and nurse, designs the resident's ROM exercise program depending on their needs, capabilities, and motivation.

Active Range of Motion Exercise (AROM). In active ROM (AROM) exercises, the person moves the body part using their own muscle power. Exercise is active when the resident can do it independently. Depending on the resident's needs, you still might help in some way. They may just need someone to remind them to do the exercises. They may need you to read the exercise program aloud as they are doing it, or they may need you to cue them for how to move each body part correctly.

Active Assistive Range of Motion Exercise (AAROM). In active assistive (AAROM) exercises, you help move the body part. Some residents need you to help them physically with some or all parts of the ROM exercise. Doing active exercise may be too strenuous for an injured body part that is healing. A resident may simply need your help to move that part of their body.

Passive Range of Motion Exercise (PROM). With passive (PROM) exercises, you do the exercise for a resident, usually because they cannot move that part of the body at all or enough to help with the exercise (Fig. 27-18). Some

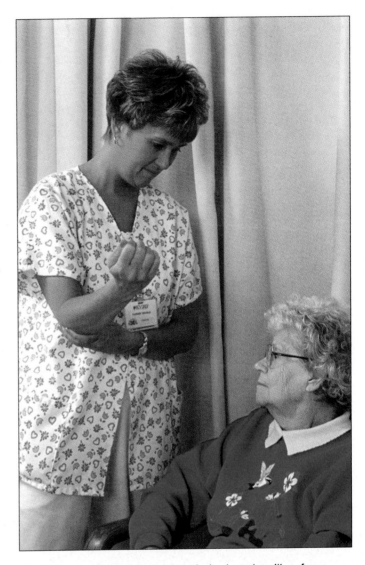

Fig. 27-18 – A nurse assistant demonstrates how she will perform passive ROM exercise.

residents may be recovering from an injury or surgery and could move the body part but should not so that it can heal better. Always ask the charge nurse or therapist if you are not sure.

Many residents perform different types of ROM exercises. They may be able to move some parts of their body better than others, while not being able to move other parts at all. For example, you may need to help a resident move their right arm (active assisted ROM exercise), yet they can move the left arm independently (AROM exercise). The same person may be unable to move their legs at all (PROM exercise).

Guidelines for ROM Exercises

Following are general guidelines for ROM exercises:

- Know what type of exercise a resident needs for each part of their body, the position they should be in during each exercise, and the amount of assistance required during each exercise. If the therapist has written the exercise program, follow the written plan.
- Remove any obstacles in the way of movement. Move pillows, sheets, and blankets out of the way. Accidentally banging a frail elderly resident's body part against something can cause bruising, skin tears, or a more severe injury.
- Explain to the resident what you would like to do and why.
- Help the resident into the correct position for each exercise.
- Remember your own body mechanics (Box 27-1) and pay attention to your body position. Experiment with different standing positions, hand placement, and bed heights to find the best position for you to avoid back strain while helping residents. Sometimes it helps to stand on one leg with your other knee on the bed. Ask the resident first and put down a bed protector before lifting your knee onto the bed.

BOX 27-1.
PRINCIPLES OF BODY MECHANICS WHEN DOING ROM EXERCISES

- Maintain a broad base of support by keeping your feet 10–12 inches apart.
- Always bend at your knees and not at your back.
- Keep your back in a neutral position.
- Turn your whole body as a unit, instead of twisting.

- Keep both hands on the person's **extremity** (if possible) during each exercise for the best support and guidance.
- When moving a joint, have one hand above and the other hand below the joint. Generally, the hand above the joint stabilizes the extremity (holds it in place), and the hand below the joint brings the part through the range of motion. For example, for ROM exercise of the elbow joint, hold the resident's upper arm (above the elbow) with one hand, and with the other hand positioned below the elbow, move the forearm up and down.
- When moving a resident's extremity, be gentle and never force the joint. Pushing or pulling too hard can cause severe damage. You might cause pain or swelling, rupture a tendon, pull a muscle, tear the skin, or even break a bone. Many residents have osteoporosis or other conditions that cause weakened bones, muscles, tendons, or ligaments. They may have fragile skin or unstable joints. The most easily damaged joints are in the neck, hands, wrists, and feet.
- Make sure to tell the resident what you are doing before each movement. During exercise, ask the resident often how they are doing, if they feel any pain from a motion, and if your hand pressure on their arm or leg is OK. Watch the person's facial expressions because they may not always tell you when they are uncomfortable.
- Do the full exercise routine at least once a day. Also encourage residents to use their arms and legs throughout the day. If a resident has an exercise program from the therapist for independent exercise, motivate them to do these throughout the day. You may need to remind them, set them up to start the exercise, or cue them during the exercises. Take advantage of this time to spend quality time with the resident.

Which Joints To Exercise

A resident may have a special exercise program designed by the therapist for problem areas. Follow this program. Ask the therapist about any other exercises for this resident.

A resident who is not seeing a therapist for special needs usually benefits from a daily general ROM exercise program. A general ROM program exercises most joints of the body, including the shoulder, elbow, wrist, hand (fingers), hip, knee, ankle, and foot (toes).

Ask your supervisor or the therapist if the resident has any restricted joints. If there are no restrictions, move each joint through its full available range at least once a day. Based on the resident's ability to help you, the resident may move some joints actively, some actively with your assistance, and some passively with you doing the motion. Let the resident do as much as possible, and help them with the rest. Give the resident time to respond to what you are asking them to do.

Extremity – a limb of the body

How Joints Move

The motion of each joint depends on the structure of the joint. Box 27-2 lists the specific motions of each joint for a general ROM exercise program. Procedure 27-1 (next page) shows these motions.

Starting a ROM Program

You can complete an entire ROM exercise program with a resident in about 15 minutes when you use a system (Procedure 27-1, next page).

Think about each motion, and try to do nursing care activities that use these motions. ROM exercises can be incorporated into the resident's ADLs. For example, help move a shoulder joint through its ROM while the resident is putting on their shirt or blouse. This is effective as well as functional. As another example, when bathing under the resident's arm, you can flex and abduct the shoulder. If you lift each shoulder up a few times or have a resident do it while bathing, this adds to the daily exercise routine. You will still need to perform the separate exercise program.

Develop a system for using every joint in an exercise routine. With this system, use the same order of exercises for each resident. You may have to change specific exercises depending on the resident's needs.

BOX 27-2.
MOTIONS OF MAJOR JOINTS

SHOULDER
Flexion: bringing the whole arm up toward the resident's head in front of the body
Extension: bringing the arm straight back to their side
Abduction: moving the arm away from the body out to the side
Adduction: bringing the arm back toward the side
Internal rotation: turning the shoulder in
External rotation: turning the shoulder out

ELBOW
Flexion: bending the elbow
Extension: straightening the elbow
Supination: turning the palm up
Pronation: turning the palm down

WRIST
Flexion: bending the wrist up
Extension: bending the wrist back
Ulnar deviation: with the hand held at the same level as the forearm, moving the hand toward the little finger side
Radial deviation: with the hand as above, moving the hand toward the thumb side

HAND
Finger abduction/adduction: spreading fingers apart and then together
Finger flexion: bending the fingers at each of the finger joints (three on each finger, two on the thumb)
Finger extension: straightening the fingers out at the finger joints
Opposition: touching each fingertip to the thumb

HIP
Flexion: bringing the knee toward the chest
Extension: lay the leg down flat
Abduction: bringing the hip out to the side by moving the leg
Adduction: bringing the hip back toward the side by moving the leg
Internal rotation: turning the hip inward by moving the leg
External rotation: turning the hip outward by moving the leg

KNEE
Flexion: bending the knee
Extension: straightening the knee

ANKLE
Dorsiflexion: bending the top of the foot up toward the face
Plantarflexion: pointing the foot down, like stepping on a gas pedal
Inversion: turning the bottom of the foot inward
Eversion: turning the bottom of the foot outward

FOOT
Toe flexion: bending the toes down
Toe extension: straightening the toes back up

PROCEDURE 27-1.   RANGE-OF-MOTION EXERCISES

▶ **REMEMBER: BE AWARE**

Note: *Do each exercise 5-10 times, depending on the resident's comfort level with each extremity.*

THE ARM
Start with the shoulder and work your way down to the hand. For each exercise help the resident move the joint or move it yourself, depending on how much they can do independently.

THE SHOULDER
Place one hand under the resident's elbow and the other under their wrist. Allow the resident's forearm to rest on your body as you move the arm. If the resident is on their back, stand close to the side of the arm you are moving.

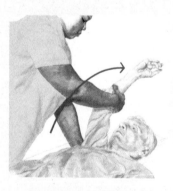

1. Help the resident to lift their arm up toward the head of the bed with the elbow straight (flexion).

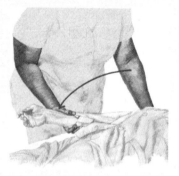

2. Bring the arm back down to the bed (extension).

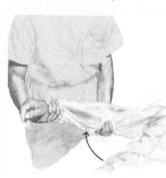

3. Help the resident to lift their arm out to the side with the elbow straight (abduction).

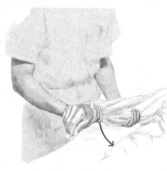

4. Bring the arm back toward the side (adduction).

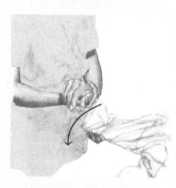

5. Help the resident lift their arm halfway out to the side. With the elbow bent rotate the arm down (internal rotation) and up (external rotation).

THE ELBOW
Place one hand above the resident's elbow and use your other hand to support the wrist. The wrist position should be neutral, not bent forward or backward.

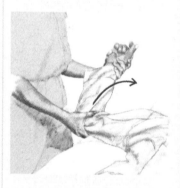

1. Help the resident bend the elbow by bringing the hand toward the upper arm with the palm facing up (flexion).

2. Help the resident straighten the elbow by bringing the hand down toward the bed until the elbow is as straight as possible (extension).

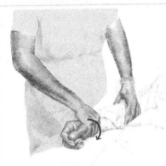

3. Help the resident turn their palm over with the elbow fairly straight and the wrist neutral (pronation).

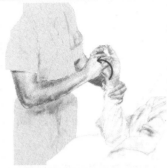

2. Help the resident bend their wrist back (extension).

THE HAND

Use your fingers to help the person move their fingers one by one.

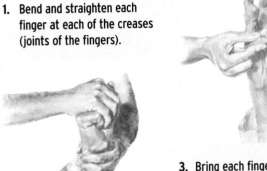

and then back together one at a time (adduction).

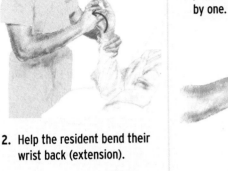

1. Bend and straighten each finger at each of the creases (joints of the fingers).

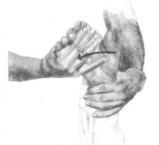

3. Help the resident move their hand toward the little finger side of the wrist (ulnar deviation).

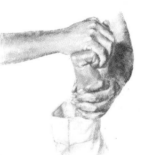

3. Bring each finger across the palm to the thumb and back out (opposition).

Then curl the hand into a fist, and straighten the fingers back out (flexion and extension).

4. Help the resident turn their palm back up with the elbow fairly straight and the wrist neutral (supination).

THE WRIST

Place one hand around the resident's forearm just above the wrist and your other hand in their hand.

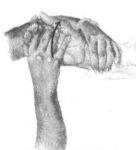

4. Help the resident move their hand toward the thumb side of the wrist (radial deviation).

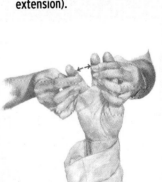

2. Spread the fingers away from each other one at a time (abduction)

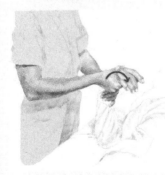

1. Help the resident bend their wrist down (flexion).

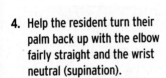

THE LEG

Start with the hip and work your way down to the foot.

THE HIP

Place one hand under the thigh and the other hand below the knee around the calf. Adjust your hand placement as needed to be comfortable for both you and the resident.

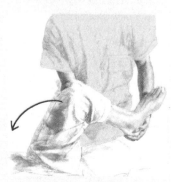

1. Help the resident bring their leg up toward the chest with the knee bent (flexion).

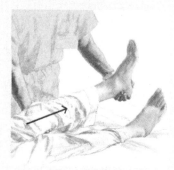

2. Bring their leg back down toward the bed (extension).

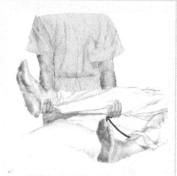

3. Help the resident bring their leg out to the side (abduction).

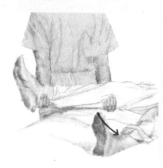

4. Bring their leg back toward the other leg (adduction).

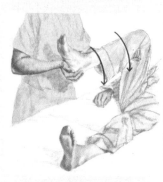

5. Help the resident bring the leg partly up toward the chest with the knee bent. Now gently turn the leg in (internal rotation) and out (external rotation).

THE KNEE

Place one hand above the resident's knee under or on their thigh and one hand below their knee around the calf.

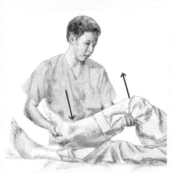

1. Help the resident bend the leg up toward the chest slightly. From this position, help them bend the knee (flexion).

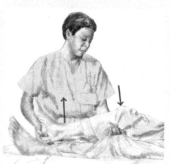

2. With the hip in the same position as described above, help the resident straighten the knee (extension).

THE ANKLE

Place one hand above the resident's ankle around the lower part of the calf and the other hand around the bottom of their foot.

1. Help the resident bend the foot up toward the head while the knee is held straight (dorsiflexion), and then point the foot downward (plantarflexion).

2. Help the resident turn the bottom of the foot outward (eversion) and then inward (inversion).

THE FOOT

As with the hand, place your fingers around each of the resident's toes and

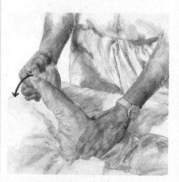

gently bend (flexion) and

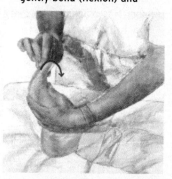

straighten each toe at each of the joints (extension). You can also bend and straighten all the toes at once.

▶ **REMEMBER: UNDERSTAND**

Walking With a Resident

Walking is another important restorative activity that helps the resident maintain their independence. It is an effective and excellent way for a resident to exercise and maintain optimal function (Fig. 27-19). Walking is also called ambulation. The term "gait" refers to how someone walks. If a resident needs assistance or supervision when walking, use a gait belt around their waist. Before you begin walking with a resident, you need to know the following:

• Do they use an assistive device?
• Do they need a brace, prosthesis, or other equipment?
• How much weight can they place on their legs while walking?
• How much help do they need to walk, if any?
• Do you need another staff person to help?
• How much cuing do they need to stay safe?
• How far can they walk safely?

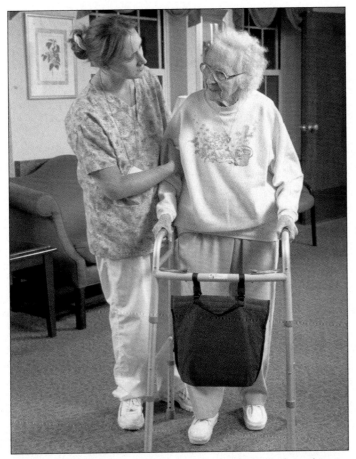

Fig. 27-19 – Walking promotes independence and is a great way to exercise.

Once you have determined a resident's situation and abilities, you can help them walk. Combine short walks with other activities such as getting out of bed, walking to and from the bathroom, walking to meals, activities, etc. Encourage residents who can walk on their own to do so throughout the day. For example, a resident who has just used the toilet needs to get back into their chair. If this resident can walk a short way without becoming tired, place the chair outside the room or down the hall instead of next to the bathroom, and have them walk to the chair. Procedure 27-2 (next page) describes the steps for assisting a resident to walk. If the physical therapist or nurse has assigned the resident to a facility ambulation program, make sure to follow the daily ambulation schedule. Record your results as requested by your supervisor. It is very important for the resident to maintain their function and mobility by ambulating as assigned as well as whenever possible. Muscles need to be used to keep their strength and function. Remember the saying, "If you don't use it, you lose it." Since it takes only a short time for a resident to lose their mobility skills, it is critical to help your residents keep moving.

Certain situations may occur when you assist residents with walking. Here are four common situations and the actions to take:

1. A resident questions why they have to walk. You explain that walking will help them get stronger or stay strong.
2. A resident who usually walks a lot during the day does not feel well today. Respect the person's right not to walk this day. Try again when they feel better.
3. The resident is on oxygen. Ask the nurse or therapist if it is OK for this person to walk. Find out if they need oxygen when they walk and how much. Ask the nurse to put this resident on a portable tank for the walk. You may need another staff person if they need help to walk. The other person pulls the oxygen tank and brings along a wheelchair in case it is needed, while you walk holding onto the guard belt and resident's walker (if used).
4. A resident sometimes acts unpredictably when walking. Their legs may get tired and give out easily. They may become confused and sit without telling you. Place a gait belt securely (not too tight or too loose) around their waist, and position your hand on the belt, usually at their back. Try not to hold onto their arm because their joints may be arthritic, frail, and painful. In such cases, have another person follow you with a wheelchair as you walk with the resident. Have the chair ready for them if they suddenly need to sit.

PROCEDURE 27-2. ASSISTING WITH WALKING

▶ **REMEMBER: BE AWARE**

Items Needed
• guard (gait) belt
• assistive device (if used)

1. Ensure that the resident is wearing shoes that fit properly before assisting with walking. Put the guard belt on the resident.
2. If the resident walks without an assistive device, stand at their side so that you can watch their face as you hold onto the belt from behind. If the resident uses a walker or cane, stand on that side with one hand on the back of the belt and the other on the walker (or cane if the resident needs help with the cane). Most residents who use a cane can hold it by themselves, so you can stand on the other side. Make sure that the resident holds the cane in the correct hand.
3. Walk with the resident. Have them take small steps and slowly progress to larger ones. When walking in hallways, encourage residents not using a walker to use the safety bars for added support. Always stand on their other side so they may use the bars.

▶ **REMEMBER: UNDERSTAND**

IN THIS CHAPTER YOU LEARNED HOW TO:
• Promote independence
• Help with various kinds of equipment that promote independence
• Perform restorative activities including range-of-motion exercises
• Assist a resident with walking

SUMMARY

As a nurse assistant, you are like a coach helping residents learn or relearn information and skills to regain or maintain their level of independent functioning. You work with residents in restorative activities and help them use special equipment and devices. With your mindful attention to residents' physical and emotional needs and your knowledge, you can promote their independent functioning and thus improve their quality of life.

In restorative activities, use everything you have learned about residents to teach, prompt, and encourage them to care for themselves. When you focus on restorative activities, your work with residents gives them many benefits.

PULLING IT ALL TOGETHER

As a nurse assistant, you need to be patient with residents as they try to regain or maintain their independence. To save time you may be tempted to move the resident in a wheelchair instead of letting them slowly walk down the hall, or you may want to feed someone who can do it themselves if given enough time.

Sometimes it is difficult to balance promoting residents' independence with your need to get the job done. Remind yourself that if you do not let the residents do their activities of daily living independently, they will become dependent on you. Eventually, they will become more difficult to care for. Then this would create more work for you.

Think about this:

Manage your time wisely to accomplish your daily assignment. When you begin your shift, decide what tasks will take the resident the longest. Think about other tasks that you can do while the resident is doing these lengthy tasks. For example, Mr. Jones prefers to shave himself. He is very slow at shaving and after having a stroke sometimes cuts himself because his right arm is weak. The physical therapist gave him a shaver with a thicker handle that is easier to hold. When you begin his morning care, you discuss with him when he wants to shave. Together you decide he will bathe first and then move to his chair. You set him up to shave in the chair. During this time, you make his bed, clean up his bathing supplies, and have a nice conversation with him while he independently shaves under your supervision. With this creative approach you can use your time with the resident to its best advantage and promote their welfare while doing your assigned duties.

1. **What is the goal of restorative activities?**
   A. To help the resident look better.
   B. To help residents and staff get along better.
   C. To help the resident regain function and independence.
   D. To help staff avoid back strain.

2. **A resident's daughter complains to you that you ask her mother to bathe herself. How should you answer the daughter?**
   A. You don't have time to care for everyone.
   B. You suggest the daughter care for the mother herself.
   C. You ask the daughter file a formal complaint.
   D. You explain you are helping her mother maintain her independence.

3. **Which of the following may be a key element in a restorative program?**
   A. Helping residents use assistive devices.
   B. Leaving residents alone until they learn to care for themselves.
   C. Asking family members to help the resident instead of you helping.
   D. Using a mechanical lift to move residents.

4. **A resident says she feels uncomfortable using the cane the physical therapist gave her. What should you do?**
   A. Tell the resident to keep trying.
   B. Suggest she try using her roommate's cane instead.
   C. Put the cane away and help the resident walk with a guard belt.
   D. Call the physical therapist to discuss the resident.

5. **Mrs. Jackson, who is on oxygen, asks you to assist her to walk. How can you help her walk safely and comfortably?**
   A. Show her how to walk holding onto the oxygen tank the way she would use a walker.
   B. Teach her to walk in circles around the oxygen tank without kinking the tubing.
   C. Explain to her that residents who are on oxygen must use a wheelchair with the tank strapped in beside them.
   D. Ask a co-worker to follow you with the oxygen tank while you assist the resident to walk.

6. **The charge nurse asks you to assist a resident using a walker. You notice that one of the rubber stoppers is missing from the walker. What should you do?**
   A. After the walk fill out an equipment maintenance form to have the stopper replaced.
   B. Borrow another resident's walker.
   C. Call the maintenance department to repair or replace the stopper.
   D. Assist the resident to walk using a cane instead.

7. **Which of these items is a prosthetic device?**
   A. Splint.
   B. Quad cane.
   C. Artificial arm.
   D. Reclining chair.

8. **If the resident does not have any restricted joints, you should move each joint through its full available range:**
   A. At least once a week.
   B. At least once a day.
   C. Before every meal.
   D. Whenever the resident says they feel stiff.

9. **When you give ROM exercises, it is important to:**
   A. Wear gloves and a gown.
   B. Exercise the resident at least until they begin to sweat.
   C. Follow the therapist's written plan.
   D. Move each joint just to the point where it begins to be painful.

10. **Mrs. Nixon has orders for passive ROM to her left arm. You should:**
    A. Explain what she needs to do and then come back later and ask if she did it.
    B. Exercise her left arm for her.
    C. Support her as she does her exercise by holding her right hand.
    D. Stand beside her bed ready to help her if she needs it.

(Answers to "Check What You've Learned" are in the Instructor's Manual.)

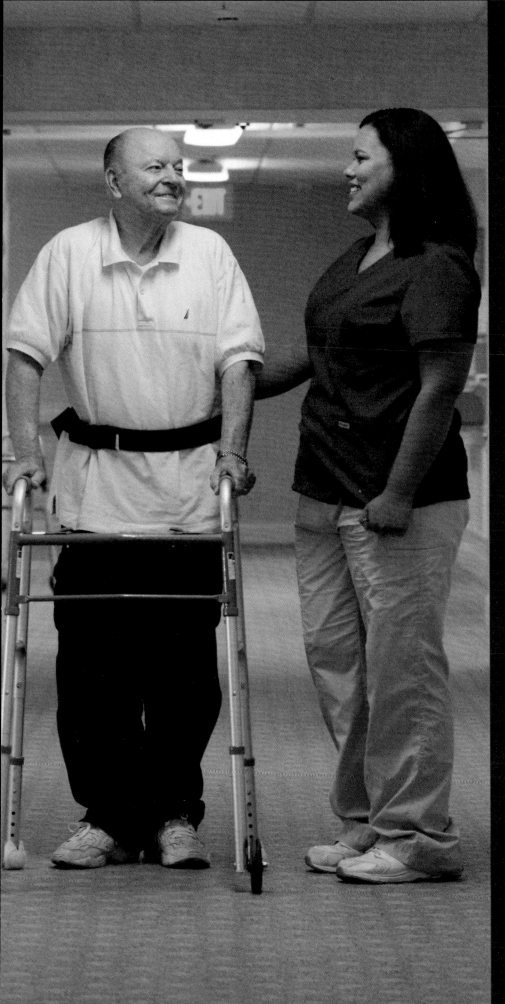

Chapter 28

PULLING IT ALL TOGETHER

Throughout your career as a nurse assistant you will hear about the importance of being organized. You need to prioritize tasks to organize your day. It is important to develop time management skills, a theme of care you learned in Chapter 12, so that you can meet all your residents' needs and enjoy your job.

Time management skills usually do not come naturally. When you first read about time management as a theme of care, it probably did not make much sense to you. But as you begin your job as a nurse assistant, you will learn quickly that you need good time management skills to do a great job.

This chapter describes a typical day in a facility. You will learn what factors influence how you organize your day. You will see how to incorporate time management in your daily work. You will learn how to organize and prioritize your tasks while you care for residents.

OBJECTIVES
- State how nurse assistants contribute to quality care
- Give examples of things that influence how tasks are prioritized
- Describe the theme of time management

MEDICAL TERMS
- **Shunt** – surgical passage created between two blood vessels to move blood from one part to another

"I love to watch my nurse assistant at work.

She is so well organized and professional it makes me feel good to be in her care."

Have you ever put together a jigsaw puzzle? You may have looked at the picture on the cover of the box and thought it looked easy, but then you opened the box and found hundreds of little pieces. Maybe you felt overwhelmed and thought, "I can't do this. I don't have the time. This is impossible."

Most people who enjoy jigsaw puzzles make a plan to avoid being overwhelmed by everything all at once. You might group all the pieces that are the same color together, or sort out all the edge and corner pieces first. You need a plan—some way to organize the pieces. Otherwise, you won't know where to begin.

Earlier chapters in this book have taught you many ideas and skills. You have learned to care for a resident mindfully, to assist with meals, and to maintain residents' independence. You may feel overwhelmed by all this information, and you may feel it will be difficult to do it all. But all you need to do is to organize these pieces of information as if they were pieces of a puzzle. Once you do this, you will feel organized and you will have a plan to put the pieces together. When you put it all together, you will see the whole picture: your job as a nurse assistant.

THE NURSE ASSISTANT'S CONTRIBUTION TO CARE

You have learned that nurse assistants give about 80% of the care for residents in long term care facilities. Nurse assistants usually make up the largest number of staff (Fig. 28-1). You have more contact with residents than anyone else on the health care team. You are closest to residents, and you know more about them than anyone else. Does this sound familiar? You have already learned this in earlier chapters.

You should now understand better what this all means. Your job description makes more sense now that you're completing this course. Think of your job description as the picture on the cover of the puzzle box: It shows you what the completed puzzle looks like. The information and skills you have learned are the puzzle pieces, and each of them is important. Leaving out even one piece creates a hole in your picture. Putting the pieces together is a challenge but is well worth the effort (Fig. 28-2).

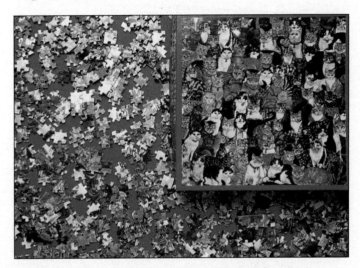

Fig. 28-2 – All aspects of being a nurse assistant are important. Putting the pieces together lets you see what's important.

Once again consider your responsibilities to residents and your employer. As you read the list of nurse assistant responsibilities in Box 28-1 (next page), think of these as the most important aspects of your job.

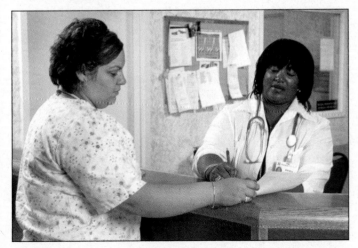

Fig. 28-1 – Nurse assistants make up the largest number of staff in the facility.

BOX 28-1.
NURSE ASSISTANT RESPONSIBILITIES

1. Recognize residents as individuals.
   - Learn their likes and dislikes.
   - Ask how they want things done. Get to know their routine.
   - Learn about their cultural background.
   - Find out if they have cultural preferences for their care.

2. Promote residents' autonomy and independence.
   - Know, respect, and support their rights.
   - Encourage them and work with them to maintain their optimal level of functioning.
   - For personal care:
     - Be sure you give residents choices.
     - Let them participate in care decisions.
     - Maintain their privacy and dignity.

3. Provide mindful caregiving.
   - Balance the skill and the art of caregiving.
   - Observe residents closely.
   - Watch for any change in their attitudes, behaviors, or condition.
   - Let the residents determine their own routines.
   - Report any changes in their condition to the charge nurse immediately.

4. Be a good employee.
   - Be reliable.
   - Be accountable.
   - Be healthy.
   - Be considerate of others.
   - Be caring.
   - Cooperate with other team members.
   - Be efficient with your time and supplies.
   - Follow all personnel policies.
   - Dress appropriately: neat and clean.
   - Pay attention to personal hygiene.
   - Do not use drugs or drink alcohol.

Also think about Chapter 12, Themes of Care, where you learned the concept "It's not what you do, but how you do it." Think about the following:
- Who is the first person you see every day?
- Who is the last person you see before you go to sleep? Is it the same person?
- What kind of influence does this person have on your day, on how you sleep?

If you always saw the same person the first thing in the morning and the last thing at night, what would you want them to be like? Doesn't your day begin more pleasantly when someone says "Good morning!" and smiles at you (Fig. 28-3, next page)? Don't you find it easier to sleep if the last person you talk to treats you well? This is true also for residents. You influence the quality of their care like no other person in the facility because you are the one who spends the most time with them. You and other nurse assistants are the first person a resident sees each day, and the last. Read the following example and think about how that nurse assistant influences that resident's day.

It is 6 a.m. and most of the residents in the facility are just waking up. The night-shift nurse assistants are making their rounds, recording measurements on intake and output sheets and starting a.m. care for residents who want an early start. One of the nurse assistants, Mary, decides to weigh residents before the next shift arrives. She checks the weight chart and makes a list of residents to be weighed.

When Mary arrives at the first room on her list, she knocks on the door and introduces herself. As she walks in, she tells Mr. Sinclair she wants to weigh him. Mr. Sinclair wakes to find Mary in his room with the scale. Without apologizing for waking him or even saying "Good morning," Mary again says that she wants to measure his weight. He hesitantly agrees and climbs out of bed onto the scale.

How would you feel if someone awakened you this way? Would you think that the person who woke you this way cared about you? Is this a pleasant way to start the day?

Mary had good intentions: to help the day staff with some of their work, but she did not consider this resident's needs. Mary was not thinking of Mr. Sinclair as a person—but as a task to check off on a list. It cannot be overemphasized that residents should be treated with respect and dignity. Although Mary was trying to use her time wisely, she did not consider the resident's preferences or needs.

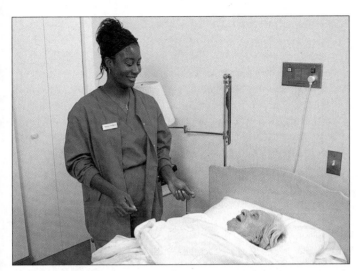

Fig. 28-3 — Being pleasant to residents all the time can make a difference in their quality of life.

TIME MANAGEMENT

Time management requires an ability to organize your activities and perform them efficiently. When you use time management skills in your work and life, you take control and prioritize your tasks. You decide what tasks are most important and what are the best ways to do things. With time management skills, you become more efficient but do not compromise quality.

In Chapter 12, Themes of Care, you read an example of helping a resident, Mrs. Jones, with a shower. Look back at that example and you will see how important planning is for time management. In the first scenario, you planned and incorporated all the themes of care. In the second example, poor planning resulted in the resident being injured. Think about that example. Imagine the rest of your day if that happened to you. You would have to call the charge nurse. Mrs. Jones' injury would be evaluated. You would have to monitor her very closely, at least once an hour. The charge nurse would call her physician and her family. You would have to prepare her to go to the hospital for X-rays. Several staff members would be involved in moving her. You would have to write an incident report. You would have to explain what happened to the charge nurse, the director of nursing, and the facility's administrator. The incident would have to be reported to the state.

While you are doing all of these things, what do you think is happening to the other residents you care for? Are their needs being met?

Time management is the theme of care that uses planning and prioritizing skills. It is **critical** to learn time management skills to ensure that you meet each resident's needs. You need to determine how much time it takes to complete the tasks you must accomplish during your shift and incorporate those tasks into the daily schedule. You need to prioritize these tasks based on the schedule and the residents' needs. By doing so, you can effectively manage your time to make sure you complete your assigned tasks by the end of your shift.

Prioritizing resident care is important. For example, the first thing you should do after you receive the report from the previous shift is walk around and see each resident. When making your rounds, see these residents first:

- ill residents
- residents with tubes or **shunts**
- residents who have recently had surgery or medical treatments
- residents whose condition has changed, such as residents experiencing falls, residents with infections, residents with behavior changes that raise concerns, and residents with poor appetite or weight loss

After you make your rounds, determine which residents require the most time to care for, which will be independent after you help them to get up, and which require total assistance. Then prioritize your tasks accordingly.

Critical — very important; a turning point or especially important period
Shunt — surgical passage created between two blood vessels to move blood from one part to another

A DAY IN A FACILITY

Nursing care is continuous 24 hours a day, 7 days a week, 365 days a year. Care in a long term care facility is typically organized into a day of three shifts. These shifts are the day shift (usually 7 a.m. to 3:30 p.m.), the evening shift (usually 3 p.m. to 11:30 p.m.), and the night shift (usually 11 p.m. to 7:30 a.m.). The shifts overlap to allow the staff who are leaving to communicate with the staff who are beginning their shifts and to ensure that residents are never without someone to care for them. Most staff are assigned to one of the three shifts. Some may rotate between two or more shifts. Some facilities offer "flex hours" such as 9 a.m. to 1 p.m. or 6 p.m. to 10 p.m. for staff who have child-care concerns.

Day Shift: 7 a.m. to 3:30 p.m.

The day shift is often very busy because most other team members work during the day shift. On this shift you are responsible for many of the personal care needs of residents. You assist with two meals, scheduled appointments, recreational activities, hydration, food supplements, and snacks. Most staff meetings, care plan meetings, and physicians' visits occur during the day. New equipment and care procedures are first tried and evaluated on the day shift. Visitors often start arriving before lunchtime (Fig. 28-4).

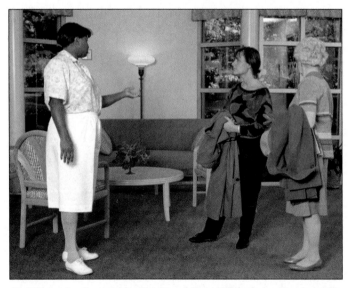

Fig. 28-4 – Family and friends often visit residents during the day shift.

Evening Shift: 3 p.m. to 11:30 p.m.

During the evening shift family members and friends often visit. Fewer staff are on duty, and scheduled appointments are fewer. Residents relax. The evening meal is served, and p.m. care is given to prepare residents for bed. This care includes undressing, partial bathing, scheduled showers, oral hygiene, toileting, evening snacks and hydration, and comfort measures for residents. Comfort measures may include straightening out or changing linens, providing back rubs, reading to residents, turning on soft music, and dimming the lights. On this shift you have an opportunity to spend more time with residents and their families (Fig. 28-5).

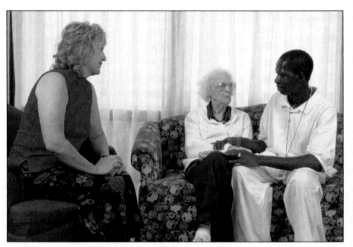

Fig. 28-5 – When family members visit a resident in the evening, you may have more time to get to know them.

Night Shift: 11 p.m. to 7:30 a.m.

This shift is often considered the quiet shift, but that's not always the case. During the night most residents sleep, but some nap during the day and are awake at night. The night shift has specific duties, such as completing tasks the evening shift could not complete: helping residents with toileting, checking supplies, comforting residents who cannot sleep, and dealing with unexpected problems and emergencies. Another night shift responsibility is a.m. care. For residents who rise early, a.m. care includes helping them wash their face and hands, brush their teeth, and go to the bathroom.

You may also be responsible for preparing paperwork for the next 24 hours (Fig. 28-6, next page). You may total input and output sheets, collect vital signs and bowel movement charts, and replace them with new ones. You may make a list of residents who need showers or tub or whirlpool baths. You have important tasks to prepare for the next day's activities. For example, you may have preoperative orders for a resident who will have a surgical procedure the next day. The most common preoperative order is keeping a resident "NPO p MN," which means a resident cannot eat or drink anything after midnight.

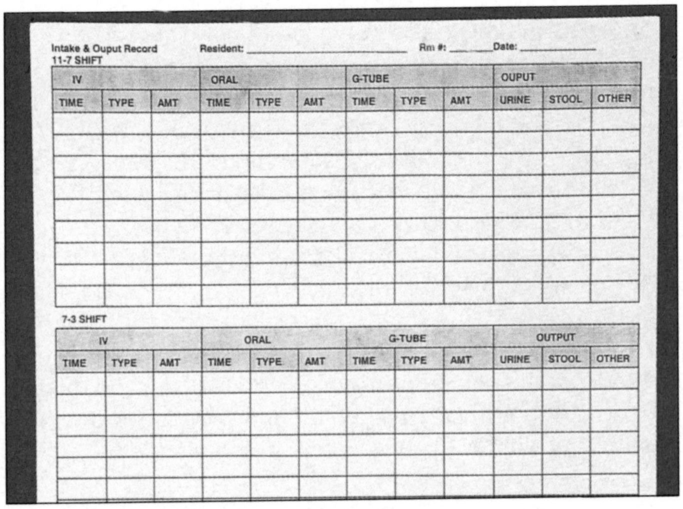

Intake & Ouput Record 11-7 SHIFT	Resident: _____		Rm #: ___	Date: ___						
IV			ORAL			G-TUBE			OUPUT		
TIME	TYPE	AMT	TIME	TYPE	AMT	TIME	TYPE	AMT	URINE	STOOL	OTHER
7-3 SHIFT											
IV			ORAL			G-TUBE			OUTPUT		
TIME	TYPE	AMT	TIME	TYPE	AMT	TIME	TYPE	AMT	URINE	STOOL	OTHER

Fig. 28-6 – The night shift is often responsible for preparing paperwork for the next day or completing paperwork begun on previous shifts.

All Shifts

At all times, on all shifts, consider each resident's needs. The shifts themselves are only a framework for care—not an absolute rule for what to do or not do. Although each shift has its specific duties, never insist on doing something if a resident does not want it done at that time. Similarly, if a resident wants you to do something that is normally scheduled for the next shift, make every effort to help.

MANAGING YOUR TIME: THE BALANCE OF ART AND SCIENCE

To begin to learn how to manage yourself and your time, consider the following pieces of the nurse assistant "puzzle." These are three sets of responsibilities you will learn to balance.

1. Residents' Preferences and Routines

As this book discusses in many different chapters, resi-

dents should always have a say in their own care. Let residents do as much of their own care as they can. Also let residents choose how they want things done. Learn about the residents' past routines and try to incorporate them into their present routine.

2. Shift Responsibilities

On your shift you have set duties. For example, on the day shift you get residents ready for an X-ray or appointments. On the evening shift you serve dinner. On the night shift you total the 24-hour intake and output records. You will learn your tasks and responsibilities during your orientation to the job.

Get to know your shift duties. Learn how to prioritize tasks and manage your time to complete your shift responsibilities during your shift. Identify which residents need baths, showers, weighing, intake and output measurements, and special turning as well as which residents have special equipment such as feeding tubes, oxygen, intravenous lines, shunts, splints, or a prosthesis.

3. Daily Assignment

You receive your daily assignment from the charge nurse. You should then ask the following questions:
• Do residents have any special needs I should know about? For example, Mrs. Brown in room 6, bed A, is going for a minor surgical procedure, and therefore she is NPO p MN and needs to be up and ready by 9 a.m.
• Do I need to call the charge nurse for any treatments? For example, Mr. Glass has a wound on his left leg. The charge nurse will clean the wound and apply the medication and dressing. The charge nurse wants to be called after Mr. Glass' shower.
• Does the charge nurse want certain activities done first? For example, the charge nurse wants you to help Mrs. Brown with personal care first so that she is ready for her 9 a.m. departure to the hospital for surgery.
• Do residents have any specific appointments? For example, Mrs. Smith has physical therapy at 10 a.m., Mrs. Cruz has physical therapy at 10:30 a.m., and Mrs. Smith has a hair appointment at 1 p.m.

These three sets of tasks help you make a plan for giving care. You are giving quality care when you balance all three responsibilities. The following case study shows how you can organize the residents' preferences, the shift responsibilities, and your daily assignments.

Case Study

You are working the 3 p.m. to 11:30 p.m. shift. The charge nurse assigns you to care for the six residents listed below. Your assignment also includes other shift responsibilities. The charge nurse gives you the following information at report time (Fig. 28-7). Getting and giving reports on each shift is very important so that you know how to care for your residents.

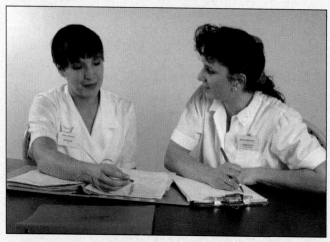

Fig. 28-7 – Getting and giving reports helps you know how to care for residents.

Residents

- Room 1, Mrs. Green—Had an uneventful day so far. Her daughter visited her at lunch. Her appetite has been poor, and she has eaten less than 60% of her meals for the last three days, but today she ate 75% of both breakfast and lunch. Her dinner intake needs monitoring.
- Room 2A, Mrs. Rose—Had a chest X-ray today at local hospital for her cough and shortness of breath, which she has had for 1 week. She seems anxious about the results. She has a history of congestive heart failure, and she has had some swelling in her feet the past two days. She is on oxygen. She was started on coughing medication today after her X-ray, and she is coughing less this afternoon.
- Room 2B, Mrs. Brennan—Slept all day because she "did not sleep the night before." She has no other complaints. She was restless last night and called out for her husband. She did not eat much during the day

shift because she was "too tired." She ate only 50% at lunch with encouragement.
- Room 3A, Mr. Gilbert—Had an uneventful day so far. Day 6 post-op; abdominal dressing dry and intact. He received pain medication once at 2 p.m.
- Room 3B, Mr. Goldberg—Is scheduled for removal of his prostate in the a.m. He seemed withdrawn during the day shift. He will be NPO after midnight.
- Room 4, Mrs. Beck—New admission to facility. She lived with her daughter who can no longer take care of her because of Mrs. Beck's deteriorating Alzheimer's condition. She is forgetful at times and wanders. She is incontinent sometimes but can walk to the bathroom when reminded. She feeds herself and is on a regular diet but needs encouragement. A meeting has been scheduled with family members and the social worker this evening.

Additional Assignments
- Add up all intake and output sheets at the end of shift.
- Supervise unit residents in the dining room at dinner.
- Take your dinner break at 7-7:30 p.m.

With this information and a clear understanding of your shift responsibilities, you can plan the order of your tasks, which give a sense of direction for your caregiving. You are prioritizing your responsibilities. You decide what to do first and what is the most important thing you must do. Prioritizing begins with making a list and then ordering the tasks on the list by what to do first, second, third, etc. The residents' preferences and routines primarily determine the order of your tasks, but you must also consider the shift responsibilities and the timing of some of these. For example, you can prioritize things to be done before dinner, things in preparation for dinner, and things after dinner but before bedtime.

Following is detailed information about these six residents, including information from the charge nurse's report, questions to ask the charge nurse, and the residents' preferences and routines.

Room 1, Mrs. Green
Information from report:
- Her daughter visited this afternoon instead of this evening, when she usually does.
- Her appetite has improved, and she is eating 75% of her meals.

Questions for charge nurse:
- Was Mrs. Green's appetite poor because she was ill, or was it something else?
- Should I talk to Mrs. Green about what foods she wants to eat?
- Does she have an intake and output sheet?
- Has she had an unintended weight loss?
- How much fluid should she be getting?

Resident's preference and routine:
- You know that Mrs. Green usually likes to get ready for bed after her daughter visits.
- She needs help with p.m. care.
- She eats by herself and is on a regular diet

Room 2A, Mrs. Rose
Information from report:
- Mrs. Rose has been short of breath and has had a cough for one week.
- Today she had a chest X-ray and is very concerned about the results.
- She is on oxygen.
- She has a diagnosis of congestive heart failure.
- She has had some swelling in her legs.
- She is taking a cough medicine.

Questions for charge nurse:
- When will the results of the chest X-ray be given to Mrs. Rose?
- Is there anything I can do to relieve her shortness of breath, like encouraging deep breathing, encouraging frequent rest periods, offering fluids, and elevating the head of her bed?
- Are there any special requirements for the oxygen?
- Should I let you know if she has swelling in her feet? Do her feet need to be elevated? Can she be out of bed?
- When is she due for her next dose of cough medicine?
- Can you explain to me what congestive heart failure is?
- What changes should I look for?

Resident's preference and routine:
- Mrs. Rose enjoys hot tea before bedtime.
- She has a favorite TV show that she watches with other residents every evening at 7:30.
- She likes her bed turned down by 9 p.m. so she can go to bed without help.
- She likes some assistance with her p.m. care.

Room 2B, Mrs. Brennan
Information from report:
- Mrs. Brennan slept all day.
- She had trouble sleeping the night before.
- She was restless and calling out for her husband.
- She did not eat much because she said she was too tired and required encouragement to eat.

Questions for the charge nurse:
- Did something happen to cause Mrs. Brennan to have trouble sleeping? An infection, change in mental status, or new medications?
- Is she not feeling well?
- Should I spend time with Mrs. Brennan to find out what is bothering her?

Resident's preferences and routine:
- Mrs. Brennan is usually independent and does not ask for help.
- She likes toast with jelly before bedtime.
- She likes to read in the lounge after dinner.

Room 3A, Mr. Gilbert
Information from report:
- Mr. Gilbert is doing well after surgery.
- He has an abdominal dressing, which is dry and intact.
- He received pain medication at 2 p.m.

Questions for the charge nurse:
- Is Mr. Gilbert in any pain? When is he due for the next dose of pain medication?
- Can he get up in a chair?
- What can he eat?
- When should I call you for the dressing change?

Resident's preference and routine:
- He needs complete assistance with p.m. care.
- He can get from his bed to his chair with help.
- He needs encouragement with eating.

Room 3B, Mr. Goldberg
Information from report:
- Mr. Goldberg is being transferred to the hospital for surgery in the morning.
- He seemed withdrawn during the day shift.
- He will be NPO after midnight.

Questions for the charge nurse:
- Is there anything I should do for this resident this evening?
- What is the surgery?
- How can I comfort him?

Resident's preferences and routine:
- He needs complete assistance with p.m. care.
- He can get from his bed to his chair with help.
- He loves to listen to the radio after dinner.

Room 4, Mrs. Beck

Information from report:
- She is a new admission.
- She lived with her daughter, who can no longer take care of her due to her deteriorating Alzheimer's condition. She is forgetful.
- She can walk and eat by herself with encouragement.
- She is on a regular diet.
- A meeting has been scheduled with the family and social worker tonight.

Questions for charge nurse:
- What is Mrs. Beck like?
- What is her level of independence?
- Does she need any supplies?
- Has she been oriented to the facility or her room and roommate?
- What time is the meeting with the family and social worker scheduled for?
- Has she eaten?
- Does she need to be monitored because of wandering?

Resident's preference and routine:
- Not known. You will begin to gather information tonight.

Organizing Care

You use each of these pieces of information to put together your plan for the evening. Following is an example of how you can organize the care you need to give.

1. Review your assignment. Determine who needs showers or baths, who requires complete assistance with eating, and who requires special attention during the shift. Prioritize the care you will give in order to accomplish all required tasks during your shift.
2. Make your rounds and say hello to all the residents you are caring for this evening, introducing yourself to the newly admitted Mrs. Beck. You now find out how residents are feeling this evening, what needs they have, and whether any resident has a particular need that becomes a top priority.
3. If no resident has a pressing need, begin to prepare residents for dinner. At this time you can ask residents about their day, focusing on any information that is a concern to them. For example, you say to Mrs. Rose, "I understand you had a chest X-ray today. How was it?" This gives her an opportunity to talk about her feelings. You tell Mrs. Rose that the charge nurse said she'll learn the result tomorrow. Maybe you offer her a cup of tea before dinner to encourage fluid intake, knowing how much she enjoys it. This gesture also shows Mrs. Rose you care about her.

   You continue to gather other information about residents' preferences and routines. For example, you could ask Mrs. Rose when she would like to get ready for bed after the 7:30 show tonight. As you follow this procedure with each resident, you will find what care you need to do and when to do it. Encouraging Mrs. Rose to take deep breaths, checking Mr. Gilbert's dressing and reporting to the nurse if it is dry or wet, and talking to residents are part of your before-dinner care.
4. Staff dinner breaks are scheduled either before or after the residents' meal. Knowing you are responsible for the unit supervision in the dining room, the nurse scheduled your break for after this time. It is important to take your break and eat so you will stay healthy and be able to keep giving the best care possible (Fig. 28-8).

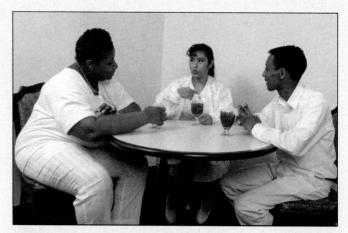

Fig. 28-8 – Taking your scheduled breaks helps you stay healthy and happy on the job.

5. The planning you did before dinner helps you organize the care you give after dinner and in preparation for bedtime. Because Mrs. Green's daughter visited during the day, she might want to go to bed earlier tonight. Checking on what she ate at dinner and talking about her likes and dislikes are very important for Mrs. Green's care, because her appetite has been poor lately.

   Knowing when and what residents like to do and how much assistance they need helps you in your planning. For example, both Mr. Gilbert and Mr. Goldberg, who are in the same room, need complete assistance with p.m. care. You need to plan a lot of time for their care and still make sure that while you're caring for them your other residents are taken care of. You need to remind the charge nurse when to come in for Mr. Gilbert's dressing change. You want to talk to Mr. Goldberg about his surgery because letting him talk about his fears will help him a lot.

6. When you have completed p.m. care for all these residents, you can now complete your other assignments. You can assist other staff members and discuss any questions you may have with the charge nurse.

7. Before ending your shift, you make rounds again. You complete all the I & O sheets and make sure that each resident's needs are met, your assignments are completed, and that you have reported to the charge nurse and have recorded necessary information.

This example shows you one way to organize your time by prioritizing your three responsibilities:
1. the residents' preferences
2. your shift responsibilities
3. your assignment to complete resident care activities

IN THIS CHAPTER YOU LEARNED:
- How nurse assistants contribute to quality care
- Things that influence how tasks are prioritized
- The theme of time management

SUMMARY
In this chapter you learned how to pull it all together using the time management theme of care. Meeting the needs of all the residents in your care requires careful planning and organization. You also learned about the three shifts and what routinely happens on these shifts in addition to resident care. In order to manage yourself and your time, you need to balance the assignments the charge nurse gives you, the residents' preferences and routines, and the shift responsibilities.

PULLING IT ALL TOGETHER
Have you ever heard the saying "Prior proper planning prevents poor performance"? This is exactly what you must do in order to do a good job. This chapter helps you learn to plan by using time management skills. Remember: Time management is the ability to organize and plan your activities and perform them efficiently. Think about everything you do, both in your job and in your life. Do you remember times when you felt more organized than at other times? When things did not go smoothly in your life, think about why. Do you think that if you had a plan in place during those times, you could have improved the outcome?

Mastering time management skills will help you to balance the art of caregiving with the science and skills of nursing. This balance is needed to ensure both quality of care and quality of life for residents. Be patient with yourself as you begin your job. Talk with other team members and the charge nurse about organizing and prioritizing your work. Their experience will be very helpful.

CHECK WHAT YOU'VE LEARNED

1. **Who has more contact with a resident than any other member of the health care team?**
   - A. The charge nurse.
   - B. The nurse assistant.
   - C. The director of nursing.
   - D. The resident's physician.

2. **To treat a resident as an individual, you must:**
   - A. Have them wear a name tag.
   - B. Learn their likes and dislikes.
   - C. Check on them at least twice an hour.
   - D. Try to become their best friend.

3. **How can you promote a resident's independence?**
   - A. Encourage them to read a book instead of watching television.
   - B. Tell them frequently that they are independent.
   - C. Give them choices in their care.
   - D. Make them do all their own personal care.

4. **How can you demonstrate your desire to be a good employee?**
   - A. Be late to work no more than once a week.
   - B. Record care activities in the resident's medical record even before you have done them.
   - C. Cooperate with other team members.
   - D. Offer to share your lunch with other nurse assistants.

5. **Why are time management skills important?**
   - A. To make more overtime pay.
   - B. To plan all residents' showers before the hot water runs out.
   - C. To be able to meet each resident's needs.
   - D. To have a fuller, more satisfying day off.

6. **Remember that mindful caregiving involves:**
   - A. Making your daily rounds within the first two hours of your shift.
   - B. Balancing the skills of nursing and the art of caregiving.
   - C. Asking every resident how their roommate is doing.
   - D. Getting lots of exercise.

7. **Which of these residents should you attend to first?**
   - A. A resident who recently lost their spouse.
   - B. A resident expecting family visitors this day.
   - C. A resident who is very ill.
   - D. A resident who recently transferred to your unit.

8. **After you make rounds, you prioritize your tasks based on:**
   - A. Which tasks require the most supplies.
   - B. Which tasks can be completed most quickly.
   - C. What tasks you'll have to leave for the next shift.
   - D. Which residents require the most assistance.

9. **Employees on the night shift have responsibility for:**
   - A. Scheduling resident appointments.
   - B. Helping residents get ready for bed.
   - C. Serving food supplements and snacks.
   - D. Giving a.m. care to residents who rise early.

10. **You are giving quality care when you balance residents' preferences and routines with:**
    - A. Routine reporting and documentation.
    - B. Your break times.
    - C. The costs to the facility for equipment and supplies.
    - D. Your assignment and shift responsibilities.

(Answers to "Check What You've Learned" are in the Instructor's Manual.)

Chapter 29

PROMOTING YOUR OWN HEALTH

Every year someone seems to come up with a new "Hollywood diet." These diets often claim that you can easily lose weight "the way movie stars do." Many people believe this and rush to try the new diet. Sometimes they work, but often the effect is only temporary. Usually people regain the weight they lost and add some more. This up and down weight loss and gain is called yo-yo dieting. It can cause your body more harm than good. For weight loss to become permanent, changes in lifestyle choices are needed.

Taking care of your health involves much more than dieting. To maintain or improve your health, you need to understand what it really means to have a healthy lifestyle. Then you must evaluate what is needed to maintain this lifestyle and make a plan to achieve your goals.

People in good health enjoy their life and their job much more than people who are tired or sick. You will also give residents better care when you feel healthy and rested and have a positive attitude. In addition, other staff can count on you not to call in sick, which would add to their workload.

Actions you take to maintain or improve your health are called health promotion. These include eating a healthy diet, getting regular exercise, managing stress, and a having positive attitude. These concepts are important for both you and the residents you work with. Improving the quality of your own life helps you improve the quality of life for others. In this chapter you will learn the benefits of good health as well as the factors that influence health.

OBJECTIVES
- List the factors that influence health
- Explain why having a positive attitude is important
- Describe general guidelines for good nutrition
- State the benefits of exercise

MEDICAL TERMS
- **Aerobic** – steady exercise that increases your heart rate and the amount of oxygen delivered to body tissue
- **Anaerobic** – exercise that does not increase the supply of oxygen to body tissue

"My nurse assistant is a model of healthy living. She motivates all those around her to take better care of themselves."

What does health really mean to you? Take a minute to visualize a healthy person. What image comes to mind? Do you see someone involved in a physical activity such as walking or jogging (Fig. 29-1)? What kind of body language do you see? What is their facial expression—are they smiling? What does their skin look like? How does someone with a healthy lifestyle make you feel when you are around them?

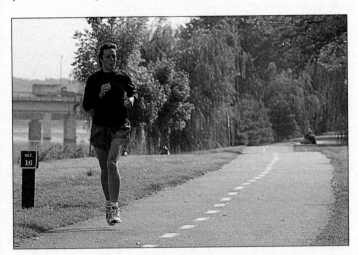

Fig. 29-1 – Healthy people usually include exercise in their life.

Health is more than just the absence of disease. Good health involves a number of factors and lifestyle choices. Together these contribute to your physical, mental, and social well-being.

Health promotion often involves changes in one's lifestyle choices. You must make a commitment to yourself and to your health. There is no magic pill or quick fix to ensure good health, just consistent healthy choices. Things that influence health affect the mind as well as the body.

YOUR HEALTH CHOICES

Many factors influence our health. Box 29-1 lists some of the most common factors. As you read that list, think about which factors you can control, which you already have in your life, and which you do not. Are there any areas where you can improve? Simple changes can sometimes make a great difference in how you feel.

There are many reasons why not everyone lives a healthy lifestyle. Often people do not recognize how their lifestyle choices affect their life and job. Think about what your day would be like and how you would treat residents if you came to work feeling terrible because you stayed up too late or drank too much alcohol. Your lifestyle choices

should not influence how you care for residents. Therefore it is important to understand the influence of your lifestyle on how you feel about your job. This knowledge can help you make the right lifestyle choices.

BOX 29-1.
FACTORS THAT INFLUENCE YOUR HEALTH AND WELL-BEING

- Your family history
- Your economic status
- Good nutrition
- Getting enough exercise
- Maintaining a healthy weight
- Getting adequate sleep
- Staying drug free
- Limiting the alcohol you drink
- Avoiding tobacco
- Using sunscreen
- Wearing your seatbelt (Fig. 29-2)

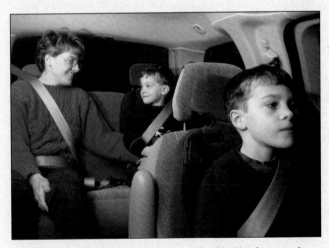

Fig. 29-2 – Many factors influence your health. Wearing a seat belt has saved many lives.

- Practicing safe sex
- Managing your stress
- Maintaining a positive attitude
- Seeing a health care provider regularly and having recommended screenings to prevent disease, such as blood tests, etc.
- Learning and paying attention to the early warning signs of cancer and diabetes

GOOD HEALTH

We all benefit from good health. Good health lets us lead a full, active life and achieve our maximum potential. This is true for you as well as for residents. Consider the following two examples of nurse assistants. As you read these descriptions, think about which one you would most like to be like. Think about what makes these two nurse assistants similar and different.

Maria is a 38-year-old mother of two. She is full of energy, always smiling and offering to help her co-workers. She has formed a walking group at lunchtime and every month organizes a potluck dinner to which everyone brings a healthy dish. Maria is also setting up an employee weight loss program at lunchtime for staff and residents.

Nancy is also a 38-year-old mother of two. She is always late for work. She never smiles but complains constantly about work. If you ask her to help, she does, but you never hear the end of it. She is overweight and eats junk food for lunch. She never participates in social activities.

Which would you like to work with?

Of all the factors listed earlier that combine to influence good health, perhaps the most important for all nurse assistants are:

- A healthy attitude
- Good nutrition
- Exercise

This chapter focuses on these three factors, although the other factors listed in Box 29-1 are also very important for a healthy lifestyle. Staying drug free, not using tobacco, and using alcohol only in moderation help you reach a higher level of health. These substances negatively affect people's lives and job performance. Drugs can impair one's mental and physical functioning. Tobacco use is linked to many diseases such as lung cancer, heart disease, and emphysema. Alcohol abuse can lead to malnutrition, impaired mental and physical abilities, and cirrhosis of the liver. It is also linked to certain cancers such as breast cancer and cancer of the esophagus.

Managing stress is also important for good health. In Chapter 2, Starting Your Job: What To Expect, you learned what you can do to help manage your stress. Stress can affect your health in many ways. It contributes to high blood pressure, heart disease, and diabetes. It can also decrease your immune system's ability to fight disease or heal from injury, and can contribute to the overall aging process. Stress can also increase your risk of getting into an accident or forgetting an important task. It is far too important to ignore.

No one can avoid stress, but we can learn to manage it more effectively. Some people exercise to reduce stress. An invigorating yoga practice or a calming meditation class might work for you. Laughter is still the best medicine, so take time to smile, increase your social interaction, talk with a trusted friend, and listen to music or participate in your favorite hobby to give your body and mind a chance to calm down. Even just taking a few deep breaths in a demanding situation can often relieve stress and anxiety. If things become unmanageable, consult a medical professional for further advice or treatment—don't go it alone.

DEVELOPING A POSITIVE ATTITUDE

One of the easiest things you can change is your attitude. A healthy attitude begins with a positive outlook. When people look at a glass half filled with water, some will say it is half-empty and some will say it is half-full. People have different attitudes and often see things differently. Those who describe the glass as half-full may have a more positive attitude than those who describe it as half empty. A positive attitude influences how you live your life, how you view your job, and how you treat residents.

It is easier to have a positive outlook when you feel good about yourself. A good attitude is also easier to maintain when you are well rested. Get plenty of sleep. It is recommended that you sleep seven to nine hours per night (Fig. 29-3).

A positive attitude can brighten your day as well as the residents'. Try to follow these guidelines:

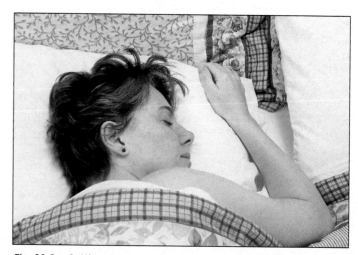

Fig. 29-3 – Getting enough sleep is important for feeling good.

- Every day think how important you are to yourself and others.
- Maintain a cheerful attitude—smile, it can be contagious!
- Be mindful of and open to others' points of view. Avoid negative criticism.
- Stay calm when things get hectic or a crisis occurs. Don't forget to breathe deeply.
- Try to think through difficult situations before you react.
- Maintain a compassionate, caring attitude.
- Emphasize the positive. See the glass as half-full, not half-empty.

- Accept yourself instead of judging yourself. Be the best you can be.
- Take charge of your life. Visualize what you want for yourself and your family, and work to achieve it.
- Refrain from gossiping. Refuse to contribute and remove yourself from a conversation moving in that direction.

A positive attitude improves your self-image and increases your happiness and well-being. This in turn helps you cope with stress and sadness. With a healthy attitude, you can also nurture this attitude in others. As a nurse assistant, your day-to-day attitude will have a direct impact on residents' attitude and quality of life.

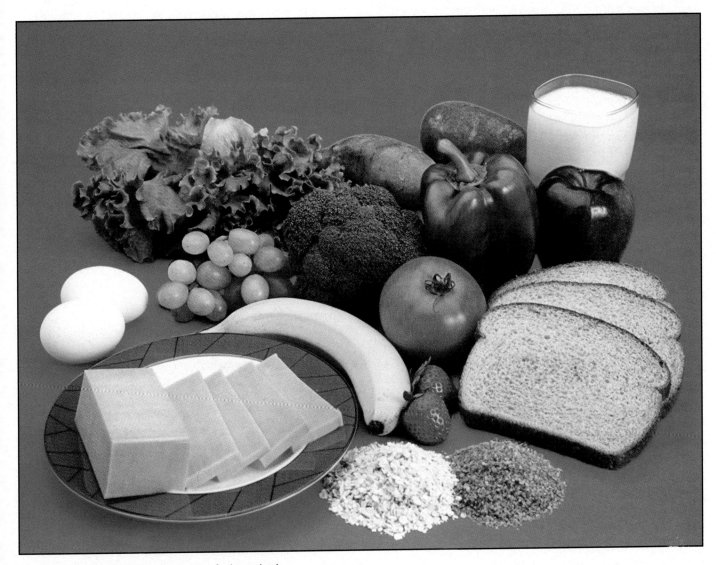

Fig. 29-4 — Eating healthy foods help you feel your best.

GOOD NUTRITION

Nutrition affects everyone's quality of life. Nutrition is even more important for a frail, elderly person. As a nurse assistant, one of your most important roles is helping residents with meals and monitoring their food intake (see Chapter 17, Assisting with Nutrition). With an understanding of what foods are needed, and in what amounts, to maintain health, you can encourage residents to make healthy food choices and make healthy choices yourself (Fig. 29-4, previous page).

What is good nutrition? Good nutrition involves eating a variety of healthy foods in appropriate amounts. This promotes maintaining a healthy body weight. Variety in your food choices helps ensure that you get all the nutrients your body needs. Some people can function for a while with poor nutrition but do not feel as good or function as well as they could. Not feeling well influences how you feel about your job. Many people eat a diet that is high in empty calories—those that fill you up but have little nutritional value. They often eat large portions and, if feeling stressed, may eat compulsively. They may function for years in this way, but eventually the results of poor choices will lead to poor health.

Guidelines for Healthy Eating

The U.S. Department of Agriculture (USDA) and Department of Health and Human Services have issued guidelines for good nutrition. These guidelines help us understand what we should eat to maintain good health. In general the guidelines recommend balancing good nutrition with physical activity to maintain an appropriate weight. They recommend a diet with plenty of whole grain products, fresh fruits, and vegetables—and only a small amount of foods high in fat, sugar, or salt.

These guidelines help you choose healthy foods for yourself and your family as well as your residents. The key is to discover what combinations of foods make you feel best. Before starting a weight loss program, you may want to see your health care provider. Read the nutrition facts on food labels, which will help you know what is in the foods you eat. Take advantage of the USDA nutritional resources offered online at www.myplate.gov. These can help you find the correct balance of food intake and exercise for you as an individual. Figures 29-5A and B, on the next two pages, provide some tips on healthy eating.

In addition, consider the following:
- Use sugar only in moderation.
  - Sugars and sugar-laden foods are high in calories and low in nutrients.
  - Sugar may be listed on food labels as fructose, glucose, maltose, lactose, molasses, high-fructose corn syrup, honey, and fruit juice concentrate.
  - Sugar contributes to tooth decay. To keep teeth and gums healthy, brush and floss regularly, and use a fluoride toothpaste.
- Drink soda (even diet soda) and coffee in moderation.
- Drink about eight glasses of water each day.
- Use salt and sodium only in moderation.
  - Use little or no salt in cooking and at the table. You can substitute herbs and spices for salt.
  - Eat only a minimum amount of salted snacks like chips, crackers, pretzels, and nuts.
  - When planning meals, consider that:
    – Fresh and plain frozen vegetables prepared without salt are lower in sodium than canned ones.
    – Cereals, pasta, and rice cooked without salt are lower in sodium than ready-to-eat cereals.
    – Milk and yogurt have less sodium than most cheeses.
    – Fresh meat, poultry, and fish have less sodium than the same foods that are canned or processed.
    – Most frozen dinners and combination dishes, packaged mixes, canned soups, and salad dressings contain a lot of sodium (salt). So do condiments such as soy sauce and other sauces, ketchup (or catsup), mustard, pickles, and olives.
- If you drink alcoholic beverages, do so in moderation (no more than two drinks a day for men and no more than one drink a day for women). One drink is considered to be:
  - 12 oz of regular beer
  - 5 oz of wine
  - 1 oz of distilled spirits (sometimes called hard liquor) (80 proof)
- Women who are pregnant or trying to become pregnant should not drink at all because alcohol may harm the fetus.

Dietary Guidelines 2010
Selected Messages for Consumers

Take action on the Dietary Guidelines by making changes in these three areas.

Choose steps that work for you and start today.

Balancing Calories

- Enjoy your food, but eat less.
- Avoid oversized portions.

Foods to Increase

- Make half your plate fruits and vegetables.
- Make at least half your grains whole grains.
- Switch to fat-free or low-fat (1%) milk.

Foods to Reduce

- Compare sodium in foods like soup, bread, and frozen meals—and choose the foods with lower numbers.
- Drink water instead of sugary drinks.

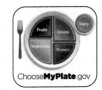

Fig. 29-5A — The USDA provides dietary guidelines to help you develop healthy eating habits.

Serving Sizes   Nutritional guidelines sometimes refer to "servings" of different foods. It can be difficult to judge exactly what is a serving. Following are some examples of serving sizes:

For grains such as bread, cereal, rice, and pasta, one serving means:
- 1 slice of bread
- 1 oz of ready-to-eat cereal
- 1/2 cup of cooked cereal, rice, or pasta (Fig. 29-6)
- 3 or 4 small plain cracke

For vegetables, one serving means:
- 1 cup of raw leafy vegetables
- 1/2 cup of other chopped vegetables, cooked or raw
- 3/4 cup of vegetable juice

For fruits, one serving means:
- 1 medium apple, banana, or orange
- 1 cup of chopped, cooked, or canned fruit
- 3/4 cup of fruit juice

For dairy such as milk, yogurt, and cheese, one serving means:
- 1 cup of milk or yogurt
- 1 oz of natural cheese
- 2 oz of processed cheese

For protein such as meat, poultry, fish, dry beans, eggs, and nuts, one serving means:
- 2-3 oz of cooked lean meat, poultry, or fish (Fig. 29-7)
- 1 cup of cooked dry beans
- 1 egg counts as 1 oz of meat
- 2 tablespoons of peanut butter equals 1 oz of lean meat

How much is an ounce of meat? Here's a guide (Fig. 29-8) to estimate the weight of a piece of meat, chicken, fish, or cheese:
- 1 oz is the size of a small matchbox.
- 3 oz is the size of a deck of cards.
- 8 oz is the size of a small paperback book.

10 tips
Nutrition Education Series

choose MyPlate

10 **tips** to a great plate

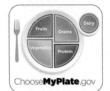
Choose**MyPlate**.gov

Making food choices for a healthy lifestyle can be as simple as using these 10 Tips.
Use the ideas in this list to *balance your calories*, to choose foods to *eat more often*, and to cut back on foods to *eat less often*.

1 balance calories
Find out how many calories YOU need for a day as a first step in managing your weight. Go to www.ChooseMyPlate.gov to find your calorie level. Being physically active also helps you balance calories.

2 enjoy your food, but eat less 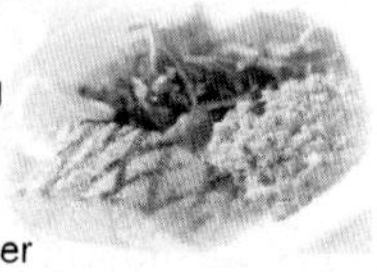
Take the time to fully enjoy your food as you eat it. Eating too fast or when your attention is elsewhere may lead to eating too many calories. Pay attention to hunger and fullness cues before, during, and after meals. Use them to recognize when to eat and when you've had enough.

3 avoid oversized portions
Use a smaller plate, bowl, and glass. Portion out foods before you eat. When eating out, choose a smaller size option, share a dish, or take home part of your meal.

4 foods to eat more often
Eat more vegetables, fruits, whole grains, and fat-free or 1% milk and dairy products. These foods have the nutrients you need for health—including potassium, calcium, vitamin D, and fiber. Make them the basis for meals and snacks.

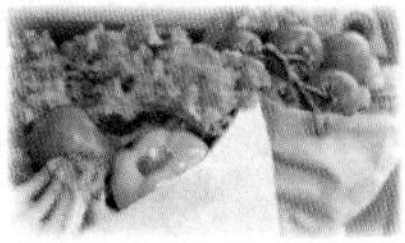

5 make half your plate fruits and vegetables
Choose red, orange, and dark-green vegetables like tomatoes, sweet potatoes, and broccoli, along with other vegetables for your meals. Add fruit to meals as part of main or side dishes or as dessert.

6 switch to fat-free or low-fat (1%) milk
They have the same amount of calcium and other essential nutrients as whole milk, but fewer calories and less saturated fat.

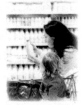

7 make half your grains whole grains
To eat more whole grains, substitute a whole-grain product for a refined product—such as eating whole-wheat bread instead of white bread or brown rice instead of white rice.

8 foods to eat less often
Cut back on foods high in solid fats, added sugars, and salt. They include cakes, cookies, ice cream, candies, sweetened drinks, pizza, and fatty meats like ribs, sausages, bacon, and hot dogs. Use these foods as occasional treats, not everyday foods.

9 compare sodium in foods 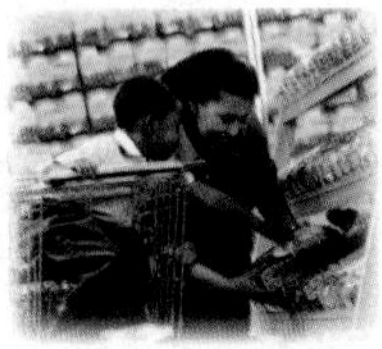
Use the Nutrition Facts label to choose lower sodium versions of foods like soup, bread, and frozen meals. Select canned foods labeled "low sodium," "reduced sodium," or "no salt added."

10 drink water instead of sugary drinks
Cut calories by drinking water or unsweetened beverages. Soda, energy drinks, and sports drinks are a major source of added sugar, and calories, in American diets.

USDA
Center for Nutrition
Policy and Promotion

Go to www.ChooseMyPlate.gov for more information.

DG TipSheet No. 1
June 2011
USDA is an equal opportunity provider and employer.

Fig. 29-5B — Tips like these are available from the USDA.

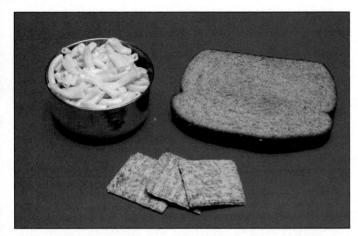

Fig. 29-6 – To have a healthy diet, you need to understand serving sizes. Each of the items shown is one serving.

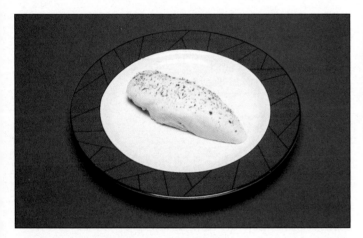

Fig. 29-7 – Recommended serving size of meat.

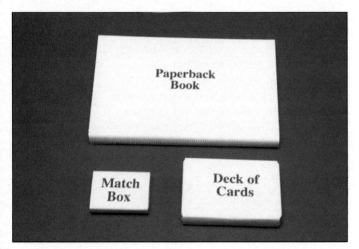

Fig. 29-8 – Understanding serving size helps you plan meals.

EXERCISE AND HEALTH

Exercise and physical activity are a vital part of life. Exercise can help you stay healthy and independent. Exercise can also help bring most people back to health.

There are two basic types of exercise. One is aerobic, which means "with oxygen." It is called this because this type of exercise requires increased breathing to supply more oxygen to the muscles over time. Walking, jogging, swimming, and cycling are examples of aerobic exercise (Fig. 29-9).

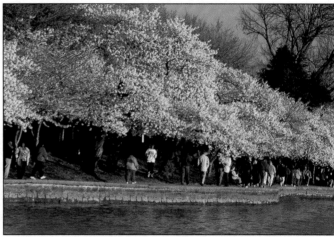

Fig. 29-9 – Walking briskly is a good form of aerobic exercise.

The other form of exercise is anaerobic, meaning "without oxygen." This is an activity of high intensity and short duration, such as weight lifting or sprinting (Fig. 29-10, next page).

It is best to get both types of exercise. Your physician can help you determine what specific exercise is best for you, including how to exercise and for how long. Exercising for 30 minutes three or four times a week can help you become more physically fit. You are never too young or old to benefit from exercise! Exercise improves the health of a 19-year-old or a 90-year-old. It benefits both you and residents

Aerobic – steady exercise that increases your heart rate and the amount of oxygen delivered to body tissue

Anaerobic – exercise that does not increase the supply of oxygen to body tissue

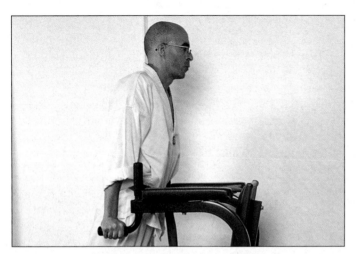

Fig. 29-10 – Weight lifting is an example of anaerobic exercise.

Find an activity that you truly enjoy and incorporate it into your daily routine. You will be more likely to stick with something that you enjoy. Walking, running, tennis, basketball, bicycle riding, hiking, yoga, or any other another activity that gets your heart beating, your blood circulating, and your muscles working will help improve your health and well-being. Be creative in finding ways to add exercise into your daily routine. For example, walk up the stairs instead of taking the elevator, or park your car far away from the entrance to the building and walk. If you find you have difficulty being consistent with an activity or routine, don't give up completely. Instead, try something different or vary your activity, but keep yourself involved.

Remember the healthy person you imagined at the beginning of this chapter. Most people visualize an active person with a strong body and good muscles. Exercise is necessary for anyone to build and maintain a healthy body. The specific health benefits of exercise are listed in Table 29-1.

TABLE 29-1
HEALTH BENEFITS OF EXERCISE

EXERCISE HELPS:	WHICH HELPS TO PREVENT:
Increase muscle strength	Muscle weakness
Maintain joint mobility and flexibility	Contractures, osteoporosis
Improve coordination	Falls
Improve self-image	Anxiety, depression
Maintain or reduce weight	Obesity
Improve circulation	Vascular disease, leg ulcers caused by poor circulation
Reduce many factors that contribute to heart disease	Heart disease
Reduce tension	Stress

TIPS FOR GETTING STARTED

Just as good nutrition and exercise help improve your health, so do other lifestyle choices. Follow these guidelines to make positive changes:

- Drink about 2 quarts of water every day, or about 8-10 glasses.
- Snack on unbuttered, unsalted popcorn, unsalted pretzels, fruit, or raw vegetables instead of candy and sweets.
- Bring your lunch to work instead of ordering fast food or buying snacks from the vending machine. Emphasize fruit, vegetables, and grains.
- Begin an exercise routine.
- Go for a walk at lunchtime or after work.
- Take the stairs instead of the elevator.
- Remember the overall principles of the USDA guidelines: To have a longer, better, and healthier life, eat a nutritious diet and be physically active everyday.

IN THIS CHAPTER YOU LEARNED:
• Factors that influence health
• Why having a positive attitude is important
• General guidelines for good nutrition
• The benefits of exercise

SUMMARY
In this chapter you learned what it means to have a healthy lifestyle. Many factors influence health, including nutrition, daily exercise, and managing stress. Some other factors you can control, and others you cannot. This chapter focused on three primary factors you can control: your attitude, nutrition, and exercise. These are important to maintain good health. You can start on the road to good health by following the helpful tips given in this chapter.

PULLING IT ALL TOGETHER
Part of being a good health care employee is making good choices about your own health. You cannot give quality care if you do not have a quality lifestyle. Think about the two nurse assistants described earlier in the chapter. Maria, who has a positive attitude, exercises, and eats a well-balanced diet is the nurse assistant everyone wants to be with. Like her, you will find that you will enjoy your work much more if you have a healthy lifestyle. If you do not, you should realize that you will be less able to manage your stress and feel good about your work. People with unhealthy lifestyles often blame their work for their stress, illness, or unhappiness—not recognizing that in fact it is their lifestyle choices that are causing their problems. Remember that the choice to promote your good health is in your own hands.

CHECK WHAT YOU'VE LEARNED

1. **How much water should you drink every day?**
   A. 1-2 glasses.
   B. 3-4 glasses.
   C. 5-7 glasses.
   D. 8-10 glasses.

2. **Alcohol abuse can lead to:**
   A. Lung cancer.
   B. Pressure ulcers.
   C. Cirrhosis of the liver.
   D. Bone disease.

3. **To become or stay physically fit you should:**
   A. Exercise only if your doctor says you need to.
   B. Exercise one minute per pound per day that you are overweight.
   C. Exercise at least 30 minutes 3 or 4 times a week.
   D. Exercise a minimum of an hour every day.

4. **Tobacco use is linked to:**
   A. Alzheimer's disease.
   B. Emphysema.
   C. Chicken pox.
   D. Brain damage.

5. **It is easier to maintain a positive attitude when you:**
   A. Be mindful of and open to others' point of view.
   B. Avoid hearing news stories on the television or radio or reading newspapers.
   C. Try not to think about difficult situations—act quickly before your mood is spoiled.
   D. Let family and co-workers make difficult decisions for you.

6. **Which is considered a healthy food choice?**
   A. Spinach.
   B. Canned fruit.
   C. Potato chips.
   D. Cold cuts

7. **What should your total intake of calories not be based upon?**
   A. Your age.
   B. Your height.
   C. Your desire.
   D. Your activity level.

8. **Glucose, maltose, lactose, and molasses are all names for:**
   A. Salt.
   B. Sugar.
   C. Sodium.
   D. Spreads.

9. **The USDA recommends which of the following as the key to good nutrition?**
   A. Become a vegetarian.
   B. Completely avoid all fats, oils, and sweets.
   C. Eat a variety of healthy foods.
   D. Put lots of salt on vegetables to make them taste better.

10. **What is an example of an anaerobic activity?**
    A. Basketball.
    B. Swimming.
    C. Weight lifting.
    D. Long distance running.

(Answers to "Check What You've Learned" are in the Instructor's Manual.)

Chapter

30

HOW TO BE A SUCCESSFUL EMPLOYEE

At the end of each chapter in this textbook, the section entitled "Pulling It All Together" is provided to help you understand key ideas and organize your time to do your job the best you can. In any profession, you first build a foundation of knowledge and then add to it with experience. In this way, you become a successful employee. You have learned much about how to successfully meet residents' needs. The information presented in these closing chapters is essential for you to know as you begin your first job as a nurse assistant.

Experience will help you incorporate additional knowledge and skill into your work. Referring back to this textbook throughout your career will help you perform procedures correctly and stay mindful in performing your job responsibilities.

Remember that in Chapter 2, Starting Your Job, you learned that you must be open, honest, and willing to learn and change. To be successful in your job you also must be mindful. If you become mindful in your life and in your care giving, you will find it easy to be a successful employee.

This chapter focuses on four topics to help you get started and then stay successful: preparing for the state competency evaluation, applying for a position, getting a successful start, and having ongoing success.

OBJECTIVES
- Describe what you can do to ensure that you pass the state competency evaluation
- Explain how to find a job
- Describe what you can do to be successful when you start your new job
- List what you can do to stay motivated on the job
- Describe how you can resolve problems on the job
- Describe the importance of inservice education

"It takes special qualities, knowledge, and skills to be a successful nurse assistant. I feel so fortunate to be cared for by such caring and dedicated people."

Have you ever gone to a party where you were supposed to meet someone, but when you arrived, they were not there and you did not know anyone else? How did you feel? Did you feel alone and uncomfortable? Did you want to leave? Did you try to hide in a corner, hoping that your friend would show up soon? Or did you introduce yourself to the host and explain you came alone but were invited by one of their guests? Did you try to mingle and fit in with the others at the party?

Sometimes starting a new job can feel the same as walking alone into a stranger's party. It is important for you to be prepared to start a new job where you do not know anyone. You should also think about how you can welcome and help others who are starting their new job at your facility.

PREPARING FOR THE STATE COMPETENCY EVALUATION

To work in a long term care facility, you must complete a state-approved training program and take a state competency evaluation, usually called "the state test." You are eligible to take the state test after you successfully finish your nurse assistant training. Your state may also allow certain employment and training experiences to substitute for training. Check with the state office in charge of nurse assistant testing or certification to learn more about eligibility and documentation requirements. That office can also provide specific information about taking the nurse assistant test. Most states have sample tests you can use to help prepare for the test.

Following are questions you should ask about the state test. Knowing the answers will help you will feel more confident.

- How do I apply for the state test?
- What type of test is given?
- How should I prepare for the test?
- When and where do I take the test?
- How do I get the results of my test?
- Can I apply for a job before taking the test?

The state test has two parts: skills and knowledge. In the skills part, you demonstrate your knowledge of clinical skills such as transferring residents, hand washing, and dressing a resident. The knowledge part, often called the written test, is usually a paper-and-pencil, multiple-choice test. The best way to prepare for the test is do well in your nurse assistant training. All the information you need to succeed on this test is in your training materials. Study your textbook before taking the test. Practice skills until you know them well. Ask your instructor to describe what you should expect on the test. Finally, be sure to arrive on time for the test so that you have time to relax before you start.

Following are some tips for taking the clinical skills part of the test:

- Review all the skills you learned in your nurse assistant training program. Ask your state office if they can give you a list of skills that you should review.
- Practice each skill with other students or family members. Ask your instructor, charge nurse, or staff developer to help you with anything you are having difficulty with or do not understand. Always remember to include the common preparation steps and common completion steps.

Here are tips for taking the written test:

- Review what you have learned in your nurse assistant training program.
- Ask for a sample test and become familiar with the types of questions on the test.
- Answer the questions to the best of your ability.
- Avoid guessing—usually your first instinct is the best choice.

General tips before you take the test:

- Get a good night's sleep before the test.
- Eat a well-balanced meal before the test.
- Make sure you know the correct address and directions to the test site. Drive there ahead of time if you have doubts or are anxious about finding the location.
- Be on time. Be prepared with all the necessary documents and tools needed to take the examination.
- Before starting, take a few deep breaths to help release stress and tension

Remember: The best thing you can do to prepare is to do well in your nurse assistant training program. Most nurse assistant students who do well in training also do well on their state examination.

GETTING A JOB AS A NURSE ASSISTANT

You should consider a number of things before beginning your search for a position as a nurse assistant. The better prepared you are, the more successful you will be in your job search. Consider the following factors:

Competency – legally qualified or demonstrating adequate abilities

CHAPTER 30 / HOW TO BE A SUCCESSFUL EMPLOYEE

- Where would you like to work? What location is best for you? Can you get to the facility by public transportation?
- What work shift is best for you?
- How many hours per week can you work?
- Can you work different shifts, or do you need one permanent shift?
- If you have children, have you arranged for childcare, and do you have a backup plan?

After doing this planning, you can take many different steps to find a nurse assistant position. Check the help-wanted ads in your local newspaper. Attend health worker job fairs. Ask the facility where you had your clinical experience if they have any openings. Ask friends, neighbors, or relatives if they know about good facilities in your area. Do an Internet search. Many newspapers also list job ads on their web site.

Once you have found a position that interests you, call or drop by the facility for an employment application and ask for an interview. Make sure you are dressed appropriately when you arrive to fill out your application. Have your current license or certificate of completion with you. The person hiring employees or a future supervisor might take that opportunity to interview you on the spot, so be prepared. Fill out the application neatly and accurately, using blue or black ink. Check your spelling. Be prepared and bring the names and phone numbers that you would like to list as references. Write down and take with you the dates, addresses, and phone numbers of previous employers and training programs, so you can list them neatly and accurately on you application. Include your dates of school attendance. Remember that the application form is often your first contact with an employer, so try to make a good first impression.

On the day of the interview, plan to arrive at least 15 minutes early (Fig. 30-1). Dress neatly and act professionally. Be open, honest, and confident during the interview. Consider asking these questions in your interview:
- What is the ratio of nurse assistants to residents at this facility?
- How long is the orientation program?
- Will I have a mentor or a buddy to help me get started—someone I can ask questions and learn from? How long does the mentoring program last?
- What type of benefits does the facility offer? Are there educational benefits?
- What shifts have job openings?
- Do staff members work on an every-other-weekend rotation?

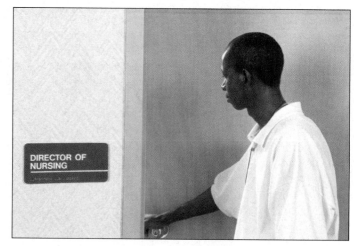

Fig. 30-1 – Arrive at your interview at least 15 minutes early.

- What do nurse assistants here wear to work?
- What type of screening will I have? (such as a background check for a criminal history or drug testing)

GETTING A SUCCESSFUL START AT YOUR JOB

Before you start your job, make sure everything in your daily life is in order. Arrange for childcare if needed, and have a backup plan in case your child or child-care provider is ill or has an emergency. Write your work schedule on your calendar to make it easier to keep track of the days and shifts you are on duty. Arrange for transportation if necessary, and arrive a few minutes early to orient yourself and settle in.

If you will wear uniforms, make sure they are clean and neat. Wear comfortable shoes that fit well and provide good support, because you will be on your feet much of your working day. Do not wear extravagant jewelry, make-up, or perfume. Keep your nails neatly manicured.

Remember how you felt alone among strangers at that party, waiting for your friend to arrive? You may experience similar feelings on your first day on the new job. Starting a new job can make you nervous and anxious. Keep in mind that you will be an asset to the care-giving team and that most staff are open and very eager to have new nurse assistants come on board. You will soon stop feeling nervous because other staff are happy to meet you and have you get started (Fig. 30-2, next page).

As a new employee, you may find that some staff members have been working together for many years. At first, you may feel left out. This is a common situation in all work settings. Soon you will stop feeling like the new

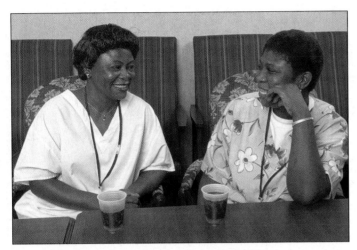
Fig. 30-2 — Other staff will welcome you to the facility.

employee, so be patient. Do not take it personally if you see other nurse assistants going to lunch together or helping each other. Eventually you will be part of the group (Fig. 30-3).

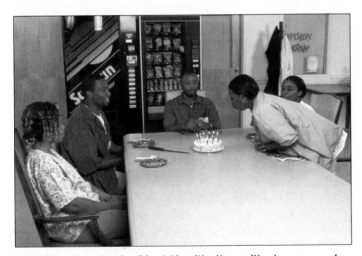
Fig. 30-3 — You will enjoy friendship with others with whom you work.

Give Yourself Time To Grow

No matter who you are or how much you know, you can always learn something new. Regardless of your experience, or how long you have been a nurse assistant, every new facility and every resident has something to teach you. Most important is being flexible and open to learning new and different information.

As a new nurse assistant, you may wonder how you will

ever be able to manage everything you have learned to properly care for each resident. Most important, remember the philosophy of mindfulness and the themes of care you have learned in this textbook. If you remember and apply these, you will not go wrong. You will be giving individualized care thoughtfully while treating residents with the dignity and respect they deserve.

When you first start your job, you may get an assignment that seems overwhelming. You may ask yourself how you can care for so many residents in the time that you have. At first, you may need to ask many questions. Be patient with yourself. Write things down. Ask the charge nurse when you have questions or need to review a procedure. Check with the charge nurse to be sure that this is a good time to talk and that they are the one you should be asking. It is important to find the right resource for information on your first day on the job. However, never feel that you cannot ask questions.

Think about what you learned in Chapter 28, Pulling It All Together, about time management and the factors that influence care. This information will help you be successful. In addition, ask yourself questions like these after your first week on the job:

- Do I know where everything is located?
- Do I know how all the equipment works, like mechanical lifts and scales?
- Do I know my shift responsibilities?
- Have I met the director of nursing, assistant director of nursing, and staff developer?
- Do I feel I've learned something new about the residents I cared for every day?

Every day as you leave the facility, think about your work experience that day. Some days you will be so busy that you will wonder where the time went. As you reflect on the day, write down any questions you have.

ONGOING SUCCESS

Managing Yourself and Staying Motivated

Managing yourself is as important as managing your time. When you are managing yourself, you are taking care of yourself. Part of managing yourself is staying motivated in your job.

If you look at each day as a new opportunity to learn and grow, you are less likely to get bored or feel discouraged. It is easy to become bored if you do not have a positive attitude toward your job or if you engage in nonproductive activities like gossiping. To stay motivated and happy in your job, do things that make you feel good and avoid certain pitfalls (Fig. 30-4). Think about the lists in Box 30-1. If you keep these things in mind, you will stay motivated and enjoy your job more.

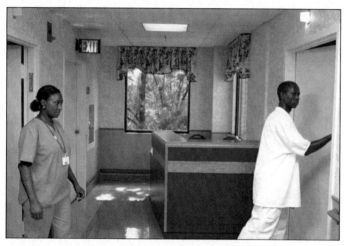

Fig. 30-4 – Helping co-workers care for residents makes you feel good about yourself.

If you feel you're falling into a negative mindset or behavior patterns or you find yourself thinking, "I don't want to do this any more," take some time and review the lists in Box 30-1. Check to see if you have slipped into behaviors that you should avoid or have forgotten things you should do. This self-evaluation can help you identify what is wrong. Discuss your concerns with a close friend or, if necessary, with the charge nurse.

Sometimes just talking out loud about your problems can help you identify the real issue. Making changes and solving problems are easier if you address them promptly. However, if you do find it necessary to take action about a concern you have regarding your job, be sure to communicate through the proper channels.

Effective Communication and Problem Resolution

Communicating through proper channels is important for all employees in a facility. Because you work in the facility's nursing department, you should understand its chain of command, which begins with the director of nursing.

If you have any grievances, complaints, concerns, or questions about your care giving or that of a co-worker or team member, first discuss the issue with the charge

BOX 30-1.
STAYING MOTIVATED AND HAPPY ON THE JOB

Things to do:
1. Take advantage of all opportunities to learn.
2. Ask questions; get involved.
3. Be open to change, and be willing to offer change.
4. Participate in evaluation exercises.
5. Try new products and techniques.
6. Stay healthy.
7. Find a balance between work and home.
8. Work with others to help them grow (Fig. 30-5).

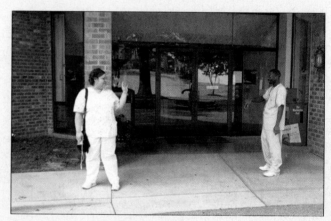

Fig. 30-5 – Working with others helps you to get to know them better.

Things to avoid:
1. Avoid cutting corners—like feeding two residents at the same time, skipping assignments, guessing about information, or not following all the steps in a procedure.
2. Do not gossip about residents or staff.
3. Avoid ignoring people or being uncooperative with co-workers.
4. Do not bring personal problems into the facility.
5. Do not discuss your frustrations with residents or their family members.
6. Avoid not being open to trying different things or to change.
7. Do not have a negative attitude about your work or residents.

nurse. Be clear about what you think the issue is, describe it accurately, and give as many examples as possible. If necessary, put your concerns in writing. Be willing to discuss different solutions.

If the charge nurse is unavailable but immediate action is necessary, you can go directly to the nursing office and ask to meet with the director of nursing. For example, incidents of resident abuse or injury require immediate attention. However, the charge nurse can handle most complaints. Give the charge nurse every opportunity to deal with your concerns before going to the director of nursing. If you find it necessary to go to the director or facility administrator, be sure you have all the information and can state the facts, give examples, and suggest solutions.

For example, you may have to go directly to the director of nursing if you need extended time off due to a family crisis or illness. In this case, the director of nursing would give you a leave of absence and inform the charge nurse of this decision.

At some point, it may be necessary for you to file a formal grievance or complaint about something related to your job or care practices you are concerned about. If so, be sure to follow your facility's policy for grievances. The procedure is in your facility's personnel policy manual. Follow each step accurately. Grievance policies are designed to give all staff members a way to state their complaints and find solutions that will lead to improvements in quality care.

Assertiveness: How To Accomplish What You Think Is Important

Assertive behavior is sometimes necessary to accomplish something you think is important without hurting other people. Being assertive means speaking up for yourself or saying no when asked to do something you are not comfortable doing. In your work, you need to communicate assertively every day. You need to be assertive to do what is best for both residents and yourself. Do you ask for what you want, or do you expect others somehow to read your mind? Can you say no without feeling guilty if someone asks you to do something you cannot do? Do you look for solutions to problems or just complain about them?

These are all types of assertive behavior. However, being assertive is different from being **aggressive**. Aggressive behavior hurts other people or makes them angry. Aggressive behavior usually does not accomplish the right things.

If you do not assert yourself and do not speak up, but keep your feelings and needs inside, you are being passive. If you do not speak up for yourself, you miss opportunities. For example, the charge nurse may ask you to do

something you have not yet learned to do. Compare these possible responses:

Assertively you would say, "I do not know that skill. If you show me how, maybe I can do it next time" (Fig. 30-6).

Passively you might say, "If you really want me to, I'll try to do it."

Aggressively you might say, "No way. That's not my job."

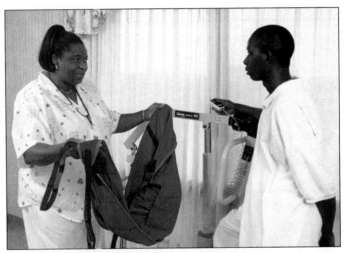

Fig. 30-6 – Saying you do not know something and asking for help are ways to be assertive.

Even when you act assertively, you still may not get the result you want. Others may still say no. Your supervisor may not let you work a different shift, or a resident may not want your help. The important thing is to stand up for yourself and try to accomplish what is important for you and the residents you work with.

📖

aggressive – behavior that is hurtful to others and may make them angry

Evaluating Your Work: Learning To Grow

This textbook often refers to the concept of quality care. Quality care is individualized resident care that you give mindfully. When you consider a resident's needs, incorporate the themes of care, and treat residents with respect, patience, and compassion everyday, you are giving quality care. You can keep improving the quality of the care you give by seeking feedback from residents, their families, your co-workers, and your supervisor. Feedback tells you how well you are doing and helps you improve your work.

In addition to evaluating yourself, you can also ask your supervisor how you are doing. Following are some of the things supervisors look at when they check your work:

- Do you complete all your assigned work?
- Do you ask questions?
- Are all your residents comfortable?
- Do you check often on all residents?
- Do you report changes in residents immediately?
- How do your co-workers feel about your work?
- Are you a team player?
- Do you arrive at work on time? (Fig. 30-7)

In addition to considering these questions yourself, you can take the initiative to ask your supervisor questions such as the following:

- Did you check my work today? How did I do?
- Could I show you how I do this to see if there is a better way?
- I seem to have a problem in this area. Can you help me?

Your open communication with other staff will help you grow as a nurse assistant. You will also feel better about your work if you seek feedback. Ask residents questions like "Have I met all your needs? Is there anything else I can do for you?" Ask a resident's family members how they think their loved one is responding to your care. Do they like the schedule for activities and other aspects of your care?

Most important, accept the feedback you receive in a positive way. Make changes when you can, and get help in any areas you find difficult. In most facilities, employees are also given a formal evaluation periodically. Ask your supervisor about the evaluation schedule (Fig. 30-8).

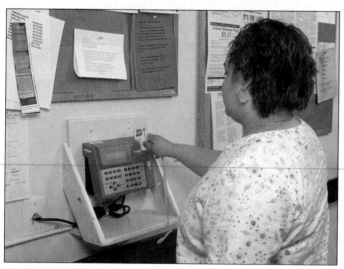

Fig. 30-7 – Arriving on time gets your work day off to a good start.

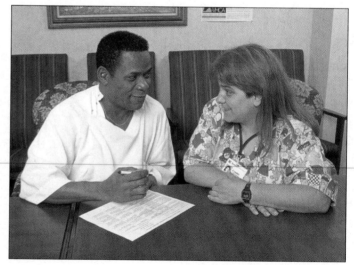

Fig. 30-8 – Your supervisor may evaluate your work either formally or informally.

📖

Initiative – introductory action, such as the first step in an attempt to resolve an issue

Improving Care Through Inservice Education

Inservice education is an important part of quality care. Inservice education involves a learning process that may be either formal or informal. Residents' needs change, technology improves, and nursing care practices are updated. Long term care facilities are required to offer nurse assistants at least 12 hours a year of inservice education. Your staff educator will inform you about future classes. Take advantage of what your facility has to offer.

Inservice education gives you an opportunity to grow, change, and improve. It is a good way to stay challenged and motivated. It is one of your most valuable employee benefits. Attending inservice education classes in your facility is the most efficient way to gain new hands-on information. Taking additional classes, subscribing to professional magazines, and joining professional organizations are other ways to continue your education and improve the quality of your care.

IN THIS CHAPTER YOU LEARNED:
• Tips for passing the state competency evaluation
• How to find a job
• What you can do to be successful when you start your new job
• What you can do to stay motivated on the job
• How to resolve problems on the job
• The importance of inservice education

SUMMARY
This chapter discusses how to be a successful employee. The employment process begins with preparing for the state test and then seeking the job you want. You also learned about how to begin your new job successfully. You must be patient with yourself when you begin. As you grow as a nurse assistant, you must always stay mindful in your care. You need to ask for feedback and be willing to change. Continuing your education through inservice will help you to grow in your career.

PULLING IT ALL TOGETHER
Have you ever met someone who even on their first day at work seemed to know everything? This is very rare. Typically, people need time to grow in their chosen profession, whether it is their first job or simply their next job. It is important to recognize that you need time to adjust to a new environment so that you are not frustrated when you start your career as a nurse assistant. You must also be willing to ask questions so that you learn things the right way from the first day.

Always remember that you are the person who spends the most time with the residents. You can make the difference in how the resident feels about their life while living in a long term care facility. Think back to the introductory paragraph in Chapter 1, which asked you what you think makes life worth living. Always remember that how you treat the residents' influences whether they feel life is worth living.

Give them the best care you have to offer.

1. **What is the best way to prepare to take the state nurse assistant exam?**
   A. Spend a day volunteering and helping nurses in a hospital.
   B. Study your Nurse Assistant textbook and review the skills you learned.
   C. Read three or four other nursing textbooks.
   D. Ask an experienced nurse assistant if they remember what was on the test.

2. **How should you answer questions during your job interview?**
   A. Tell the interviewer what you think they want to hear.
   B. You can avoid having to answer uncomfortable questions if you ask questions back instead.
   C. Offer no more information than exactly what is asked for.
   D. Be honest and open in answering questions.

3. **When you interview for a nurse assistant position, which question should you ask?**
   A. Will I have a mentor to help me get started?
   B. Do you have a smoking lounge for employees?
   C. How long do lunch breaks last?
   D. Do I really have to empty bedpans?

4. **On your first day of work you feel overwhelmed by everything you have to do. What should you do about this?**
   A. Just do your best and don't worry if not everything gets done.
   B. Be sure to do what you think are the most important things, and leave everything else for the next shift.
   C. Talk to the charge nurse.
   D. Help only those residents who use their call lights.

5. **As you become more experienced in your job you'll learn when you can safely:**
   A. Save time by feeding two residents at once.
   B. Ignore certain co-workers who would never say anything to the charge nurse.
   C. Skip steps in a procedure as long as the resident will not be injured.
   D. Try new products and techniques.

6. **In the chain of command, to whom do you report?**
   A. The charge nurse.
   B. The administrator.
   C. The staff developer.
   D. The director of nursing.

7. **Whenever you have a concern or complaint about an issue at work, who should you talk to first?**
   A. A resident you can trust.
   B. The charge nurse.
   C. The ombudsman.
   D. The director of nursing.

8. **You are communicating assertively when you:**
   A. Feel guilty after saying you cannot volunteer for an extra shift.
   B. Share your complaints with residents.
   C. Speak up for yourself without hurting others.
   D. Say what you think other people will want to hear.

9. **Which of the following statements is an example of an aggressive remark?**
   A. "I don't have time right now to help you finish your work."
   B. "I'm not able to help you today; maybe I can do it next time."
   C. "If you weren't so lazy you could get your work done yourself."
   D. "If you want me to, I'll try to do it, but I really don't have time."

10. **Inservice education is important because:**
    A. It prepares you for the nurse assistant exam that you have to take every year.
    B. You get paid more for every hour of inservice you take.
    C. The nurse assistants with the most hours of inservice get to pick their shifts.
    D. It gives you an opportunity to grow, change, and improve.

(Answers to "Check What You've Learned" are in the Instructor's Manual.)

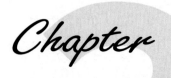

Chapter 31

CUSTOMER SERVICE is just what it sounds like: service to a customer. Serving a customer is what defines your job as a nurse assistant. People enter health care professions because they want to help people. Most of the people that you will serve are having problems with failing health or are trying to recover to a healthy way of life. Everything that you do in health care is centered on the principle of service. Customer service is not just a task—it has to be part of who you are. You will use this skill with your residents, families, supervisors, peers, and guests. It is important that you look at what customer service means to you as a nurse assistant as you discover who your customers are and what they all expect of you in your role.

CAN I HELP YOU?

Have you ever gone into a store to buy new clothes and received really poor customer service from a sales clerk? What did that person do that you did not like? Did they treat you rudely or act like they really did not want you in their store? Now think about a time when you felt like you got great customer service. How were you treated in that situation and what were the differences in those two experiences? As you read this chapter, think about customer service in a positive way. Relive that first negative event and think about what could have made that experience better for you. How would you have liked that situation to have been different? What would have made it the perfect customer service experience? These are things that you would want to include in your own actions toward others on your job as a nurse assistant.

In this chapter you will learn what it takes to provide good customer experiences through the use of communication skills, understanding customers' expectations, and being attentive to their needs. You will understand the effect of customer service on the quality of care for residents and the impact that it will have with your co-workers.

OBJECTIVES
- Define customer service
- Understand what customer service means in long term care
- Understand the importance of providing good customer service to residents and co-workers
- Describe how poor customer service affects the satisfaction of residents and families
- Explain how to give good customer service as a part of excellent resident care

KEY TERMS
- **Customer service –** the quality of a service given a customer
- **External customers –** individuals not employed within the organization, such as residents, family members, vendors, and guests
- **Internal customers –** customers who are within the same organization, such as supervisors, peers, and other co-workers
- **Empathy –** the ability to identify with and understand somebody else's feelings or difficulties

"I don't expect everything to be perfect, I am just so glad that you try."

546

This chapter focuses on two types of customers. External customers are those who seek services from you outside of your organization. External customers include residents, families, vendors, and guests. You will also serve internal customers within the organization where you work. Those include supervisors, peers, and people in other departments within your organization. Good internal customer service has as much effect on care as it does on your organization's image within the community. Organizations in which everyone provides good customer service have greater job satisfaction, lower absenteeism, higher morale and engagement, and less turnover. All people want to work where they are happy and are treated with respect and enjoy being with people who they work with as partners. Every individual employee has an important part to play in giving good service, which also improves the quality of the organization.

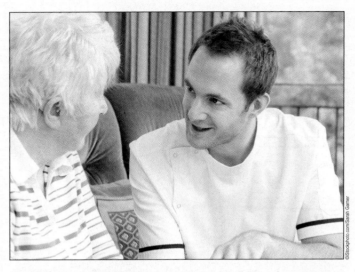

Fig. 31-2 – Employees who develop a service mentality are a valuable asset to the organization.

WHY CUSTOMER SERVICE IS IMPORTANT

Serving customers is a key part of every job in every organization (Fig. 31-1). It also has a definite impact on the overall success of every type of organization. Successful facilities have fewer complaints from residents and their family members, as well as from employees in the facility. Every organization needs customers to succeed, just as long term care facilities do. Many employees in long term care think they work only in health care, but that is only partially true. You are also in the *people care* business. It is part of the job of the whole health care team to be the people care team. You must be willing to take care of not

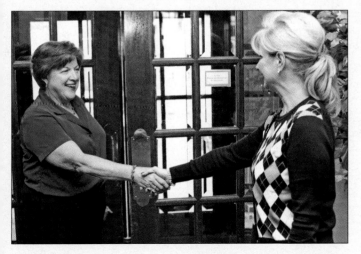

Fig. 31-1 – The first impression is made when the customer enters the facility.

only residents but also their families, visitors, and guests. How you treat them and react to their concerns will affect how they talk about the facility. You need to make sure that you have satisfied customers. You can do this by developing a service mentality (Table 31-1).

Satisfied customers have their needs met, but the best customer service makes sure that customers get what they need and more than they want, within reason. Great customer service includes making an extra effort and giving more than what is expected or needed. A service mentality shows empathy in every encounter with both internal and external customers. Excellent customer service includes passion that will spread to everyone around you. Your service attitude shows in your patient care and in the pride you show in all that you do. You will have a "whatever it takes" attitude that can be easily seen by others. You should be responsible and respectful of your peers and what they do within the team, and you will be able to make changes with a positive attitude and friendly face. When you fully understand the service mentality, you can balance many different needs and make good decisions. Nurse assistants who can master all or most of these skills are a valuable asset to the organization (Fig. 31-2).

In recent years long term care services have increased to include home health, home- and community-based programs, assisted living, senior housing, retirement communities, etc. Long term care is no longer the only option. Customers can select the long term care environment that best suits their needs. For your organization to be the top choice for residents and families, you must

TABLE 31-1 SERVICE MENTALITY

SERVICE MENTALITY	DEFINITION	EXPLANATION
Empathy	The ability to understand, be aware of, and be sensitive to the feelings, thoughts, and experiences of others	• Customers need to know that we care • A caring tone lets customers hear your concern • Customers need to know they are heard and understood
Enthusiasm	Bringing a strong interest and energy to a project or service situation	• The enthusiasm people show affects how the world perceives their willingness to help • Enthusiasm influences effectiveness • Truly enthusiastic people do not discriminate between activities • Enthusiastic people enjoy thinking ahead and going the extra mile
Ownership	Being committed to solve a problem or take it to someone who will	• It only takes one person to provide a good customer experience • Ownership is partnering with the customer to address their need and solve their problems • When we own the problem, we are more committed to solving it
Responsibility	Living up to the responsibilities one accepts	• Important to internal customer service • Important to be as considerate and responsible to our co-workers as to our customers
Adaptability	Being flexible to effectively deal with different customers and situations	• Adapters can handle all types of customers and situations positively • Adaptability is changing your approach with each customer's needs • Serving each customer respectfully and effectively
Balance	Being able to satisfy the customer while considering the resources and needs of the organization	• Finding a balanced solution to meet the challenge of the customer and also meet the needs of the organization • Helping customers feel they are heard and treated fairly • Acknowledging the feelings of the customer even if you disagree
Resiliency	Being able to bounce back from adversity	• Remaining calm in adverse situations, recovering quickly, and not showing signs of discouragement • Speaking in a controlled, unemotional manner • Handling life's setbacks by bouncing back emotionally and professionally • Never taking it out on the next customer or co-worker

deliver good customer service. Great customer service by nursing assistants will:
- Increase the quality of care for residents
- Improve the overall quality and reputation of the organization as a place where people will want to go or send their loved one
- Improve the opportunities for professional growth and opportunities within the organization

In most communities, families have several choices to make before their loved one moves into in a long term care setting. Customer care and service can be the key in their choosing your organization for the care of their loved ones. Superior customer service skills help you be seen as an excellent employee and caregiver. If your organization is to succeed, you must help create an environment where your customers get more than they expect from you (Fig. 31-3). This goes past great customer service. You want families to say: "We are so glad we brought our Mom here!"

WHAT CUSTOMERS EXPECT

What residents expect today is not the same as even 10 years ago. People are better informed and have more choices available to them. They know how to use the Internet to research their options. Residents are more independent and want more input into their care. The generation now entering long term care is used to things being convenient for them. They require more than ever before to have their needs met. It is up to you to assist them in ways so they feel they are important and are

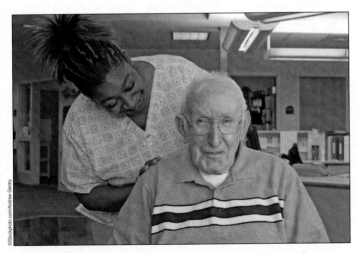

Fig. 31-3 – You must create an environment that gives the customer more than what they expect.

BOX 31-1.
EXPECTATIONS OF RESIDENTS FOR CUSTOMER SERVICE

Residents expect nurse assistants to:
- Be friendly
- Be confident
- Build relationships and rapport
- Smile when you ask questions
- Find solutions for problems quickly
- Be accountable
- Assure that they can provide needed help
- Be consistent in what they say and do, and how they provide care

getting the very best care. Excellent customer service means giving your residents the care they want and need. It also means providing less obvious services, such as really listening to residents and responding with empathy to unhappy customers. It may also mean doing what you can when you can't give them exactly what they want. How customers are treated can make the difference in decisions regarding where they choose to be cared for. Box 31-1 outlines expectations residents may have for customer service.

To provide the best service possible, you must know the expectations customers have for your work. Customer expectations go beyond basic service. Positive customer relationships and loyalty come from what it is like doing business with you. A family cares about issues like these: How does my loved one like you? How well do the staff know my mother? How are messages delivered? How are problems resolved? Feelings of trust build as small things add up. These factors can make or break the customer service relationship over time.

"Average" is not good enough anymore. Average care and customer service are not what residents and families are looking for. Residents and their families want excellent care, and this has become the new minimum standard.

Simply satisfying your customer is not enough. You must go beyond average levels of satisfaction to improve the quality of your residents' lives. People do not talk to others about average service, but they do talk about exceptional service. The facility develops its reputation based on the customer service it provides.

GIVING GOOD CUSTOMER SERVICE

Self-Image and First Impressions

Customer service begins with the first contact. We only have one opportunity for a first impression, and that sets the tone for anything else that follows. When a negative impression is made, we must try much harder to get our customers to trust us. But when we manage our first impressions, we set a positive tone for everything that we do from that point on.

Greeting staff members, visitors, and residents is key for giving good customer service. Everyone who enters the facility deserves a hello from staff members, and especially from nurse assistants caring for residents. If you ignore or fail to greet or speak to family members, this sends a non-verbal message that they are not important to you.

When you see a new face in the facility, be friendly. This person may be a visitor who is deciding whether to reside in the facility. A visiting potential resident and his or her family will share their decision with other people they know. Offer to escort the visitor or give directions. Make eye contact and introduce yourself. Smile. When greeting a frequent guest, remember and use his or her name. The impression that facility staff members make on visitors contributes to the facility's overall reputation.

Customer service is not a system, but a way of being that everyone should practice. We know that we should treat our residents and families the way we would want to be treated ourselves. That means that we have to be flexible to do what we can to make the resident and family happy. We need a "whatever it takes attitude."

MINDFUL CAREGIVING

Mindful Caregiving

Mindful caregiving is important in everything that you do, especially as you observe and attend to customer service needs. You need to understand what the resident and the family want, need, and expect, so that you will know how to respond. You need to be flexible and open to what is going on with every resident with whom you work everyday. What residents wanted yesterday may not be what they want today. Just because someone wanted eggs for breakfast last week does not mean that they will be excited to get them every day.

Customer service skills play a big role in mindful caregiving. As you give care to residents, *observe* what they say

and notice changes in them (Fig. 31-4). Always then report your observations to your supervisor. Sometimes you may not be able to explain why you think a resident is "different" today, but all changes can be significant. You are the person who has the closest contact with each resident on a daily basis. Often you are the first to notice even the slightest change in their behavior or actions. Sometimes these small changes are very important because there is a serious underlying reason. If a resident becomes more confused than normal, for example, this may be an early sign of a serious medical condition that needs attention. You can play a big role in their care by observing and reporting all changes you see.

Sometimes routine caregiving can have a negative customer service effect. If you get into an automatic routine for feeding, bathing, grooming, and dressing your residents, your customer service skills will probably suffer. Mindful caregiving is needed for maintaining great customer service skills.

Consider the Resident a Customer

Customer satisfaction for a resident involves their perception of the quality of the care and services they receive. To be successful in your caregiving, always consider how the resident feels about the care and service they are receiving. Remember that the facility is the resident's home, and they should direct their care just as they did when they lived in their previous home.

Today more than ever your attitude should be that they give you permission to help them. You understand that the resident should control their own care. You under-

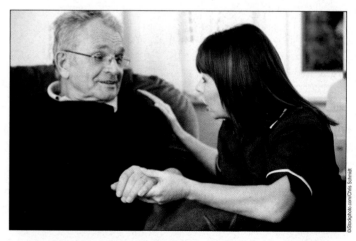

Fig. 31-4 – Customer service skills play an important role in mindful caregiving.

stand that meeting their needs is the most important part of your job. Staff who understand and accept this are the most successful.

Think about different times when you are a customer, such as when you order food at a restaurant or buy something new. What makes the experience positive for you? Doesn't it please you when someone looks at you, smiles, and asks, "May I help you?" Think about what makes one customer experience positive and another negative. To promote customer satisfaction, you must understand three things:

• what is important to the resident
• your role and ability to meet the resident's needs
• your ability to solve problems that may occur

Most residents do not expect everything to be perfect every day and at every minute, but they have a right to expect that their care team is making every effort to meet their needs. They expect that when they mention a problem, staff will truly try to solve it.

Think again about your own experiences as a customer: Has a waiter ever brought you the wrong food in a restaurant? If the waiter made you feel you were a burden and sighed when they took your plate back to the kitchen, you would be upset. On the other hand, if they apologized and said, "Let me take that back and get you what you ordered," you would be happy they respected your need for better service and would go to that restaurant again.

Remember always to ask residents what they want, and give it when you can (Fig. 31-5). Do your best to grant difficult requests if possible, and do it with a smile. You are expected to provide high-quality care and services and do whatever it takes to make the answer "Yes." Adopt the attitude that you will always try to do the job right the first time. These simple actions are important for building trust with your residents.

You also need to keep your promises. Ask for and encourage input from family members. Go out of your way for all your residents. Strive to make "extra effort" your standard effort! Remember: *If you over-deliver, you will become a great nurse assistant with excellent customer service.*

Customer Service During Mindful Caregiving

To incorporate customer service into your caregiving, first you must understand your role in meeting residents' needs and solving residents' problems. Ask the charge nurse how to handle any problem a resident tells you

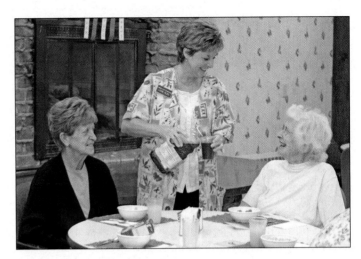

Fig. 31-5 – Good customer service includes offering choices and making sure residents get what they want.

about, if you do not know the answer. Listen to the resident. Learn what is important to them and communicate their needs to other staff members.

If you do not know how to handle a problem, discuss it with someone who does. Tell the resident what you are doing to solve it and then make your best effort. Although not every issue has a solution, customer satisfaction depends on the effort you make to solve the problem and meet the resident's needs.

You can tell which nurse assistants believe in customer service. They have a certain way about them. They are the ones who have a smile on their face, who greet you in the hall, and who are always helpful. These nurse assistants listen to residents and communicate their needs to other team members. (Chapter 7, Communication, describes good listening skills.)

When you have a customer service focus, you use good listening skills when talking with the resident. You never make up excuses for poor service or care. You try to solve problems with a positive approach. You are mindful and never let caregiving tasks become routine. Balancing your technical skills with the art of caregiving in everything you do shows residents they are important to you. (Chapter 2 offers more ideas about this.)

ADL Care
Good customer service during care for the activities of daily living helps make the resident feel more comfortable. During ADL care residents may feel embarrassed and

ashamed at having to have others to care for their basic needs, which they have done for themselves for most of their lives. It is important to maintain their dignity while also making them as comfortable as possible. Good customer service skills play a key role. Asking them about their preferences, letting them have choices, and making accommodations to meet their requests help establish a good relationship. Often it is simple things that make a difference for residents. Make sure their hair is combed and styled the way they like it, that women have their nails done and polished if they choose, and that you take time to apply their favorite lotions and perfumes. Most residents are used to wearing makeup and having pedicures and manicures, and these gestures can make all the difference in how the residents perceive you.

Always give residents a choice in their care. They need to be involved in choosing how and when they are bathed or showered and dressed.

Appropriate Socialization During Meals and Dining

Meals and dining experiences are another time when customer service gestures are very important. Meals are a traditional time for socialization, when we want to engage with others on a more intimate level (Fig. 31-6). Think about how when you want to treat someone, you take them out to eat. You invite family and friends over for a meal. Most of our holidays and special occasions involve the sharing of good food that has been lovingly prepared

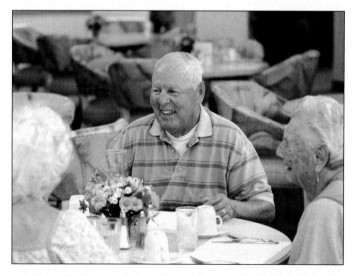

Fig. 31-6 – Meals are an important time for the residents to connect and socialize with others.

and served in an appealing manner. All these things play a part in the dining experience.

Consider different aspects of customer service related to meals. Is the food presented in a way that you would want to eat it? Is this when, where, and what the resident likes to eat? Who do they want to eat with, or do they prefer to eat in their room while watching an old movie? Remember to be a mindful caregiver who considers what the resident likes and wants. Do they want butter on their bread, or do you even ask? Residents have preferences about their diets and when they are served and where. Many individuals have very different cultural requests for meals. For example, tofu may soon be a common long term care menu item. Individual choice and resident-centered care are now expected in long term care facilities.

Residents' Activities and Environments

Activities are more than the afternoon bingo games. Residents want to be involved in recreational activities that they have chosen and that make them happy. Customer service should include making sure that residents want to participate in the activity. Asking and honoring each resident's requests for their activities is a big part of customer service. Being mindful of the activities they enjoyed before coming to the facility and trying to recreate those help meet that resident's needs. It is important for residents' overall well-being to maintain as much quality of life as they can for as long as they can. This includes engaging in activities of their choice. Sometimes, of course, they cannot continue activities after entering the facility, but with careful planning by the family and the health care team, ways can be found to keep the resident as involved as they would like to be in preferred activities.

CUSTOMER SERVICE IN DIFFICULT SITUATIONS

Sometimes, no matter how hard we try, problems happen. Customers can be difficult to deal with. This is especially true after a negative customer service experience. When people are upset, they get emotional. Your ability to respond to the emotional needs of your residents is one of the best skills for trying to correct a situation. The customer needs to know that you understand what they are trying to tell you and how they feel about the service that they want you to provide. There are three things to remember: (1) listen, (2) don't take it personally, and (3) be aware of your responses. These are discussed in the following sections.

Listen

Listening is a key skill for nurse assistants. Residents, families, and your team all make requests, and it is important that you understand what is being said and sometimes what is not being said. As you learned in Chapter 7, people communicate in two ways:
• Verbally - a spoken message
• Nonverbally - an unspoken message

Examples of verbal communication are requests from your supervisor or residents. "Can you help me?" "Will you go and get…." We hear and understand these kinds of communications and can respond to them easily. Sometimes a verbal request may be loud or harsh, or it can be sad and spoken tearfully, but they are all verbal communication.

When you listen well, you will be able to:
• Determine what the customer wants and needs
• Prevent misunderstandings and errors
• Gather clues about ways to improve the service you provide
• Build long-term trusting relationships

The first step in identifying a resident's need is listening to what they say. Let them present the issue, and hear their message about what is really on their mind. Be sure not to interrupt before they are finished. If you offer an answer, solution, or statement too early in the conversation, the person may stop listening. They think that your mind is already made up. Therefore, listen first and solve problems second.

Nonverbal communication can be harder to understand. It includes simple body language that shows that you are being attentive, such as leaning in toward a resident when they are speaking and maintaining eye contact. Nonverbal messages might also show that you are not being attentive, such as rolling your eyes, looking away, or doing other things when another person is speaking. Nonverbal expressions can communicate both positive and negative emotions, so it is important that you as a caregiver pay close attention to your nonverbal responses to others (Fig. 31-7).

Don't Take It Personally

Try not to take things personally. Becoming defensive is a very natural response in a difficult and emotional situa-

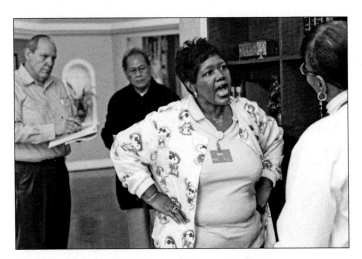

Fig. 31-7 - Nonverbal expressions can communicate either positive or negative emotions.

tion—especially if you feel that you are being attacked or accused wrongly. But defensiveness prevents any real communication from happening. Instead, try to be objective about the information the resident is providing. This helps you respond more openly and identify their real issues and concerns. Here are some ways to avoid reacting emotionally:
• Slow down
• Listen attentively
• Take notes to record the facts correctly
• Ask clarifying questions

These techniques can help you be emotionally aware and sensitive without becoming personally affected. When you respond with empathy, you stay calm and in control. Only then are you at your absolute best. You can then be ready, willing, and able to help your customer.

Be Aware of Your Responses

People who successfully manage difficult situations use good communication skills. They listen carefully for nonverbal messages expressed in emotions, and understand how their own behavior and language affect other people.

Another way to manage difficult situations is to avoid trigger words and be very aware of your responses to what residents say. Trigger words are words that can make the situation worse by making the customer even angrier. Examples are saying: "Calm down!" "Please be quiet!" "You need to listen!" or "You do not understand." All these phrases can annoy the customer or give the impression that you are talking down to them. This only makes the situation worse, so watch out for such trigger words when speaking with angry customers. How you physically react is also important. Do not roll your eyes or turn your head while others are talking. Pay attention to what is being said, and keep an empathetic attitude. Maintain eye contact. Acknowledge what is being said with phrases like "I hear your concern" or "I see this is very upsetting to you." Responses like these show compassion. Just knowing they are heard will go a long way to helping the overall situation.

Everyone needs help from time to time with managing difficult family members or situations. The following are examples of what to look for in family members who may have unmet needs or unrealistic expectations:

- Being openly hostile about admitting their loved one to the facility
- Expressing hostility toward staff
- Being critical of most aspects of care provided
- Requesting the physician be called in frequently
- Demanding special treatments that are not needed or wanted by the resident
- Overreacting to situations
- Insisting on new or unusual treatments and being upset when the physician does not agree
- Making numerous complaints
- Frequently asking to see the medical record
- Keeping a diary or frequently taking photos
- Threatening legal actions

You should know that some people may be hoping to "catch you" or have other reasons for finding fault. Be sure to keep in close communication with the entire health care team about any situation that arises with these individuals. If you inform your supervisor about family members' actions and inquiries, then they can take appropriate measures and set up a meeting to help address any concerns.

Your Role with the Family

Residents usually enter a long term care facility because family members and their health care provider have determined that the resident needs more support and care than they can receive at home or in the community. Family members often choose the facility. Most try to find a facility close by.

Earlier in this chapter you learned that the resident is your customer. The resident's family is also your customer.

How you greet family members, how you talk to them about the resident, and how you address their concerns all affect how they think their loved one is cared for (Fig 31-8).

Consider the family in the same way as the resident. Think of the family as your partner. With a partner you share common goals and decision making. Family members who are well informed will support the resident's goals for care. Keep them informed, treat them with respect, and they will usually support your efforts.

Residents and their family members want to trust the people who care for them or their loved one. Trust is needed for good customer service. Customers who trust the caregiver are happier and spread positive feelings in the community. To gain the trust of a customer, you need a consistent approach, which includes the following:

- **Use common language**. The average health care customer does not understand medical terms and abbreviations. Use language that the average person will understand. Staff may try to impress a family member by using technical words, but instead this may lead to confusion and mistrust. Family members who do not understand might not ask for clarification for fear of seeming uneducated or embarrassed.
- **Keep the customer informed.** Talk to the resident's family members often. Tell them what you are doing and why. Relay positive information to family members regularly. You don't need to write formal progress notes to the family, but you can foster trust with a brief conversation. Making family members aware of the progress of

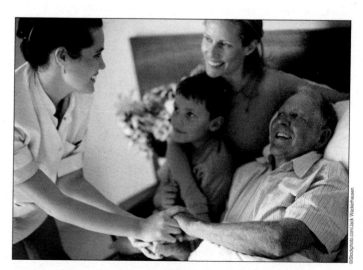

Fig. 31-8 – How you relate to family members and address their concerns affects how they think their loved one is being cared for.

their loved one helps build confidence in your service. For example, say something such as, "When your father first got here, he could only take a few steps—now he can walk all the way down the hall. He is doing very well." Let family know that you are aware of who they are and who they are visiting. Always tell them about their loved one's progress. Be careful not to share confidential information, but tell about things that can comfort the family, such as "At breakfast today your mother really enjoyed telling me about your vacation to the beach. We had the best talk." Family members are reassured when you can share information with them that shows that you know and care about their loved one.

- **Honor commitments**. If you make a commitment, you should do all that you can to keep it and to do it on time. If for some reason you cannot carry out a commitment right away, then it is important to let the family know that you will get to it as soon as you can. Remember that we are catering to their needs—not making them adhere to our schedule.

Open and honest communication with the family as soon as the resident is admitted goes a long way to build a lasting positive family-facility relationship. Answer family members' questions with appropriate answers. Center your conversations on the needs of the resident. Assure the family that the staff is there to help. These are all ways that nurse assistants can maintain that positive relationship while also reducing a potential threat of a lawsuit. When family members are updated about how the resident is eating, socializing, and mobilizing, they do not feel as disconnected from their loved one's care.

Your Role with Supervisors, Peers, and Guests

Customer service is not just how you relate to the residents and their families. It also involves how you relate to your supervisors, peers, and the rest of the health care team (Fig. 31-9). Working as a team requires respect for all individuals as well as the team. You can develop the skill of showing respect on a daily basis by following these guidelines:

1. **Do not gossip**. Gossip hurts people. It is insulting and abusive. Avoid sharing negative information about other people. You should also refuse to listen to gossip. Gossip can destroy an organization and the positive customer service built by a facility. Gossiping about co-workers, residents, and their families is one of the most destructive things anyone may do. Never tolerate gossip. If

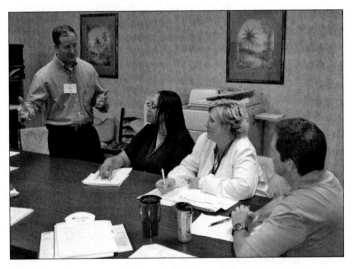

Fig. 31-9 – Working as a team requires respect for all individuals.

someone brings gossip to you, don't spread it. Tell that person that gossip is not part of your work ethic. It will only take a couple of times for others to know where you stand on this issue, and they will respect you for it.

2. **Begin with a greeting.** A simple smile and a warm greeting go a long way for developing positive relationships with your peers and making a more positive work environment. It will help to develop a positive environment among your peers. How you treat your peers and supervisors reflects how satisfied you are with your job and life. You have known people who always seem grumpy and have a guarded and unhappy attitude. They always seem negative. Nothing is ever right. How do you feel when you encounter these individuals? You need to pay attention to your attitude and make sure that you are greeting and addressing people with an attitude of service and caring. Peers, supervisors, and customers know a genuine response and will recognize you as having a service attitude.

3. **Remember to individualize.** Ask people how they would like to be addressed. People feel honored when they are called by their name, and feel good when someone remembers it. Remember to call a person by their real name unless they ask you to use a nickname. Always refer to staff by their name when talking with others. If you don't know a person's name, ask. Saying "I'm sorry, but I've forgotten your name" is better than not using the person's name at all. Refer to vendors, delivery people, and visitors by name.

4. **Provide respect.** Respect for your peers and supervisors is vital in the long term care environment. You will be sharing many details and observations with the other members of your team. If your relationship with them does not include mutual respect, the working relationship will be difficult. Quality of care can suffer as a result of a poor working relationship among team members. Remember to always speak in a kind manner and to convey honesty and caring for your fellow workers. Maintain your professionalism at all times. Always treat your co-workers with the same respect that you want for yourself (Fig. 31-10). It is very important for the organization to have a healthy and respectful work environment at all levels.

CO-WORKERS

Resolving Concerns

Problem solving is important when meeting our residents' and families' needs. How we respond when something bad happens affects how much the resident and family trust us to care for them. Strive to preserve good relationships even in difficult situations. You will be working with these people in the future, so you will need to maintain a professional relationship in order to give the best possible care. Use the following strategies when working to resolve problems:
- Assume that the other person has good intentions, even if that is not your impression.

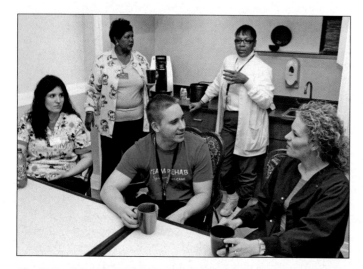

Fig. 31-10 - It is important to have a healthy and respectful relationship with your co-workers.

- Turn a negative into a positive by asking the customer what they think the best possible solution might be.
- Don't assume the situation is personal just because you have a difference of opinion.
- Be supportive of the other's ideas and show interest in their opinion.
- Be open to ideas that others have to offer.

The ability of the health care team to resolve conflicts quickly and improve the situation for the customer should be everyone's goal. This leads to the customer's final judgment about how good we really are.

TABLE 31-2 - GOLDEN RULES OF CUSTOMER SERVICE

PRINCIPLES OF CUSTOMER SERVICE	HOW TO ACT
People come first	• Give the resident your complete attention
Don't rush	• Take time to get information • Remember speed is not success
Be friendly always	• Treat everyone equally • Remember their behavior mirrors how they are treated
Don't be too busy to be nice	• Don't give short answers • Keep your sense of humor
Don't use technical language	• Use easy, understandable words • Explain unfamiliar words
Remember your manners	• Don't slip into slang • Good manners never go out of style • "There ya go" is not "Thank you" • "Uh huh" is not "You're welcome"

IN THIS CHAPTER YOU LEARNED:

- The meaning of customer service
- What customer service means in long term care
- The importance of providing good customer service to residents and co-workers
- How poor customer service affects the satisfaction of residents and families
- How to give good customer service as a part of excellent resident care

SUMMARY

Providing excellent customer service is one of the most important responsibilities of nurse assistants. Residents and their families want to know that they will be treated in a respectful, honest, and courteous manner at all times—and you can be the key to make that happen. You can take away from this chapter the skills and tools that will help you provide great customer service. Making customer service a priority is not only the right thing to do for the residents you care for, but it will have a positive and long-lasting effect on your success in health care. When you develop and use your excellent customer service skills, your supervisor, residents, and families will definitely notice and appreciate it.

PULLING IT ALL TOGETHER

Mr. Hood was admitted to the nursing home two days ago. He is alert and oriented. He is neatly groomed and dressed in business attire. He is very close to his three daughters. They are all present at his admission. He is on hospice, and they were taking care of him previously at home. His wife was ill, and he knew that his cancer was worsening, so he chose to be admitted to the nursing home because he did not want to be a burden to his wife or daughters.

He has had cancer for 8 years, which has now spread to his bones. He is on a constant morphine pump and requires assistance to transfer only because of the pain. He still insists on getting up everyday and getting dressed and being taken to the lobby to wait for the visit of his daughters and grandchildren.

One of his daughters is a nurse who has worked in long term care for several years. His wife is quite anxious about him being in the facility, saying that they have never been apart for 50 years. She asks a lot of questions and is constantly at the nursing station with questions and concerns. She insists on doing his laundry and taking him out for lunch when he feels like it.

Today Mr. Hood requests to have a private phone in his room so that he can call his family easily when he chooses. He says that he is willing to pay the cost so that it will not be an imposition on the nursing home.

This is your first day working with this new resident. How do you think that you should interact with Mr. Hood? After reading this chapter, how should you interact with his family? On entering his room, you introduce yourself to Mr. Hood and ask if there is anything that he needs immediately. You explain to him and his family that you will be caring for him for today and reassure him that you are there to help make him comfortable. You also reassure the family that if they need anything, you will be glad to help them as well. Ask Mrs. Hood about her concerns. You are beginning to develop a relationship with Mr. Hood, his wife, and other family members.

Being proactive and seeking answers before they become problems will be important. You realize that his wife's anxiety and questions also involve her own grieving and the loneliness she feels while away from her husband. How can you best reassure her that he will be cared for? What kind of assistance can you engage from the daughters to help with his wife's concerns? What is the key part of this customer service experience?

It is important to let your supervisor know right away that Mr. Hood requests a phone—and to let him know when it will be installed. His ability to speak with his wife on the telephone at any time is important to ease some of the anxiety they both are feeling.

Make sure to take notes about the time that she expects him to be ready to go out for lunch everyday so that you can relay that information to other staff who also will be caring for him. There is nothing worse than ignoring an issue when emotions are already running high. Talk with the daughters to learn about their requests and expectations for their father. It is important to clarify these to prevent misunderstandings and avoid unrealistic expectations. Family members who are informed are happier with care than those who develop their own expectations without understanding the resident's situation.

CHECK WHAT YOU'VE LEARNED

1. **Who has responsibility for customer service?**

   A. The receptionist only.
   B. The administrator only.
   C. The Director of Nursing only.
   D. It is everyone's job.

2. **Which of the following is part of a service mentality?**

   A. Empathy.
   B. Resiliency.
   C. Enthusiasm.
   D. All of the above.

3. **Which are examples of internal customers?**

   A. Housekeepers.
   B. Residents.
   C. Family members.
   D. Volunteers.

4. **Which are examples of external customers?**

   A. Supervisors.
   B. Activity staff.
   C. Vendors.
   D. Dietary staff.

5. **Which of the following is an example of good nonverbal customer service?**

   A. Explaining what you are doing.
   B. Smiling at visitors.
   C. Rolling your eyes.
   D. Ignoring requests.

6. **Which is an example of verbal customer service communication?**

   A. Not rushing.
   B. Cheerfully helping a resident get dressed.
   C. Explaining what you are about to do.
   D. Time management.

7. **Which of the following is most likely to show that a family member has unrealistic expectations?**

   A. Wanting a phone in the room.
   B. Demanding doctor visits twice daily.
   C. Visiting frequently.
   D. Bringing in outside food.

8. **Which of these phrases could trigger a negative reaction?**

   A. "I can see this is upsetting you."
   B. "I hear that you are very unhappy."
   C. "Is there something wrong?"
   D. "I don't think you understand."

9. **Which is a technique for dealing positively with a customer's emotional response?**

   A. Hurrying them so that you can get it resolved.
   B. Asking questions.
   C. Telling them to calm down.
   D. Ignoring their behavior.

(Answers to "Check What You've Learned" are in the Instructor's Manual.)

Chapter 32

UNDERSTANDING THE SURVEY PROCESS

Have you ever had visitors come to your home unannounced? What did you think? If you are like most people, you may have wished you had spent more time cleaning and preparing. You want them to know that you take pride in your home and you want that to show. The same is true in your job as a nursing assistant. You want the quality work that you do everyday to show when the surveyors arrive. Surveyors are inspectors who visit to make sure the facility is giving good care. The best way to make sure of this is to treat every day like a survey day.

Have you ever thought that you actually are being inspected everyday? People are observing everything that you do. Your work is seen daily by your residents. How your residents look and feel, and how they feel about their care, reflects the service you give them. Think about these questions to know what surveyors are looking for when they visit your facility:

•   Are residents dressed appropriately?

•   Are their clothes clean, especially after meals?

•   Are they bathed and groomed and well fed?

•   Are their emotional needs being met? Do they feel loved and cared for in a gentle, "patient" manner?

•   Are you keeping them safe and nourished?

•   Are they confident in the care that you provide for them?

•   Are their families and visitors also happy with the care?

Everyone who comes in contact with the residents that you care for is surveying your work. Residents, families, physicians, supervisors, administrators, and visitors all consider all these factors. This daily evaluation is very important. It may be more important than what the surveyors observe.

OBJECTIVES
- Distinguish among different types of surveys
- Know the purpose of surveys
- Understand the steps of a survey
- Learn common survey questions
- Learn what types of questions residents will be asked
- Understand your role in surveys
- Know how to identify problem areas within your own facility

KEY TERMS
- **Quality Indicator Survey (QIS)** – new process for annual evaluation of facility quality of care
- **Life Safety Codes** – rules for safety in a facility
- **Regulatory survey** – required of every facility that accepts Medicaid or Medicare payments from the government for care
- **Deficiency** – a weakness in a program, system, or process that has been identified as needing improvement during a survey

"I don't mind when surveyors are here, since they just want to make sure that we are doing our jobs and taking care of our residents."

xcellence in care starts with caring about the fragile individuals that have been entrusted to your care. Always think of how you would want your grandmother or grandfather to be cared for, even when a resident's behavior or actions may be difficult for you to address at the moment.

When you realize that every day is a survey day, you will have discovered the secret to not being fearful about surveys. As you give care throughout the day, realize that others can observe or audit your performance at any time. When you are giving quality care daily, you have no reason for concern when you are being surveyed.

WHAT IS A SURVEY?

The purpose of surveys is to verify that residents are receiving proper care. The main focus is to observe residents and to evaluate their condition. Surveys help make sure that the facility is following state and federal guidelines for operation. If the facility is following these rules, state surveyors assume the facility is giving good care. This should be evident in your residents.

As you learned in Chapter 1, all skilled nursing facilities participating in Medicare and Medicaid must meet certain specified requirements. These requirements serve as the basis for survey activities. The purpose of a survey is to determine whether a facility meets the requirements of Medicare and Medicaid, following state and federal regulations for long term care facilities. Written survey guidelines are used to ensure that surveys are conducted in a fair manner. All facilities are measured by the same set of rules so that the process is clear to everyone.

The survey process involves many different areas of review. As a nurse assistant, you will have an active role in some of these steps. Other steps involve the other members of the health care team. During the survey process, information is gathered from many sources:
• The resident
• The family
• The staff
• The doctor
• The records
• The MDS
• The physical environment

Remember you learned about the MDS and quality indicators in Chapter 8. They are used as indicators of potential problems or concerns that need further investigation during the survey process. These quality indicators measure information about the facility's residents' health and well-being. Your facility's results are compared to other facilities in your state, and then nationally, to determine if there is a potential problem.

Many areas are assessed in a survey, and they are all important. The number of staff on each shift is as important as giving medications at the right time. The survey examines how clean kitchen vent hoods are and the temperatures of refrigerators. The cleanliness and condition of residents' equipment are checked, including wheelchairs, shower chairs, oxygen filters, tube feeding poles, etc. The surveyors look at how laundry is done and how you handle residents' soiled laundry (linens, towels, washcloths, and personal items). The surveyors want to see that you understand infection control. They want to see that you know handwashing is the most important thing we all do to prevent the spread of infection (Fig. 32-1). All areas are examined in the survey process.

Surveyors look at the physical structures of the facility to see that they meet what are referred to as **Life Safety Codes**. Life Safety Codes are rules for safety in a facility. These standards reduce the risk of damage in case of fire and other disasters. These inspections include fire drills and safety checks in a variety of areas (Fig. 32-2). All of the Life Safety regulations focus on the physical plant, maintenance, and the operation of systems within the facility. Examples include fire doors and kitchen equipment.

In addition to the Life Safety inspection, the surveyors observe residents, review charts, and ask staff questions about the care being provided. The facility is toured to observe safety and cleanliness. Surveyors review employee records to ensure staff have the right credentials. Surveyors want to make sure that you are qualified

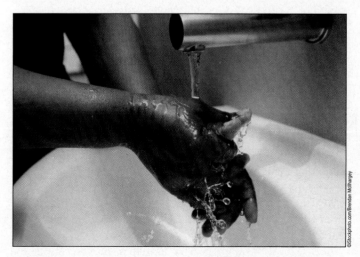

Fig. 32-1 – The surveyors look at all areas of care, including infection control.

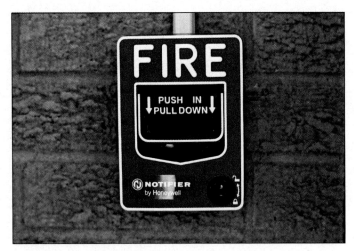

Fig. 32-2 – Life safety inspections are performed to ensure that all systems are in working order.

for the work that you do. Surveyors make sure that everyone has received the in-service education and health screenings required by each state. Surveyors watch the staff at work to verify that all regulations are being closely followed. They interview residents and families to find out how they perceive the care they are receiving.

The survey process leaves out no areas within the facility. Every department must meet a set of standards when inspected. All the staff must work together as a team in order to make the survey process a success.

TYPES OF SURVEYS

There are several types of surveys. The regulatory survey is required by every facility that accepts Medicaid or Medicare payments from the government for care. This type of survey is conducted every 9 to 15 months. This visit can occur at any time of the day or night, and survey-ors sometimes come on the weekend. Surveyors come to the facility unannounced and spend several days or up to a week. The length of the survey depends upon the size of the facility and any areas of concern found in their first few days. If surveyors find severe care issues, they can stay even longer. An extended survey can potentially be very serious for the facility, and the surveyors will explore their focus areas in more depth to ensure resident safety. In this case, the facility may no longer be eligible to conduct nurse assistant classes in the facility after an extended survey.

Other, optional surveys are conducted by accrediting organizations. Facilities choose to be reviewed by other organizations in order to receive an additional stamp of approval. Facilities get this accreditation to be viewed as having a higher quality. These surveys are usually sched-uled and are known in advance, but there still may be an unannounced visit. In addition, some surveys are required if a facility has a contract with an agency, such as the Veteran's Administration. These surveys are only done if the facility has a contract for services to their members.

This chapter focuses on the required governmental survey. All long term care facilities are surveyed by state agencies, which check to see that both state and federal rules are being followed (Fig. 32-3).

Currently two different regulatory survey processes are used in long term care: the traditional survey and the Quality Indicator Survey (QIS). Not all states are using the same process, but soon all states will use the QIS process. Individual states must follow set guidelines to implement the newer QIS survey process. States have to be certified and trained to use this process. Following are differences in the two processes:

QIS	Traditional
Larger sample of residents and staff	Smaller sample of residents and staff
More deficiencies expected	Fewer deficiencies expected
Interview focused	Observation focused
Longer survey time	Shorter survey time

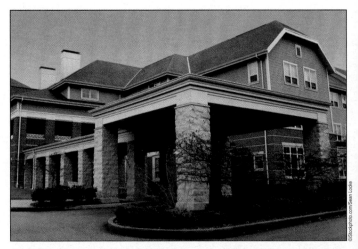

Fig. 32-3 – All long term care facilities are surveyed to make sure that both state and federal regulations are being followed.

REASONS FOR SURVEYS

A facility can receive a survey for three main reasons. First, an annual survey is required in every state for all facilities that provide long term care services. These surveys are conducted by employees in the state's Department of Health and Human Services. A second reason for a survey is a complaint about the facility. If a family member, staff, or visitor files a complaint, the state agency will assign surveyors to investigate. Complaints can occur for a variety of reasons, such as suspected abuse of a resident or a fracture that cannot be explained. If anyone makes a complaint, even anonymously, the state agency sends surveyors to investigate. This kind of survey is unannounced and is usually a day visit at the facility.

The third reason that surveyors visit is a follow-up to the annual survey. Usually about 30 to 45 days after the annual survey, a follow-up visit is conducted. Follow-up visits are to ensure that any deficiencies found in the annual survey have been corrected and that compliance is being maintained.

STEPS IN THE SURVEY PROCESS

Several steps are involved in the survey process. Some happen before the survey team arrives, and others are conducted on site. The following sections describe these steps and how they may involve you as a nurse assistant.

Survey Preparation

Getting ready for a survey is very difficult but necessary process. Facility routines should be no different with surveyors present than at any other time. This is why surveyors do not tell the facility when they are coming. They want to see what care is like on a normal day. Facility staff should know to act as if every day is survey day (Fig. 32-4). The facility must remain clean, the residents must have their needs continually met, and the documentation must be to date and accurate. If these processes are consistently maintained, the results will be positive.

Before coming to the facility, the surveyors review the facility's history and quality indicator documents. These reports give much information about the type of residents who live in a facility. The reports also show complaints that have been made and past problems. Surveyors look for issues that may show a pattern of concern, such as weight loss trends, falls, or pressure ulcer development. They explore all these areas to make sure there is not a more serious problem, such as not having enough staff to provide good care. All this is done before the surveyors come to the facility.

Initial Interview

Once in the facility, the surveyors first see the administrator. They introduce the members of their team and explain their roles (Fig. 32-5). They explain the reason for the survey, such as a recertification survey (commonly called the annual survey), a complaint survey, a review of a self-report incident, a follow-up survey, or a combination. You may be asked to show the surveyors to the administrator's office or to gather additional staff together. Remember to greet everyone with a smile, and offer to show them where the restrooms are located or other areas of the facility. Offer to bring a drink of water or anything else they may need as they settle into the location where they will be working. Your customer service skills will be very important during this time.

During the initial interview, the surveyors explain the reason for their visit and any complaints that they will be reviewing. One surveyor may conduct this interview while other team members begin rounds to inspect the nursing units.

It is important that you keep providing care to residents as you normally do. Keep doing frequent rounds and answering call lights and requests promptly. Make sure your residents are clean, happy, and content as always.

Surveyors typically post a sign in the facility to let everyone know they are available. They will make time to speak with anyone who wants to meet with them to discuss care in the facility.

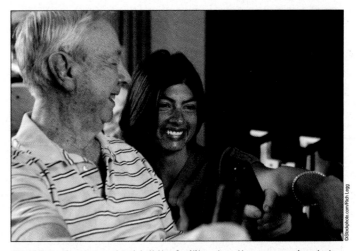

Fig. 32-4 – Surveyors don't tell the facility when they are coming, but when you provide care as if every day is a survey day, you will have nothing to worry about.

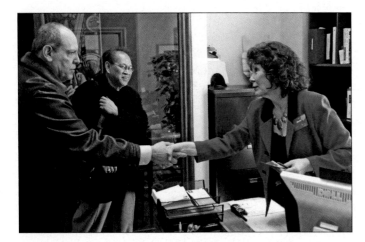

Fig. 32-5 – The surveyors will meet with the administrator for the initial interview.

Facility Tour

Surveyors usually begin their facility tour almost immediately (Fig. 32-6). In their initial tour of the facility, they will observe residents and the environment. They will take notes as they split up and tour different areas of the building to see separate units. This prevents staff from trying to correct any problems before the survey begins.

The surveyors will take notes and later compile them to look for areas of concern. Their first impressions are very important! What they see, hear, smell, and feel on that first round will set the tone for the rest of their visit. The initial tour is designed to:

• make an initial review of the facility, residents, and staff
• make an initial evaluation of the environment, the residents' equipment, and the facility's kitchen
• confirm or resolve any pre-survey concerns based on the earlier reports and new concerns they develop once in the facility

During their tour, the survey team will focus on the following **quality of life** issues:

• residents' grooming and dress, including cleanliness and appropriate shoes and slippers
• the staff's interaction with residents in regard to residents' dignity, privacy, and care needs, including the availability and responsiveness of staff to residents' requests for assistance
• how staff talk to residents, the nature and the manner of their interactions, and whether staff speak with residents when giving care

• scheduled activities that take place and how appropriate they are for residents
• equipment in proper working order and good repair
• alarms used for residents' safety in proper position and functioning

Another focus is the **residents' emotions and behaviors** and reactions and interventions of staff:

• resident behaviors such as crying out, disrobing, acting agitated, rocking, or pacing, and how staff address these behaviors, including the manner of staff behavior, response time, availability, and methods of dealing with residents who are experiencing behavioral reactions

The third focus of the surveyors is care issues: how care is provided as well as the nature of special care needs such as these:

• skin conditions, such as being too dry or wet
• mouth care, including clean teeth and moist lips
• skin tears, bruising, or evidence of fractures that need investigation
• dehydration risk factors, including the availability of water for most residents, and other factors such as the amount and color of the urine in tubing and collection bags, how much residents depend on staff, strong urine odors, and residents' complaints of dry mouth and lips
• clinical signs such as edema, emaciation, and contractures
• functional risk factors such as poor positioning and use of physical restraints

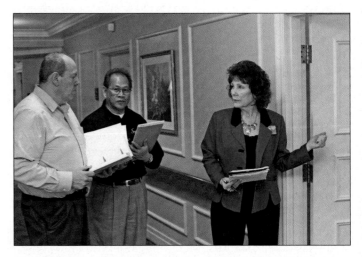

Fig. 32-6 – During the rounds surveyors will focus on many of the aspects of care as well as the environment that the residents live in.

- side effects of any antipsychotic drugs
- the presence of any infections, including antibiotic-resistant strains of bacteria such as methicillin-resistant Staphylococcus aureus (MRSA), vancomycin-resistant Enterococcus (VRE), and Clostridium difficile (C-DIFF); other infections, urinary tract infections, skin rashes (especially if they are spreading, undiagnosed, or not responding to treatment), respiratory infections, gastroenteritis (including diarrhea), etc.
- medications given correctly as ordered by the doctor
- perineal and catheter care performed correctly
- pressure sores, old scars from pressure sores, or evidence of surgical repair of pressure sores
- amputations
- significant weight loss
- use of feeding tubes or improper positioning for feeding
- use of ventilators, oxygen, and intravenous therapies

The fourth focus involves **facility environment and safety issues**:
- infection control practices, such as handwashing, glove use, and isolation procedures
- functioning, clean equipment, including kitchen equipment
- maintenance of a homelike, clean environment (Fig. 32-7)
- availability, use, and maintenance of assistive devices
- staff knowledge of disaster and emergency preparedness plans

It is important that you know the facility's policies and procedures related to all these focus areas. How you

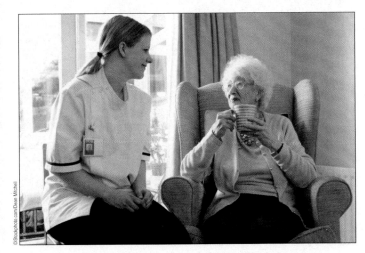

Fig. 32-7 – The physical environment should convey a homelike atmosphere for the residents that can be observed by the surveyors.

handle your care and interactions with residents will play a major roll in the survey outcome. If the initial tour reveals problems, the surveyors may immediately begin an extended survey. As a nursing assistant, your actions will be examined throughout the survey, so it is important that you are prepared.

After the tour, the surveyors will interview residents and more closely examine information and documentation in the resident records. They want to ensure that what is being recorded is accurate.

Resident Interviews

Surveyors will interview residents individually and in groups. The group interview usually happens during a meeting with the resident council. This is another reason why it is important to always pay attention to concerns raised in the resident meetings. If the facility has been responsive and has taken care of issues reported by residents, that positive service will be seen in this interview.

Surveyors measure the facility's care standards in part by this resident interview. They want to know how residents feel about the care that they are being given. You can never be sure how residents will answer the surveyors' questions, so it can be helpful to know what questions may be asked. Common questions include the following:
- Can you choose your food preferences?
- What choices do you have about when you get up in the morning and go to bed at night?
- Can you choose what you wear?
- Have you ever been treated roughly by staff?
- Have you ever felt afraid here?
- Do you go to activities when you wish to?
- Do you have any problem getting to activities?
- Is the food served the way you like it?
- Do you get things to drink between meals?
- How do staff members act toward you when they take care of you?
- Do you have choices about when and how your care is provided?
- Do you feel that staff treat you with respect and dignity?
- Have you lost any personal items? Did you tell a staff member? What did he or she do?
- How promptly do staff members come to assist you when you use your call signal?
- During evenings and at night, are sounds too loud and distracting? If yes, have you told a staff member about this? How did he or she respond?

- How do staff members react to residents who repeatedly ask for help?
- Is your mail sealed when you get it?
- Do you have privacy when you want to use the telephone?
- Can you meet with your visitors in private?
- Do you have enough light in your room to read?
- Is your room cool enough in the summer and warm enough in the winter?
- Have you seen any bugs or rodents in the facility or in your room?

These are just a few of the questions that residents may be asked during a survey. As a nurse assistant, you can have a positive impact on the survey by helping make sure that residents can answer all of the above questions positively (Fig. 32-8). That is done by assuring that residents are respected and well cared for every day.

The best way to ensure that residents respond positively to these questions is to always be polite and friendly and to provide the highest quality care. When consistent quality care is given, resident interviews will reflect that fact.

Family Interviews

Family interviews are also an important part of the survey process. The surveyors will ask family members many of the same questions they ask residents. They want to ensure that families have a choice in the care that their loved one is getting. It is important that family members have had positive interactions with staff that they can talk about with the surveyors. If you and other staff are responsive to the needs and concerns of the family, then those actions will become known to the surveyors. You should always pay attention to their concerns and solve problems as they arise (Fig. 32-9).

Staff Interviews

Be proud of what you do everyday, and when asked about your work be confident in your answers. If you are asked a question that you do not know the answer to, don't guess. It is OK for you to say that you are not sure. If you do not understand the question, then say so. Trying to make up an answer will only cause a bigger problem. Be sure to tell the surveyor that you will be glad to find the answer for them. Report these questions to your charge nurse, who can help you find the answers.

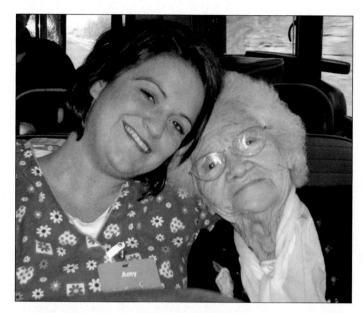

Fig. 32-8 – The best way to ensure a positive survey is to get to know your residents and provide them with quality care.

Surveyors may ask you questions like these:
1. What would you do in case of a fire?
2. How do you know what your facility's policies are?
3. What would you do if you thought a resident was being abused?
4. What can you tell me about your facility's quality improvement program?

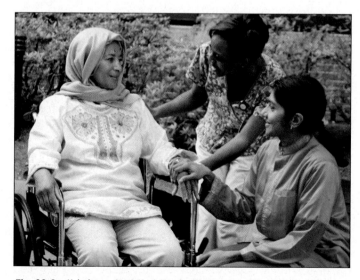

Fig. 32-9 – It is important that the family have positive interactions with staff that they can share with the surveyors.

5. How are changes in residents' care communicated to you? How do you communicate changes in residents?
6. How do you know what equipment (such as splints, lifts, restraints, bed or chair alarms) is needed to care for your residents?
7. How do you know if a resident is on special isolation precautions?

Make sure that you know your facility's policies and procedures for abuse, fire safety, disaster plans, and reporting issues.

Always try to avoid making certain negative responses when speaking with a surveyor:

- Avoid over-sharing. If the surveyor asks a question, answer it simply. Do not try to discuss everything you know about a resident. Just stick to the facts.
- Don't try to impress. Speak to the surveyor in the same way you do to any other visitor. Be professional and polite, and use appropriate language. Do not try to impress them with all that you know.
- Don't blame others. This is not the time to talk about problems that you may have had with laundry, for example. Don't blame other people or departments for an issue that a surveyor may have found.
- Avoid complaining. If you have a problem finding supplies, for example, you should talk about this with your supervisor, not the surveyor. Don't complain about facility policies or staffing concerns. You do not want surveyors to think there may be other problems.

Here are some ways to reinforce your positive responses to a surveyor:

- Smile. Smiling is good for you, residents, and your peers. Surveyors like to see nursing assistants who are smiling and interacting with residents and families.
- Be polite. This should be a daily habit. How you interact with residents, families, and visitors is always part of good customer service.
- Keep your attitude in check. When you feel stressed or anxious, take a minute to get refocused. Take your breaks so that you can give yourself some time. Think good and happy thoughts.
- Reward yourself. Carry keepsakes, photos, or candy in your pocket to give yourself a reward after stressful tasks.

Your positive attitude will give the surveyors a better understanding of how valuable you really are (Fig. 32-10). Maintaining these positive habits everyday will pay off during a survey.

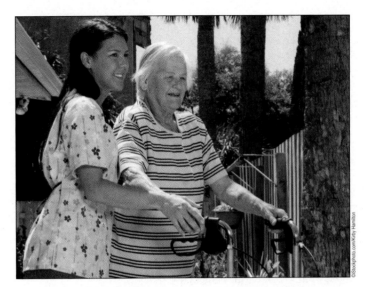

Fig. 32-10 – The surveyors will notice your positive attitude and see how valuable you are to the facility and its residents.

Resident Monitoring and Reviews

Surveyors will carefully review residents' medical records and plans of care (Fig. 32-11). Surveyors may also ask you specific questions about a resident you are caring for. You should know what is documented in your residents' record and care plans. Surveyors will watch staff to ensure that activities in the care plan are actually being done.

The surveyors also review incident reports, fall records, and injury reports. From this they will determine whether staff are doing all they can to prevent injuries and maintain safety for residents. The surveyors also want to make sure that staff protect residents' rights during care giving.

Surveyors will also observe many care activities such as range of motion exercises, splinting, and special feeding techniques. They will take note of how staff communicate with residents while giving this care. Surveyors are always looking for the outcome of all care activities. They want to make sure the facility is offering services that will maintain residents' current level of functioning and improve residents' conditions. Any decline in function needs to be prevented if at all possible.

Meal service is another focus of this monitoring. The surveyors inspect the cleanliness of the kitchen but also review the documentation about meals. They will examine menus, temperature logs for refrigerators, dietary assessments, and weight records. They will watch staff serve the food to ensure correct portion size and consistency of

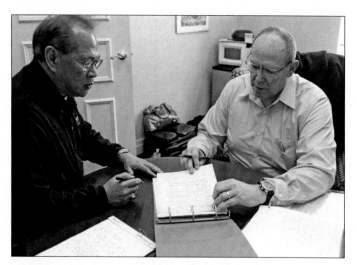

Fig. 32-11 – Surveyors will carefully review resident records and plan of care.

food (such as a puree or soft consistency) is provided as ordered for specific residents. The surveyors will monitor food temperatures, as well as safe techniques and positive staff interactions with residents. If a resident does not eat the provided food, the staff should request alternatives for the resident. The food must be appealing. The surveyors will taste items. They will observe for any breaks in infection control techniques. They will make sure that residents' hands are cleaned before and after meals. They want to observe that any spilled foods are removed, and that clothing is changed after meals if needed. They will watch meals being served at different times and in different areas of the facility. They want to ensure that meal service is consistent throughout the building.

The surveyors also observe specialty items and procedures, such as use of catheters, oxygen, restraints, or special dressings. They will also pay special attention to pressure ulcers, tube-fed residents, IV solutions, and tracheotomy care. They will want to see how these specialty care procedures are performed. In these observations they will review techniques used, the safety of procedures, and infection control practices. You must maintain the resident's dignity in all of these difficult procedures, and surveyors will watch to ensure that this is happening. If the procedure should be done in private, such as when the nurse gives an injection, the doctor listens to a resident's heart, or a nursing assistant provides any personal care, the resident should be taken to their room or a private area.

Exit Conference

At the end of the survey, the surveyors will hold an exit conference. In this meeting they describe any items of concern that they found (Fig. 32-12). This serves as a preliminary verbal report. The later written report will describe in more detail any areas that do not meet the minimum standards for long term care facilities.

Final Report and Follow-Up

The term used for problems found in a long term care survey is "deficiencies." Deficiencies in the areas of resident rights, quality of care, and quality of life are the most serious.

After leaving the facility, the surveyors produce a report of their findings (Fig. 32-13). They use standard measures for the level of deficiencies that they will cite. Both monetary factors and point systems are used in the rating system, which is standard measure for all facilities.

If the survey found a number of serious problems, the facility may not be allowed to admit new residents, may be fined, or even may be closed—depending on the seriousness of problems found.

This final, official report is sent to the facility. The facility's interdisciplinary team then develops a plan to correct the problems and notifies the surveying agency about this plan. The survey agency may accept the facility's plan, may ask for revisions, or may reject it outright. If this happens,

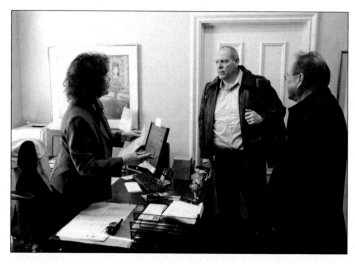

Fig. 32-12 – At the end of the survey, the surveyors discuss any concerns they have.

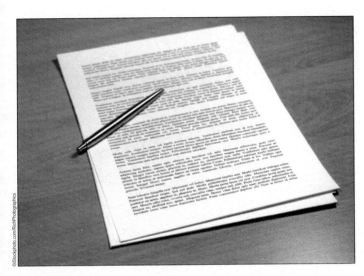

Fig. 32-13 – The surveyors will produce a report and send it to the facility.

the facility has to start over and make an alternate plan for correction.

When the facility's plan is accepted, a time frame is set for the correction of problems. At the end of that time, the facility has a follow-up visit to ensure that the facility has corrected problems.

The results of the survey are calculated with a rating system. Long term care facilities are rated from one to five stars. The stars are determined by the survey results, staffing patterns, and quality indicators for each facility. Every facility has the goal of having a five-star rating. In addition, all survey results are a matter of public record and are published for everyone to see on Medicare's "Nursing Home Compare" website. The facility must also post a copy of the most recent survey results in an accessible area where the public and residents can view it. Since this report does not contain corrections later made to the problems found, the problems can be seen by everyone who visits. You want it to be as good as possible.

YOUR ROLE IN THE SURVEY PROCESS

You may be asked questions by the surveyors, or asked to gather information to help with the survey process. Your exact role in this process depends on the surveyors' requests. Follow these general guidelines during the review process:

- Do not call in sick (unless you *really* are sick)
- Look professional at all times
- Smile and say hello
- Carry out your assignments as usual
- Be confident in yourself when you are asked questions
- Do not try to tell the surveyors what you think they want to hear
- Help housekeeping by notifying them of any spills
- Keep work areas neat and clean, even if they are not your areas
- Make sure the break room is not cluttered
- Be very observant of everything going on around you
- Make sure you know your facility's policies

If you have any questions before, during, or after the survey, be sure to talk to the charge nurse. If you are not certain about a policy or process, it is very important to let your supervisor know before the survey. Your supervisor will be glad to explain it to you to prevent any confusion or questioning during the survey.

You can also request a copy of your facility's survey results. Remember, you are a vital part of the health care team. Your role in any survey is very important and can make a huge difference in the results.

IN THIS CHAPTER YOU LEARNED:

- How to distinguish among different types of surveys
- The purpose of surveys
- The steps of a survey
- Common survey questions
- The types of questions residents will be asked
- Your role in surveys
- How to identify problem areas within your own facility

SUMMARY

During a survey, you and other staff may become anxious and may feel uncertain even about things you easily do everyday. Learning to view every day as survey day really helps prevent this anxiety. Following standards for care and documentation everyday helps ensure a positive survey outcome.

Preparing for a survey is not something that begins just before the surveyors enter the building. Survey preparation really is what you do every day. If you give the highest possible level of care, are attentive in your work, and know your residents, then you should feel proud. Those are exactly the qualities surveyors want to see during their visit.

PULLING IT ALL TOGETHER

Have you ever heard it said that for every action there is a reaction? This is very true also of your work as a nurse assistant. You care for residents and their families, and they react to how you give this care. You should always act with great care and attention to detail. These details are reviewed in the survey process. All these observed details add up to a measurement of quality. You should ask yourself questions daily about the details of your work to make sure you maintain the highest level of quality. You need to do this every day.

We all know that the survey is important. Still, no matter how well you do your job, knowing that someone is watching you is stressful. But when you have positive habits you use everyday to give quality care, survey day should not feel any different. In reality, every day is a survey day!

1. **What is the purpose of the survey?**

   A. Verify residents get proper care
   B. Make sure that payments for services are received
   C. Ensure that family members stay involved with care
   D. Make sure that staff are present at work

2. **What is the newest survey process?**

   A. Traditional Survey
   B. Follow-up Survey
   C. Quality Indicator Survey (QIS)
   D. Complaint Survey

3. **Which of the following is a reason for a survey?**

   A. Reported abuse of resident
   B. Complaint by family
   C. Complaint about an unexplained fracture
   D. All of the above

4. **Which of the following is a care issue included in the survey?**

   A. Skin condition of resident
   B. Staffing and scheduling
   C. Previous survey results
   D. Kitchen inspection

5. **Which of the following is an environmental issue included in the survey?**

   A. Dehydration
   B. Positioning
   C. Cleanliness of rooms
   D. Weight loss

6. **What is considered a dignity issue during the survey?**

   A. Clean equipment
   B. Emergency drills
   C. Use of privacy curtains
   D. Staffing shortage

7. **Who may surveyors do interviews with?**

   A. Staff
   B. Confused and demented residents
   C. Delivery personnel
   D. None of the above

8. **When should you maintain a resident's dignity?**

   A. Only during procedures and treatments
   B. Only during bathing
   C. Only during meal service
   D. All of the time

9. **A deficiency in which area is considered more severe?**

   A. Quality of life or care
   B. Staff in-service documentation
   C. Environmental services
   D. Admission process

10. **What kind of system is used to rate long term care facilities?**

    A. QIS
    B. 1 to 5 star system
    C. Annual survey
    D. Family satisfaction

(Answers to "Check What You've Learned" are in the Instructor's Manual.)

Appendix A

MEDICAL TERMINOLOGY

Abduction – moving away from the body

Abuse – to hurt, injure, or damage

Accredit – to recognize or vouch for as conforming with a standard

Activities of daily living – tasks needed for daily living, like dressing, hygiene, eating, toileting, and bathing

Acupuncture - a medical therapy that originated in ancient China

Acute – problem that begins rapidly and typically lasts 7-10 days; then the person recovers

Adapt – change to fit new conditions

Adaptive skills – skills people use every day to live, work, and play

Adduction – moving toward the body

Adjustment – a correction or modification for actual conditions

Admission – administrative procedure for entering a facility; opposite of discharge

Adrenal gland – located on top of the kidneys, this gland secretes hormones that regulate metabolism, increase blood sugar, control blood vessel constriction, and help us react in emergency situations

Advocate – someone who takes the side of another person and speaks for them

Aerobic – steady exercise that increases your heart rate and the amount of oxygen delivered to body tissue

Agenda behavior – tending to follow a certain agenda, often a past routine

Aggressive – behavior that is hurtful to others and may make them angry

Agitation – movements that are irregular, rapid, or violent; state of excitement, often troubled

Airborne transmission – route of infection that occurs when the reservoir coughs microorganisms into the air and a susceptible host breathes them into the lungs

Alert – quick to perceive and act

Alignment – to put in a straight line

Allegation – a person's statement or intended legal action

Alternative – a choice, a different possibility

Alveoli – air sacs in the lungs

Alzheimer's disease – a progressive, incurable disease that affects the brain and causes memory loss and eventual death

Ambulation – moving about; walking

Amniotic sac – membrane that encloses the fetus inside the uterus; it contains amniotic fluid that cushions and supports the fetus during development

Amputation – cutting a limb (for example an arm or leg) from the body

Anaerobic – exercise that does not increase the supply of oxygen to body tissue

Analyze – to study, to determine chemical parts or the presence of disease

Anatomy – study of body structures, such as body systems

Anesthesia – state of being unaware or unable to feel; anesthesia can be general (whole body) or local (a specific body part or region)

Anesthetic – the medication given to a person before surgery to induce anesthesia; administered in different ways depending on whether general or local

Anti-embolism stockings – elastic stockings often worn after surgery to help prevent blood clots

Antibiotics – drugs that reduce or kill microorganisms

Antibody – type of protein that the body produces to fight infection or illness

Antibody – type of protein that the body produces to fight infection or illness

Antiseptic – a substance that reduces the growth or action of microorganisms

Anus – the posterior opening of the large intestine (rectum)

Anxiety – an uneasiness in the mind

Aorta – large artery by which blood leaves the heart

Apgar scale – a tool for assessing the health status of a newborn

Apical pulse – pulse measured at the heart through auscultation

Aphasia – condition in which a person has difficulty putting thoughts into words

Arteries – blood vessels that carry oxygenated blood to all parts of the body

Arthritis – joint inflammation that causes pain and limits movement in affected joints

Artificial airway – a tube placed into the trachea of a person's respiratory system, through the nose, mouth, or surgically through a stoma in the neck, to assist in breathing

Artificial limb - human-made leg or arm

Aspirate – to breathe in or draw in by suction

Assault – to touch the body of another person without consent

Assertive – being confident

Assess – to evaluate or determine a person's strengths and limitations

Assessment – an evaluation of a patient or condition

At risk – has a probability of having some type of medical incident (for example, falls, seizures, allergies, asthma, heart condition)

Aura – a subtle sensation that often precedes a seizure

Auscultate – to listen to body system sounds with a stethoscope

Auscultation – a technique of listening through a stethoscope to sounds produced by organs (such as heart, lungs, or bowels) to evaluate a body area

Autism – rare, severe disorder in which the child withdraws from the world; the cause is not known, and there is no cure

Autoclave – a machine used to sterilize instruments and supplies with steam under pressure

Autonomy – making decisions for oneself

Avoidance – escaping from an issue rather than dealing with it

Axillary – armpit

Bacteria – one-celled microorganisms that may cause infection (bacterium is the singular form)

Barrier – something that protects, or separates, a person from an infectious microorganism

Baseline – beginning observations used for later comparisons

Battery – unlawful beating or use of force—or even touching someone without their consent

Behavioral symptoms – actions that are caused by a disease or condition

Belittle – to make a person feel smaller or less important

Bereavement – period of grief after a loved one dies

Biceps – strong arm muscles used for lifting

Biohazardous – anything that is harmful or potentially harmful to humans or the environment; contaminated material

Biologicals – medical products made from living organisms, such as vaccines or blood components

Bladder – sac inside the body that holds urine

Bladder training – a care plan to help a resident regain voluntary control of urination

Blindness – the inability to see

Blister – elevated area of epidermis (skin) containing watery liquid

Blood pressure – pressure of blood in the arteries

Blood sugar – measures the amount of one type of sugar (glucose) in the blood

Body fluids – natural fluids in the body, such as blood, semen, and secretions which may transmit disease

Body Mass Index (BMI) – a measurement of a person's body fat

Body mechanics – principles of using your body efficiently to do something

Bowel – large and small intestines

Brace – device that supports and strengthens a body part

Bronchi – left and right airway passages to the lungs (bronchus is the singular)

Bronchioles – branches of each bronchus

Callus – a thickened or hard area of skin

Capability – being able to do something

Capillaries – tiny blood vessels that connect arteries and veins, where oxygen is exchanged for carbon dioxide inside organs

Cardiac – involving the heart

Cardiac arrest – the stoppage of the heart

Cardiopulmonary resuscitation (CPR) – procedure to maintain breathing and circulation in a person experiencing cardiac arrest

Care plan – a written, interdisciplinary document developed for each resident, listing the resident's needs and goals as well as the actions and approaches that staff will take to help the resident to meet their goals

Cataract – cloudy film that develops in the lens of the eye and reduces sight

Catheter – a small tube used to drain fluid

Cerebral palsy – condition resulting from damage to the central nervous system before, during, or after birth

Cerebral vascular accident (CVA) – condition that occurs when blood flowing to the brain is interrupted (also called stroke)

Cervix – the opening of the uterus into the vagina

Cesarean section – giving birth through a surgical incision made through the abdomen into the uterus

Challenge – something that is difficult but important

Charge nurse – nurse who has the day-to-day responsibility for supervising nurse assistants and resident care

Chart – a summary of the resident's medical records, routine care, treatments, drugs, etc.

Chemical restraint – medication used to sedate a resident or slow their muscle activity

Chemotherapy – use of chemical agent to treat or control disease

Chicken pox – contagious disease caused by a virus; one early symptom is a low-grade fever

Circumcision – surgical removal of the foreskin at the head of the penis

Cholesterol – a substance present in animal cells and body fluids

Chronic – an ongoing illness or condition that does not have a cure, usually has a gradual onset, and lasts for a long time

Chronic carrier – someone with an infectious disease such as hepatitis B and hepatitis C who never gets well

Chronic obstructive pulmonary disease (COPD) – chronic inflammatory disease of bronchial passages and lungs; three most common types of disease are bronchitis, emphysema, and asthma

Circulation – flow of blood throughout the body

Circulatory system – body system that includes the heart and blood vessels that carry oxygen and nutrients to the body and remove carbon dioxide

Clarify – make sure something is clearly understood

Clean – free of germs that cause infection or disease

Coercion – making someone do something against their will, often by a threat

Cognitive impairment – disruption in knowledge, memory, awareness, or judgment

Collaboration – the act of working together

Colostomy – surgical opening of the colon or bowel on the surface of the abdomen where fecal contents collect in an external appliance

Colostrum – the watery "first milk" that appears from a newborn mother's breasts

Comatose – describes someone in a coma, unconscious

Commode – a box-like structure with a chamber pot under an open seat; usually portable

Communicable disease – disease that is spread from one person to another

Communication – sending and receiving messages verbally and nonverbally

Competency – legally qualified or demonstrating adequate abilities

Competition – trying to beat another person to some goal or in a game

Complementary – nondrug or alternative treatments

Compress – cloth or pad folded to press against part of body

Compromise – an agreement in which both sides give up something

Concentrated – less diluted, more intense in color

Condolences – expressions of sympathy or sorrow

Condom – a thin, flexible covering commonly made of latex rubber, worn over the penis to reduce the risk of pregnancy and susceptibility to or transmission of sexually transmitted diseases

Confidentiality – keeping information private

Conflict resolution – use of effective communication to resolve problems

Confront – to face with a challenge

Congestive heart failure (CHF) – condition that occurs when the heart muscle weakens and the heart becomes ineffective in moving blood through the body

Constipation – condition in which bowel movement is delayed and feces are difficult to expel from the rectum

Contaminated – impure or unclean

Context – the whole situation, background, or environment that gives meaning to someone's words

Continent – able to control elimination of urine and stool

Contracture – deformity caused by a permanent shortening of a muscle or by scar tissue

Contusion – a type of wound made by blunt force, causing bruising and swelling but usually the skin is not broken

Convalescent – recovering health and strength gradually after sickness or weakness

Corn – a local hardening and thickening of the epidermis (as on a toe)

Coronary artery disease (CAD) – condition that results from reduced flow through the coronary arteries, which nourish the heart

Corporal punishment – physical punishment

Critical – very important; a turning point or especially important period

Cuing – telling or showing a resident the steps in a task

Culture – the customary beliefs, social forms, and traits of a racial, religious, or social group

Curtness – being so short or brief that you are not polite; brusque

Cyanosis – bluish or purplish discoloration of the skin caused by deficient oxygenation of the blood

Decubitus ulcer (pressure ulcer) – an opening, or wound, that appears in pressure areas of skin overlying a bony area in an immobile person

Defecate – to have a bowel movement, to pass stool

Dehydration – a serious condition that can occur if a resident does not have adequate fluid intake

Delivery – the act of giving birth

Delusion – thinking that one's false thought is real

Dementia – loss of mental functions such as memory, thinking, and reasoning

Dentures – false teeth

Dermatitis – inflammation of the skin; contact dermatitis is a skin reaction resulting from coming in contact with something you are allergic to

Dermis – second layer of the skin

Deteriorate – to grow worse

Developmental disability – chronic, severe condition that a person develops from various causes, which prevents them from living independently without assistance

Diabetes – a common disease involving a problem in the body's production or use of insulin

Dialysis – a method used to artificially remove waste from the blood when the kidneys are not functioning well

Diaphragmatic breathing – deep breathing that uses muscles of the abdomen

Diarrhea – very frequent and liquid stools

Diastolic – pressure the bottom number in the blood pressure reading; reflects the pressure of blood in vessels when the heart is at rest

Digestive system – body system that provides the body with a continuous supply of nutrients and fluid and removes waste products

Dignity – a feeling of pride and self-respect

Direct transmission – direct transfer of microorganisms from one person to another

Dirty – contaminated with germs

Disability – lack of a full physical or mental function

Discharge – administrative procedure for leaving a facility; opposite of admission

Discrimination – a prejudiced or unfair action because of some characteristic of the person

Disinfectant – an agent that inactivates microorganisms on inanimate objects

Distraction – something that directs the resident's attention away from something or eases mental confusion

Diversion – anything that distracts a person's attention

Documentation – written reports that the facility maintains

Door card – a sign on or beside the door to a resident's room containing their name and other information

Down syndrome – condition in which a person is born with an extra chromosome, causing some level of mental retardation, abnormal features, and often other medical problems; also known as mongolism and trisomy 21 syndrome

Drape – to cover

Dry cold – dry cold application

Dry heat – dry warm application

Dysphagia – a condition that causes a problem chewing or swallowing food, liquid, or medication

Dyspnea – difficulty breathing

Edema – swelling because of fluid gain, most commonly observed in the legs and ankles

Eden Alternative – an alternative environment in which a long term care facility is transformed from an institution that treats residents into a home

Elimination - process of ridding the body of urine and stool

Emesis – related to vomiting, as in an emesis basin

Endocrine system – body system made up of many glands that secrete hormones

Endorphins – natural morphine-like substances released by the brain during exercise, which can alter one's feeling of pain

Endotracheal tube – a tube placed through the mouth or nose into the trachea for breathing

Enema – procedure that introduces fluid into the rectum to stimulate a bowel movement

Engorgement – a postpartum mother's breasts being swollen with milk, which may be uncomfortable or painful

Enteral nutrition – providing liquid nourishment through a tube passed into the nose and down to the stomach (a nasogastric tube, or NGT) or a tube surgically inserted through the abdominal wall into the stomach (a gastrostomy tube, or G-tube)

Epidermis – top or first layer of the skin

Epidural – a type of anesthetic given by injection to minimize the pain of childbirth

Epilepsy – disorder of the nervous system that causes seizures and may also cause a developmental disability

Episiotomy – a surgical incision made to enlarge the vaginal opening for childbirth

Ergonomics – the study of relationships between workers' physical capabilities and their job tasks

Esophagus – the muscular tube that leads from the mouth to the stomach

Ethics – knowledge, awareness, or study of good and bad, right and wrong, and moral duty

Exposure – a condition of being in direct or indirect contact with an infectious microorganism

Express – technique used by breastfeeding mother to remove breast milk to a container to be used later for bottle feeding

Extension – straightening of an extremity

External evacuation – moving residents out of the facility to another site for safety

Extremity – a limb of the body

Fallopian tubes – two tubes that carry egg cells from the ovaries to the uterus

Family – a group of persons of common ancestry or associated by marriage; significant others, or persons important to the resident

Fasting blood sugar (FBS) – test of blood glucose level using a blood sample (from a prick in a finger or ear or through a needle from a vein) taken at least eight hours after last eating

Fecal impaction – condition that may occur when constipation is not treated; hard feces are packed in the rectum

Feces – stool, bowel movement

Feedback – information received that is corrective or evaluative

Flexion – bending of an extremity

Force fluids – encourage fluid intake

Foreskin – a fold of skin that covers the tip of the penis in an uncircumcised male

Fortified – strengthened by adding some additional ingredient

Fowler's position – sitting upright

Fracture – broken bone

Fracture pan – a type of bedpan that is smaller and has a lower front lip so it is easier to slide under a resident. It is usually used for residents with hip or back problems, or a broken hip or leg.

Fragile – easily broken or destroyed, delicate

Frailty – weakness

Frequency – how often something happens, an habitual pattern

Function – key action(s) of an organ or body system

Functional nursing – a nursing approach in which nurse assistants have specific tasks rather than specific residents as the focus of care

Fungus – a type of microorganism like yeast and mold (fungi is the plural form)

Gastrointestinal – related to the stomach and intestines

Generativity – ability to produce or create something

Gerontology – a branch of knowledge dealing with aging

Glaucoma – disease of eye that can cause gradual loss of vision

Gonorrhea – contagious bacterial venereal infection that is sexually transmitted

Grievance – a formal complaint

Gross motor skills – abilities in the larger physical skills (running, catching a ball, etc.) vs. fine motor skills (drawing a picture, writing, etc.)

Gross negligence – any action that shows no concern for the resident's well being

Guaiac test – procedure for checking blood in the stool or vomit

Guard belt – belt used for safety to transfer and ambulate residents (also referred to as a gait belt, transfer belt)

Guided imagery – relaxation technique using words and music

Guilt – negative feelings experienced by someone who has committed an offense or believes they have done something wrong to another person

Habilitation plan or model – philosophy of care in which an individual with a developmental disability is educated or trained to participate as fully as possible in all aspects of life, including interaction with their family and community, and to have a satisfying social life

Habitat – a place where plants and animals are found growing naturally

Hallucination – seeing or hearing things that are not really there

Hat – device placed in toilet to collect urine; also called collection hat or urine hat

Hearing (legal sense) – initial examination in a criminal procedure

Heimlich maneuver – technique used to free a foreign object from the airway when a resident is choking

Hemodialysis – a process for removing waste and fluid directly from the person's blood through a tube that has been surgically implanted; the tube is connected to an artificial kidney machine that filters and returns the blood to the person

Hemorrhage – excessive loss of blood in a short period of time

Hemorrhoids – enlarged blood vessels at the anus that look like flat or swollen tags of skin

Hepatitis – infection or inflammation of the liver

Hierarchy – a specific, organized order or ranking

History – A record of a person's medical background, including lifestyle and social information

Hospice – program with a specially trained interdisciplinary team that cares for a terminally ill resident who is expected to die within 6 months

Human immunodeficiency virus (HIV) – viral infection transmitted by contact with blood and other body fluids such as semen and vaginal secretions

Hydration – maintaining adequate fluid in the body

Hydrocephalus – a build-up of fluid in the brain, possible cause of cognitive impairment

Hyperglycemia – blood sugar level that is too high

Hypertension – high blood pressure; leading cause of stroke

Hypodermis – lining beneath the epidermis

Hypoglycemia – blood sugar level that is too low

Hypoxia – a state in which the blood oxygen level shows that the body is not getting enough oxygen

Ileostomy – surgery that leads the opening of the ileum to the stoma. The ileum is a part of the small intestine.

Imminent – about to take place

Immobilize – to prevent freedom of movement

Immunization – administration of a vaccine to make the person immune (not susceptible) to a specific infection

Impairment – loss, something made worse

Incentive spirometer – a device that measures and shows how deeply a person breathes; seeing the result helps to encourage deep breathing

Incident – Something happens that is unusual; it could be medical or behavioral

Incision – a type of wound with straight edges, made by a sharp instrument or object, including surgical incisions

Incontinence – inability to hold urine or stool

Independence – not subject to control by others, not requiring something else

Indirect transmission – transmission of infection by an intermediate object, such as food, water, medical equipment, or a person's hands, into the portal of entry of a susceptible host

Individual service plan or individual program plan – plan of care that provides special accommodations and sets the priorities of care for the resident; also called an individual habilitation plan

Indwelling catheter – a plastic tube inserted into the body to drain fluids (usually urine)

Infection – condition produced when an infective agent becomes established in or on a suitable host; infections usually have signs and symptoms

Infection control – methods used to prevent the transmission of infection

Influenza (flu) – contagious viral disease which has a sudden onset, fever, and severe aches and pains

Initiative –introductory action, such as the first step in an attempt to resolve an issue

Inservice – educational programs taught to staff while on the job

Insomnia – inability to sleep enough

Insulin – hormone involved in breaking down carbohydrates in the body; it can be given as a shot to control diabetes

Integrity – being whole or complete

Integumentary system – body system made up of the skin, nails, and hair

Intellectually disabled – a person with impaired mental skills, characterized both by a significant below average score on a test of mental ability or intelligence and by limitations in the ability to function in areas of daily life; sometimes called cognitive disability or mental retardation

Interdisciplinary – involving two or more academic, scientific, or artistic disciplines

Interdisciplinary team – a group of caregivers from all departments in a facility

Interference – act of obstruction; preventing a person from doing something

Internal evacuation – moving residents to another section within the facility for safety

Intestines – part of the digestive tract through which food passes after leaving the stomach that help digest food and eliminate waste

Intravenous – entering through a vein

Invasion of privacy – an interruption of a resident's right to privacy or intimacy

Invasive – something that enters the body

Involuntary seclusion – isolation of a resident against their will

IQ test – test of a person's intelligence (IQ means intelligence quotient)

Isles of Langerhans – cells in the pancreas that secrete insulin

Isolation – set apart from others

Labia – the outer and inner fatty folds around the vulva

Labor – stages of expulsion of the fetus from the uterus through the vagina, beginning with contractions and the release of amniotic fluid and ending with delivery

Laceration – a type of wound made by an object causing an irregular, jagged wound

Lactation – the production of breast milk

Lather – foam or froth when shaving cream or soap is mixed with water

Localized response – a response to infection that occurs in a specific body area

Legal – according to law

Limb – arm or leg

Linen – bed linen: sheets, pillow cases, mattress covers

Living will/advance directive – legal document used by a resident to communicate their wishes about the care they want if they become incapacitated and cannot make decisions

Lochia – vaginal discharge that occurs after childbirth

Long term care facility – part of the health care system that provides rehabilitation, continuous supportive, high level nursing, respite, or hospice care

Lubricant – a slippery substance such as petroleum jelly, which facilitates passage of instruments into body orifices

Macular degeneration – eye condition that causes loss of central vision

Maintain – to keep something in its existing state

Malignant – refers to a tumor or condition that tends to spread abnormal cells (especially cancer cells)

Mask – protective covering for the face

Material safety data sheets (MSDS) – written information sheets describing chemicals used in a facility

Maximize – to increase to the maximum

Maximizing capabilities – working with a resident's own capabilities to their fullest

Measles – contagious disease caused by a virus, which produces red spots on the skin

Mechanical ventilator – a machine used to assist or replace spontaneous breathing when a person cannot breathe on their own

Medical history – a record of a person's medical background, including lifestyle and social information

Melanocytes – cells that give color to the skin

Mental abuse – any action that makes a resident fearful

Mental retardation – condition in which the individual has significantly below-average intelligence and minimal adaptive skills

Mercury – a heavy, silvery, poisonous, metallic element that is liquid at ordinary temperatures, used in scientific instruments

Metabolism – the body's process of producing energy

Microorganisms – viruses, bacteria, or fungi that cannot be seen with the naked eye; also called germs

Mindful – continually being aware

Minimum Data Set (MDS) – resident information on the RAI, including levels of physical functioning and bowel and bladder continence

Mobility – capable of moving or being moved

Moist cold – moist cold application

Moist heat – moist warm application

Mole – a colored spot on the body

Mongolism – another (older) name for Down syndrome

Multidisciplinary team – another name for the interdisciplinary team

Multi-infarct – damage to blood vessels that may cause a loss of function in a tissue or organ

Multiple sclerosis – progressive disabling disease that affects nerve fibers

Muscle atrophy – muscle wasting

Musculoskeletal system – body system made up of bones, muscles, tendons, ligaments, and joints

Nasal cannula – two-pronged tube inserted into the nostrils to deliver oxygen

Need – something necessary for a person

Neglect – failure to do something that should have been done

Negligence – failure to act in the same way that a reasonable person with the same training would act in the same situation

Neonate – the newborn infant up to one month of age

Nervous system – body system made up of the brain, spinal cord, and nerves

Nickname – a familiar name that family and friends use

Nonpathogenic – microorganisms that do not cause infection

Nonpathologic – not disease-causing

Nonverbal communication – sending and receiving messages without the use of words

Normalization – creation of an environment for individuals with developmental disabilities that is as close to normal as possible

Nurse assistant – a trained member of the health care team who provides the majority of hands-on resident care

Nutrition – the act of nourishing or being nourished

Objective – information that can be observed; factual; not subjective

Observation – recognizing and paying attention to details

Occult – cannot be seen

Occupational therapist – works with fine motor skills to help residents to keep using their hands and arms for activities

Occupational transmission – the transmission of an infection while on the job

Occupied bed – the resident is in the bed

Ombudsman – person required by law to investigate complaints by residents or other violations of rights

Onset – beginning (of a disease or condition)

Open-ended – questions that encourage residents to talk, rather than questions with "yes" or "no" answers

Optimal – most desirable or satisfactory; highest

Oral – by mouth

Orientation – to be shown something new (as a new job); ability to accurately identify person, place, and time

Oropharyngeal tube – a tube placed through the mouth into the pharynx for breathing

Orthotic device – supportive equipment made for a resident, such as a brace or splint

Osteoarthritis – joint inflammation caused by wear and tear of the joint

Osteoporosis – condition in which bones become weak and brittle due to loss of minerals, especially calcium

Ostomy – a surgical opening from the intestine to outside the body

Outbreak – sudden, dramatic increase in cases of a particular disease or harmful organisms

Ovaries – organs in the female's pelvic area that secrete hormones involved in sexual function and becoming pregnant

Oxygen – an odorless, tasteless, and colorless gas

Pain – bodily sensation that causes suffering and distress

Palliative – care focused on comfort and symptom relief rather than cure

Palpate – use of touch to assess

Palpitations – strong, rapid heartbeats

Pancreas – digestive system organ located near the stomach; its cells secrete insulin

Paralysis – loss of voluntary movement

Parasite – an organism living in or on another organism

Parkinson's disease – neurological disease that affects motor skills

Pathogenic – microorganisms or substances that can produce disease

Pathological – caused by disease

Penis – male organ of sexual intercourse and urination

Perception – a mental image of something

Percussion – tapping on a body area and listening to the sound produced, used to determine if tissue is air-filled, solid, or fluid-filled

Perfectionist – someone who insists you do everything in a certain way

and the same way every time

Perineal – area of body between the anus and the external genitals

Peripheral vascular disease (PVD) – condition that causes diminished blood flow to the arms and legs

Peritoneal dialysis – process used for removing waste and fluid from the blood through a surgically placed catheter in the abdominal (peritoneal) cavity

Permission – the act of giving formal consent

Personal – private, or referring to a person's body

Perspiration – a saline fluid secreted by sweat glands

Philosophy – a belief about quality care

Physical abuse – any action that causes actual physical harm

Physical examination – an organized approach to learn about a resident's health status and needs by looking, listening, feeling, and smelling.

Physical restraint – any mechanical device that restricts a resident's movement or access to their body

Physical therapist – works with residents to improve functional mobility so residents can maintain or increase their physical abilities, such as walking

Pica – having an appetite for nonfood items of no nutritional value

Pituitary gland – gland located in the brain that secretes hormones and regulates other glands

Pivot – to turn on

Placenta – a temporary organ that develops in the uterus during pregnancy to transfer oxygen and nutrients to the fetus and remove carbon dioxide and some waste products; commonly called "the afterbirth"

Plaque – fatty deposits on blood vessel walls

Pneumonia – lung infection

Podiatrist - physician specializing in the care and treatment of the feet

Policy – a high-level plan for meeting goals, acceptable procedure

Portal of entry – natural openings in the body where microorganisms can enter

Portal of exit – a route by which microorganisms leave the body, such as in blood or through the natural openings of the body

Positioning – an act of placing or arranging

Postmortem – after death

Postoperative – time after surgery

Postpartum – the period after childbirth

Postural hypotension – reduced blood flow (blood pressure) upon sitting or standing, causing   dizziness

Precipitating factors – factors that cause pain to occur

Preferences – personal choices or favorites

Premiums – payments for insurance policies

Prenatal – the period of pregnancy before childbirth

Preoperative – time before surgery

Primary nursing – a nursing approach in which a registered nurse or licensed practical nurse has the primary responsibility for residents'

needs and nurse assistants work with the nurse and care for the same residents each day

Primary site – the first system or organ affected by a cancer

Prompting – moving a person to action, helping a person remember something

Prone – lying flat, face down

Prosthesis – a device that substitutes and functions in the place of a missing body part, such as dentures

Prosthetic device – device made to replace a missing body part or function

Protein – combination of amino acids that are essential for all living cells

Protocol – a facility's official way of doing something, usually put in writing

Psychosocial – involving psychological and social aspects of mental health

Pubic – the region of pubic hair, genital area

Pulse – measure of heart rate

Puncture – a type of wound down into the skin, made by something pointed

Purulent – infected, such as secretions or drainage

Pus – a yellowish-white fluid formed when an infection is present

Quality indicators – outcomes or a summary of the entire facility's MDS information, which indicate the quality of care provided by a facility

Radial pulse – pulse felt at the inner wrist

Radiation – medical treatment using X-rays

Range of motion – extent to which a joint can be moved safely

Reality – an actual event, thing, or situation; a fact

Recognition – to be acknowledged as important

Recreational therapy – working with residents to help them stay active

Rectal – by rectum

Regain – to gain or reach again

Rehabilitation – the process of restoring to a former state

Rehabilitative – restoring to former health

Reincarnation – rebirth in another form of life

Reinforce – to strengthen by additional assistance

Relocation stress syndrome – reaction of an unprepared resident entering a long term care facility

Reprisal – retaliation against or punishment of a person for doing something

Reproductive system – body system that provides sexual pleasure and allows for human reproduction

Reservoir – a person, animal, or environment in which an infectious agent lives

Resident Assessment Instrument (RAI) – an assessment tool used in long term care facilities to document key information about residents including their care plans and outcomes

Resident Assessment Protocols (RAPs) – section of the RAI that includes a more detailed assessment of problem areas

Residential – long term care facility in which people live

Residents' rights – legal protections ensuring residents' physical and mental well-being

Respect – to consider worthy of high regard

Respiration – exchange of oxygen and carbon dioxide in the lungs

Respiratory system – body system that takes in oxygen (inhaling) and expels carbon dioxide (exhaling)

Respite – an interval of rest or relief (in this case, rest or relief for family who have been providing care)

Restorative – designed to help one return to health and be as independent and functional as possible

Restraint – device used to restrict movement

Resuscitate – to revive from apparent death

Retaliation – getting revenge or punishing a person for doing something

Rheumatoid arthritis – inflammatory joint disease

Right – something one has a just or legal claim to

Risk management – process of limiting legal liability, especially in reducing liability insurance risk

Role – the part that one plays in relationship to others

Routine – pattern of activities you set with each resident individually; something repeated on a schedule

Sacrum – bottom part of the spine

Safety – being free from harm or risk and secure from threats or danger

Sanitation – the promotion of hygiene and prevention of disease by maintaining clean conditions

Scrotum – the external pouch in males that contains the testes

Sebaceous glands – glands that are located in the dermis and secrete oil

Secretions – substances such as saliva, mucus, perspiration, tears, etc. that come out of the body

Securing – making something safe

Sedate – to calm with drugs

Seizure – a condition resulting from an abnormality in the brain

Self-determination – freedom to make your own choices and choose your own actions

Sensory system – body system of sense organs that gain information from the world outside the body

Sentimental value – the value of the object comes not from the money it could be sold for, but because of the associations and memories it has for the owner—perhaps it was a present from a parent, child, or spouse

Sexual abuse – sexual acts with a resident including touching in an intimate or suggestive manner, making sexual comments, or allowing another resident to do such acts

Sexuality – the quality of being male or female

Sexually transmitted diseases (STDs) – diseases are acquired through sexual activity with an infected partner, such as genital herpes, gonorrhea, chlamydia, and AIDS

Shift − scheduled period of work for a group of people (day shift, evening shift, night shift)

Shingles − viral inflammation that affects the nerves in the skull and spine

Shock − a condition in which vital organs in the body are not getting enough blood and oxygen to maintain good function

Shunt − surgical passage created between two blood vessels to move blood from one part to another

Sign − body characteristic that can be observed objectively, such as a red rash or bruising

Significant other − a person who is very close and important to another person, but who is not related by a traditional family relationship or marriage; usually refers to a sexual partner outside of marriage

Silent response − an infection that causes no signs or symptoms in the body

Single-minded − an attitude of seeing someone or something in only one way

Sitz bath − special basin, often attached to a toilet, which is filled with water to allow a person to sit down to wash or soak their genital and perineal areas

Smirking − smiling in a way that gives the impression you are superior to or making fun of another person

Sodium − salt

Speech therapist − works with residents who have difficulty with speech

Sphygmomanometer − instrument for measuring blood pressure (cuff and gauge)

Splint − device to use to support or immobilize a body part

Sputum − mucus from the lungs

Standard precautions − activities based on recommendations of CDC for facilities to use in handling blood, body fluids, secretions, excretions (except sweat), nonintact skin such as cuts and wounds, and mucous membranes to prevent infection

Status − position, rank, or prestige in relation to other people; state, situation

Sterile − free of all germs

Sterilization − elimination or destruction of all microbial life

Sternum − breastbone

Stimulate − to arouse a function

Stoma − a surgically created opening

Stool − human waste, feces from the bowel

Stress − physical or emotional reaction that causes mental tension

Stress incontinence − a leakage of urine that happens when the person coughs, sneezes, or laughs hard

Structure − definite pattern of organization (as of organs in a body system)

Stump − the amount of an extremity remaining after the rest is removed

Subacute care − care provided to residents who do not need to be in the hospital but are not ready to be at home

Subcutaneous − under the skin

Subjective − guess or hunch about what you observe, or something a resident feels inside and tells you about; not objective

Sundown syndrome − situation later in the day when a resident may become irritable, combative, tearful, or withdrawn, or wander or become confused

Supine − lying on the back

Supplement − a concentrated form of nutrition given to a resident in addition to their meals

Surgery − operation; procedure done to the body

Surname − last name or family name

Susceptible host − a person who is not resistant to infection by a microorganism

Symptom − any condition that accompanies or is caused by a disease or medical disorder; may be something observable or something reported by the patient

Syphilis − a chronic, contagious venereal infection that is sexually transmitted

Systolic pressure − the top number of the blood pressure, reflects pressure in vessels when the heart is beating

Tact − the art of saying the appropriate and polite thing at the right time

Tarry stool − stool that looks black and sticky, usually because of bleeding

Team nursing − a nursing approach in which the charge nurse is the team leader and makes nurse assistant assignments based on the needs for the shift and the team cares for the whole group of residents in a unit or a wing

Technique − a method for reaching a desired goal

Temperature − a degree of heat that naturally occurs in the body

Temporal scan − measurement of temperature of the forehead

Testes (testicles) − the two oval glands that manufacture sperm cells and the male sex hormone testosterone

Theme − something practiced continually

Theory − a set of ideas or principles offered to explain something observed

Therapeutic − referring to a treatment

Therapeutic diet − special diet that is a treatment for a disease or condition

Thyroid gland − gland located in the neck that secretes hormones that help regulate metabolism

Time management − ability to organize activities and perform them efficiently

Tolerate − to put up with, to endure

Total parenteral nutrition (TPN) − nutrition administered intravenously

Tracheostomy or tracheotomy − a stoma through the trachea into the respiratory airway

Tracheostomy tube − a breathing tube placed directly into the trachea through a surgical opening (stoma) in the person's neck

Transfer − move to another room in the facility; a process that occurs when a resident moves from one area to another; to move a resident from one surface to another, such as from bed to chair, chair to toilet, bed to commode, and so on

Transmit − transfer an infectious agent from one person or place to another

Trapeze − a short horizontal bar suspended by two parallel ropes, used to pull oneself up in bed

Trauma − a physical injury such as hitting head in a fall

Trimester − one third of the normal period of pregnancy, which is divided into three trimesters

Trisomy 21 syndrome – another name for Down syndrome

Tuberculosis (TB) – infectious, bacterial, communicable disease that primarily affects the lungs

Turgor – a characteristic of skin that indicates hydration: tight skin that does not "tent" shows good hydration

24-hour urine specimen – a collection of all urine a resident voids in a 24-hour period

Tympanic temperature – measurement of temperature of the eardrum

Umbilical cord – a tube connecting the fetus to the mother's placenta.

Uncircumcised – not circumcised, the foreskin remaining at the tip of the penis

Unoccupied bed – the bed is empty

Ureterostomy – a stoma through the skin into the kidney ureter, done to divert a resident's urine

Urethra – the canal in males and females that carries urine from the bladder; in males also serves as the duct for sperm

Urinary system – body system that helps maintain fluid balance and eliminates liquid wastes

Urinate – to pass urine

Urine – fluid waste formed by the kidney and excreted from the bladder

Uterus – muscular reproductive organ in which the fetus develops during pregnancy; it sheds its lining during menstruation

Vagina – muscular canal in the female leading from the uterus; involved in sexual intercourse, childbirth, and passage of menstrual flow

Validate – prove to be valid, sound, or effective

Validation – confirmation of something

Values – beliefs people have about what is important to them

Veins – blood vessels that carry deoxygenated blood from the body back to the heart and lungs

Ventilation – process of moving air in and out of the lungs

Verbal abuse – using profanity to a resident, calling a resident names, yelling at a resident in anger, making oral or written threats, or teasing a resident in an unkind manner

Virus – a type of microorganism that survives only in living things

Vital signs – necessary for life: temperature, pulse, respiration, and blood pressure

Void – to eliminate liquid or solid waste from the body; commonly used to describe urination

Vulva – external structure of the female sex organs

Wandering – aimless movement from one place to another

Wart – horny bump on the skin caused by a virus

Wing – separate section of a building attached to the central section

Appendix B

COMMON MEDICAL ABBREVIATIONS

ā before
abd abdomen
a.c. or āc before meals
ADL activity of daily living
ad lib as desired
Adm administrator
AM morning
amb ambulate
amt amount
AP apical
ASAP as soon as possible
bid 2 times a day
BM bowel movement
B/P or BP blood pressure
BR bedrest
BRP bathroom privileges
BSC bedside commode
c̄ with
cath catheter
cc cubic centimeter
c/o complains of
CPR cardiopulmonary resuscitation
CVA cerebrovascular accident; stroke
DC or D/C discontinue, stop
DNS Director of Nursing Service
DON Director of Nursing
drsg or dsg dressing
dx diagnosis
F Fahrenheit
FF force fluids
ft. foot, feet
h or hr hour
H_2O water
HA or H/A headache
HOH hard of hearing
hs hour of sleep; bedtime
ht height
I&O intake and output
ICP interdisciplinary care plan

IV intravenous
kg kilogram (2.2 kg = 1 lb)
L or lt left
lb pound
MD medical doctor
midnoc midnight
ml milliliter (1 ml = 1 cc)
NA sodium (salt)
NAS no added salt
neg. negative
noc night
NPO nothing by mouth
OD right eye
OOB out of bed
OS left eye
OT occupational therapy
p̄ after
p.c. or p̄c after meals
PM afternoon or evening
PO by mouth
PR per (or by) rectum
PRN as needed
PT physical therapy
q every
qd every day
qhs every hour of sleep
qid four times a day
qod every other day
q2h, q3h, etc. every 2 hours, 3 hours, etc.
R or rt right (R can also mean rectal)
RCP resident care plan
res resident
ROM range of motion
s̄ without
SOB shortness of breath
spec specimen
Stat immediately
tid three times a day
TPR temperature, pulse, respiration

u/a or U/A urinalysis
VS vital signs
W/C wheelchair
wt weight
x times

Appendix C

COMMON MEDICAL PREFIXES AND SUFFIXES

PREFIX/ SUFFIX	TRANSLATION	EXAMPLE
a-, an-	without, lack of	anemia (lack of blood)
ab-	away from	abduct (move extremity away from body)
ad-	toward, near	adduct (move extremity toward the body)
-al	pertaining to	dermal (pertaining to the skin)
-algia, -algesia	pertaining to pain	myalgia (muscle pain)
ante-	before, forward	antecubital (before or in front of the elbow)
anti-	against	antidepressant (drug to counter depression)
arter-	artery	arteriosclerosis (hardening of arteries)
auto-	self	autoinfection (infection by organism already in the body)
bi-	twice, double	bifocal (two points of focus)
bio-	life	biology (study of living things)
brady-	slow	bradycardia (slow heart rate)
-cele	herniation, pouching	mucocele (cavity containing mucus)
cent-	hundred	centimeter (hundredth of a meter)
-centesis	puncture and aspiration	thoracentesis (puncture through thoracic cavity to remove fluid)
-cid(e)	cut, kill	germicide (kills germs)
-cise	cut	incise (cut into)
circum-	around	circumcision (incision removing foreskin around penis)
con-	with	concurrence (agree with)
contra-	against, opposite	contraception (against conception)
-cyte	cell	erythrocyte (red blood cell)
de-	down, away from	dehydrate (remove water)
dia-	across, through	diameter (distance across a circle)
dis-	apart from, separate	disinfection (apart from infection)
dys-	difficult, abnormal	dysfunctional (not functioning normally)
ecto-	outer, outside	ectoderm (outer layer of tissue)
-ectasis	dilation	telangiectasis (dilation of capillaries)
-ectomy	removal of	tonsillectomy (removal of tonsils)
-emia	blood condition	anemia (lacking iron in blood)
en-	in, into, within	enclave (tissue enclosed inside other tissue)
endo-	inside	endoscope (instrument for looking inside the body)
epi-	over, on	epidermis (outer layer of skin)
eryth-	red	erythrocyte (red blood cell)
-esthesia	sensation	paresthesia (abnormal sensation)
ex-	out, out from	extract (to remove)
extra-	outside of	extracellular (outside the cell)
-genesis	development	pathogenesis (development of disease)

PREFIX/ SUFFIX	TRANSLATION	EXAMPLE
-genic	producing	pathogenic (disease-causing)
-gram	printed recording	arteriogram (diagnostic picture of an artery for visualization)
-graph	instrument for recording	audiogram (device to evaluate hearing)
hemi-	half	hemiplegia (half of body paralyzed)
hyper-	over, excessive	hypertension (high blood pressure)
hypo-	below, deficient	hypoglycemic (low blood sugar)
-iasis	condition of	nephrolithiasis (condition of having kidney stone)
il-	not	illegible (not readable)
in-	into, within or not	injection (forcing liquid into)
inter-	between	intercostal (between the ribs)
intra-, intro-	within	intravenous (within the veins)
-ism	a condition	rheumatism (condition of having rheumatoid arthritis)
-itis	inflammation	appendicitis (inflamed appendix)
-logy	the study of	psychology (study of the mind)
-lysis	destruction of	hemolysis (destruction of blood cells)
leuk-	white	leukocyte (white blood cell)
macro-	large	macromastia (abnormally large breasts)
mal-	illness, disease	malabsorption (inadequate absorption of nutrients)
-megaly	enlargement	acromegaly (enlargement of head, hands, and feet)
-meter	measuring instrument	spirometer (instrument that measures breathing)
-metry	measurement	telemetry (measurement using remote transmitter)
micro-	very small	microorganisms (very small organisms)
mono-	one, single	monoplegia (paralysis of one extremity)
neo-	new	neoplasm (tumor growing new cells)
non-	not	noninflammatory (not causing inflammation)
olig-	small, scanty	oliguria (low excretion of urine)
-oma	tumor	granuloma (tumor consisting of granulation tissue)
-oscopy	look into	gastroscopy (look into the stomach)
-osis	condition	fibrosis (condition of fibrous tissue formation)
-ostomy	opening into	colostomy (opening into the colon)
para-	abnormal	paralgesia (abnormal painful sensation)
-pathy	disease	myopathy (disease of muscle)
-penia	lack	leukopenia (lack of enough white blood cells)
per-	by, through	perfusion (passage of fluid through an organ)
peri-	around, covering	pericardium (the sac around the heart)
-phasia	speaking	aphasia (speaking or language disorder)
-phobia	exaggerated fear	hydrophobia (fear of water)
-plasty	surgical repair	myoplasty (repair of a muscle)
-plegia	paralysis	quadriplegia (paralysis of arms and legs)
poly-	much, many	polyuria (much urine)
post-	after, behind	postoperative (after surgery)
pre-, pro-	before, in front of	preoperative (before surgery)
-ptosis	falling, sagging	ptosis (drooping eyelid)
re-	again, back	reinjure (injure again)
retro-	backward	retrograde (moving backward)
-rrhage	excessive flow	hemorrhage (heavy bleeding)

PREFIX/ SUFFIX	TRANSLATION	EXAMPLE
-rrhaphy	suturing	colporrhaphy (surgical suturing of vagina)
-rrhea	profuse discharge	diarrhea (heavy discharge of watery stool)
-scope	examination instrument	microscope
-scopy	examination using a scope	endoscopy (looking inside body with endoscope)
semi-	half, part	semi-reclined (partly lying down)
-stasis	control, stop	hemostasis (stopping bleeding)
-stomy	creation of opening	colostomy (opening of bowel to abdomen)
sub-	under	subcutaneous (under the skin)
super-	above, excessive	superinfection (excessive infection occurring during the treatment of another infection)
tachy-	fast, rapid	tachycardia (fast heartbeat)
-tomy	incision	sinusotomy (incision of a sinus)
trans-	across	transdermal (across the skin)
uni-	one	unilateral (one side)
-uria	condition of the urine	polyuria (passing abnormally large amount of urine)

Appendix

D

EMERGENCY TRANSFER TECHNIQUES

Blankets are the most useful of all the evacuation equipment available, for several reasons:
- They can serve as a stretcher for moving residents quickly.
- They can be used to smother fires.
- They can be used in different evacuation techniques.

EVACUATION TECHNIQUES

There are six different evacuation techniques you should know. Which you use in an evacuation depends on the particular situation and the availability of help from others.

One Nurse-Blanket Carry

This carry should be used for a resident who is smaller than you when you are doing the carry alone.
1. Fold the blanket diagonally with the point downward and the long ends on either side of the resident.
2. Help the resident into a sitting position on the bed.
3. Wrap the blanket around the resident's back and under the arms (like a shawl), and then tie the ends of the blanket in a knot. Cross the resident's arms.
4. Insert your right arm between the knotted blanket (below knot) and resident's chest.
5. Turn your back to the resident, bend your knees, and adjust the blanket comfortably over your right shoulder.
6. Straighten your knees to lift the resident from the bed with a minimum amount of strain or effort. Carry the resident on your back. Support the resident's legs with your left arm.
7. Carry the resident to safety.

Blanket Drag

1. Unfold the blanket on the floor.
2. Help the resident onto the blanket diagonally.

Note: *If the resident is wearing shoes, remove them. This eliminates the possibility of the heels catching on stairs and floor obstructions.*

3. Lift the corner of the blanket nearest the resident's head. This keeps the resident's head off the floor.
4. Using one or both hands, pull the resident, head first, to a place of safety.

Pack Strap Method

1. Help the resident to a sitting position.
2. Grasp the resident's right wrist with your left hand and left wrist with your right hand.
3. Place your head under the resident's arms without releasing their wrists and turn, placing your back against the resident's chest so that your shoulders are lower than their armpits.
4. Then pull the resident's arms over your shoulders and across your chest for leverage. Keep the resident's wrists firmly grasped.
5. Lean forward slightly, straighten your knees, and transport the resident to safety.

Hip Method

1. Turn the resident on their side facing you, sit on the bed, and place your back against the resident's abdomen.
2. Grasp the resident's knees with one arm and slide your other arm down and across their back.
3. Begin to stand while drawing the resident up onto your hips.
4. Carry the resident to safety.

Cradle Drop (To Blanket)

1. Unfold the blanket on the floor; face the side of the bed. the resident should be in the supine position.
2. Lift under the resident's knees with one arm and under their shoulders with the other. Guide the resident toward you.
3. Bend one knee at a right angle, and press it against the bed, keep your foot firmly on the floor.
4. Lower the resident to the floor by bending your back leg to the floor. Keep your other knee against the bed.
5. Pull the resident toward you and ease them onto the blanket.

Note: *Your raised knee will support the resident's knees and legs, and your arm will support their shoulders and head. The cradle formed by your arm and knee will protect their shoulders and head.*

Kneel Drop

1. Unfold the blanket on the floor. the resident should be in the supine position.
2. Face the side of the bed and lower your body to both knees in a kneeling position.
3. Grasp the resident's knees with one arm, and their head and shoulders with the other.
4. Pull the resident straight out from bed until their body contacts your chest, and allow the resident to slide down your body to the cushion formed by your knees.
5. Ease the resident to the blanket and move to safety.

Appendix

E

ENGLISH-SPANISH/SPANISH-ENGLISH GLOSSARY OF BASIC LONG TERM CARE TERMS

ENGLISH-SPANISH GLOSSARY

abdomen abdomen
ache dolor
afternoon tarde
angry enojado
ankle tobillo
arm brazo
back espalda
bandage venda
bathroom cuarto de baño
bathtub bañera
bed cama, lecho
bedpan chata
black negro
blanket manta
blood sangre
blouse blusa
blue azul
bottom fondo
bread pan
breakfast desayuno
brother hermano
brown castaño
butter mantequilla
cane bastoón
chair silla
chest pecho
chew masticar
child niño
chin barbilla
clean (adjective) limpio
clear transparente
clothes ropa; men's suit: traje, woman's dress: vestido
coffee café
cold (adjective) frío
comfort consuelo
constipation estreñimiento
cough (noun) tos
cream crema

cup taza or vasa
dark oscuro
daughter hija
day día
depressed depresivo
dinner cena
dirty enlodado
disease enfermedad
doctor doctor
door puerta
dress (clothing) vestido
drink (verb) beber
drink (noun) bebida
dry seco
ear oreja
eat comer
eggs huevos
elbow codo
emergency emergencia
exercise ejercicio
eye ojo
eyeglasses lentes
face cara
family familia
fever fiebre
finger dedo
fire fuego
floor suelo
flu influenza
foot pie
forehead frente
fork tenedor
friend amigo
fruit fruta
green verde
hair pelo
hairbrush cepillo (para el pelo/cabello)
hallway pasillo
hand mano

hat sombrero
head cabeza
hearing aid audífono
help! ¡socorro!
here aquí
hot caliente
hungry hambriento
husband marido
ice hielo
infection infeccíon
juice jugo
knee rodilla
knife cuchillo
left izquierdo
leg pierna
light luz
lonely solitario or solo
lunch almuerzo
man hombre
meat carne
medicine medicina
milk leche
morning mañana
mouth boca
move mover
music música
neck cuello
need (noun) necisidad
night noche
nightgown camisón
no no
noon mediodía
nose nariz
nothing nada
nurse enfermera
oxygen oxígeno
pain dolor
painkiller analgésico
pajamas piyamas
pants pantalones
pantyhose media
pardon me perdóneme
pepper pimienta
pillow almohada
plate plato
please por favor
potatoes papas
preference preferencia
priest sacerdote
red rojo

right (opposite of left) derecho
roommate compañero de cuarto
sad triste
salt sal
sheet sábana
shirt camisa
shoes zapatos
shoulder hombro
shower ducha
sister hermana
sit sentarse
skin piel
skirt falda
sleep (noun) sueño
sleep (verb) dormir
snack bocado
sneeze (noun) estornudo
socks calcetínes
son hijo
sorry lo siento
spoon cuchara
spouse cónyuge
stand estar de pie
stomach estómago
stool (feces) excremento
sugar azúcar
sunlight luz del sol
swallow tragar
table mesa
talk hablar
teeth dientes
telephone teléfono
television televisión
thanks gracias
thermometer termómetro
thirsty sediento
toast tostada
today hoy
toes dedos del pie
toilet taza
toilet paper papel higiénico
tomorrow mañana
toothbrush cepillo de dientes
toothpaste pasta dentífrica
underclothes ropa interior
urinal orinal
urinate orinar
urine orina
vegetable verdura(s), vegetal(es)
vomit (noun) vómito

wake **(verb)** despertar
walk **(verb)** andar, caminar
walker andador
want (verb) desear
wash (verb) lavar
water agua
weigh pesar
wet mojado
wheelchair silla de ruedas
when? ¿cuando?
where ¿donde?
white blanco
wife esposa
window ventana
woman mujer
wound herida
wrist muñeca
yellow amarillo
yes sí

SPANISH-ENGLISH GLOSSARY

abdomen abdomen
agua water
almohada pillow
almuerzo lunch
amarillo yellow
amigo friend
analgésico painkiller
andador walker
andar walk (verb)
aquí here
audífono hearing aid
azúcar sugar
azul blue
bañera bathtub
barbilla chin
bastoón cane
beber drink (verb)
bebida drink (noun)
blanco white
blusa blouse
boca mouth
bocado snack
brazo arm
cabeza head
café coffee
calcetínes socks
caliente hot
cama bed

caminar walk (verb)
camisa shirt
camisón nightgown
cara face
carne meat
castaño brown
cena dinner
cepillo (para el pelo/cabello) hairbrush
cepillo de dientes toothbrush
chata bedpan
codo elbow
comer eat
compañero de cuarto roommate
consuelo comfort
cónyuge spouse
crema cream
¿cuando? when?
cuarto de baño bathroom
cuchara spoon
cuchillo knife
cuello neck
dedo finger
dedos del pie toes
depresivo depressed
derecho right (opposite of left)
desayuno breakfast
desear want (verb)
despertar wake (verb)
día day
dientes teeth
doctor doctor
dolor ache
dolor pain
¿donde? where
dormir sleep (verb)
ducha shower
ejercicio exercise
emergencia emergency
enfermedad disease
enfermera nurse
enlodado dirty
enojado angry
espalda back
esposa wife
estar de pie stand
estómago stomach
estornudo sneeze (noun)
estreñimiento constipation
excremento stool (feces)
falda skirt

familia family
fiebre fever
fondo bottom
frente forehead
frío cold (adjective)
fruta fruit
fuego fire
gracias thanks
hablar talk
hambriento hungry
herida wound
hermana sister
hermano brother
hielo ice
hija daughter
hijo son
hombre man
hombro shoulder
hoy today
huevos eggs
infeccíon infection
influenza flu
izquierdo left
jugo juice
lavar wash (verb)
leche milk
lecho bed
lentes eyeglasses
limpio clean (adjective)
lo siento sorry
luz del sol sunlight
luz light
mañana morning, tomorrow
mano hand
manta blanket
mantequilla butter
marido husband
masticar chew
media pantyhose
medicina medicine
mediodía noon
mesa table
mojado wet
mover move
mujer woman
muñeca wrist
música music
nada nothing
nariz nose
necisidad need (noun)

negro black
niño child
no no
noche night
ojo eye
oreja ear
orina urine
orinal urinal
orinar urinate
oscuro dark
oxígeno oxygen
pan bread
pantalones pants
papas potatoes
papel higiénico toilet paper
pasillo hallway
pasta dentífrica toothpaste
pecho chest
pelo hair
perdóneme pardon me
pesar weigh
pie foot
piel skin
pierna leg
pimienta pepper
piyamas pajamas
plato plate
por favor please
preferencia preference
puerta door
rodilla knee
rojo red
ropa clothes
ropa interior underclothes
sábana sheet
sacerdote priest
sal salt
sangre blood
seco dry
sediento thirsty
sentarse sit
sí yes
silla chair
silla de ruedas wheelchair
¡socorro! help!
solitario lonely
solo lonely
sombrero hat
suelo floor
sueño sleep (noun)

tarde afternoon

taza or vasa cup

taza toilet

teléfono telephone

televisión television

tenedor fork

termómetro thermometer

tobillo ankle

tos cough (noun)

tostada toast

tragar swallow

traje men's suit

transparente clear

triste sad

vegetal(es) vegetable

venda bandage

ventana window

verde green

verdura(s) vegetable

vestido woman's dress

vómito vomit (noun)

zapatos shoes

Bibliography

AARP Research: *The 1987 nursing home reform act*, www.research.aarp.org/health/fs84-reform.html, 1995, 2002.

AARP: *Federal and state enforcement of the 1987 nursing home reform act*, www. research.aarp.org/health/fs83-reform.html, February 2001.

Abraham I and Neudorker M: *Alzheimer's disease: a decade of progress, a future of nursing challenges*, Geriatr Nurs (New York) pp 116-119, May/June 1990.

ADA: *Blood sugar levels and diabetes*, April 14, 2007 www.webmd.com.

Administration on Aging: *Aging into the 21st century*, www.aoa.dhhs.gov/aoa/stats/aging21/summary.html, May 31, 1996.

Administration on Aging: *The older americans act nutrition programs*, www.ada.dhhs.gov/aoa/pages/nutreval.html, July 30, 2001.

Age Works: *Normal aging*, www.ageworks.com/information-on-aging/cha.../aspects.htm, April 30,2002.

Aging changes in the male reproductive system: www.health central.com, August 13, 2002.

Agitation: www.adrc.wustl.edu/Alzheimer/fdts/agitation.html, 2002.

Alzheimer's Association Massachusetts Chapter: *Alzheimer's disease progressive stages statistics*, Cambridge, MA, 2002, Alzheimer's Association Massusetts Chapter.

Alzheimer's Association: *Facts, statistics about Alzheimer's disease*, Oct. 2001 www.alzmass.org.

Alzheimer's Association: *Key elements of dementia care*, Chicago, IL, 1997, Alzheimer's Association.

Alzheimer's Association: *People with Alzheimer's disease, providing quality care, cognitive and behavioral symptoms, treating behavior symptoms, treating cognitive symptoms, cause, ten warning signs,diagnosis, treatment options, current research*, www.alz.org/people/understanding/cognitive.htm March 12, 2002.

Alzheimer's Association: *Research on improving care, research on the causes of alzheimer's disease*, www.alz.org/research/current/care, 2001.

Alzheimer's Association, Paul Raia: *Common Problems in Early Alzheimers's Disease*, www.alzmass.org/common-problems.htm, December 14, 2000.

Alzheimers Association: *Key elements of dementia care*, www.alz.org/hc/qcare/dementia.htm,October 1, 2002.

American Academy of dermatologist FAQS: *Aging skin*, www.derm-infonet.com/aginhskinnet/Q&Ahtml, 2001.

American Academy of Dermatology: *What is aging skin*, www.derm-infonet.com/agingskinnet/basic facts.html, 2001.

American Association on Mental Retardation: *Fact sheet aging, older adults and their aging caregivers*, Washington, DC, March 6, 2001.

American Association on Mental Retardation: *Fact sheet what is mental retardation*, Washington, DC, December 2001.

American Diabetes Association: *All about Diabetes*, www.diabetes.org/about-diabetes.jsp

American Health Care Association Memorandum: *Comment on barriers to community-based alternatives*, Washington, DC, August 30, 2001.

American Health Care Association/American Association of Homes and Services/ National Center for Assisted Living: *Draft voluntary ergonomics guidelines for long term care*, Washington DC.

American Health Care Association: *Nutrition and hydration in long term care*, Washington DC, 1999.

American Health Care Association: *A consumer guide to nursing facilities*,Washington DC.

American Health Care Association: *A family guide to making the transition to nursing home life*, Washington DC, 2002.

American Health Care Association: *A new view of end of life care*, Provider, May 1999.

American Health Care Association: *Facts and trends: assisted living source book*, Washington DC, 2001.

American Health Care Association: *Comment letter on the proposal to permit nursing facilities use of feeding assistants*, Washington DC May 23, 2002.

American Health Care Association: *Consumer information a guide for families*, Washington DC, April 2,2002.

American Health Care Association: *Family questions: the first thirty days*, Washington DC, 2002.

American Health Care Association: *Governors urged to transition disabled out of nursing homes*, Washington DC, August 15, 2002.

American Health Care Association: *Hazard communication*, Washington DC, May 2002, AHCA OSHA workgroup.

American Health Care Association: *How to pay for nursing home care*, Washington DC, 1996.

American Health Care Association: *Long term care resident assessment instrument*, Washington DC, June 2006.

American Health Care Association: *The Long Term Care Survey*, Washington DC, September 2007.

American Health Care Association: *Managed care and*

sub-acute care, an update # 5112, Washington DC, 1997.

American Health Care Association: *Practical approaches to reducing falls in nursing facilities*, Provider l2 (11) November 2001.

American Health Care Association: *Quest for quality* ed 2, Washington DC 1991.

American Health Care Association: *Retrain don't restrain*, Washington DC, 1991.

American Health Care Association: *Tips on visiting friends and relatives*, Washington DC, 2002.

American Medical Directors Association, American Health Care Association: *Altered mental status clinical practice guideline*, Washington DC.

American Medical Directors Association: *Caring for the ages*, www.amda.com/caring/november2001/falls.htm, October 15, 2002.

American Medical Directors Association: *Chronic pain management in long term care setting*, Columbia, MD, April, 2002.

American Medical Directors Association: *Pressure ulcer therapy companion clinical practice guidelines*, Washington DC, 1999.

American National Red Cross: *Nurse assistant training*, Washington, 1989.

American Red Cross: *Instructor Candidate Training Participants'* Training Manual, 1990.

American Social Health Association: *Prevention*, www.iwannaknow.org

American Social Health Assoc\iation: *Puberty*, www.iwannaknow.org

American Stroke Foundation: *Stroke Test*, www.americanstroke.org/content/view/36/56/

Arking R: *Biology of aging*, Englewood Cliffs, NJ, Prentice-Hall Inc., 1991.

Assessment of work and energy transfers in nursing aides lifting patients, Ergonomics.

Association for Protection of the Elderly: *Advocacy and information network for nursing home residents*, www.apeape.org/index.html April 17, 2002.

Back tips for health care providers, Daly City, Calif, 1986, Krames Communications.

Back to backs: a guide to preventing back injury, San Bruno, 1988, Krames Communications.

Batshaw, M: *Children with disabilities*, Baltimore, MD., 1999, Paul H. Brookes Publishing Co.

Benensori AS, editor: *Control of communicable diseases in man*, ed 15, Washington, DC, 1990, American Public Health Association.

Bennett JV and Brachman PS, editors: *Hospital infections*, ed 3, Boston, 1992, Little Brown and Co.

Brown M: *Nursing assistants' behavior toward the institutionalized elderly*, QRB, pp 15-17, Jan 1988.

Brubaker TH: *Aging, health, and family long-term care*, Newbury Park, NJ 1987, Sage Publications.

Burgener S and Barton D: *Nursing care of cognitively impaired, institutionalized elderly*, J Geriatr Nurs 17:37-43, 1991.

Burger S: (1993) *Avoiding physical restraint use: new standards in care*, 1993, The National Citizens' Coalition for Nursing Home Reform.

Casey, G.: *Modern wound dressings*, Nursing Standard, Sept. 7, 2000 pp 47-51.

Casey M: *How to be a nurse assistant inservice education series unit 3 quality of life restorative care*, Unit 1, Washington DC, 1995, AHCA.

Casey M: *Managing difficult behavior symptoms*, Washington DC, 1996, AHCA/NCAL.

Casey M: *National center for assisted living quality of life student manual*, Washington DC, 1996, AHCA.

Caudill M and Patrick M: *Nursing assistant turnover in nursing homes and need satisfaction*, J Gerontol Nurs 15:24-30, 1989.

CDC, MMWR (morbidity and morality weekly report): *U.S. public health service guidelines for the management of occupational exposures to HBV, HCV, and HIV and recommendations for post exposure prophylaxis*, www.cdc.gov/mmwr/preview/mmwrhtml, June 29, 2001.

CDC: *Protecting Patients from Infectious Diseases* 2007 http://www.cdc.gov www.cdc.gov

CDC: *Recommendations and universal precautions for the preparation of the transmission of HIV, hepatitis b and other blood-borne pathogens in health care settings*, National Prevention Information Network, vol.36 (25).

CDC: *Healthy aging for older adults*, www.cdc.gov/nccdphp/aging/index.htm.

CDC: *Healthy aging for older adults*, www.cdc.gov/nccdphp/aging/listerv.htm, October 16, 2002.

CDC: *National center for injury prevention and control falls and hip fractures among older*, www.cdc.gov/ncipc/factors/falls.htm, March 6, 2002.

CDC: *Physical activity and good nutrition*, www.cdc.gov/nccdphp/dnpa/dnpaaag.htm, September 7, 2002.

CDC: Reducing falls and resulting fractures among older women, recommendations and reports, www.cdc.gov/mmwr/preview/mmwrhtml/rr4902a2.htm, March 31, 2000.

CDC: *Report 5 a day fruits and vegetables*, www.cdc.gov/nccdphp/dnpa/5a day/index.htm, August 5, 2002.

CDC: *Summary recommendations of the physical fitness and exercise working group*, www.cdc.gov/mmwr/preview, October 20,1989 reviewed May 2, 2001.

CDC: *Surveillance for morbidity and mortality among older adults*, www.cdc.gov/mmwr/preview/mmwrtml/ss4808a2.htm, December 19,1999.

CDC: *Surveillance of health care workers with HIV/AIDS*, www.cdc.gov/ncidod/hip/isolat/isotab-1htm, updated October 2001.

CDC: *TB: the connection HIV what health care workers should know*, Washington DC, 2002, CDC Booklet

CDC: *Youth Risk Behavior Survey* 2005, www.cdc.gov/HealthyYouth/asthma/index.htm

Centers for Disease Control: *CDC Guideline for isolation precautions in hospitals*, Infection Control 4(4) :245-325, July/August 1983.

Centers for Disease Control: *Guideline for prevention of transmission of HIV and HBV to health-care and public-safety workers*. MMWR 38(Suppl S6):l-37, 1989.

Centers for Disease Control: *Intellectual/Developmental Disabilities*, Oct. 2005 www.cdc.gov/ncbddd.

Centers for Disease Control: *Recommendations for prevention of HIV transmission in health-care settings*, MMWR 36(Suppl 2S):1-18, 1987.

Centers for Disease Control: *Update: universal precautions for prevention of transmission of HIV, HBV, and other bloodborne pathogens in health-care settings*, MMWR 37(24):377-388, 1988.

Charnes LS and Moore PS: *Meeting patients' spiritual needs: the Jewish perspective*, Holistic Nurs Pract 6(3):64-71, 1992.

CMS media Release: *HCFA asks nursing homes to join education*, www.cms.hhs.gov/media/press/release.asp?counter=134, June 30,1999.

CMS: *Accidents & Supervision revised guidelines, F323* Aug. 6, 2007.

CMS: *Restraint information*:www.cms.gov/providerupdate/regs/cms, October 2, 2002.

Columbia University School of Nursing: *Skin hygiene and infection prevention more of the same or different approaches*, New York, June18, 1999.

Consultant Dieticians in Health Care Facilities: *Dining skills*, 1992, funded by The Retirement Research Foundation.

Convatec: *Caring for your Stoma*, www.convatec.com.

Coons D, editor: *Specialized dementia care units*, Baltimore, 1991, Johns Hopkins University Press.

Cronin, Colleen: *Nutrients and normal blood sugar control*, Oct. 3, 2005 www.healthline.com

Cruz, V: *Criteria to receive services developmental disability denver working with families with children/parents with developmental disabilities*, Denver, Co., 2000, The Social Work Program, Metropolitan State College of Denver.

Davis, Jeanie L: *Type 2 Diabetes treatment options* http://diabetes.webmd.com/features/new-type-2-diabetes-treatment-option, October 2006.

Dawson P et al: *Preventing excess disability in patients with Alzheimer's disease*, Geriatr Nurs, pp 298-301, Nov/Dec 1986.

Defined Terms: *Aerobic or anaerobic? quick activity*, www.plu.edu/~chasegu/terms.html, 1995.

Diseases, Springhouse, PA, 1996, Springhouse Corporation.

Diabetes Forecast: Urine Testing, 2007 Resource Guide

Drugay M: *Influencing holistic nursing practice in long-term care*, Holistic Nurs Pract.

Easter Seals Central: *Pa success stories*, www.visit Easter seals.org/success.htm, 2001, 2003.

Elder Care Online: *Nursing home resident rights*, www.ec-online.net/knowledge/articles/resrights.html, 1998.

Long term care regulatory guide to Obra regulations and interpretive guidelines, Miamisburg, Oh., 1999, Heaton Publications.

Elias M: *Sexuality: late love life*, Harvard Health Letter 18(l):l-3, 1992.

Evans Land Strumpf N: *Tying down the elderly*, J Am Geriatr Soc 37:65-74, 1989.

F.A. Davis Co., Wilkinson & Van Leuven: *Procedure Checklists for Fundamentals of Nursing* 2007.

Federal Register: *The proposed rule feeding aid*, www.frwebgate.access.gpo.gov, March 29, 2002.

Fraser D: *Patient assessment: infection in the elderly*. In Jackson MM, guest editor.

Gagnon M, Sicard C, and Sironis JP: *Evaluation of forces on the lumbosacral joint*.

Gallagher-Allred CR: *OBRA: a challenge and an opportunity for nutrition care*, Columbus, OH, 1992, Ross Laboratories.

Garg A, Owen BD, and Carlson B: *An ergonomic evaluation of nursing assistants' jobs in a nursing home*, Ergonomics 35(9):979-995, 1992.

Gillogly, B: *The new nurse assistant, fifth edition*, Cypress

Ca., Medcom Trainex, 2002.

Gould J and Davies GS: *Orthopaedic and sports physical therapy*, St. Louis, 1985, Mosby.

Gwyther LP: *Care of Alzheimer's patients: a manual for nursing home staff*, ed 2, Washington, DC, AHCA and Alzheimer's Association, 2001.

Havens, Lila: *Hemodialysis information and resources*, Nov. 2005 www.webmd.com/a-to-z-guides/hemodialysis-20667.

Havens, Lila: *Peritoneal dialysis information and resources*, Nov. 2005 www.webmd.com/a-to-z-guides/peritoneal-dialysis-4391.

HCFA/CMS: *Restraint definition*: www.hcfa.gov/medicaid/1+csp/q%26a, July 15, 1997.

HCFA: *National restraint reduction newsletters*: www.hcfa. gov/ pub forms /newsletter/restraint, January 22, 2001.

Health Care Financing Administration, Department of Health and Human Services: *Nutrition and hydration care information pack*, HCFA.

Health Care Financing Administration: *Interpretative Guidelines*, Washington, DC, 1989.

HealthDay News: *Chest Compressions Key to Revised CPR Guidelines*, www.medlineplus.com, Oct. 2007.

Health on the Net Foundation: *Top 10 Causes of Death Among Adults Over Age 65*, June 2007 seniorhealth.about.com.

Hegland A: *Resident assessment: means justifies ends*, Contemporary Long Term Care.

Hegner B: *Nursing assistant: a nursing process approach*, ed 8, Albany, NY, 1999, Delmar Publishers.

Herbert R: *The normal aging process reviewed*, Int Nurs Rev 39(3):93-96, 1992.

Heriot C: *Spirituality and aging*, Holistic Nurs Prac 7(1):22-31, 1992.

HFCA: *Nutrition/hydration clinical practice guidelines*, www.cms.hhs.gov, October 28, 1999.

Hiatt-Snyder L, et al: *Wandering*, Gerontologist 18:272-80, 1978.

Hirst S and Metcalf B: *Why's and what's of wandering*, Geriatr Nurs pp 237-238, Sept/Oct 1989.

Hoffman SB and Platt CA: *Comforting the confused*, Owings Mills, Maryland, 1990, National Health Publishing.

Holleman J and Mayfield E: *Dehydration and fluid maintenance clinical practice guideline*, Washington DC, 2001, American Medical Directors Association.

Hussian R: *Severe behavioral problems*. In Terri L and Lewinsohn P, editors: Geropsychological assessment and treatment, New York, 1985, Springer.

i Village: *Alzheimer's disease*, www.ivillagehealth .com/library, March 12, 2002.

Institute of Medicine: *Approaching death, improving care at the end of life, a profile of death and dying in america, caring at the end of life, educating clinicians and other professionals, the health care system and the dying patient, accountability and quality in end of life care*, www.4.nationalacademeies.org/news.nsf, June 4, 1997.

Jackson MM and Lynch P: *An alternative to isolating patients*. Geriatr Nurs 8:308-311, 1987.

Jackson MM and Lynch P: *An attempt to make an issue less murky: a comparison of four systems for infection precautions*. Infect Control Hosp Epidemiol 12:448-450, 1991.

Jackson MM and Lynch P: *In search of a rational approach*. Am J Nurs 90(lO):65-73, 1990.

Jackson MM and Lynch P: *Infection control: too much or too little?* Am J Nurs 84:208-210, 1984.

Jackson MM and Schafer K: *Identifying clues to infections in nursing home residents: the role of the nurses' aide*. J Gerontol Nurs 19(7):33-42, July 1993.

Jackson MM et al: *Clinical savvy: why not treat all body substances as infectious?* Am J Nurs 87:1l37-1139, 1987.

JCAHO: *Standards for long term care*, Oakbridge Terrace, IL, 2002-2003, Joint Commission on Accreditation of Healthcare Organizations.

JCAHO Committee: *Abbreviations do-not-use list*, 2007 www.jcaho.org.

Jernigan AK: *Nutrition in long term care facilities*, Chicago, IL, 1987, The American Dietetic Association.

Jewish Home and Hospital: *Retrain don't Restrain*, prepared for the National Restraint Minimization Project at The Jewish Home and Hospital for Aged under a grant from the Commonwealth Fund, 1991.

Johnson-Pawlson J: *How to be a nurse assistant*, ed 2, Washington, DC, 1990, American Health Care Association.

Joint Commission on Accreditation of Health Care Organizations: *ORYX The next evolution in accreditation*, Oakbridge Terrace, IL, 1997, JCAHO.

Journal of the Southern Orthopaedic Association: *Sequential Compression Devices*, Nov. 15, 2002 www.medscape.com/viewarticle/444065.

Kantor, M.D., Daniel: *Seizures*, www.medlineplus.com, Aug. 6, 2007.

Kass M: *Sexual expression of the elderly in nursing homes*, Gerontol 78(18):372-378, 1992.

Kisner C and Colby LA: *Therapeutic exercise: foundation and techniques*, Philadelphia, 1985, FA Davis.

Lancaster E: *Tuberculosis comeback: Programs for long-term care*. 3 Gerontol Nurs, l9(7):l6-21, July 1993.

Langer: *Mindfulness*, Reading, MA, 1989, Addison-Wesley.

Larson E: *APIC guideline for use of topical antimicrobial agents*. Am J Infect Control 16(6):253-266, December 1988.

Levy L: *Psychosocial intervention and dementia: part I: state of the art, future directions*, Occupational Therapy in Mental Health 7:69-107, 1987.

Lewis CB and Knortz KA: *Orthopedic assessment and treatment of the geriatric patient*, St. Louis, 1993, Mosby.

Lewis CB: *What's so different about rehabilitating the older person*, Clinical Management 4(3)l0-13, 15, 1984.

Lift With Care (videodisc), Redwood City, CA,1987, VISU-COM Productions, Inc., for Beverly Enterprises.

LTC-Resource. com: *Your rights in a nursing home*, www.ltcresources.com/Rights.html, April 5, 2002.

Lucero M: *Products for Alzheimer's self-stimulatory wanderers, Phase I Final Report*, Bethesda, MD, National Institute on Aging Research Project (1R43AGO7759-O1A1), 1990.

Lyman K: *Bringing the social back in: a critique of the biomedicalization of dementia*, Gerontologist 29:597-605, 1989.

Lynch P et al: *Implementing and evaluating a system of generic infection precautions: body substance isolation*. Am J Infect Control 18:1-12, 1990.

Lynch P et al: Letter: *handwashing versus gloving*. Infect Control Hosp Epidemiol.

Lynch P et al: *Rethinking the role of isolation practices in the prevention of nosocomial infections*. Ann Intern Med 107:243-246, 1987.

Marton WJ and Garner JS, guest editors: *Proceedings of the third decennial international conference on nosocomial infections*. Am J Med 91 (special issue 3B), pp. 15-35, September 16, 1991.

Maslow A: *Toward a psychology of being*, New York, 1962, D. Van Nostrand.

Mayo Clinic: *Burns First-Aid Guide*, www.mayoclinic.com Dec. 2, 2006

Mayo Clinic: *Choking First-Aid Guide*, Jan. 9, 2006.

Mayo Clinic: *Electrical Burns First-Aid Guide* Jan. 5, 2006.

Mayo Clinic: *Prevention and management geriatric medicine*, www.mayo .edu/geriatrics-rst/pv.ntml, November 13, 2002.

McCaffery M and Pasero C: *Pain clinical manual*, second edition, St Louis, 1999, Mosby.

McCracken A and Fitzwater J: *The right environment for AD*, Geriatr Nurs (New York), pp 243-244, Nov/Dec 1989.

Medicare: *Medicare nutrition and hydration alert*: www.Medicare.gov/nursing/campaigns/ nutricare alerts.asp, updated January 6, 2003.

MedicineNet: *Biological therapy definition*, Jan. 2004, www.medterms.com/script/main/art.asp?articlekey=2465

Mery B: *Healthy aging: why we get old*, Harvard Health Letter 10(9):9-12, 1992.

Midwest College of Oriental Medicine: *The layman's guide to oriental medicine*, www.acupunture.edu/laymans/faq.htm.

Morris J Lipsitz, L Murphy, K Belleville, Taylor P: *Quality care in the nursing home*, St Louis, MO, 1997, Mosby Lifeline.

Mourad LA and Droste MM: *The nursing process in the care of adults with orthopedic conditions*, ed 2, New York, 1988, Wiley Medical.

MSN: *Recognizing Alzheimer's disease*, www.content.health.msn.com/content/article/1626.50837?z=1626-50804-6510-00-03, March 06, 2000.

MSN: *Understanding alzheimers*, www.content.health.msn.com/content/article/54/61451htm, June 1, 2002.

National Council on Aging, Beattie B and Whitelaw N: *Assessment of a Falls Prevention Program*, www.ncoa.org/publications.inno/01/untoward.html, 2001.

National Council on the Aging, James Hood: Growing awareness of falls threat, www.ncoa.org/publications.innol-01/falls.html, 2001.

National Guideline Clearinghouse: *Pressure ulcers*, www.guideline.gov/index, January 2001.

National Institute for Health: *Skin integrity* chapter 4, www.nih.gov/ninr/reseach/vol3/skin.html, 1992.

National Institute of Health: *Infections in long term care*, www.nih.gov/ninr/research/vol3/infection.html, May 07, 2002.

National Institute of Health: *Problems associated with the use of physical restraints chapter 5*, www.nih.gov/ninr/research/vol.3/Restraints.html, June 18, 2002.

National Institute of Nursing Research: *End of life care*, www.nih.gov/ninr/about/legislation/eolbreifing.htm, March 16, 1998.

National Institute of Nursing Research: *Treating symptoms in terminal illness*, www.nih.gov/ninr/wnew/symptoms-in-terminal-illness.html, September 22,1997.

National Library of Medicine: *Highlights of patient management*, www.hstat2,nlm.nih.gov, December, 1994.

National Library of Medicine: *Pressure ulcers in adults*, www.hstat.nlm.nih.gov/hq www.ahrg.gov/clinic/

cpg online.htm, August 19, 2001.

National pressure Ulcer Advisory Panel: *Pressure Ulcer definition and stages,* Feb. 2007 www.mpuap.org.

Nettina, Sandra: *Manual of Nursing Practice,* 8th Edition, Ambler, Pennsylvania: Lippincott, Williams and Wilkins 2006.

Newsburn VB: *Failure to thrive: a growing concern in the elderly,* 3 Gerontol Nurs 18(8):21-25, 1992.

Newsweek: *My World Now, Life in the Nursing Home from the Inside,* with permission from her son Richard H. Seaver, Sr. June 27 1994.

Nichols, Ronald: *Preventing Surgical Site Infections: A Surgeon's Perspective,* Emerging Infectious Diseases vol. 7, No.2 March-April 2001.

Niemoller J: *Change of pace for AD patients,* Geriatr Nurs (New York), pp 86-87, March/April, 1990.

NIH Guide: *Managing the symptoms of cognitive impairment,* www.grants.nih.gov/grants/pa-files/PA-97-050.html, March 7, 2002.

Northern Michigan University: *Skin integrity,* www.instruct.nmu.edu/nursing, November 11, 2002.

Novitis Nutrition U.S.: *Novartis article an overview of the role of nutrition support in wound care,* www.novartis nutrition.com, 2002.

Nursing Home Abuse Resource: *Signs of nursing home abuse, nursing home regulations-history, growing numbers are alarming,* nursing home abuse faq, www.nursing-home-abuse-resource.com/html/definitions.html , 2000.

Nursing Home Medicine, MacLean, Duncan: *Preventing abuse and neglect in long term care part I legal and political aspects,* www.mmhc.com/nhm/articles/NHM9912/mclean.html, updated 2003.

Nutrition interventions manual for professionals caring for older Americans, Washington, DC, 1991, Greer, Margolis, Mitchell, Grunwald & Associates, Inc.

OSHA: *Exposure control plan and compliance guide,* Washington DC, 2001, Heaton Publications Inc

Parke F: *Sexuality in later life,* Nurs Times 8/(50):40-42, 1991.

Perspectives on dysphagia, Evansville, IN, 1990, Bristol-Myers Squibb Company. pp 54-56, Jan 1991.

Pritchard V: *Infection control programs for long-term care.* J Gerontol Nurs, 19(7), July 1993.

ProCare: *Body mechanics* (videodisc), Atlanta, 1991, Interactive Health Network.

ProCare: *How to be a nurse assistant* (videodisc), Atlanta, 1990, Interactive Health Network.

Pueschel, S: *Down Syndrome,* Silver Spring, MD, 1990, The ARC National Headquarters.

Pugliese G, Lynch P, and Jackson MM, editors: *Universal precautions: policies, procedures, and resources,* Chicago, 1990, American Hospital Publishing.

Rader J, Doan J, and Schwab M: *How to decrease wandering behavior: a form of agenda behavior,* Geriatr Nurs, pp 196-99, July/Aug 1985.

Rader J: *Magic, mystery, modification and mirth: the joyful road to restraint free care,* Mt. Angel, OR, 1991, The Benedictine Institute for Long Term Care, under a grant from the Robert Wood Johnson Foundation.

Rader J: *Magic, mystery, modification, & mirth.* Mt. Angel, OR, 1992, Benedictine Institute for Long Term Care.

Reed PG: *Spirituality and mental health in older adults: extant knowledge for nursing,* Fam Comm Health 14(2):14-25, 1991.

Regional Education Center: *Anonymous Poem,* Geriatric Nurse Assistant Manual, City College, Seattle Washington, 1978.

Reid M.D., Tony: *Congestive Heart Failure,* www.noblemed.com/heart.htm.

Reisberg B and Ferris S: *The global deterioration scale for assessment of primary degenerative dementia,* Am J Psychiatry 139:1136-1139, 1982.

Reisberg B et al: *Stage specific incidence of potentially remediable behavioral symptoms in aging and Alzheimer's disease,* Bull Clin Neurosci 54:95-112, 1989.

Reuters Health: *Insulin Administration,* www.reutershealth.com/atoz/html/Insulin.htm.

Rutala WA: *APIC guideline for selection and use of disinfectants.* Am J Infect Control 18(2):99-ll7, April 1990.

Saunders DH and Melnick MS: *Self help manual: save your back,* Minneapolis, 1987, Educational Opportunities Publishers.

Science Daily: *Mild cognitive impairment appears to be Alzheimer's disease,* www.Science daily.com/releases/2001/03/010315075517.htm, March 3, 2001.

Senior Living: *Managing cognitive dysfunction important definitions,* www. the doctor will see you now.com/article/senior-living/cogdys-6/.

Sherman S with Sherman vC: *Total customer satisfaction,* San Francisco, 1999, Jossey-Bass Inc.

Sine R et al: *Basic rehabilitation techniques. a self instructional guide,* Rockville, MD, 1988, Aspen Publishers.

Smith PW and Rusnak PG: *APIC guideline for infection prevention and control in the long-term care facility.* Am J Infect Control l9(4):l98-215, August 1991.

Smith PW, editor: *Infection control in long-term care*

facilities, ed 2, New York: 1993, John Wiley and Sons.

Sorrentino S: *Textbook for long term care* assistants, third edition, St. Louis, 1999, Mosby.

Spechko PL: *Bloodborne pathogens: can you become infected from your older patient?* In Jackson MM, guest editor: *Special issue: infection in the elderly*. J Gerontol Nurs 19(7), 12-15, July 1993.

Special issue: *infection in the elderly*, J Gerontol Nurs 19(7), July 1993.

Stolley J, Buckwalter K, arid Shannon M: *Caring for patients with Alzheimer's disease*, J Gerontol Nurs 17:34-38, 1991.

Sundowning: www.adrc.wustl.edu/Alzheimer /fdts/ sundowning.html, 2002.

Sunshine Terrace Foundation Policy Manual: *Policy & procedures for safeguarding residents' belongings*, Logan, UTAH, June 1992.

Swartz K: *Abuse prohibition program* , Des Moines, IA, 2000, Briggs Corp.

Taylor J Brown A Meredith S Ray W: *The fall prevention program a comprehensive program for prevention of falls and injuries in long term care residents*, Nashville, TN, 1998, Department of Preventive Medicine, Vanderbilt University School of Medicine.

Taylor, M: *The direct support workforce*, Cambridge, Ma, 1999, Human Services Research Institute.

Tellis-Nayak V and Tellis-Nayak M: *Quality of care and the burden of two cultures*, Gerontologist, 29:307-313, 1989.

The 7 habits of highly effective people, New York, 1989, Simon & Schuster.

The American Dietetic Association: *Nutrition fact sheet*, Chicago, IL, 2002, ADA.

The ARC National Headquarters: Introduction to mental retardation, ARC Publication # 101(2), 1999.

The eden alternative: www.morningsidemin.org/manor/t.htm, 2002.

Theraputic Resources Volicer L and Bloom C: Enhancing the quality of life in advanced dementia, www. theraputicresources.com, 1997,1999.

Thomas W: *Life worth living*, Acton, Ma, 1996, VanderWyk and Burnham.

Thornbury J: *Cognitive performance on Piagetian tasks by Alzheimer's disease patients*, Res Nurs Health 15:11-18, 1992.

Tideiksaar R: *Fall prevention in the home, Topics in Geriatric Rehabilitation* 3(1):57-64, 1987.

Totonto Star: *"Aging"*, www.baycrest.org/column/Gordon.html, February 22, 2002.

Tripod: *Erikson's theory: 8 stages*, www.members.tripod.com, June 26, 2002.

Troya SH et al: *A survey of nurses' knowledge, opinions, and reported uses of the body substance isolation system.* Am J Infect Control 19:268-276, 1991.

Tufts Nutritional Commentator: *A modified food guide for people over 70 years old*, www.commentator.tufts.edu/archive/pyramid.html, March 3, 1999.

University of Kentucky: *Non-Mercury thermometers*, http://ehs.uky.edu/hmm/thermo_facts.html.

University of Pittsburgh Medical Center: *Managing your Colostomy*, www.upmc.com.

U.S. Dept. Health & Human Services: *Avian Influenza*, Pandemicflu.gov.

U.S Dept. of Health and Human Services: *What you need to know about HIV and AIDS, changing symptoms, providing emotional support, giving care*:www.hivatis.org/caring/care3.html, December 1, 2002

U.S. Department of Health and Human Services/Administration on Aging: Long-term Care Ombudsman Program, Washington DC, www.aoa.gov.

U.S. EPA: *Mercury thermometers/toxic*, Apr. 2001 www.epa.gov/NE/pr/2001/apr/010428.html.

U.S. FDA/Center for Food Safety and Applied Nutrition HHS,USDA: *Nutrition and your health*, www.usda.gov/cnpp/dietgd.pdf, December 23, 2002.

U.S. Department of Labor, Occupational Safety and Health Administration: *Occupational exposure to bloodborne pathogens*: final rule (29 CFR Part 1910.1030). Federal Register 56(235), December 6, 1991.

U.S. Department of Labor, Office of Health Compliance Assistance. OSHA Instruction CPL 2-2.44C: *Enforcement procedures for the occupational exposure to bloodborne pathogens standard*, 29 CFR 1910.1030, March 6, 1992.

United States Federal Register: *Rules and Regulations*, Vol. 56, No. 187, Sept 26, 1991.

USDA: *Dietary guidelines for americans*, www.nal.usda.gov/fnic/dga/dguide95.html, 2000.

USDA: *Eat a variety of foods*, www.nal.usda.gov/fnic/dga/95/variety.html, December 1995.

USDA: *Food Guidance System, replaces 12 year old food guide pyramid*, mypyramid.gov 2005.

USDA: *Nutrition and your health dietary guidelines for americans*: www.Health.gov/dietary guidelines/dga 2000/do, May 30, 2000.

USDA: *Pyramid guidelines*, www.Health.gov/ dietary guidelines/dga 2000/do, May 17, 2001.

USDA: *What counts as a serving*, www.nal.usda.gov/fnic/dga/dga95/box02.html, 1995.

USFDA/Center for Drug Evaluation/Research: *Drugs FDA glossary terms.*

Walker B: *Fire and safety in long term care*, Washington DC, 2002, AHCA.

Wandering: www.adrc.wustl.edu/Alzheimer/fdts/ wandering.html, 2002.

Waxman H et al: *How nurse aides perceive quality care*, Nursing Homes, pp 12-16, Sept/Oct 1990.

WebMD: *Diabetes Complications* www.webmd.com/solutions/diabetes-complications/complications-checklist October 2006.

WebMD: *Diabetes Guide* http://diabetes.webmd.com/guide/diabetes-overview.

Web MD: *Genital herpes*, www.content.health.msn.com/content/article/ 1680.51307, May 29,2002.

Web MD: *Health topics a-z gonorrhea*, www.content.health.msn.com/content/article/1680.51324May 29,2002.

WebMD: *Heart Disease and Diabetes* http://diabetes.webmd.com/heart-blood-disease July 2007.

WebMD: *Infections linked to Diabetes* www.webmd.com/solutions/diabetes-wound-care/infection June 2007.

WebMD: *Information and resources/blood clot in legs* www.webmd.com/a-z-guides/blood-clot-legs, September 2005.

Web MD: *Sexual conditions bacterial vaginosis*, www.content .msn.com/encyclopedia/article/2953.2047, May 29, 2002.

WebMD Health: *Nourishing your skin*, www.WebMD.com/content/article 1689 50438, May 29, 2002.

WebMD Health:*Pressure ulcer/ skin integrity*, www.WebMD.com/content/asset/miller-keane-30554, 1996, 2002.

WebMD: *End of life care*, www.my.WebMD.com/ encyclopedia/article, 1996, 2002.

WebMD: *Women's conditions vaginal yeast infections*, www.content.health.msm.com/encyclopedia, May 29, 2002.

WebMD: *Your guide to prostate cancer*, www.content.health.ms/1688.50814?z=1688-00000-6502-rl, May 29,2002.

Wenzel RP (editor): *Prevention and control of nosocomial infections*, ed 2. Baltimore, 1993, Williams & Wilkins.

What is guided imagery: www.senenity music.com/ whatisgim.html, November 2002.

Will-Black,C,and Eighmy, J: *Being a long term care nurse assistant, fifth edition*, Upper Saddle River,NY, 2002, Prentice Hall.

Williams CO'B and Feldt K: *A nursing challenge: methicillin-resistant Staphylococcus aureus in long term care*, J Gerontol Nurs 19(7), 22-27, July 1993.

Wolgin F., American Hospital Association: *Being a nurse assistant, eighth edition*, Upper Saddle River, NY, 2002, Prentice Hall.

Yurick A et al: *The aged person and the nursing process*, ed 3. Norwalk, CT, 1989, Appleton & Lange.

Index

Page numbers in **bold** mean this is the major reference for the term (rather than an incidental mention).